NURSING INFORMATICS
for the
Advanced Practice Nurse

Susan McBride, PhD, RN-BC, CPHIMS, FAAN, is a clinical nursing informaticist at the Texas Tech University Health Sciences Center. As a professor at Texas Tech, she teaches DNP courses, including statistics, informatics, epidemiology, and population health at the organizational and public policy level. She is also the director of the master's and postmaster's nursing informatics programs. Dr. McBride's clinical expertise also includes perioperative and cardiovascular nursing, with a research focus on methods development for implementing, evaluating, and utilizing large health care datasets and health information technology (HIT) to improve patient safety and quality within the health care delivery system. She has developed and deployed software and services with executive oversight in the for-profit and not-for-profit arenas. Most recently, she supported operational activity and administrative oversight of the West Texas Health Information Technology Regional Extension Center (WTxHITREC) under the F. Marie Hall Institute for Rural and Community Health in a senior leadership role. Her focused activities include advising practices and hospitals on workflow redesign, clinical decision support, strategies to assist providers in meeting meaningful use of electronic health records (EHRs), quality measures, and analytics using certified EHR technology. Her current research involves an EHR-enhanced simulation program to develop best-practice competencies in the use of EHRs for interprofessional teams and evaluation of the use of social media initiatives in improving population health.

Mari Tietze, PhD, RN-BC, FHIMSS, is an associate professor at Texas Woman's University College of Nursing, where she teaches nursing research and informatics. She also supports the statistics component of capstone projects. Previously, she worked as senior manager, Center for Research and Innovation, VHA Inc., in Irving, Texas. She also served as director of nursing research and informatics in the Dallas–Fort Worth Hospital Council's Education and Research Foundation. In that role, Dr. Tietze was responsible for deployment of the Council's 3-year technology implementation project on behalf of the Small Community, Rural Hospitals Research Grant, a National Institutes of Health grant funded by the Agency for Healthcare Research and Quality. She was a key member on a team that was awarded an $8.4 million grant for a Regional Extension Center in North Texas. Dr. Tietze directed workforce center nursing research and data initiative informatics projects, and is board certified by the American Nurses Credentialing Center in informatics nursing. She is fellow of the Healthcare Information and Management Systems Society (FHIMSS) certified by the Health Information Management Systems Society. Since 2010, Dr. Tietze has been an associate professor at the Houston J. and Florence A. Doswell College of Nursing at Texas Woman's University. In 2014, she became the program director of the graduate certificate program in interprofessional informatics at Texas Woman's University.

NURSING INFORMATICS
for the
Advanced Practice Nurse

Patient Safety, Quality, Outcomes, and Interprofessionalism

Susan McBride, PhD, RN-BC, CPHIMS, FAAN

Mari Tietze, PhD, RN-BC, FHIMSS

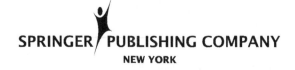

SPRINGER PUBLISHING COMPANY

NEW YORK

Springer Publishing Company, LLC
11 West 42nd Street
New York, NY 10036
www.springerpub.com

Acquisitions Editor: Joseph Morita
Production Editor: Kris Parrish
Composition: Westchester Publishing Services

ISBN: 978-0-8261-2488-3
e-book ISBN: 978-0-8261-2489-0

Instructor's Manual ISBN: 978-0-8261-2512-5
Instructor's PowerPoints ISBN: 978-0-8261-2482-1
Instructor's Test Bank ISBN: 978-0-8261-2499-9
Student Study Guide ISBN: 978-0-8261-2519-4

Instructor's materials are available to qualified adopters by contacting textbook@springerpub.com.
A student study guide is available at springerpub.com/mcbride.

16 17 18 / 5 4 3 2

The author and the publisher of this Work have made every effort to use sources believed to be reliable to provide information that is accurate and compatible with the standards generally accepted at the time of publication. Because medical science is continually advancing, our knowledge base continues to expand. Therefore, as new information becomes available, changes in procedures become necessary. We recommend that the reader always consult current research and specific institutional policies before performing any clinical procedure. The author and publisher shall not be liable for any special, consequential, or exemplary damages resulting, in whole or in part, from the readers' use of, or reliance on, the information contained in this book. The publisher has no responsibility for the persistence or accuracy of URLs for external or third-party Internet websites referred to in this publication and does not guarantee that any content on such websites is, or will remain, accurate or appropriate.

Library of Congress Cataloging-in-Publication Data
Nursing informatics for the advanced practice nurse : patient safety, quality, outcomes, and interprofessionalism / Susan McBride, Mari Tietze, authors.
    p. ; cm.
Includes bibliographical references and index.
ISBN 978-0-8261-2488-3 (hard copy : alk. paper) — ISBN 978-0-8261-2489-0 (ebook)
I. McBride, Susan, 1957– , editor.   II. Tietze, Mari, editor.
[DNLM: 1. Nursing Informatics.   2. Advanced Practice Nursing.   WY 26.5]
RT50.5
610.730285—dc23
                                                                                2015026693

XV, 234, 303, 305

Printed in the United States of America by Bradford & Bigelow.

To my amazing family, who always stand in support of all the work I am committed to doing to improve health and the health care delivery system. Thank you, dear family!

—Susan McBride

To my Mom, Pauline L. Bruschi, who was proud to be on my right side . . . through it all. Thanks, Mom!

—Mari Tietze

CONTENTS

Section V: New and Emerging Technologies

CONTRIBUTORS

Cindy Acton, RN, DNP
Associate Professor
Texas Tech University Health Sciences Center School of Nursing
Lubbock, Texas

Elaine Ayres, MS, RD, FAC-PPM III
Deputy Chief, Laboratory for Informatics Development
NIH Clinical Center, National Institutes of Health
Bethesda, Maryland

Itara K. Barnes
Senior Associate
Healthcare & Life Sciences Data and Analytics
KPMG, LLP
Greenville, South Carolina

David M. Bergman, MPA
Founder and Principal
Healthcare Intelligence Partners, LLC
New York, New York

Carol J. Bickford, PhD, RN-BC, CPHIMS, FAAN
Senior Policy Fellow, Department of Nursing Practice & Work Environment
American Nurses Association
Silver Spring, Maryland

Richard Booth, MScN, RN
Assistant Professor
Arthur Labatt Family School of Nursing
Western University
London, Ontario, Canada

Georgia Brown, RRT
Vice President and Chief Operating Officer
CareCycle Management
Dallas, Texas

Stacey Brown, RN, BSN
Vice President of Operations
CareCycle Management
Dallas, Texas

Lisa A. Campbell, DNP, RN, APHN-BC
Executive Director
Population Health Consultants, LLC
Associate Professor
Texas Tech University Health Sciences Center School of Nursing
Lubbock, Texas

Helen Caton-Peters, MSN, RN
Senior Health Information Privacy Program Analyst
Office of the Chief Privacy Officer/ONC/HHS
Washington, DC

Sharon Decker, PhD, RN, ANEF, FAAN
Associate Dean for Simulation and Professor
School of Nursing
Covenant Health System Endowed Chair in Simulation and Nursing Education
Executive Director of the F. Marie Hall SimLife Center
Texas Tech University Health Sciences Center
Lubbock, Texas

Susan H. Fenton, PhD, RHIA, FAHIMA
Associate Dean for Academic Affairs
Principal Investigator, Gulf Coast Regional Extension Center
The University of Texas Health School of Biomedical Informatics
Houston, Texas

Robert D. J. Fraser, BScN, MN, RN
President
Rob D. Fraser & Associates Inc.
Toronto, Ontario, Canada

Richard Gilder, MS, RN-BC, CNOR
Nursing Analysis Champion, Office of Patient Safety
Baylor Scott & White Health
Dallas, Texas

Tony Gilman
Chief Executive Officer, Texas Health Services Authority
HIETexas
Austin, Texas

George Gooch, JD, LLM
Associate Director of Policy & Planning
Texas Health Services Authority
HIETexas
Austin, Texas

Stephanie H. Hoelscher, BSN, RN, CHISP
Chief Clinical Analyst
Department of Clinical Transformation
Texas Tech University Health Sciences
Lubbock, Texas

Maxine Ketcham, RN, MBA, CPHIMS, CPHQ
Clinical Decision Support
Texas Health Resources
Arlington, Texas

Anne Kimbol, JD, LLM
General Counsel
Texas Health Services Authority
HIETexas
Austin, Texas

Andrea Lorden, PhD, MPH
Assistant Professor
University of Oklahoma Health Sciences Center
College of Public Health
Oklahoma City, Oklahoma

Susan McBride, PhD, RN-BC, CPHIMS, FAAN
Professor and Program Director, Master's and Postmaster's Nursing
Informatics Program
Texas Tech University Health Sciences Center School of Nursing
Lubbock, Texas

Deb McCullough, DNP, RN, FNP
Administrator and Family Nurse Practitioner
Andrews County Health Department
Andrews, Texas

Mary Beth Mitchell, MSN, RN-BC, CPHIMS
Chief Nursing Information Officer
Texas Health Resources
Arlington, Texas

Susan Newbold, PhD, RN-BC, FAAN, FHIMSS
Newbold Consulting/Nursing Informatics Boot Camp
Franklin, Tennessee

Diane Pace, PhD, APRN, FNP-BC, NCMP, FAANP
Associate Professor, Department of Advanced Practice and Doctoral Studies
Director, DNP Program
Family Nurse Practitioner/Methodist Teaching Practice
University of Tennessee Health Science Center
College of Nursing
Memphis, Tennessee

Joni Padden, MSN, APRN, ACNS-BC, CIN-BC, CPHIMS
Clinical Education Specialist
Texas Health Resources
Arlington, Texas

Billy U. Philips, Jr., PhD, MPH
Sr. Vice President and Executive Director, F. Marie Hall Institute for Rural
and Community Health
Texas Tech University Health Sciences Center
Lubbock, Texas

Sue Pickens, MEd, PCMH, CCE
Director, Population Medicine
Parkland Health & Hospital System
Dallas, Texas

Cynthia Powers, DNP, MS, RN
Director of Ambulatory Workflow Standardization
University of Texas MD Anderson Cancer Center
Houston, Texas

Terri Schreiber, MS
Consultant
Westat
Arlington Heights, Illinois

Diane C. Seibert, PhD, ARNP, FAANP, FAAN
Professor, Chair/Director Family Nurse Practitioner Program
Uniformed Services
University of the Health Sciences
Washington, DC

Trish Smith, MPH, MS
President, Chief Executive Officer
Taurus Performance, LLC
Austin, Texas

Annette Sobel, MD, MS
Associate Professor
Executive for Critical Infrastructure Protection and Health Security Initiatives
Texas Tech University and Texas Tech University Health Sciences Center
Lubbock, Texas

John Terrell, MS, SSBB
Senior Industrial Engineer
University of Texas MD Anderson Cancer Center
Houston, Texas

Laura Thomas, PhD, RN, CNE
Assistant Professor
Texas Tech University Health Sciences Center School of Nursing
Lubbock, Texas

Mari Tietze, PhD, RN-BC, FHIMSS
Associate Professor
The Houston J. and Florence A. Doswell College of Nursing
Director, Graduate Certificate in Interprofessional Informatics Program
Texas Woman's University
Dallas, Texas

Patricia Hinton Walker, PhD, RN, FAAN, PCC, CMC
Vice President for Strategic Initiatives and Professor, Nursing
Uniformed Services University of the Health Sciences
Bethesda, Maryland

Cristina Winters, DNP, FNP-C, CCRN
Practitioner, Ambulatory Clinic
San Antonio, Texas

FOREWORD

As a nurse whose career began at the patient bedside, and now, 33 years later, as a clinical informatics officer for one of the country's leading and most comprehensive health care services companies, I have experienced the highs and lows of overseeing the advancement of health information technology (HIT), both at the bedside and with performance analytics, both retrospective and prospective. As such, I have been a strong advocate for nursing informatics as a science, as an effective role within professional teams, and as a critical component of the successful deployment and use of HIT.

There are two main themes in this book and they align perfectly with my needs as an informaticist:

1. Federal policy is driving health care information technology initiatives; however, it does not lend itself to promoting innovative thinking, which is up to us.

2. It is innovative thinking, making sense of the federal policy, that moves us toward our goal of *improved patient care.*

As you explore the information provided in these pages, you have the opportunity to gain knowledge leading to innovation, "thinking out of the box," teaching others, encouraging new approaches, opening minds to the power of information, and improving our nation's health care through our actions. Join Susan, Mari, and myself as leaders in using informatics as a powerful tool in providing better patient care now and in the future.

As the authors state in the Preface, the intent of this book *is to think in an expansive, open, innovative, and "out-of-the-box" way about how we can use technology as another tool in our toolkit for improving the quality of care that we deliver.*

As students of clinical informatics who will play an important role in the effective and efficient deployment of HIT, readers of this book will benefit from this well-organized, well-illustrated primer. I commend the authors for providing the readers with the necessary foundational content essential to understanding the national HIT strategy. So often it is simply assumed that the issues about which a book is written are well known and well understood.

Whenever I am engaged in dialogue about the challenges inherent with HIT and the use of electronic information in the health care setting, I remind myself and others to think back to a time when other industries had to choose between becoming technology-enabled and becoming obsolete. Reflect back 30 years and think about how you planned your travel, did your banking, accessed your newspapers or books, listened to your music, or watched a movie. Technology has changed everything about the ways businesses and individuals operate and live. Enormous amounts of time and money are being saved; convenient and constant communication now prevails, including the ability to receive answers in an instant for just about any question we might have. I suspect that, even today, you "Googled" an answer to an inquiry ranging from "How did my sports team fare today?" to "What are the side effects of the drug just prescribed for my parent?" How did all that happen? Consumer demand certainly played a part in spurring on the momentum, but it was the "out-of-the-box" thinkers, the innovators, and the visionaries who embraced technology and made it possible for all of us to enjoy many facets of our world at the touch of a button.

In comparison, momentum for advancing HIT and building an electronic infrastructure to support patient safety, quality, and population health initiatives stems largely from federal policy and not from the consumer (i.e., the patient). Recognize the fact that health care is an extremely regulated, policy-driven, compliance-governed business, where "out-of-the-box" and "innovative thinking" are not typically phrases and adjectives that characterize the industry. This environment creates challenges that potentially impede the full adoption and use of digital information to improve health care delivery.

Given the complexity of the U.S. health care system and the ongoing development of HIT to support the goals of safety, quality, and efficiency, the foundational aspects behind this movement need careful explanation. This book expertly provides that knowledge, with additional sections covering point-of-care technology; data management and analytics; patient safety, quality, and population health; and new and emerging technologies. The authors provide the reader with a unique perspective in aligning the national goals with the achievement of safe, efficient quality of care through use of technology.

It always seems impossible until it is done.
—*Nelson Mandela*

Liz Johnson, MS, BSN, RN-BC, FCHIME, FHIMSS, CPHIMS
Chief Information Officer, Acute Care Hospitals & Applied Clinical Informatics
Tenet Healthcare Corporation
Dallas, Texas

PREFACE

The health care industry is undergoing a major transformation that requires advanced practice nurses to rethink practice, leadership, and educational approaches. "In order to improve health care outcomes, the National League for Nursing's new vision statement calls for nursing programs to teach with and about technology to better prepare the nursing workforce" (National League for Nursing, 2015, p. 1). Fundamentals of practice are changing in terms of workflow, decision making, and management of information. These changes, to a large degree, are motivated by a federal policy-driven health care industry focused on building an electronic infrastructure within the United States that will support patient safety, quality, and population health initiatives. These changes, and those discussed in this book, are then guided by the nation's *National Strategy for Quality Improvement* report (U.S. Department of Health and Human Services, 2012).

Health information technology (HIT) has been promoted as a key element in the National Quality Strategy to achieve three aims: better care, affordable care, and healthy populations and communities (U.S. Department of Health and Human Services, 2012). In fact, each year the U.S. Congress receives a report on the national health care trends toward achieving these three aims (U.S. Department of Health and Human Services, 2014). Nurses will play an important role in the related transformation of the health care delivery system and are critical to the success of this overall strategy, particularly as it relates to the effective and efficient deployment of HIT (Institute of Medicine [IOM], 2011). This book addresses that role and provides information and tools that nurses can utilize practically to serve in prominent roles within interprofessional teams to align with our National Quality Strategy (U.S. Department of Health and Human Services, 2012) supported by HIT.

We have taught informatics and analytic methods for many years, and our approach is grounded in application of informatics using HIT as a tool for improving the care we deliver and the health of populations served. Since we were beginning nurses, both of us have had a natural inclination to use analytic methods of various types to answer questions about data. For most nurses, the analytic process comes naturally because it is very similar in approach to what we do every day in the nursing process to assess, analyze, and intervene, and to evaluate outcomes on behalf of patients.

Solving problems on behalf of patient care is thrilling for us, and we believe that with strong analytic techniques and use of technology nurses can "take it to the bank." We have discovered that the teams we were on could use the answers to improve health care delivery. It felt powerful to provide them, we felt powerful, and patients benefited. Over the years, we have solidified our approaches and "packaged" our methods for using HIT, data, and analytics in the business setting, in for-profit industry, and not-for-profit health care association work. We elected to take this into the academic setting and began teaching it in master's, DNP, and PhD programs.

We believe that the book represents a unique perspective tying into the national goals of achieving safe, efficient quality of care through use of technology. It emphasizes the advanced practice nursing informatics (NI) role and the importance of the NI nurse working within interprofessional teams to address patient safety and quality through the deployment of successful HIT implementation.

Major themes and concepts include patient safety and quality, point-of-care applications, data management, and analytics with emphasis on the interprofessional team. The goal of this text is to position it as a "must have" text for all health care professionals practicing in the Health Information Technology for Economic and Clinical Health (HITECH) Act age of health care, primarily targeted for nursing but applicable to medicine, health information management, occupational therapy (OT), physical therapy (PT), and other disciplines. We have designed a model that we utilize as a foundation for teaching clinicians nursing informatics (McBride, Tietze, & Fenton, 2013). The Nursing Education Health Informatics (NEHI) model, reflected in Figure P.1, includes three core domains: (a) point-of-care technology, (b) data management and analytics, and (c) patient safety and quality. We begin the text with an introductory section laying the foundation for these three core domains, and conclude with a fifth section discussing the exciting and emerging technologies that will further transform the way we deliver care, including areas such as genomics, nanotechnology, and deployment of social media in health care.

This textbook is designed to be complementary to many of the nursing informatics textbooks currently used in nursing programs throughout the nation. The intent is to create a way of thinking about technology that is expansive, open, and innovative, often referred to as "out-of-the-box" thinking, to consider technology as yet another tool in our toolkit for improving the quality of care we deliver.

Although a concept-based curriculum is an emerging trend in academics today, the authors believe that HIT is a very competency-laden area of health care that lends itself to the use of a concept-based educational pedagogy and approach. We have threaded concepts aligned with the six domains within the Quality and Safety Education in Nursing (QSEN) approach to nursing education, and use practical examples to drive home the competencies recommended within QSEN. Examples of the practical application

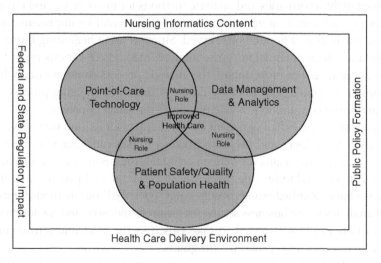

FIGURE P.1. NEHI model. Framework for development of curriculum to align with IOM and essentials.

Source: McBride et al. (2013).

include exercises and case studies with concepts threaded throughout the book, including patient safety, quality, patient-centered care, evidence-based practice, interprofessionalism, and, of course, technology. Additional concepts equally as important for nursing informatics include health care policy, population health, data management, and privacy and security.

Practical examples are weaved into the content of the chapters and are followed with case studies and exercises reflective of the material within the chapter, thereby incorporating active learning into use of technology solutions presented. We find that to fully grasp some of the information it is important to provide real-life examples of how the tools and information relate to the current health care environment. For example, in the Computers in Health Care chapter, we provide a case study of effective selection and deployment of an electronic health record (EHR) in a rural local public health department, and questions reflect issues unique to rural provider's experience. In the Workflow Redesign chapter, we present a case study of a clinic with issues in ePrescribing and the associated workflow diagram relating the current situation in the clinic. Details relating to the assessment of the clinic are provided and the reader is asked to use an interprofessional team approach and design a strategy for addressing the problems presented. The Quality Improvement chapter presents two case studies relating to a hospital's materials management challenges and a computer provider order entry and barcoding patient safety challenge. All of the chapters are designed with an eye on what the industry is experiencing with respect to the rapid deployment of HIT, and we provide the reader with tools and information to address those issues to fully optimize HIT.

We caution the industry that although we stress the amazing capabilities we have through HIT, we need to be cautious that we do not rely too much on technology and fail to think as clinicians. The text emphasizes, in several chapters, the unintended consequences that can occur when technology is implemented poorly, resulting in unsafe practices. We provide clinicians with recommendations on what to do in the event one experiences HIT deployed unsafely and provide tools that a nurse can apply to optimize technology for patient-centered quality care.

Throughout the text, we have included contributors with domain expertise on the chapter content. We have intentionally selected a wide area of expertise representing a truly interprofessional team approach to the content within the book, believing that it will take a team approach to fully realize the benefit of HIT for patients and health care consumers. Authors include nurses, physicians, epidemiologists, engineers, dieticians, and health services researchers, as well as a significant array of HIT content experts. Within the HIT expertise represented by chapter coauthors are informatics content experts in areas such as EHR adoption and implementation, privacy and security, cyber security, public health, workflow redesign, data management, and advanced analytics.

The American Association of Colleges of Nursing's (AACN) *The Essentials of Master's and Doctoral Education* for advanced nursing practice (American Association of Colleges of Nursing, 2006, 2011) is addressed throughout the text, including emphasis on not only the essentials of informatics and health care technology, but also those essentials that relate to patient safety, quality, integrating evidence into practice, population health, and policy. All of these graduate nursing essentials are addressed in this text, positioning HIT as an integral component of most, if not all, of the graduate AACN essentials of education in nursing. ***Qualified instructors may obtain access to ancillary materials,*** *such as an instructor's manual, PowerPoints, and a test bank, by contacting textbook@ springerpub.com. A student study guide is available at springerpub.com/mcbride.*

   To address these essentials of education for nursing, this textbook strives to offer a practical application of tools and information needed by advanced practice graduate-level nurses to fully understand *what is happening* in the United States, and *why it is occurring*, and to provide the reader with what is needed to effectively play a role within interprofessional teams *to make it happen*. This textbook provides nurses with the tools and information to lead, as is called for in the IOM report: *The Future of Nursing: Leading Change, Advancing Health* (IOM, 2011). To lead within the teams, we will need the information, tools, and expertise outlined and stressed within this text.

Susan McBride
Mari Tietze

REFERENCES

American Association of Colleges of Nursing. (2006). *The essentials of doctoral education for advanced nursing practice.* (No. AACN2006). Washington, DC: Author.

American Association of Colleges of Nursing. (2011). *The essentials of master's education in nursing.* Retrieved from http://www.aacn.nche.edu/education-resources/MastersEssentials11.pdf

Institute of Medicine. (2011). *The future of nursing: Leading change, advancing health.* Washington, DC: National Academies Press. Retrieved from www.iom.edu/Reports/2010/The-Future-of-Nursing-Leading-Change-Advancing-Health.aspx

McBride, S. G., Tietze, M., & Fenton, M. V. (2013). Developing an applied informatics course for a doctor of nursing practice program. *Nurse Educator, 38*(1), 37–42. doi:10.1097/NNE.0b013e318276df5d

National League for Nursing. (2015). *A vision for the changing faculty role: Preparing students for the technological world of health care.* A living document from the National League for Nursing (NLN) board of governors, January 2015 (No. NLNvisionSer2015). Washington, DC: Author. Retrieved from http://www.nln.org/aboutnln/livingdocuments/pdf/nlnvision_8.pdf

U.S. Department of Health and Human Services. (2012). *National strategy for quality improvement in health care.* (Congressional Report No. DHHS-2012). Washington, DC: Agency for Healthcare Research and Quality.

U.S. Department of Health and Human Services. (2014). *2014 Annual report to Congress: National strategy for quality improvement in health care* (No. AHRQ-2014). Washington, DC: Agency for Healthcare Research and Quality.

SECTION I

Introduction to the
National Health Information
Technology Strategy

CHAPTER 1

Introduction to Health Information Technology in a Policy and Regulatory Environment

Susan McBride and Mari Tietze

OBJECTIVES

1. Provide explanation of the national agenda for transformation of the health care system.

2. Explain why technology is essential to driving down costs and improving quality.

3. Outline key components of regulation and policy driving the change underway in the U.S. health care system.

4. Explain meaningful use, the Medicare Incentive program and the other programs under the Health Information Technology for Economic and Clinical Health Act, including the Regional Extension Centers, health information exchange, and the workforce development.

5. Discuss the diverse role of nurses in health information technology advancement.

KEY WORDS

patient safety, quality, population health, Accountable Care Act, HITECH Act, National Strategy for Quality, meaningful use, HIE

CONTENTS

INTRODUCTION

The health care environment in which advanced practice registered nurses are currently practicing is a complex setting with rapid change underway driven by a need to transform the health care delivery system by focusing on improving patient safety, quality, and population health, while at the same time decreasing the overall cost of health care. Health information technology (HIT) has been promoted as a key element in the National Quality Strategy (NQS) to achieve three aims: better care, affordable care, and healthy populations and communities (Department of Health & Human Services, 2011). Nurses will play an important role in the transformation of the health care delivery system and are critical to the success of this overall strategy, particularly as it relates to the effective and efficient deployment of HIT. This chapter focuses on regulatory requirements underway to implement the U.S. health care system's strategic plan, the importance of HIT to the strategy, and the diverse role that nurses will play in this transformation.

POLICY AND REGULATION TO TRANSFORM THE DELIVERY SYSTEM

In order to implement the National Strategy for Quality Improvement in Health Care, several legislative components have been implemented. The Patient Protection and Affordable Care Act (PPACA) focuses on providing all Americans with access to quality and affordable health care (Patient Protection and Affordable Care Act, 2010). As a component of the federal plan, HIT plays a critical role in ensuring transparency, increasing efficiency, engaging consumers, and providing data to effectively manage the cost and quality of care in the United States (Patient Protection and Affordable Care Act, 2010). The Health Information Technology for Economic and Clinical Health (HITECH) Act was passed as part of the American Recovery and Reinvestment Act (ARRA). Under the HITECH Act there are two sets of standards established as regulatory requirements by the Office of the National Coordinator for Health Information Technology (ONC-HIT) to help providers meet the meaningful use (MU) of electronic health records (EHRs) and to assure that the EHRs across the nation meet an adequate standard for performance. The first standard defines the MU of EHRs and the second specifies how EHRs are to be developed and certified to meet the MU criteria (Health Information Technology for Economic and Clinical Health Act, 2009). The Centers for Medicare & Medicaid Services (CMS) couples this infrastructure regulation with an EHR incentive program to encourage providers and hospitals to adopt and implement certified technology (CMS, 2013a, 2013b).

Affordable Care Act

Health care costs in the United States are escalating at unprecedented levels despite efforts to contain them. Health care expenditures are consuming approximately 18% of the gross domestic product (GDP), and are expected to rise to 20% by 2020 (Keehan et al., 2011). The nation had to contain the costs and despite significant bipartisan political controversy, legislation was passed in 2009 to implement the Affordable Care Act (ACA). Health care reform under the ACA puts into place several mechanisms to improve care and decrease cost, including the implementation of the accountable care organizations (ACOs). Shared savings accounts under Section 3022 of the ACA create savings accounts to support at-risk contracts in which provider organizations take on the responsibility of patient populations for which they provide care at a fixed rate per person. In addition to the at-risk contracts, ACA establishes metrics to measure success with improving quality and creating efficiencies. The measures are organized under five domains to monitor performance in key areas, including (a) patient/caregiver experience, (b) care coordination, (c) patient safety, (d) preventive health, and (e) at-risk population/frail elderly health. In order for organizations to achieve the 65 measures required to perform as an ACO, systems that take on these contracts must have significant technology implemented. HIT infrastructure will be required to succeed within the health care delivery system under ACA, including EHRs and health information exchange (HIE) data translated to actionable information with extensive data management and reporting capability on which providers can manage and improve care.

HITECH Act

The U.S. Strategic Plan for Health & Human Services addresses several critical objectives emphasizing improvements in the health of the nation, a safer and more effective health care delivery system, transparency, and consumer engagement. To achieve the plan for the United States, a key objective for the plan is to promote the adoption and meaningful use of HIT (Department of Health & Human Services, 2011). HIT has the potential to support the transformation of a safer and a more effective health care delivery system. To establish the HIT infrastructure, the HITECH Act was passed in 2009 as part of the ARRA (Health Information Technology for Economic and Clinical Health Act, 2009). Several programs were implemented under the HITECH Act, which includes the following:

► Sixty-two Regional Extension Centers (RECs) providing HIT assistance to smaller health care organizations (small hospitals, federally qualified health care clinics, and small provider practices)

► Eighty-four community college programs offering HIT training

► Seventeen Beacon Community projects, demonstrating how HIT can help address local health needs through the use of HIEs

► Grants to states to support development of statewide HIEs (ONC-HIT, 2013b)

The HITECH Act lays out three phases of "meaningful use" to achieve the goals necessary under the national strategy with each phase of MU escalating in what the technology is designed to achieve, ultimately resulting in sufficient infrastructure and information to result in improved outcomes (see Table 1.1). Phase one is focused on the implementation of certified EHRs meeting basic requirements such as electronic exchange of information through ePrescribing (electronic prescriptions) and ability to capture and report quality metrics. Phase two of MU focuses on consumer engagement also termed "patient centeredness" and increases the capacity within the certified product to capture and exchange data. Phase three will further expand the requirement to capture more structured data, better quality reporting, and better capacity to exchange data using HIEs within and across states and regions. Phase three will also emphasize technical standards that support population health management and outcomes measurement while continuing to emphasize patient-centered care. These phases and the evolution of the technical capability are reflected in Table 1.1.

EHR Incentive Program

Throughout the MU phases, providers and hospitals that implement EHRs meeting federal standards outlined under the meaningful use regulatory requirements are financially incentivized with payments from CMS. The incentive program started in 2011 and extends over several years with the time table determined by whether a provider elects to access the Medicaid or Medicare incentive program. Hospitals can access both Medicaid and Medicare incentives, and in many cases these incentives equate to millions of dollars.

Under the Medicaid incentive program, incentives available for adopting, implementing, and meaningfully utilizing a certified EHR can be as much as $63,750 per provider and includes nurse practitioners. Medicare incentive payments can be as much as

TABLE 1.1 Stages of Meaningful Use		
Stage 1	Stage 2	Stage 3
Meaningful use criteria focus on basic data capture and sharing	Meaningful use criteria focus on advancing clinical processes	Meaningful use criteria focus on improved outcomes
Electronically capturing health information in a standardized format	More rigorous HIE	Improving quality, safety, and efficiency, leading to improved health outcomes
Using that information to track key clinical conditions	Increased requirements for ePrescribing and incorporating lab results	Decision support for national high-priority conditions
Communicating that information for care coordination processes	Electronic transmission of patient care summaries across multiple settings	Patient access to self-management tools
Initiating the reporting of clinical quality measures and public health information	More patient-controlled data	Access to comprehensive patient data through patient-centered HIE
Using information to engage patients and their families in their care		Improving population health

HIE, health information exchange.

Adapted from ONC (ONC-HIT, 2013b).

$44,000 per provider, and do not include nurse practitioners in the program. However, providers must select either Medicare incentives or Medicaid incentives. As of October 2014, CMS had paid out more than 100,000 eligible Medicaid providers, more than 200,000 Medicare providers, and more than 4,200 hospitals with approximately $17.2 billion in Medicare incentives paid and with more than $8.7 billion in Medicaid EHR incentive program payments since January 2011 (when the first set of states launched their programs; CMS, 2014). This indicates that the update of technology over a very short period of time (2009–2014) has been extensive under this incentive program.

The HITECH Act had two components requiring that vendors providing EHRs develop products in accordance with criteria that have been laid out in the statutory rule-making process as "certified" products (ONC-HIT, 2013a). The second component of the Act required that providers effectively use these systems in a meaningful way measured by detailed metrics that determines that the provider meets "meaningful use" criteria. These measures are outlined in Appendix 1.1, comparing and contrasting Stages 1 and 2 measure sets for hospitals and eligible providers. Eligible providers are defined as providers that meet the criteria under the CMS EHR incentive program for the incentive dollars. These measures are described in more detail in Section II of the text, which addressed the use of point-of-care technology and implications for advanced practice registered nurses.

The ACA and HIT

Although the PPACA is not directly tied to the use of information technology in health care delivery, it is indirectly connected through the mandate of MU standards for care delivery. Examples of this include population health management and quality measures required under ACA without which EHRs would be unattainable. At this point in time, providers in this country are incentivized to deliver care that includes Stage 1 and subsequently Stage 2 of MU standards, with Stage 3 planned in the near future (CMS, 2013b). The incentive program will be followed by penalty reductions in Medicare and Medicaid reimbursement for providers and hospitals that fail to adopt EHRs. Appendix 1.1 compares MU Stage 1 and Stage 2 measures (core and menu metrics) that address patient engagement and exchange of information, such as the ability to access lab values and conduct interactive communication with primary care providers (CMS, 2013c).

Patient engagement is an important aspect of how these guidelines will ultimately impact population health in the long term. The consumer emphasis as a partner in the health care delivery process is believed to be one of the most important aspects of how technology and care will be transformed over time. Evidence suggests that patient engagement in the care plan is essential to fundamentally realizing the full impact of technology to improve the health of the nation, particularly when addressing the increasing load of chronic illness within the United States. The expanded use of advanced practice registered nurses and new models of care utilizing technology to support patient engagement are important predictors of success (Cumbie, Conley, & Burman, 2004). Chapter 5 further expands on this important aspect of the federal strategic plan to impact the long-term health of the nation by discussing consumer engagement, activation, and how consumer engagement can be enhanced by technology.

NURSING'S ESSENTIAL ROLE IN HEALTH CARE REFORM

This section discusses the important role that nurses will play in the transformation of the health care system and the various roles nurses will play in nursing informatics (NI). Figure 1.1 illustrates three components needed for the reformation of the health care delivery system in which the goal of MU can be fully realized. These components include (a) technology for lowering cost and improving safety, (b) assurance of patient safety and quality in a technology-driven environment, and (c) nursing's diverse role as HIT advances. Ultimately, the MU of HIT for continuity of care and safety becomes *the* definition of advancing health care through nursing.

Technology for Lowering Costs and Improving Safety

The use of technology for lowering costs and improving safety during health care delivery has long been advocated. Recent studies have reported the impact of HIT on patient safety and quality outcomes. For example, one study assessed the output of grants funded by the Agency for Healthcare Research and Quality (AHRQ), the federal government's highest agency focused on the safe use of technology in health care. Bibliographic analysis of the 2010 articles, citations, and journal titles was performed along with a qualitative review of the full-text article and grant document. Findings indicated that the 75 qualifying articles represented a broad range of HIT topics from the role of health care

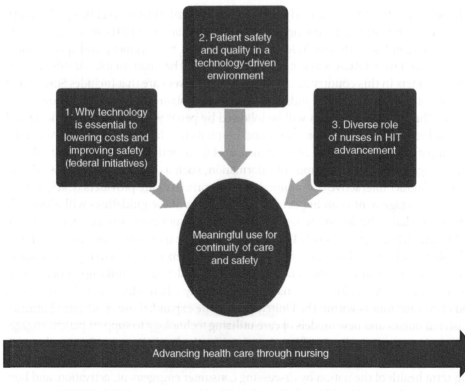

FIGURE 1.1. Key components for nursing involvement in health care reform.
HIT, health information technology.

professionals in HIT, to patient engagement using HIT, to the cost analysis of HIT use. Authors concluded that this set of AHRQ-funded research projects addressed the goals and priorities of AHRQ, indicating notable contributions to the scientific knowledge base on the impact of information system use in health care (Whipple, Dixon, & McGowan, 2013).

Another comprehensive study exploring the impact of HIT on patient care delivery focused on the structured and/or coded EHRs and the associated direct patient care benefits or value noted. The researchers searched for evidence of direct patient care values from the use of structured and/or coded information within EHRs by exploring nine international databases from 1990 to 2011. Value (benefit) was defined using the Institute of Medicine's (IOM) six areas for improvement for health care systems: effectiveness, safety, patient-centeredness, timeliness, efficiency, and equitability (Kalra, Fernando, Morrison, & Sheikh, 2013). In this study on the benefits of EHRs for patient care delivery, 5,016 potentially eligible papers were considered. Of those, 13 studies satisfied the criteria focusing on effectiveness, safety, and improved clinical outcomes if a structured and/or coded EHR was combined with alerting or advisory systems. No studies were found reporting value in relation to patient-centeredness, timeliness, efficiency, or equitability. Authors indicated that evidence for the impact of this EHR-based structured data is not well documented. Authors concluded that there have been patchy efforts to investigate empirically the value from structuring and coding EHRs for direct patient care. They further noted that future investments in structuring and coding of EHRs should be informed by robust evidence as to the clinical scenarios in which patient care benefits may be realized (Kalra et al., 2013).

Assurance of Patient Safety and Quality in Technology-Driven Environments

One aspect for consideration in technology-driven environments is the assurance of patient safety and quality during the continued rapid deployment of EHRs across the nation. It is a common understanding among informaticists that, although there was the ability to harm patients prior to the use of technology for health care delivery, there is potentially more serious harm that can be done to patients with the use of technology for health care delivery (Institute of Medicine [IOM], 2012).

As a result of observing a trend in unintended consequences of HIT in delivery of patient care, the federal government's Department of Health and Human Services, published a guide on how to implement safe HIT systems for better care (IOM, 2012). The recommendations centered on the premise that the departments in the federal government must work together, communicate together, and share knowledge and experience together to safely and effectively deploy HIT across the nation. Important details on unintended consequences and patient safety with respect to HIT adoption and implementation of point-of-care technology are further addressed in Section II of this book.

Nursing's Diverse Role in HIT Advances

The role of nurses in patient care has evolved and so has their role in the use of technology to improve health care delivery. Now informatics nurses and informatics nurse specialists provide important direction in the leadership and practice arenas related to

HIT. The American Nurses Association (ANA) recognized NI as a nursing specialty in 1992. Numerous scope and standards documents have reflected the evolution of this specialty practice, the most recent being the 2015 *Nursing Informatics Nursing: Scope and Standards of Practice,* Second Edition. That resource includes the revised definition of nursing informatics:

> Nursing informatics (NI) is the specialty that integrates nursing science with multiple information and analytical sciences to identify, define, manage, and communicate data, information, knowledge, and wisdom in nursing practice. NI supports nurses, consumers, patients, the interprofessional healthcare team, and other stakeholders in their decision-making in all roles and settings to achieve desired outcomes. This support is accomplished through the use of information structures, information processes, and information technology. (ANA, 2015, p. 1)

According to this definition, the "multiple information and analytic sciences" include "A listing of sciences that integrate with nursing informatics includes but is not limited to: computer science, cognitive science, the science of terminologies and taxonomies (including naming and coding conventions), information management, library science, heuristics, archival science, and mathematics" (ANA, 2015, p. 1).

Research addressing the relationship among nursing informatics, increased patient safety, and reduced health care-associated costs is challenging to identify (Carrington & Tiase, 2013). This reflects the need for the nursing informatics community to study and publish these types of articles broadly so that health care institutions may benefit from this body of work. With the involvement of informatics nurses in the development of EHR products, the interface (integration) of the EHR with the flow of direct patient care delivery can be realized, yielding an improved and safer product (Carey, 2013). Many of the influential studies on the role of the NI in HIT involve medication administration, prediction of patterns to predict changes in patient conditions, and nursing documentation within an EHR (Carrington & Tiase, 2013).

IOM's Report on the Future of Nursing

The IOM has long been interested in quality of patient care delivery. The institute is known for its 1999 report, *To Err Is Human: Building a Safer Health System*, which pointed out that approximately 48,000 patients die each year due to errors encountered during health care delivery in the United States (Kohn, Corrigan, & Donaldson, 1999). Other books followed as part of the 11-book Quality Chasm Series. *Crossing the Quality Chasm: A New Health System for the 21st Century* provided a focus on a definition of quality in the context of the aforementioned medical error epidemic (Committee on Quality of Healthcare in America, 2001). Ann Page edited one of the next books opening the discussion for the reality of the work environment of nurses, where the pivotal role of nursing in quality of care was emphasized (Page, 2004).

In 2004, the same year of the book on the work environment of nurses, the book *Patient Safety: Achieving a New Standard of Care* was released. It is appropriate that a book on safety became available shortly after the publication on the environment of nurses. More recently, prevention of medication errors was the topic of concern, to which the description of an ideal medication administration system was born (Committee on Identifying and Preventing Medication Errors, Aspden, Wolcott, & Bootman, 2007).

In 2010, the IOM, in partnership with the Robert Wood Johnson Foundation, published its landmark report, *The Future of Nursing: Leading Change, Advancing Health* (IOM, 2010). This book focuses on the expansion of affordable health care and how it will bring thousands of new patients into the health care system. Advanced practice registered nurses will shoulder most of the primary care delivered to those patients with the assistance of various types of information technology, including the EHR (IOM, 2010). The remainder of this book includes additional content from these IOM reports and their influence in the transformation of health care delivery in this country.

Nursing Education for the Healthcare Informatics Model

As noted, the role of the nurse is expanding to include information technology. This is also true of the doctor of nursing practice (DNP) role (McBride, Tietze, & Fenton, 2013). The authors developed a conceptual framework, which addresses the major roles that advanced practice registered nurses play within the information technology environment. This framework is the Nursing Education for the Healthcare Informatics (NEHI) Model. The framework is targeted to advanced practice care delivery and is composed of three main content domains: (a) patient safety/quality, (b) data management and analytics, and (c) point-of-care technology. These domains align well with the DNP Essentials, and has been discussed in previous publications by the authors (McBride et al., 2013).

The model was originally developed for a DNP informatics and statistics course and has subsequently been used in different venues to develop master's courses in informatics, design a master's nursing informatics program, and various educational workshops developing competencies for advanced practice registered nurses in HIT (see Figure 1.2

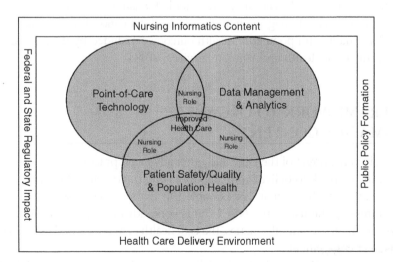

FIGURE 1.2. The NEHI model. Framework for development of curriculum to align with IOM and essentials.
Source: McBride et al. (2013).

for schematic representation). Examples of these programs include the use of EHRs in MU, unintended consequences in use of HIT, and workflow redesign boot camps.

The first domain of the framework, *point-of-care technology*, reflects the use of technology in patient care delivery. Point-of-care technology includes technology in which data that is transformed to information is gathered as part of the technology, the most common example being the EHR. Thus, for example, the point-of-care technology content domain focuses on content in support of EHR implementations.

The second content domain of the NEHI framework, *data management and analytics*, then relates to the first content domain of the NEHI framework, namely, point-of-care technology. This second content domain, data management and analytics, reflects applied information management tools, such as business intelligence tools and statistical software programs, to transform data and information into improved health care delivery.

The third content domain of the NEHI framework, *patient safety/quality and population health*, then relates to the second content domain of the NEHI framework, namely, data management and analytics, This third content domain, patient safety/quality and population health, reflects quality-improvement tools applied to individuals, as well as to public health initiatives.

Figure 1.2 also illustrates the three content domains and their influence by environmental factors of federal and state regulatory impact and public policy formation. The three content domains are thought to constitute important foci for the transformation of the health care delivery system and the associated role DNPs and other advanced practice professions will play within that transformation.

These core content domains in the NEHI model are foundational and closely tied to both the masters essentials (American Association of Colleges of Nursing, 2011) and the DNP essentials (American Association of Colleges of Nursing, 2006; see the Appendices for a complete list of these essential guidelines for education). These three areas serve as the organizational structure for this book, focusing on point-of-care technology needed to support data management and analysis of data and ultimately addressing the patient safety/quality and population health outcomes intended by the national strategy (U.S. Department of Health and Human Services, 2014).

NEHI FRAMEWORK TO ORGANIZE INFORMATICS CONTENT

As noted, given the target of the DNP and other advanced practice professionals, and in order for this textbook to deliver content supporting those roles, the NEHI framework was used to organize the content. For example, the textbook begins with an introductory section addressing the use of the NEHI framework, advanced practice roles and interprofessionalism, theories in informatics, the U.S. health care policy, and federal landscape and consumer engagement.

The next three sections of the book outline content for the three main NEHI framework domains. Table 1.2 lists the chapters by section. For example, the point-of-care technology domain, deemed fairly fundamental to informatics, is the first of these three

TABLE 1.2 Chapters Organized by the NEHI Framework		
NEHI Framework Component	**Chapter Number**	**Chapter Title**
1. Introduction	1	Introduction to Health Information Technology in a Policy and Regulatory Environment
	2	Advanced Practice Roles in Interprofessional Teams
	3	Scientific and Theoretical Foundations for Driving Improvement
	4	National Health Care Transformation and Information Technology
	5	Consumer Engagement/Activation Enhanced by Technology
2. Point-of-Care Technology	6	Computers in Health Care
	7	Electronic Health Records and Point-of-Care Technology
	8	Systems Development Life Cycle for Achieving Meaningful Use
	9	Workflow Redesign in Quality-Improvement Modality
	10	Evaluation Methods and Strategies for Electronic Health Records
	11	Electronic Health Records and Health Information Exchanges Providing Value and Results for Patients, Providers, and Health Care Systems
	12	National Standards for Health Information Technology
	13	Public Health Data to Support Healthy Communities and Health Assessment Planning
	14	Privacy and Security in a Ubiquitous Health Information Technology World
	15	Personal Health Records and Patient Portals

(continued)

TABLE 1.2 Chapters Organized by the NEHI Framework *(continued)*		
NEHI Framework Component	**Chapter Number**	**Chapter Title**
	16	Telehealth and Mobile Health
3. Data Management and Analytics	17	Strategic Thinking in Design and Deployment of Enterprise Data, Reporting, and Analytics
	18	Data Management and Analytics: The Foundations for Improvement
	19	Clinical Decision Support Systems
4. Patient Safety/ Quality and Population Health	20	Health Information Technology and Implications for Patient Safety
	21	Quality-Improvement Strategies and Essential Tools
	22	National Prevention Strategy, Population Health, and Health Information Technology
	23	Developing Competencies in Nursing for an Electronic Age of Health Care
	24	Genomics and Implications for Health Information Technology
5. New and Emerging Technologies	25	Nanotechnology and Implications for Health Care Interprofessional Teams
	26	"Big Data" and Advanced Analytics
	27	Social Media: Ongoing Evolution in Health Care Delivery
	28	Electronic Clinical Quality Measures: Building an Infrastructure for Success
	29	Interprofessional Application of Health Information Technology in Education

NEHI, nursing education for healthcare informatics.

sections. It includes chapters for computer technology, EHR implementation for reaching MU, workflow redesign, and data privacy/security.

The second of the NEHI framework-based segments is the *data management and analytics* section. The authors believe that data analytics is one of the main reasons for the existence of the EHR. It includes a chapter for data management, advanced data analytics, and clinical decision support.

The third of the NEHI-framework-based segments is the *patient safety/quality and population health* section. Patient safety and quality should be part of any patient-care delivery educational effort along with effort to improve health of the population. As such, this section includes chapters for a national prevention strategy, quality improvement tools, and public health informatics.

The last section of the book describes *new and emerging technologies* and is intended to provide the advanced practitioner with a view for the future of health care-based informatics. It includes chapters on genomics, nanotechnology, big data and advanced analytics, electronic quality measures, social media, and interprofessionalism in education. All of these chapters, in the context of the NEHI framework, are thought to provide the comprehensive outline needed by today's advanced practice professional.

SUMMARY

The U.S. health care delivery system is under major transformation driven by policy changes that work in tandem to build regulation and structure needed to overhaul the delivery system. This transformation is needed because of escalating costs of health care in the United States and quality considerations noted in numerous reports by the IOM. Yet, the rapid deployment of EHR technology over a very short period of time sets the delivery system up for serious patient safety issues with the very technology that was established to address the quality and safety of health care. The role of nurses in supporting the national plan is critical to ensure safe effective care in the United States with respect to new payer models and use of technology to deliver care. The nation needs EHRs at the point of care to capture and collect data to report and manage care in the United States. The remaining chapters within Section I of this book expound on the need for the technology and the important role of nurses in this national strategy.

EXERCISES AND QUESTIONS FOR CONSIDERATION

Consider content covered with respect to policy changes in the United States and the strategic plan to improve care and drive down cost through the use of HIT, and respond to the following questions:

1. What are the three aims in the NQS outlined by the Department of Health and Human Services, and why is technology an important aspect of that plan?
2. How do you see your role in nursing impacted by changes related to health care reform and the HITECH Act of 2009?
3. Reflect on rapid change underway with regard to the implementation of EHRs. What are the factor(s) driving the rapid adoption of EHRs? Is this positive or negative for the health care industry?

4. Compare and contrast the Medicare and Medicaid EHR incentive program and reflect on why the two programs are different for providers and hospitals.

5. Discuss the positive and negative aspects of transformation underway as it relates to the NQS and the rapid deployment of HIT.

REFERENCES

American Association of Colleges of Nursing. (2006). *The essentials of doctoral education for advanced nursing practice* (No. AACN2006). Washington, DC: Author.

American Association of Colleges of Nursing. (2011). *The essentials of master's education in nursing.* Retrieved from http://www.aacn.nche.edu/education-resources/MastersEssentials11.pdf

American Nurses Association. (2015). *Nursing informatics: Scope and standards of practice.* Silver Spring, MD: American Nurses Association.

Carey, E. (2013). Not all nurses wear scrubs. Nursing informatics: What is it and what do they do? *Ohio Nurses Review, 88*(2), 7.

Carrington, J. M., & Tiase, V. L. (2013). Nursing informatics year in review. *Nursing Administration Quarterly, 37*(2), 136–143. doi:10.1097/NAQ.0b013e3182869deb

Center for Medicare & Medicaid Services. (2013a). *Medicare and Medicaid EHR incentive program basics: Payments and registration summary overview.* Retrieved from https://www.cms.gov/Regulations-and-guidance/legislation/EHRIncentivePrograms/DataAndReports.html

Center for Medicare & Medicaid Services. (2013b). *The official web site for the Medicare and Medicaid electronic health records (EHR) incentive programs.* Retrieved from http://www.cms.gov/Regulations-and-Guidance/Legislation/EHRIncentivePrograms/index.html

Center for Medicare & Medicaid Services. (2013c). *Stage 1 & Stage 2 comparison tables.* Retrieved from http://www.cms.gov/Regulations-and-Guidance/Legislation/EHRIncentivePrograms/Downloads/Stage1vsStage2CompTablesforEP.pdf

Center for Medicare & Medicaid Services. (2014). *Combined Medicare and Medicaid payments by state: January 2011 to November 2014.* (No. EHR2014Nov). Washington, DC: Department of Health and Human Services. Retrieved from http://www.cms.gov/Regulations-and-Guidance/Legislation/EHRIncentivePrograms/Downloads/November2014_PaymentsbyStatebyProgram.pdf

Committee on Identifying and Preventing Medication Errors, Aspden, P., Wolcott, J., & Bootman, J. L. (Eds.). (2007). *Preventing medication errors: A quality chasm series.* Washington, DC: National Academies Press. Retrieved from http://www.nap.edu/catalog.php?record_id=12610

Committee on Quality of Healthcare in America. (2001). *Crossing the quality chasm: A new health system for the 21st century.* Washington, DC: National Academies Press. Retrieved from http://www.nap.edu/catalog.php?record_id=10027

Cumbie, S. A., Conley, V. M., & Burman, M. E. (2004). Advanced practice nursing model for comprehensive care with chronic illness model for promoting process engagement. *Advances in Nursing Science, 27*(1), 70–80.

Health Information Technology for Economic and Clinical Health Act. (2009). *Public Law 111-5 American Recovery and Reinvestment Act of 2009, Title XIII Health Information Technology for Economic and Clinical Health Act.*

Institute of Medicine. (2010). *The future of nursing: Leading change, advancing health.* Washington, DC: National Academies Press. Retrieved from http://www.iom.edu/Reports/2010/The-Future-of-Nursing-Leading-Change-Advancing-Health.aspx

Institute of Medicine. (2012). *Health IT and patient safety building safer systems for better care.* Washington, DC: Author.

Kalra, D., Fernando, B., Morrison, Z., & Sheikh, A. (2013). A review of the empirical evidence of the value of structuring and coding of clinical information within electronic health records for direct patient care. *Informatics in Primary Care, 20*(3), 171–180. doi:10.14236/jhi.v20i3.22

Keehan, S. P., Sisko, A. M., Truffer, C. J., Poisal, J. A., Cuckler, G. A., Madison, A. J., . . . Smith, S. D. (2011). National health spending projections through 2020: Economic recovery and reform drive faster spending growth. *Health Affairs, 30*(8), 1594–1605. doi:10.1377/hlthaff.2011.0662

Kohn, L. T., Corrigan, J. M., & Donaldson, M. S. (Eds.). (1999). *To err is human: Building a safer health system.* Washington, DC: National Academies Press.

McBride, S. G., Tietze, M., & Fenton, M. V. (2013). Developing an applied informatics course for a doctor of nursing practice program. *Nurse Educator, 38*(1), 37–42. doi:10.1097/NNE.0b013e318276df5d

Office of the National Coordinator for Health Information Technology. (2013a). *Health IT certification program.* Retrieved from http://www.healthit.gov/policy-researchers-implementers/onc-health-it-certification-program

Office of the National Coordinator for Health Information Technology. (2013b). *HITECH programs for health information technology.* Retrieved from http://www.healthit.gov/policy-researchers-implementers/health-it-adoption-programs

Page, A. (2004). *Keeping patients safe: Transforming the work environment of nurses.* Washington, DC: National Academies Press.

Patient Protection and Affordable Care Act (2010). (No. Pub. L. No. 111–148, §2702, 124 Stat. 119U.S.C. 111–148). U.S. Government Printing Office.

U.S. Department of Health & Human Services. (2011). *Report to Congress: National strategy for quality improvement in health care.* Retrieved from http://www.ahrq.gov/workingforquality/nqs/nqs2011ann lrpt.pdf

U.S. Department of Health and Human Services. (2014). *2014 Annual Report to Congress: National strategy for quality improvement in health care.* (No. AHRQ-2014). Washington, DC: Agency for Healthcare Research and Quality.

Whipple, E. C., Dixon, B. E., & McGowan, J. J. (2013). Linking health information technology to patient safety and quality outcomes: A bibliometric analysis and review. *Informatics for Health and Social Care, 38*(1), 1–14. doi:10.3109/17538157.2012.678451

APPENDIX 1.1 STAGE 1 VERSUS STAGE 2: COMPARISON TABLE FOR ELIGIBLE PROFESSIONALS

Core Objectives (17 Total)

Stage 1 Objective	Stage 1 Measure	Stage 2 Objective	Stage 2 Measure
Use CPOE for medication orders directly entered by any licensed health care professional who can enter orders into the medical record per state, local, and professional guidelines.	More than 30% of unique patients with at least one medication in their medication list seen by the EP have at least one medication order entered using CPOE.	Use CPOE for medication, laboratory, and radiology orders directly entered by any licensed health care professional who can enter orders into the medical record per state, local, and professional guidelines.	More than 60% of medication, 30% of laboratory, and 30% of radiology orders created by the EP during the EHR reporting period are recorded using CPOE.
Implement drug–drug and drug–allergy interaction checks.	The EP has enabled this functionality for the entire EHR reporting period.	*No longer a separate objective for Stage 2.*	*This measure is incorporated into the Stage 2 clinical decision support measure.*
Generate and transmit permissible prescriptions electronically (eRx).	More than 40% of all permissible prescriptions written by the EP are transmitted electronically using certified EHR technology.	Generate and transmit permissible prescriptions electronically (eRx).	More than 50% of all permissible prescriptions written by the EP are compared to at least one drug formulary and transmitted electronically using certified EHR technology.
Record the following demographics: ▲ Preferred language ▲ Gender ▲ Race ▲ Ethnicity ▲ Date of birth	More than 50% of all unique patients seen by the EP have demographics recorded as structured data.	Record the following demographics ▲ Preferred language ▲ Gender ▲ Race ▲ Ethnicity ▲ Date of birth	More than 80% of all unique patients seen by the EP have demographics recorded as structured data.

Maintain an up-to-date problem list of current and active diagnoses.	More than 80% of all unique patients seen by the EP have at least one entry or an indication that no problems are known for the patient recorded as structured data.	*No longer a separate objective for Stage 2.*	*This measure is incorporated into the Stage 2 measure of Summary of Care Document at Transitions of Care and Referrals.*
Maintain an active medication list.	More than 80% of all unique patients seen by the EP have at least one entry (or an indication that the patient is not currently prescribed any medication) recorded as structured data.	*No longer a separate objective for Stage 2.*	*This measure is incorporated into the Stage 2 measure of Summary of Care Document at Transitions of Care and Referrals.*
Maintain an active medication allergy list.	More than 80% of all unique patients seen by the EP have at least one entry (or an indication that the patient has no known medication allergies) recorded as structured data.	*No longer a separate objective for Stage 2.*	*This measure is incorporated into the Stage 2 measure of Summary of Care Document at Transitions of Care and Referrals.*
Record and chart changes in vital signs: ▲ Height ▲ Weight ▲ Blood pressure ▲ Calculate and display BMI ▲ Plot and display growth charts for children 2–20 years, including BMI	For more than 50% of all unique patients aged 2 and above seen by the EP, blood pressure, height, and weight are recorded as structured data.	Record and chart changes in vital signs: ▲ Height ▲ Weight ▲ Blood pressure (age 3 and above) ▲ Calculate and display BMI ▲ Plot and display growth charts for patients 0–20 years, including BMI	More than 80% of all unique patients seen by the EP have blood pressure (for patients aged 3 and above only) and height and weight (for all ages) recorded as structured data.

(continued)

Core Objectives (17 Total) (*continued*)

Stage 1 Objective	Stage 1 Measure	Stage 2 Objective	Stage 2 Measure
Record smoking status for patients older than or equal to 13 years.	More than 50% of all unique patients older or equal to 13 years seen by the EP have smoking status recorded as structured data.	Record smoking status for patients older than or equal to 13 years.	More than 80% of all unique patients older than or equal to 13 years seen by the EP have smoking status recorded as structured data.
Implement one clinical decision support rule relevant to specialty or high clinical priority along with the ability-to-track compliance rule.	Implement one clinical decision support rule.	Use clinical decision support to improve performance on high-priority health conditions.	1. Implement five clinical decision support interventions related to four or more clinical quality measures, if applicable, at a relevant point in patient care for the entire EHR reporting period. 2. The EP, eligible hospital, or CAH has enabled the functionality for drug–drug and drug–allergy interaction checks for the entire EHR reporting period.
Report clinical quality measures (CQMs) to CMS or the states.	Provide aggregate numerator, denominator, and exclusions through attestation or through the PQRS Electronic Reporting Pilot.	*No longer a separate objective for stage 2, but providers must still submit CQMs to CMS or the states in order to achieve meaningful use.*	*Starting in 2014, all CQMs will be submitted electronically to CMS.*

Provide patients with an electronic copy of their health information (including diagnostic test results, problem list, medication lists, medication allergies), upon request.	More than 50% of all patients of the EP who request an electronic copy of their health information are provided it within 3 business days.	Provide patients the ability to view online, download, and transmit their health information within 4 business days of the information being available to the EP.	1. More than 50% of all unique patients seen by the EP during the EHR reporting period are provided timely (available to the patient within 4 business days after the information is available to the EP) online access to their health information. 2. More than 5% of all unique patients seen by the EP during the EHR reporting period (or their authorized representatives) view, download, or transmit to a third party their health information.
Provide clinical summaries for patients for each office visit.	Clinical summaries provided to patients for more than 50% of all office visits within 3 business days.	Provide clinical summaries for patients for each office visit.	Clinical summaries provided to patients within 1 business day for more than 50% of office visits.
Exchange key clinical information (e.g., problem list, medication list, medication allergies, diagnostic test results), among providers of care and patient-authorized entities electronically.	Performed at least one test of certified EHR technology's capacity to electronically exchange key clinical information.	*This objective was eliminated from Stage 1 in 2013 and is no longer an objective for Stage 2.*	*This measure was eliminated from Stage 1 in 2013 and is no longer a measure for Stage 2.*

(continued)

Core Objectives (17 Total) (*continued*)

Stage 1 Objective	Stage 1 Measure	Stage 2 Objective	Stage 2 Measure
Protect electronic health information created or maintained by the certified EHR technology through the implementation of appropriate technical capabilities.	Conduct or review a security risk analysis per 45 CFR 164.308 (a)(1) and implement security updates as necessary and correct identified security deficiencies as part of its risk-management process.	Protect electronic health information created or maintained by the certified EHR technology through the implementation of appropriate technical capabilities.	Conduct or review a security risk analysis in accordance with the requirements under 45 CFR 164.308 (a)(1), including addressing the encryption/security of data at rest and implementing security updates as necessary and correctly identifying security deficiencies as part of its risk-management process.
Implement drug-formulary checks.	The EP has enabled this functionality and has access to at least one internal or external drug formulary for the entire EHR reporting period.	*No longer a separate objective for Stage 2.*	*This measure is incorporated into the ePrescribing measure for Stage 2.*
Incorporate clinical lab test results into certified EHR technology as structured data.	More than 40% of all clinical lab test results ordered by the EP during the EHR reporting period whose results are either in a positive/negative or numerical format are incorporated in certified EHR technology as structured data.	Incorporate clinical lab-test results into certified EHR technology as structured data.	More than 55% of all clinical lab test results ordered by the EP during the EHR reporting period whose results are either in a positive/ negative or numerical format are incorporated in certified EHR technology as structured data.
Generate lists of patients by specific conditions to use for quality improvement, reduction of disparities, research, or outreach.	Generate at least one report listing patients of the EP with a specific condition.	Generate lists of patients by specific conditions to use for quality improvement, reduction of disparities, research, or outreach.	Generate at least one report listing patients of the EP with a specific condition.

Send reminders to patients per patient preference for preventive/follow-up care.	More than 20% of all unique patients older than or equal to 65 years or younger than or equal to 5 years were sent an appropriate reminder during the EHR reporting period.	Use clinically relevant information to identify patients who should receive reminders for preventive/follow-up care.	Use EHR to identify and provide reminders for preventive/follow-up care for more than 10% of patients with two or more office visits in the last 2 years.
Provide patients with timely electronic access to their health information (including lab results, problem list, medication lists, medication allergies) within 4 business days of the information being available to the EP.	More than 10% of all unique patients seen by the EP are provided timely (available to the patient within 4 business days of being updated in the certified EHR technology) electronic access to their health information subject to the EP's discretion to withhold certain information.	*This objective was eliminated from Stage 1 in 2014 and is no longer an objective for Stage 2.*	*This measure was eliminated from Stage 1 in 2014 and is no longer a measure for Stage 2.*
Use certified EHR technology to identify patient-specific education resources and provide those resources to the patient if appropriate.	More than 10% of all unique patients seen by the EP are provided patient-specific education resources.	Use certified EHR technology to identify patient-specific education resources and provide those resources to the patient if appropriate.	Patient-specific education resources identified by CEHRT are provided to patients for more than 10% of all unique patients with office visits seen by the EP during the EHR reporting period.
Perform medication reconciliation if the EP who receives a patient from another setting of care or provider of care believes an encounter is relevant.	The EP performs medication reconciliation for more than 50% of transitions of care in which the patient is transitioned into the care of the EP.	Perform medication reconciliation if the EP who receives a patient from another setting of care or provider of care believes an encounter is relevant.	The EP performs medication reconciliation for more than 50% of transitions of care in which the patient is transitioned into the care of the EP.

(continued)

Core Objectives (17 Total) *(continued)*

Stage 1 Objective	Stage 1 Measure	Stage 2 Objective	Stage 2 Measure
Provide summary-of-care record for each transition of care or referral when the EP transitions his or her patient to another setting of care or provider of care or refers his or her patient to another provider of care.	The EP who transitions or refers a patient to another setting of care or provider of care provides a summary-of-care record for more than 50% of transitions of care and referrals.	Provide summary-of-care record for each transition of care or referral when the EP transitions his or her patient to another setting of care or provider of care or refers his or her patient to another provider of care.	1. The EP who transitions or refers a patient to another setting of care or provider of care provides a summary-of-care record for more than 50% of transitions of care and referrals. 2. The EP who transitions or refers a patient to another setting of care or provider of care provides a summary-of-care record either (a) electronically transmitted to a recipient using CEHRT or (b) where the recipient receives the summary-of-care record via exchange facilitated by an organization that is an NwHIN Exchange participant or is validated through an ONC-established governance mechanism to facilitate exchange for 10% of transitions and referrals. 3. The EP who transitions or refers a patient to another setting of care or provider of care must either (a) conduct one or more successful electronic exchanges of a summary-of-care record with a recipient using technology that was designed by a different EHR developer than the sender's, or (b) conduct one or more successful tests with the CMS-designated test EHR during the EHR reporting period.

Submit electronic data to immunization registries or immunization information systems and actual submission except where prohibited and in accordance with applicable law and practice.	Performed at least one test of certified EHR technology's capacity to submit electronic data to immunization registries and follow-up submission if the test is successful (unless none of the immunization registries to which the EP submits such information have the capacity to receive the information electronically).	Submit electronic data to immunization registries or immunization information systems and actual submission except where prohibited and in accordance with applicable law and practice.	Successful ongoing submission of electronic immunization data from certified EHR technology to an immunization registry or immunization information system for the entire EHR reporting period.
NEW	NEW	Use secure electronic messaging to communicate with patients on relevant health information.	A secure message was sent using the electronic messaging function of certified ERT technology by more than 5% of unique patients seen during the EHR reporting period.

CAH, critical access hospitals; CEHRT, certified electronic health record technology; CFR, code of federal regulations; CPOE, computer-based provider order entry; EHR, electronic health record; EP, eligible provider; NwHIN, nationwide health information network; PQRS, physician quality reporting system.

Menu Objectives (EPs Must Select 3 of 6 Menu Objectives)

Stage 1 Objective	Stage 1 Measure	Stage 2 Objective	Stage 2 Measure
Submit electronic syndromic surveillance data to public health agencies and actual submission except where prohibited and in accordance with applicable law and practice.	Perform at least one test of certified EHR technology's capacity to provide electronic syndromic surveillance data to public health agencies and follow-up submission if the test is successful (unless none of the public health agencies to which an EP, eligible hospital or CAH submits such information has the capacity to receive the information electronically).	Submit electronic syndromic surveillance data to public health agencies and actual submission except where prohibited and in accordance with applicable law and practice.	Successful ongoing submission of electronic syndromic surveillance data from certified EHR technology to a public health agency for the entire EHR reporting period.
NEW	NEW	Record electronic notes in patient records.	Enter at least one electronic progress note created, edited, and signed by an EP for more than 30% of unique patients.
NEW	NEW	Imaging results consisting of the image itself and any explanation or other accompanying information are accessible through CEHRT.	More than 10% of all scans and tests whose result is an image ordered by the EP for patients seen during the EHR reporting period are incorporated into or accessible through certified EHR technology.

NEW	NEW	Record patient family health history as structured data.	More than 20% of all unique patients seen by the EP during the EHR reporting period have a structured data entry for one or more first-degree relatives or an indication that family health history has been reviewed.
NEW	NEW	Identify and report cancer cases to a state cancer registry, except where prohibited, and in accordance with applicable law and practice.	Successful ongoing submission of cancer case information from certified EHR technology to a cancer registry for the entire EHR reporting period.
NEW	NEW	Identify and report specific cases to a specialized registry (other than a cancer registry), except where prohibited, and in accordance with applicable law and practice.	Successful ongoing submission of specific case information from certified EHR technology to a specialized registry for the entire EHR reporting period.

CAH, critical access hospitals; CEHRT, certified electronic health record technology; CMS, Centers for Medicare & Medicaid Services; EHR, electronic health record; EP, eligible provider.

CHAPTER 2

Advanced Practice Roles in Interprofessional Teams

Carol J. Bickford, Diane Pace, and Mari Tietze

OBJECTIVES

1. Distinguish between advanced practice registered nurses (APRNs) and other advanced practice professionals.
2. Describe interrelatedness of nursing education, faculty, American Nurses Association (ANA) nursing informatics standards, Quality and Safety Education for Nurses and American Association of Colleges of Nursing essentials for master's and doctoral education.
3. Summarize the role of the APRN and other advanced-level practitioners in the report *The Future of Nursing: Leading Change Advancing Health*.
4. Indicate importance of reports, such as the *National Prevention Strategy* and *National Strategy for Quality Improvement in Health Care*, to advanced-level practitioners.
5. Discuss the role of the APRN as it relates to nursing informatics (NI) in the current HITECH environment.
6. Explain the impact of NI on health information technology deployment.
7. Explore concepts relating to the interprofessional team, such as:
   a. Patient centricity
   b. Interprofessionalism
   c. Simulation (both education and practice)

KEY WORDS

patient safety, quality, nursing, interprofessional, advanced practice

CONTENTS

INTRODUCTION

Chapter 1 introduced the importance of health information technology (HIT) in today's health care environment and described its associated legislative, regulatory, and policy initiatives, which will continue to influence the health care system and its evolution for many years. The successful implementation and integration of HIT into practice cannot be accomplished without careful preparations and the dedicated commitment of the affected stakeholders, including organizations, employees, health care consumers, and others.

Two themes are consistent in today's health care literature. One is that health care job demands are stable and in some subsectors are on the rise; the other is that *interprofessional team* is the new buzzword for success. According to the Bureau of Labor Statistics (BLS), the health care and social assistance industries are the combined largest employer in 34 states, suggesting a major shift from the retail and manufacturing industries (Bureau of Labor Statistics, 2014a) as the U.S. population is aging and associated health care needs and costs are projected to rise. Figure 2.1 illustrates the dominance of health care and social assistance employment by state in the United States.

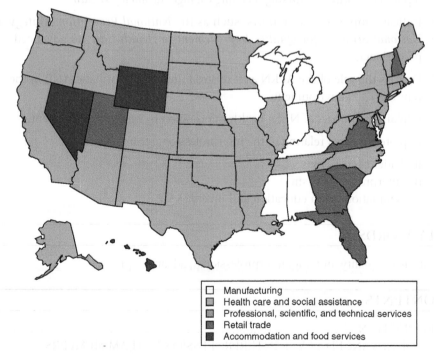

□ Manufacturing
■ Health care and social assistance
■ Professional, scientific, and technical services
■ Retail trade
■ Accommodation and food services

FIGURE 2.1. Dominant industries in the United States in 2013.
Source: Bureau of Labor Statistics.

Worsening primary care physician shortages are predicted and this has prompted calls for other clinicians to fill the gap (Bodenheimer & Smith, 2013). Similarly, the rise of accountable care organizations (ACOs) and implementation of medical homes has spiked demand to unprecedented levels for nurse practitioners (NPs), who have become important support resources in providing care to those who gained coverage under the Affordable Care Act (ACA), according to findings from a Merritt Hawkins survey (Merritt Hawkins, 2014). The consulting firm found that demand for NPs and physician assistants increased by 320% over the past 3 years, putting them into the top five most desired specialties. Neither ranked in the top 20, 3 years ago.

With the enactment of the ACA, the need for access to primary care delivery of services within the United States has increased. Advanced practice registered nurses (APRNs) are licensed, independent providers with a significant role in meeting the existing and future primary care needs of the nation by providing high-quality, patient-centered health care to a broad range of consumers (American Association of Nurse Practitioners [AANP], 2014a). Very often NPs fill this role, beginning at the time of the initial office visit and often extending into homes, long-term care and rehabilitation facilities, hospice, correctional facilities, and other settings where health care services and behavior changes are targeted.

TYPES OF ADVANCED-LEVEL INTERPROFESSIONAL TEAM MEMBERS

Although NPs have been mentioned as one group of advanced-level health care clinicians, a more detailed discussion of evolving roles of other advanced-level clinicians and other members of the interprofessional health care team follows.

Advanced Practice Registered Nurse

Registered nurses (RNs) who are considering graduate education and advanced clinical training commonly pursue an APRN (Brassard, 2013). The APRN Consensus Model (APRN Consensus Work Group and the NCSBN APRN Advisory Committee, 2008) reflects decisions associated with the nursing profession's identification and clarification of the APRN title, the expected educational preparation and credentialing process, and regulation of the four APRN roles:

- ► Certified nurse-midwife (CNM)
- ► Certified nurse practitioner (CNP)
- ► Clinical nurse specialist (CNS)
- ► Certified registered nurse anesthetist (CRNA)

Each APRN group focuses on different categories of patients and their associated health care needs.

Further detail on the number of practitioners in each type of role (Brassard, 2012) has indicated that a majority of APRNs are NPs (58.5%, $n = 158,348$) followed by CNSs (21.9%, $n = 59,242$), CRNAs (12.9%, $n = 34,821$), and CNMs (6.8%, $n = 18,492$).

According to a white paper published by AANP (2014a), more than 75% of the NPs credentialed to practice in the United States are actively practicing in primary care. Their role includes ordering, conducting, and interpreting diagnostic and laboratory tests; prescribing both pharmacologic/nonpharmacologic agents; establishing and coordinating interprofessional plans of care; and teaching and counseling about health promotion and risk reduction of disease. Other NPs have elected to practice in other specialties such as cardiovascular care, pediatrics, neonatology, women's health, neurology, and pulmonary care.

In terms of the regulatory perspectives of practice, regulation of practice and licensure of APRNs varies across states from total regulation within the state board of nursing to occasional shared regulation with the board of medicine. In addition to state licensure, APRNs obtain national board certification. The four roles of APRNs, CNSs, CNPs, CRNAs, and CNMs have varying scopes of practice. For example, the AANP identifies three types of practice environments for NPs that vary across the United States: (AANP, 2014b).

1. *Full Practice*: State practice and licensure laws and regulations provide for NPs to evaluate patients; diagnose, order, and interpret diagnostic tests; and initiate and manage treatments—including prescribing medications and other therapies—under the exclusive licensure authority of the state board of nursing. This is the model recommended by the Institute of Medicine (IOM) and National Council of State Boards of Nursing.

2. *Reduced Practice*: State practice and licensure laws and regulations reduce the ability of NPs to engage in at least one element of NP practice. The state requires a regulated collaborative agreement with an outside health discipline in order for the NP to provide patient care.

3. *Restricted Practice*: State practice and licensure laws and regulations restrict the ability of an NP to engage in at least one element of NP practice and mandate required supervision, delegation, or team management by an outside health discipline in order for the NP to provide patient care.

Multiple government and third-party payer agencies oversee or control the reimbursement structure for payment of services. One of those governmental agencies, the Federal Trade Commission (FTC), has carefully examined the potential for restraint of trade and the lack of health care consumer choice. The FTC has provided an extensive comment/report on the topic of ideal payment balanced with degree of supervision and legal risk (Gilman & Koslov, 2014). This report summarized the key points allowing for the fair trade of service by APRNs to consumers. Appendix 2.1 provides those key points in detail. Many APRNs are designated Medicare and Medicaid providers and elect to bill under their own national provider identifier (NPI).

CNMs have prescriptive authority and provide care to women during pregnancy and birth, as well as primary care health services to women from adolescence beyond menopause (American College of Nurse-Midwives, 2014). These APRNs are available to receive 100% reimbursement for approved Medicare services and are also recognized as approved Medicaid providers. The Bureau of Labor Statistics reported the number of 5,460 nurse-midwives as of 2013 (Bureau of Labor Statistics, 2014i) as an estimate based on employers' reporting that differs from the 2009 statistics available at http:// campaignforaction.org/photo/types-advanced-practice-registered-nurses.

CNSs are prepared at the master's or doctoral level as expert clinicians in a specialized area of nursing practice. The specialty may be identified in terms of population (e.g., pediatrics, geriatrics, women's health), setting (e.g., critical care, emergency room), disease or medical subspecialty (e.g., diabetes, oncology, cardiology HIV/AIDS), type of care (e.g., psychiatric, rehabilitation), or type of problem (e.g., pain, wounds, stress). In addition to providing direct patient care, CNSs influence care outcomes by providing expert consultation for nursing staff and by implementing improvements in health care delivery systems. They may provide primary care services and also have prescriptive authority in an increasing number of states. Explorehealthcareers.org identifies approximately 69,000 CNSs practicing in the United States (American Dental Education Association, 2014).

CRNAs numbered 35,430 in 2013, as reported by the Bureau of Labor Statistics (2014c). The American Association of Nurse Anesthetists identified that these anesthesia providers safely administered more than 34 million anesthetics to U.S. patients in 2012 (American Association of Nurse Anesthetists, 2014). CRNAs are the primary anesthesia providers in rural America and other medically underserved areas. Practice settings include traditional hospital surgical suites, obstetrical delivery rooms, critical access hospitals, ambulatory surgical centers, U.S. military and Public Health Services facilities, Department of Veterans Affairs health care facilities, and offices of dentists, podiatrists, plastic surgeons, ophthalmologists, and pain management specialists.

As electronic health records (EHRs) and information systems are becoming ubiquitous in today's health care delivery environments, APRNs continue to be important contributors and leaders in defining requirements; assisting with implementation decisions and activities; engaging in evaluation initiatives; and ensuring consideration and inclusion of the health care consumer's perspectives, information, contributions, and requests. It is not uncommon for the APRN in the practice or facility to become the "go to" person who engages as the "superuser" to learn the fine points of the information system architecture and operations. The APRN then teaches others "survival skills" during installation of a new health information system and provides orientation to new ways of doing business. These clinicians are often the champions for effective use and mentor colleagues, especially during the orientation to the software application for computer-based provider order entry (CPOE).

Physician Assistant

Physician assistants constitute another advanced-level clinician category of the interprofessional team and must become expert users of EHRs and HIT. The Bureau of Labor Statistics estimates that 88,110 physician assistants are employed in the United States as of May 2013 (Bureau of Labor Statistics, 2014g). This clinician cohort is expected to assume increased importance in delivery of health care services as primary care clinicians in the coming years.

Physical Therapist

More than 195,670 physical therapists are estimated to be in practice as of 2013 by the Bureau of Labor Statistics (2014f). These health care professionals, most of whom are doctorally prepared, assess, plan, organize, and participate in rehabilitative programs that improve mobility, relieve pain, increase strength, and improve or correct disabling conditions resulting from disease or injury. They may find that the mandated EHR system in their organization does not sufficiently support their practice needs so they must move into an advocacy role to effect necessary changes.

Occupational Therapist

The Bureau of Labor Statistics estimates that in 2013 more than 108,410 occupational therapists, most of whom are prepared at the master's or doctoral level, are engaged in assessing, planning, organizing, and participating in rehabilitation programs that help build or restore vocational, homemaking, and daily living skills, as well as general independence, to persons with disabilities or developmental delays (Bureau of Labor Statistics, 2014d). Like physical therapists, this professional group may find it must advocate for changes in the facility's EHR system to support its practice needs.

Dietitian and Nutritionist

The Bureau of Labor Statistics identifies that dietitians and nutritionists plan and conduct food service or nutritional programs to assist in the promotion of health and control of disease. They counsel individuals and groups, conduct nutritional research, and may supervise activities of a department providing quantity food services. An estimated 59,530 dietitians and nutritionists were available in 2013 to help address the U.S. obesity epidemic (Bureau of Labor Statistics, 2014b). Access to the patient's EHR information is often challenging, as these clinicians are not always recognized as essential interprofessional health care team members. The HIT systems may not include sufficient resources to adequately support their work processes and extensive communications and partnerships with health care consumers and their families.

Pharmacist

Pharmacists dispense drugs prescribed by physicians and other clinicians with prescriptive authority and have become important information resources for patients regarding medications and their use. Similarly, these professionals, most of whom are doctorally prepared, provide information to prescribing clinicians for decision making about the selection, dosage, interactions, and side effects of medications. The 287,420 estimated pharmacists work in diverse health care facility pharmacies, retail pharmacies, and other settings (Bureau of Labor Statistics, 2014e). Pharmacists are integral users of EHR systems and must often address issues related to interoperability and appropriate information exchange, especially when dealing with an interfaced rather than integrated pharmacy information management system.

Behavioral Health Professional

The category of behavioral health professionals includes many diverse professionals, and the numbers of these professionals are harder to quantify. Grohol identified that clinical and counseling psychologists, mental health and substance abuse social workers, mental health counselors, substance abuse counselors, psychiatrists, and marriage and family therapists comprise the mental health professionals and numbered 552,000 in 2011

(Grohol, 2011). These clinicians must address facility and organizational decisions to segregate clinical documentation of mental health information from view by other clinicians and the health care consumer. Also, they must determine the adequacy of the EHR systems to identify *Diagnostic and Statistical Manual of Mental Disorders,* Fifth Edition (*DSM-5*; American Psychiatric Association, 2013) diagnostic criteria in patient medical records.

Health Care Administration Professional

The Bureau of Labor Statistics includes health care administrators as part of the medical and health services manager's category, the group of professionals who plan, direct, and coordinate medical and health services. In 2012, BLS reported 315,500 positions for this category, with a projected growth of 23% from 2012 to 2022, identified as a much faster rate than the average for all occupations (Bureau of Labor Statistics, 2014h). Although these professionals do not engage in clinical care services, they rely on correct data and information reporting, analysis, and evaluation of these services for organizational decision making and planning. Useful information displays for these individuals vary from those provided to clinicians and may not be a focus for the operational HIT system.

HIT Professional

In terms of information technology in health care, the trend in this role is also increasing over time. In a study of HIT-related job postings, results suggested that these job postings accelerated following the Health Information Technology for Economic and Clinical Health (HITECH) Act and have grown substantially over time, tripling its number of health care job postings since 2007 (Schwartz, Magoulas, & Buntin, 2013). According to the authors, HITECH was associated with an 86% increase in monthly HIT postings, or 162,000 additional postings overall. Additionally, these HIT-related job listings had descriptions containing key phrases, such as "EHR" or "clinical informatics," emphasizing the focus on health care professionals who had EHR and clinical informatics skills.

Informatics Nurse Specialist

Description of the interprofessional health care team members would not be complete without referencing the graduate or doctorally prepared informatics nurse specialist team member. These RNs have declared NI as their nursing specialty and have completed graduate or doctoral education in an informatics program. Certification in nursing informatics is available, as are other applicable credentials. The informatics nurse specialist's work involves the identification, definition, management, and communication of data, information, knowledge, and wisdom. These advanced-level nurses support colleagues, health care consumers, patients, the interprofessional health care team, and other stakeholders in their decision making in all roles and settings to achieve desired outcomes (American Nurses Association [ANA], 2015). The informatics nurse specialist is the translator between clinical and information technology personnel and sectors. Similarly, informatics nurse specialists serve as translators and liaisons for health care consumers and patients accessing the EHR system and other HIT resources.

INFORMATICS COMPETENCIES FOR INTERPROFESSIONAL TEAMS

In addition to acquiring requisite profession-specific knowledge, skills, and abilities, all interprofessional team members must now demonstrate an acceptable informatics competence. Examination of the nursing community's approach to assuring integration of informatics competencies into all nursing curricula provides a glimpse of the magnitude of such actions.

Scope and Standards of Practice

The ANA identified NI as a nursing specialty in 1992 and published the specialty's first scope of practice statement in 1994, followed by the NI standards of practice in 1995. As the steward for the NI scope and standards of practice resource, ANA also supported the review, revision, and publication of the 2001, 2008, and 2015 editions of the NI scope and standards.

As the professional organization for all nurses, ANA, as mentioned, is the steward for the nursing scope and standards of practice that apply to all registered and APRNs in all roles and setting. Originally, each standard of practice was further explicated by accompanying measurement criteria that included some very basic informatics concepts. In the 2010 second edition of *Nursing: Scope and Standards of Practice*, measurement criteria were removed and the standards of practice and professional performance included competencies, which describe the expected level of performance that integrates knowledge, skills, abilities, and judgment (American Nurses Association, 2015). These competencies incorporate slightly more advanced informatics competencies expected of all nurses.

Education Standards

In its efforts to assure all prelicensure baccalaureate, graduate, and doctoral nursing education programs prepare students for contemporary and future practice environments, the American Association of Colleges of Nursing (AACN) publishes documents that identify and direct inclusion of essential content within all nursing curricula. *The Essentials of Baccalaureate Education for Professional Nursing Practice* (AACN, 2008), *The Essentials of Master's Education in Nursing* (AACN, 2011), and *The Essentials of Doctoral Education for Advanced Nursing Practice* (AACN, 2006) include specific sections addressing information technology and what each learner is expected to achieve. Each document is available at www.aacn.nche.edu/education-resources/essential-series.

Because of its focus on nursing educators, the National League for Nursing (NLN) released the position statement "Preparing the Next Generation of Nurses to Practice in a Technology-Rich Environment: An Informatics Agenda" in 2008 to highlight the need for nurse educators to be competent in preparing, teaching, and evaluating informatics competence and associated content at all levels. The position statement included recommendations related to the development of informatics content and competence for nurse faculty, deans/directors/chairs, and the NLN. Extensive resources and an informatics toolkit are available at http://www.nln.org/professional-development-programs/teaching-resources/toolkits/informatics-teaching.

The Quality and Safety Education for Nurses (QSEN) project, begun in 2005 by the Robert Wood Johnson Foundation, has completed three funding phases that generated quality and safety competencies and accompanying educational materials for prelicensure nursing students and the faculty teaching such content. Additional funding has been allocated to now expand the QSEN initiative to graduate and doctoral education programs. This advanced-level content addresses competencies associated with patient-centered care, teamwork and collaboration, evidence-based practice (EBP), quality improvement (QI), safety, and informatics. Although each QSEN statement describing the competency and associated knowledge, skills, and attitudes is meant for advanced-level nurses, the actual language and content are applicable to all advanced-level health care team members, including administrative and technical professionals. Details about the graduate level QSEN competencies are available at http://qsen.org/competencies/graduate-ksas/.

A grassroots collaborative effort, the Technology Informatics Guiding Education Reform (TIGER) initiative, established specific recommendations for schools of nursing to prepare nursing students and practicing nurses to fully engage in digital health care. The compendium of informatics competencies for every practicing nurse is retrievable at www.thetigerinitiative.org/docs/tigerreport_informaticscompetencies.pdf. The extensive TIGER initiative's list of associated resources and reports is available at www.thetigerinitiative.org/resources.aspx

Nursing Education for Healthcare Informatics Model-Based Role

As referenced in Chapter 1, McBride, Tietze, and Fenton (2013) developed the Nursing Education for Healthcare Informatics (NEHI) model to assist faculty and learners in organizing and understanding the important and interrelated components of (a) point-of-care technology; (b) data management and analytics; and (c) patient safety, quality, and population health associated with integration of informatics into professional education, practice, and policy.

Nursing educators are pivotal in addressing the influence of point-of-care technology on the experience of all nurses throughout their educational trajectory and professional practice continuum. Data management and analytics are foundational to practice decision making in every role and must be adequately supported with readily available and sufficiently robust technology solutions. Of key importance, adequate preparation in data, information, and knowledge management and analysis must be sufficiently detailed to enable effective application to practice. Curricular content should incorporate discussions of the specific responsibility and accountability of the RN, APRN, and other advanced-level health care team members to be informed participants, partners, and decision makers regarding these components. Such content is best described as being part of the informatics body of knowledge.

The third component—patient safety, quality, and population health—concisely categorizes the desired outcomes. These outcomes are reliant on the correct implementation and continued use of point-of-care technology and the concomitant data management and analytics activities. Again, each APRN and interprofessional health care team member cannot abdicate their responsibility and accountability to understand and focus on achieving the outcomes component within the context of interprofessional practice within a larger system. That system context is reflected in the NEHI model by the outer perimeter framed as health care delivery environment, public policy formation, federal and state regulatory impact, and NI content (Figure P.1). Although the NEHI model was created within the lens of nursing and informatics, other interprofessional health care team professionals can appreciate an architecture that promotes a patient-centric focus.

INTERPROFESSIONAL TEAMS WORKING TOGETHER

Today's health care environment includes numerous discussions of the need to implement interprofessional teams as one of the solutions that will help improve access, increase quality, and reduce the cost of health care services. Several initiatives support this evolution. The Interprofessional Education Collaborative (IPEC®) began in 2009 as a collaborative of six national education associations of schools of the health professions focused on creation of core competencies for interprofessional collaborative practice to guide curricula development at all health professions schools. Allopathic and osteopathic medicine, dentistry, nursing, pharmacy, and public health partners supported the aim to integrate the roles of health care delivery professionals to optimize care delivery. Five resource documents addressing competencies and the advancement of interprofessional clinical prevention and population health are available at https://ipecollaborative.org/Resources.html/.

The World Health Organization released its 2010 *Framework for Action on Interprofessional Education & Collaborative Practice* to enable its partners to recognize and appreciate the important contribution interprofessional education has on shaping effective collaborative practice to achieve optimal health services and improved health outcomes. The proposed health and education system collaboration includes interprofessional education that prepares present and future health workforce members who are prepared to be collaborative-practice ready and capable of addressing local health needs. This report is available at www.who.int/hrh/resources/framework_action/en/.

Cuff's published summary of two workshops funded by the IOM, *Interprofessional Education for Collaboration: Learning How to Improve Health from Interprofessional Models Across the Continuum of Education to Practice: Workshop Summary* (2013), reiterates the need for interprofessional education for and about interprofessional collaborative health care teams, includes models, provides examples of successful implementation strategies, and metrics used for evaluation of effectiveness in achieving improvements garnered in interprofessional education and practice. A key theme presented by the student participants was the tremendous importance of effective communications among all stakeholders (Cuff, 2013).

Pentland (2012), from Massachusetts Institute of Technology's Human Dynamics Laboratory, reports that patterns of communication explain the success or failure of a team. His research identified that energy, the number and nature of the exchanges among team members; engagement, the distribution of energy among team members; and exploration, communication that members engage in outside their team are three aspects of communication that affect team performance. Such human-to-human interactions and exchanges merit further attention and development for those educational and practice settings moving forward with the implementation of interprofessional teams.

Also important in the elaboration of interprofessional teamwork is information technology and the four IOM core competencies (see Figure 2.2). The key provision of

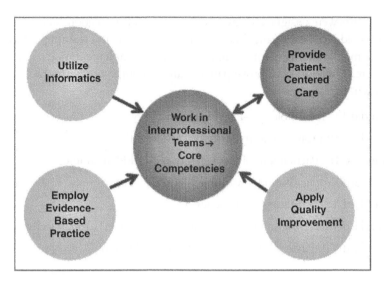

FIGURE 2.2. Interprofessional teamwork and Institute of Medicine (IOM) core competencies.
Source: Interprofessional Collaborative Expert Panel (2011).

patient-centered care is the goal of interprofessional teamwork and it increasingly relies on technology solutions to enhance patient–clinician communications, planning, and decision making. The nature of the relationship between the patient and the team of health professionals is central to competency development for interprofessional collaborative practice. Without this kind of centeredness, interprofessional teamwork has little rationale. The other three core competencies, in the context of interprofessional teamwork, identify 21st-century technologies for teamwork communication and coordination (i.e., informatics), rely on the evidence base to inform teamwork processes and team-based care, and highlight the importance of continuous improvement efforts related to teamwork and team-based health care (Interprofessional Collaborative Expert Panel, 2011, p. 14).

Reports have indicated the benefits of interprofessional education. For example, Liaskos et al. (2009) deemed patient safety is a major concern that involves a wide range of roles in health care, including those who are directly and indirectly involved and the patients themselves. They identified that developing a safety culture among health care providers, caregivers, and patients requires attention and investment in building appropriate education and training tools, especially addressing those interprofessional team members who plan patient safety activities. Their framework delineates the principles and elements of the guidance that should be provided to those who collaborate to design and implement patient safety education and training activities.

Increasing use of simulation technologies in education and practice environments has focused on development of effective interprofessional health care teams engaged in continuous improvement in patient-centric care and achievement of optimal outcomes. Development of standardized simulation experiences encompasses extensive and time-consuming faculty preparation. The International Nursing Association for Clinical Simulation and Learning (INACSL) has developed the eight Standards of Best Practice: Simulation available at www.inacsl.org/files/journal/Complete%202013%20 Standards.pdf

The standards were designed to advance the science of simulation, share best practices, and provide evidence-based guidelines for implementation and training. Adoption of the standards demonstrates a commitment to quality and implementation of rigorous EBPs in health care education to improve patient care by complying with practice standards in the following areas:

▶ Standard I: Terminology—Provide Consistency

▶ Standard II: Professional Integrity of Participants

▶ Standard III: Participant Objectives—Clear and Measurable

▶ Standard IV: Facilitation—Multiple Methods

▶ Standard V: Facilitator—Proficiency

▶ Standard VI: Debriefing Process—Improve Practice Through Reflection

▶ Standard VII: Participant Assessment and Evaluation

NATIONAL IMPERATIVES AND ROLE OF INTERPROFESSIONAL TEAMS

Several national efforts, linked by the health care improvement mission and vision for the nation, collectively guide agencies, communities, and providers in health care delivery approaches. They ranged from those specific to how the value of health care services delivery is measured to general guidelines for disease-specific efforts. Of those, many have an interprofessional framework.

National Prevention Strategy

The National Prevention Strategy reflects the U.S. goal for improving health care of the population and is reported to Congress each year (National Prevention Council, 2014). One of the six main priorities is Priority 2: Ensuring That Each Person and Family Is Engaged in Their Care (National Prevention Council, 2014, p. 14). Figure 2.3 illustrates the three key aims and lists associated priorities.

The National Prevention Strategy guides the nation in identifying the most effective and achievable means for improving health and well-being. It prioritizes prevention by integrating recommendations and actions across multiple settings to improve health and save lives. Because many of the strongest predictors of health and well-being fall outside the health care setting, the strategy envisions a prevention-oriented society where all sectors recognize the value of health for individuals, families, and society and work together to achieve better health for all Americans. The National Prevention Strategy identifies four strategic directions—the foundation for all prevention efforts—and seven targeted priorities designed to improve health and wellness for all Americans. These are illustrated in Figure 2.4 (National Prevention Council, 2014, p. 3).

The prevention strategy provides evidence-based recommendations for each strategic direction and priority and supports Healthy People 2020, a 10-year set of science-based national health objectives (National Prevention Council, 2014). The National Prevention Strategy responds to these challenges by aligning and coordinating prevention efforts across disciplines, sectors, and institutions. This report showcases how the federal

Aims

- Better Care: Improve the overall quality by making health care more patient-centered, reliable, accessible, and safe.
- Healthy People/Healthy Communities: Improve the health of the U.S. population by supporting proven interventions to address behavioral, social, and environmental determinants of health in addition to delivering higher quality care.
- Affordable Care: Reduce the cost of quality health care for individuals, families, employers, and government.

Setting priorities

- Making care safer by reducing harm caused in the delivery of care.
- Ensuring that each person and family is engaged as partners in their care.
- Promoting effective communication and coordination of care.
- Promoting the most effective prevention and treatment practices for the leading causes of mortality, starting with cardiovascular disease.
- Working with communities to promote a wide use of best practices to enable healthy living.
- Making quality care more affordable for individuals, families, employers, and governments by developing and spreading new health care delivery models.

FIGURE 2.3. National Quality Strategy: three aims and six priorities.

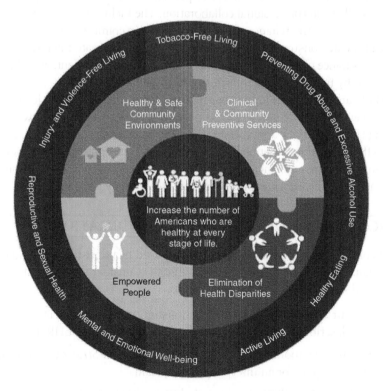

FIGURE 2.4. National Prevention Strategy framework.
Source: National Prevention Council (2014).

government and its partners are addressing ongoing public health challenges through innovation and collaboration to ensure all Americans live long and healthy lives (National Prevention Council, 2014, p. 4). IPEC suggests that interprofessional health care teams focused on collaborative patient-centric care would help achieve the target outcomes.

Meaningful Use Via the HITECH Act

Meeting the criteria for meaningful use (MU) of an EHR is one of the new methods of Medicare and Medicaid reimbursement associated with the HITECH Act. The Centers for Medicare & Medicaid Services (CMS) serves as the primary regulator, with each individual state dictating the Medicaid operations within its jurisdiction (Health Information Technology for Economic and Clinical Health Act, 2009). This statute identifies the eligible providers, primarily physicians, for the Medicare and Medicaid reimbursement structure. Such prescriptive language does not recognize, embrace, or support the interprofessional team and the critical and collaborative work completed by such an entity to improve access, improve health care, and reduce costs.

SUMMARY

Nurses must collaborate with many stakeholders in every setting to effect patient-centric care that includes identified outcomes, implementation plans, and outcomes evaluation. Such care also incorporates the concept of patient–clinician partnerships and decision making, as well as interprofessional collaboration. The inclusion of ever-increasing technology solutions and the reliance on mobile devices as communication and work tools for the health care consumer and interprofessional teams create interesting needs and problems. Assurance of positive user experiences merits greater attention and can be best accomplished by increased human factors and usability research.

The APRN and informatics nurse specialist communities are in key leadership positions to engage in the necessary discussions and decisions to move forward in safely integrating HIT and mobile applications and tools into health care practice. Such efforts mandate effective communications and collaborative interprofessional actions, all the more reason to ensure implementation of interprofessional education in all professional schools, including the information systems and technology programs.

EXERCISES AND QUESTIONS FOR CONSIDERATION

Consider content covered with respect to IPEC-based health care delivery and the U.S. strategic plan to improve care and drive down cost. Consider the use of IPEC and HIT to do that and respond to the following questions:

1. Given your understanding of the relationship between the HITECH Act and the NI role, describe the ideal team members to accomplish an EHR implementation.

2. Identify two components of the *National Prevention Strategy* report and create an education plan for an interprofessional team.

3. Using the role of APRN in managed chronic disease/population health, suggest the ideal type of collaboration between the APRN and the NI specialist.

REFERENCES

American Association of Colleges of Nursing. (2006). *The essentials of doctoral education for advanced nursing practice.* (No. AACN2006). Washington, DC: Author.

American Association of Colleges of Nursing. (2008). *The essentials of baccalaureate education for professional nursing practice.* Retrieved from http://www.aacn.nche.edu/education/pdf/baccessentials 08.pdf

American Association of Colleges of Nursing. (2011). *The essentials of master's education in nursing.* Retrieved from http://www.aacn.nche.edu/education-resources/MastersEssentials11.pdf

American Association of Nurse Anesthetists. (2014). *Certified registered nurse anesthetists at a glance.* Retrieved from http://www.aana.com/ceandeducation/becomeacrna/Pages/Nurse-Anesthetists-at-a-Glance.aspx

American Association of Nurse Practitioners. (2014a). *Nurse practitioners in primary care.* (No. AANP-2014). Alexandria, VA: Author.

American Association of Nurse Practitioners. (2014b). *State practice environment.* Retrieved from http://www.aanp.org/legislation-regulation/state-legislation-regulation/state-practice-environment

American College of Nurse-Midwives. (2014). *The nurse-midwives.* Retrieved from www.midwife.org

American Dental Education Association. (2014). *Clinical nurse specialist: Overview.* Retrieved from http://explorehealthcareers.org/en/Career/82/Clinical_Nurse_Specialist

American Nurses Association (ANA). (2015). *Nursing informatics: Scope and standards of practice* (2nd ed.). Silver Spring, MD: Nursesbooks.org.

American Psychiatric Association. (2013). *Diagnostic and statistical manual of mental disorders* (5th ed.). Arlington, VA: American Psychiatric Press.

APRN Consensus Work Group and the NCSBN APRN Advisory Committee. (2008). *The consensus model for APRN regulation, licensure, accreditation, certification and education.* (No. NCSBNJuly7_2008). Chicago, IL: National Council of State Boards of Nursing. Retrieved from https://www.ncsbn.org/4213.htm

Bodenheimer, T. S., & Smith, M. D. (2013). Primary care: Proposed solutions to the physician shortage without training more physicians. *Health Affairs, 32*(11), 1881–1886. doi:10.1377/hlthaff.2013.0234

Brassard, A. (2012). *Types of advanced practice registered nurses.* Retrieved from http://campaignforac tion.org/photo/types-advanced-practice-registered-nurses

Brassard, A. (2013). So you want to be an APRN? *American Nurse, 45*(6), 9–9. Retrieved from http://www.TheAmericanNurse.org

Bureau of Labor Statistics. (2014a). *Largest industries by state, 1990–2013.* (No. BLS2014). Washington, DC: U.S. Department of Labor. Retrieved from http://www.bls.gov/opub/ted/2014/ted_20140728.htm

Bureau of Labor Statistics. (2014b). *Occupational employment and wages, May 2013: Dietitians and nutritionists.* Washington, DC: U.S. Department of Labor. Retrieved from http://www.bls.gov/oes/current/oes291031.htm

Bureau of Labor Statistics. (2014c). *Occupational employment and wages, May 2013: Nurse anesthetists.* Washington, DC: U.S. Department of Labor. Retrieved from http://www.bls.gov/oes/current/oes291151.htm

Bureau of Labor Statistics. (2014d). *Occupational employment and wages, May 2013: Occupational therapists.* Washington, DC: U.S. Department of Labor. Retrieved from http://www.bls.gov/oes/current/oes291122.htm

Bureau of Labor Statistics. (2014e). *Occupational employment and wages, May 2013: Pharmacists.* Washington, DC: U.S. Department of Labor. Retrieved from http://www.bls.gov/oes/current/oes291051.htm

Bureau of Labor Statistics. (2014f). *Occupational employment and wages, May 2013: Physical therapists.* Washington, DC: U.S. Department of Labor. Retrieved from http://www.bls.gov/oes/current/oes291123.htm

Bureau of Labor Statistics. (2014g). *Occupational employment and wages, May 2013: Physician assistants.* Washington, DC: U.S. Department of Labor. Retrieved from http://www.bls.gov/oes/current/oes291071.htm

Bureau of Labor Statistics. (2014h). *Occupational outlook handbook: Medical and health services managers.* Washington, DC: U.S. Department of Labor. Retrieved from http://www.bls.gov/ooh/management/medical-and-health-services-managers.htm

Bureau of Labor Statistics. (2014i). *Occupational employment and wages, May 2013: Nurse-midwives.* Washington, DC: U.S. Department of Labor. Retrieved from http://www.bls.gov/oes/current/oes291161.htm

Cuff, P. A. (2013). *Interprofessional education for collaboration: Learning how to improve health from interprofessional models across the continuum of education to practice: Workshop summary.* (No. 13486). Washington, DC: National Academies Press.

Eibner, C. E., Hussey, P. S., Ridgely, M. S., & McGlynn, E. A. (2009). *Controlling health care spending in Massachusetts: An analysis of options.* Retrieved from www.rand.org/content/dam/rand/pubs/technical_reports/2009/RAND_TR733.pdf

Gilman, D. J., & Koslov, T. I. (2014). *Policy perspectives: Competition and the regulation of advanced practice nurses.* (No. FTC-2014). USA: Federal Trade Commission.

Grohol, J. M. (2011). *Mental health professionals: US statistics.* Retrieved from http://psychcentral.com/lib/mental-health-professionals-us-statistics/0009373

Health Information Technology for Economic and Clinical Health Act. (2009). Retrieved from http://www.hhs.gov/ocr/privacy/hipaa/understanding/coveredentities/hitechact.pdf

Interprofessional Collaborative Expert Panel. (2011). *Core competencies for interprofessional collaborative practice: Report of an expert panel.* (No. ICEP-2011). Interprofessional Education Collaborative. Retrieved from https://ipecollaborative.org/uploads/IPEC-Core-Competencies.pdf

Liaskos, J., Frigas, A., Antypas, K., Zikos, D., Diomidous, M., & Mantas, J. (2009). Promoting interprofessional education in health sector within the European interprofessional education network. *International Journal of Medical Informatics, 78*(Suppl. 1), S43–S47. doi:10.1016/j.ijmedinf.2008.08.001

McBride, S. G., Tietze, M., & Fenton, M. V. (2013). Developing an applied informatics course for a doctor of nursing practice program. *Nurse Educator, 38*(1), 37–42. doi:10.1097/NNE.0b013e318276df5d

Merritt Hawkins. (2014). *Trends in physician and advanced practitioner recruiting* (No. MH2014). Irving, TX: Author. Retrieved from http://www.merritthawkins.com/physician-compensation-and-recruiting.aspx

National Prevention Council. (2014). *National Prevention Council: Annual report* (No. NPC2014). Washington, DC: U.S. Department of Health and Human Services, Office of the Surgeon General. Retrieved from http://www.surgeongeneral.gov/initiatives/prevention/about/annual_status_reports.html

Pentland, A. (2012). The new science of building great teams. *Harvard Business Review, 90*(4), 60–70. Retrieved from https://hbr.org/2012/04/the-new-science-of-building-great-teams/ar/1

Schwartz, A., Magoulas, R., & Buntin, M. (2013). Tracking labor demand with online job postings: The case of health IT workers and the HITECH Act. *Industrial Relations, 52*(4), 941–968. doi:10.1111/irel.12041

APPENDIX 2.1 FTC SUMMARY DETAILS

The FTC has looked to the findings of the IOM and other expert bodies—analyses based on decades of research and experience—on issues of APRN safety, effectiveness, and efficiency.[1] Based on those expert analyses and findings, as well as our own reviews of pertinent literature and stakeholder views, the FTC staff has urged state legislators and policymakers to consider the following principles when evaluating proposed changes to APRN scope of practice.

▶ Consumer access to safe and effective health care is of critical importance.

▶ Licensure and scope of practice regulations can help to ensure that health care consumers (patients) receive treatment from properly trained professionals. APRN certification and state licensure requirements should reflect the types of services that APRNs can safely and effectively provide, based on their education, training, and experience.

▶ Health care quality itself can be a locus of competition, and a lack of competition—not just regulatory failures—can have serious health and safety consequences. More generally, competition among health care providers yields important consumer benefits, as it tends to reduce costs, improve quality, and promote innovation and access to care.

▶ Potential competitive effects can be especially striking where there are primary care shortages, as in medically underserved areas or with medically underserved populations. When APRNs are free from undue supervision requirements and other undue practice restrictions, they can more efficiently fulfill unmet health care needs.

▶ APRNs typically collaborate with other health care practitioners. Effective collaboration between APRNs and physicians can come in many forms. It does not always require direct physician supervision of APRNs or some particular, fixed model of team-based care.

▶ APRN scope of practice limitations should be narrowly tailored to address well-founded health and safety concerns, and should not be more restrictive than patient protection requires. Otherwise, such limits can deny health care consumers the benefits of competition, without providing significant countervailing benefits.

▶ To promote competition in health care markets, it may be important to scrutinize relevant safety and quality evidence to determine whether or where legitimate safety concerns exist and, if so, whether physician supervision requirements or other regulatory interventions are likely to address them. That type of scrutiny

---

[1]None of the studies in the NGA's literature review raise concerns about the quality of care offered by NPs. Most studies showed that NP-provided care is comparable to physician-provided care on several process and outcome measures (Eibner, Hussey, Ridgely, & McGlynn, 2009). Christine E. Eibner et al., RANDHealth Report Submitted to the Commonwealth of Massachusetts, Controlling Health Care Spending in Massachusetts: An Analysis of Options 99 (2009), www.rand.org/content/dam/rand/pubs/technical_reports/2009/RAND_TR733.pdf (hereafter "Eibner et al., Massachusetts Report;" "studies have shown that they provide care similar to that provided by physicians.")

can be applied not just to the general question whether the state requires physician supervision or collaborative practice agreements but also to the particular terms of those requirements as they are sometimes applied to, for example, APRN diagnosis of patient illnesses or other health conditions, APRN ordering of diagnostic tests or procedures, and APRN prescribing of medicines.

CHAPTER 3

Scientific and Theoretical Foundations for Driving Improvement

Richard Booth, Susan McBride, and Mari Tietze

OBJECTIVES

1. Define *epistemology, science,* and the *generation of new knowledge.*

2. Discuss levels of theoretical foundations and their application to health information technology (HIT).

3. Provide description of other relevant theoretical foundations to examine and evaluate HIT from a quality-improvement (QI) perspective.

4. Outline practical recommendations/implications for use of theory to inform the industry in adoption, implementation, and evaluation of technology.

5. Provide case examples related to QI, HIT, and the use of theory-driven evaluation.

KEY WORDS

epistemology, science, theory, sociotechnical, actor–network theory, quality improvement, technology, Plan-Do-Study-Act model, Donabedian-inspired models

---

CONTENTS

INTRODUCTION

The foundations of science and how they relate to work within nursing informatics are an important element in the full realization and maximization of the use of information technology in health care. In this chapter, we briefly review some fundamental aspects of science and place this discussion of theory within a practical application of health information technology (HIT) relevant to our efforts to optimize technology in health care. In-depth discussion of theory, as it relates to quality improvement (QI), is conducted in a latter section of this chapter to ground the use of theory within informatics practice to improve quality. Overall, this chapter provides the health care professional with useful considerations to support the practice setting and research efforts related to informatics and improve the delivery system with technology. We do not anticipate that this is a comprehensive overview of *all* theory relevant to HIT, but we have selected an important range of theories as examples of how theory can be applied practically to understand and intervene in HIT projects to support research, as well as improvement in patient safety, quality, and population health.

The Basic Building Blocks of Science

When exploring aspects surrounding *theory*, it is important to appreciate how people (or groups of people) view the world, and the knowledge encapsulated within their worldview. *Epistemology* is a term that attempts to elucidate how people view knowledge, and has been defined as the *nature of knowledge* and what we can actually understand and "know" (i.e., "how do we know what we know;" Samuels-Dennis & Cameron, 2013, p. 27). Ultimately, an individual's alignment with a certain epistemology informs her or his opinions and ideas surrounding a number of other important concepts, like how *science* is both conceptualized and produced. *Science* is defined by Chinn and Jacobs (1983) as "a body of knowledge including facts and theories generated by the use of controlled rigorous and precise methods within a delimited area of concern" (p. 205). A theory or theoretical framework attempts to describe, explain, or predict some phenomenon of interest. We often use theory to conceptualize a research study or area of investigation utilizing scientific methods to control for bias that may be introduced within the study. Englebardt and Nelson (2002) outline the following stages of theory development: (a) observation of some phenomenon is made; (b) explanation of the phenomenon is proposed; (c) a model is developed outlining key concepts and their relationship to the phenomenon, including processes and interaction of the concepts; and (d) the model is tested and refined. It is through this iterative inquiry that a *theory* develops and evolves.

There are different levels of theory, varying by specificity and concreteness (Fawcett, 1984, p. 24). The broadest in scope is referred to as *grand theory*, followed by middle-range (or midrange) theories. Midrange theories are traditionally defined as such by the ability to empirically test propositions within the theory. Within some midrange theories, Fawcett (1984) describes a structural hierarchy of contemporary nursing knowledge relevant to all aspects of scientific inquiry. This hierarchy is informed by an overarching epistemology that views science as a process that encourages objectivity and detailed analysis of empirical findings. This hierarchy, provided by Fawcett (1984), is reflected as follows: metaparadigm → conceptual framework → theories → empirical indicators.

Within nursing informatics, midrange theory has commonly been used to assist in the development of objective empirical indicators like variables or constructs. From a more constructivist perspective, midrange theories are also useful in building deeper understandings about processes and actions within phenomena. As outlined by Geels (2007), midrange theories can also be used to aid in the building of *enlightenment* regarding complex social processes, and similarly, offer a useful lens from which to *narratively* describe complex processes involving humans and technology. Therefore, one of the main objectives of this chapter is to describe a useful theoretical methodology for a practitioner that is compatible with development of traditional *empirical elements* (e.g., variables, constructs, etc.) commonly found within midrange theories. Simultaneously, we also advocate that a practitioner use the *enlightenment* and *narration* potentials of a specific genre of mid-range theory (i.e., the sociotechnical perspectives of actor–network theory [ANT]) to help deconstruct complex phenomena involving humans and HIT.

Nursing Informatics Specialty and Traditional Midrange Theory

In nursing informatics, we have studied and embraced several nursing informatics-based theories and/or frameworks over the past three decades (Bakken, Stone, & Larson, 2008; Carrington, 2012; Effken, 2003; Goossen, 2000; Graves & Corcoran, 1989; Matney, Brewster, Sward, Cloyes, & Staggers, 2011; Staggers, Gassert, & Curran, 2001; Staggers & Parks, 1993; Thompson, Snyder-Halpern, & Staggers, 1999; Turley, 1996). For example, both Staggers and Park (1993) and Turley (1996) developed seminal frameworks outlining their conceptions related to nursing informatics. Contained within these two frameworks is the idea that nursing informatics is a merger of various other sources of knowledge, including information science, cognitive science, computer science, various information/knowledge attributes, and technology interface characteristics. More recently, Matney et al. (2011) generated a nursing informatics model that encompasses both objectivist (post-positivist) and constructivist tenets, including the constructs of data–information–knowledge, with the recent extension of the concept of *wisdom*. In the remainder of this chapter, we propose and outline an innovative and novel theoretical methodology (not commonly used by nursing informaticians) to examine the complex phenomena of how humans and HIT interact. To do this, we advocate that a reader be sensitized past nursing informatics theory (as briefly described earlier), and also be receptive to newer theoretical approaches that are fluid, dynamic, and nonlinear. Only through this appreciation will practitioners and researchers be able to develop a deeper understanding of the complex environments in which health care, QI endeavors, and HIT exist. In order to optimize technology in the complex environment of health care for the end user, we believe different constructs and theory-base will be required.

THEORETICAL FOUNDATIONS USED TO EXAMINE HIT

Over the past few decades, the health care system has witnessed significant increases in the amount of HIT used to underpin various elements of nursing work. With the increased power and efficiency of health technology, there has also been a corresponding appreciation toward the inherent complexity of the health care environments in which humans and technology interact. Historically, health technology used in practice was evaluated in conceptual isolation from the context in which it operated. It was common for researchers in the 1990s and early 2000s to report that unplanned contextually dynamic variables influenced their study findings (e.g., organizational redevelopment, staffing changes, development of clinician workarounds, etc.), but were either not captured by the study protocols or recognized as potentially important until the end of the analysis (Brown, Cioffi, Schinella, & Shaw, 1995; Pabst, Scherubel, & Minnick, 1996; Sleutel & Guinn, 1999; Van Onzenoort et al., 2008).

During this same time period, newer perspectives within the health sciences domain that supported conceptualizing health care environments as dynamic systems containing both social and technical (sociotechnical) entities gained popularity (Berg, 1999). This body of knowledge, commonly known as sociotechnical systems, is aligned with viewing reality from a balanced perspective that appreciates the importance and agency of both humans and technology. Within this perspective, all *things* (e.g., people, technology, processes, organizations, etc.) have the potential to interact with each other, and mutually inform, influence, and generate action (Berg, 1999; Berg, Aarts, & van Der Lei, 2003; Coiera, 2004). For instance, Berg (1999) outlined that work practices in health care should be the initiation point from which health care technology is designed and implemented, and that "any potential benefit that information technology might bring to health care has to be realized at the level of concrete interaction with these tools . . . [and that] it is here that any development of evaluation process should start" (p. 89). This perspective would focus our efforts practically on workflow redesign; interaction of the technology and end users with evaluation methods focused on these intersections of influence.

Many of the perspectives currently used in nursing and health informatics research tend to subscribe to reductionist methods, valuing either socially centric or technically centric outlooks. For instance, several technology adoption models stemming from the business information systems literature have gained popularity within the health sciences literature over the past decade. Models such as the Technology Acceptance Model (TAM; Davis, 1989; Davis, Bagozzi, & Warshaw, 1989) and the Unified Theory of Acceptance and Use of Technology (UTAUT; Venkatesh, Morris, Davis, & Davis, 2003) have provided immediately usable frameworks, which predict end-user adoption and intention to use technology (Chang, Hwang, Hung, & Li, 2007; Edwards, 2006; Holden & Karsh, 2010; Rahimi, Timpka, Vimarlund, Uppugunduri, & Svensson, 2009; Zhang, Cocosila, & Archer, 2010). These frameworks attempt to control the dynamic interaction between humans and technology (Bagozzi, 2007).

Some authors (Berg, 1999; Berg et al., 2003; Coiera, 2004; Sittig & Singh, 2010) suggest that a sociotechnical lens on everyday action can help provide practitioners and researchers with a dynamic perspective from which to view processes and actions that occur in health care. This perspective is effective when examining the value or role provided by technological systems used in health care (Koppel et al., 2005; M. I. Harrison, Koppel, & Bar-Lev, 2007). For example, M. I. Harrison et al. (2007) frame their study of unintended consequences of HIT in a sociotechnical lens through the use of an interactive sociotechnical analysis (ISTA). Figure 3.1 highlights this framework and the researchers' suggested model to address unintended consequences of HIT. When viewing situations from a sociotechnical perspective, all actors within the situation are interconnected and potentially interdependent on each other to generate or perpetuate action. The ISTA model addresses various types of social, technical, and contextual interactions with HIT that can result in

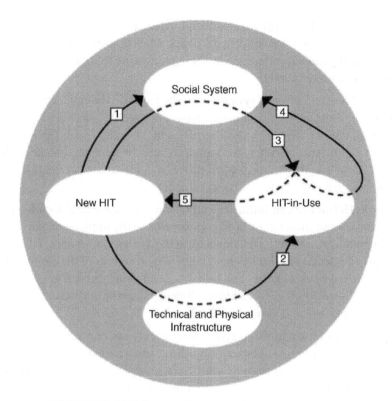

FIGURE 3.1. ISTA framework.

HIT, health information technology; ISTA, interactive sociotechnical analysis.

unintended consequences. M. I. Harrison et al. (2007) propose that the ISTA model out-lines five different interaction typologies that occur when new HIT is introduced into an established social system (e.g., hospital unit) comprised of other technical and physical features (e.g., other HIT, environmental and usability considerations related to location of equipment, etc.). The ISTA model stresses that as a collective, these interactions form a larger recursive process of various sociotechnical components, complete with feedback loops that can stimulate secondary evolution of both social and technical properties. The types of dynamic interactions are noted in Figure 3.1.

Figure 3.1 attempts to outline the recursive processes behind how a new HIT chal-lenges, modifies, and evolves an existing environment complete with social, technical, and other physical infrastructure. The authors of the ISTA model propose five types of interactions that occur when an HIT is introduced to an environment. The following interaction types correspond to the numbers denoted on the model:

- ▶ *Type 1*: Introduction of a new HIT changes the present *social system*. This may include the generation of new (or more) work for clinicians, various changes to communication patterns, and other workflow disruptions and/or changes.

- ▶ *Type 2*: Various existing technical and physical infrastructures in the environ-ment mediate *HIT-in-use*. For instance, the physical environment of the clinical area may not be suited to HIT use. Similarly, other HIT present in the environment may not be compatible with the introduced HIT. Subsequently, these technical and physical infrastructure issues can mediate how a new HIT is actually used. Often, HIT deviates from its original design when implemented into clinical areas, and in many cases is influenced by these preexisting technical and physical infrastructure considerations.

▶ *Type 3*: Preexisting *social systems* typically facilitate the reinterpretation of *HIT-in-use*. For instance, clinicians may have a preference toward using paper-based records. If an electronic medical record is implemented with the expectation to eliminate the use of paper, workarounds may be generated to keep the paper actor present within clinical work processes (due to the preexisting *social system* that preferred the use of paper records).

▶ *Type 4*: *HIT-in-use* can influence and change preestablished *social systems*. For instance, some clinician roles' may evolve due to the implementation of HIT that either adds or removes tasks previous to their roles. Sometimes, HIT can evolve preexisting *social systems* by changing power structures in the environment (e.g., force the rewriting of policy and best practices), or make clinicians overly dependent on the technology by reducing clinical judgment in certain automated situations (e.g., clinical decision support tools).

▶ *Type 5*: *HIT-in-use* and *social system* interactions can engender overall HIT redesign. Because all clinical practice by clinicians occurs within a sociotechnical environment, it is clear that the addition of a new HIT eventually influences both the social and the technical features of the environment. In this way, *HIT-in-use* and *social systems* eventually force evolution of each other in potentially asymmetric, yet reciprocal fashions, with sometimes unpredictable outcomes.

For instance, when implementing a workstation-on-wheels device in an acute care medical unit, there are thousands of potentially important social elements (e.g., workflow, staffing schedules, clinician types, usage policies, etc.) and technical elements (e.g., type and number of devices, service quality, interoperability with electronic record systems, security, interface usability, etc.) that are required to come together in a synergistic fashion. If some element(s)—whether social or technical, or both—should fail or be resistant, other elements of the implementation may also suffer. When examining research utilizing the M. I. Harrison et al. (2007) model that is precisely what these researchers focused on: *How can we mitigate unintended consequences with respect to these dynamic relationships?*

Defining and Operationalizing QI

QI science is not a new phenomena or practice. Currently, there exists a range of various epistemology and ontological perspectives of what QI science is, and what QI *should be* moving into the future (Batalden, Davidoff, Marshall, Bibby, & Pink, 2011). To date, there is no singular approach or definition of QI that is universally accepted or valid in every context. As outlined by Batalden et al. (2011), given the various epistemological interpretations of QI science, attempting to "distill a single overarching principle from the wealth of thought" related to QI is likely of little value (p. i103). However, when exploring QI science, Batalden et al. advocate taking into account the importance of the multiple epistemologies and knowledge of the domain.

Originally, development of QI within health care was highly influenced by various medically focused researchers, beginning with Codman (1916), and subsequently evolving in the latter part of the century with the works of Donabedian (Donabedian, 1980, 1989) and Berwick (Berwick, 1989, 2003, 2008; Berwick, Nolan, & Whittington, 2008). Other influential bodies of literature that evolved along with modern-day QI approaches include the rise of the evidence-based practice ideals in the 1990s (Guyatt & Drummond, 2002), and emergence of synthesized care pathways and clinical guidelines, which translated knowledge into more practitioner-friendly, usable protocols (Grinspun, Virani, & Bajnok, 2001). Similarly, business researchers have had a long history of exploring QI perspectives, as evidenced through a lineage of work examining managerial, information systems, and other manufacturing quality elements (DeLone, 2003; DeLone & McLean, 1992; Drucker, 1971; Sugimori, Kusunoki, Cho, & Uchikawa, 1977). With the increased automation of many clinical and health care environments, a trickle effect and hybridization of perspectives from the business realms began to merge wholeheartedly with health care processes and research. Change-management ideals, organizational behavior perspectives, and business process reengineering activities have become important QI perspectives within the health care environment. Correspondingly, other works from the business information systems literature and emerging health informatics literature also exerted force upon considerations related to notions of *quality* within health care, indicating it could be potentially *improved*. The culmination of this blurring, blending, and hybridization of ideas and perspectives from a variety of industries and bodies of knowledge has generated a domain of science that could be considered fragmented and largely nonsynthesized. Much like the scientific foundations of nursing informatics, QI science is also a relatively new body of knowledge challenged with the ability to truly explain and understand phenomena in the health care environment.

Quality Improvement

The definition of *QI* is largely a dynamic, nonstatic construct. Subsequently, depending on a practitioner's positioning and role within the QI endeavor, interpretations of the construct can be entertained and/or endorsed as operational definitions to assist the larger activity. Donabedian (1988) provides a practitioner-centric interpretation of quality, stating that quality within his perspective involves attributes related to how a clinician interacts with patients (including knowledge, skills, and judgment), a patient's own actions within their care, amenities offered by the care setting, and other social distribution aspects of health care. Alternatively, Hurtado, Swift, and Corrigan (2001) offer a systems-level perspective of quality, which identifies six core areas that should be addressed to fulfill a QI endeavor. These areas included elements surrounding safety and patient-centered nature of care, effectiveness, timeliness, efficiency, and equitability of services. Hurtado et al. indicate that these key constructs should be the "centerpiece . . . a commitment to care that is evidence-based, patient-centered, and systems-based" (Hurtado et al., 2001, p. 1). Although there is commonality between the Donabedian (1988) and Hurtado et al. (2001) interpretations of *quality*, there is also a significant amount of conceptual distance between the two interpretations (i.e., clinician focus vs. systems focus, respectively), both of which are important considerations.

As outlined by Boaden, Harvey, Moxham, and Proudlove (2008), QI endeavors can resemble both "approaches" and "tools" (p. 46). Many of the process-outcome models endorse the *approach* perspective of QI, on which the entire QI activity is conceptualized as a larger process that is preplanned, executed, and evaluated in a logical, stepwise fashion. For instance, the commonly utilized *Plan-Do-Study-Act* (PDSA) model by Deming (1986) would fulfill the *approach* to conceptualization of QI.

The PDSA model is based on the assumption that in order to improve downstream outcomes, upstream processes must also be improved. Within health care, in an effort to evaluate and improve quality, the PDSA model has been used on a number of occasions as a useful means from which to map the processes and outcomes of an implementation or system use (Murphy, 2013; R. L. Harrison & Lyerla, 2012). This model is discussed in more depth in Chapter 21. However, with respect to theoretical foundations, Donabedian's (1980, 1988) three-part approach to quality assessment and patient safety also fulfills the *approach* ideal, in the way he emphasizes that structure, process, and outcome are all interrelated and should be evaluated as such (Agency for Healthcare Research and Quality [AHRQ], 2005, p. 31). With respect to HIT deployment and use, all three parts are important considerations.

Sociotechnical-Compatible Conceptual Perspectives

There currently exist a number of sociotechnical perspectives that can be used to explore the dynamic relationships between humans and technology within complex environments. Table 3.1 outlines a number of sociotechnical-congruent theoretical perspectives that can be used by a practitioner/researcher to theoretically underpin a QI endeavor. For the purpose of this chapter, ANT will be operationalized as the primary sociotechnical lens of discussion for use within QI activities. The theoretical foundation of ANT encourages a practitioner/researcher to conceptualize that all *things* in an environment are individual *actors* (e.g., people, computers, pencils, chairs, patients, etc.). Actors within an environment are dynamic entities that possess the ability to modify and shape the context around them. ANT is a perspective that first originated from the sociology literature in the early 1980s through the seminal works of Callon (1986), Latour (1991, 2005), and Law and Hassard (1999). Over time, a number of different disciplines have been drawn to ANT as a prospective lens from which to view reality. Geography, sociology, business, literature, and health sciences are among a few of the various disciplines that currently use ANT to help describe and represent the complex environments that are present within each discipline's domain. One of the most contentious (yet important) attributes of ANT is the perspective's inherent assumption that *nonhuman* entities (e.g., computers, pens, chairs, automobiles, etc.) have agency and shape both social and technical processes. Proponents of ANT claim that by viewing situations through a lens in which all actors have agency and importance, a deeper understanding of the role of all actors (whether they are human or nonhuman) can be elucidated (Cresswell, Worth, & Sheikh, 2011; Greenhalgh & Stones, 2010).

ANT—The Basics

An *actor* within ANT is used to denote artifacts or entities that may be human or nonhuman in nature (e.g., pencil, computer, human, etc.), and that have the ability to perform

TABLE 3.1 Sociotechnical-Congruent Theoretical Lenses and Their Relationship to QI Initiatives

Theory Premise/Thesis	Relevant Seminal Author(s)	Summary	Relationship to QI Initiatives	Example of Use in HIT
ANT	Callon (1986), Latour (1991, 2005), Law and Hassard (1999)	Human and nonhuman actors are afforded equal privilege in analysis. Similarly, all actors have the ability to move fluidly between structures in order to translate new networks to facilitate action.	Offers an interpretative lens that affords human and nonhuman actors agency within larger networks of actors. Subsequently, any action QI activity is conceptualized as a network effect of various actors translating new networks.	Cresswell et al. (2010, 2011)
Activity Theory	Engeström (1987, 2001), Lomov (1981), Nardi (1996)	All human action is directed toward an objective (outcome) in the material world. This action is mediated by tools (material tools or other immaterial tools like language), objects, community, subjects, rules, and divisions of labor. Actions and behavior occur within an activity system that may link to other activity systems.	Offers an interpretative lens that identifies various systems-related actors and distributions of culture-work-rules that mediate the generation of an outcome in the activity system. QI strategies can be deconstructed to provide details into the various system actors at play.	Hasu (2000), Korpelainen and Kira (2013), Varpio, Hall, Lingard, and Schryer (2008)

(continued)

55

Theory Premise/Thesis	Relevant Seminal Author(s)	Summary	Relationship to QI Initiatives	Example of Use in HIT
Complexity Theory (Complex adaptive systems)	Benbya and McKelvey (2006), Lewin (1992), Lorenz (1972), Plsek and Greenhalgh (2001), T. Wilson and Holt (1996)	Agents act with freedom and are not predictable, and are interconnected with other agents. Actions of one agent inherently affect other interconnected agents in (sometimes) unpredictable fashions. Agents in systems (embedded into other subsequent systems) subscribe to internalized rules, which may be operationalized in nonlinear and unpredictable fashions.	All QI endeavors operate with complex adaptive systems that are nonlinear and possess inherent unpredictability. Subsequently, the outcome of a QI action is the result of a massive number of other agents interacting among each other (in nonlinear fashions).	Ellis (2010), Kannampallil, Schauer, Cohen, and Patel (2011), Paley (2007)
Socio-technical Systems Theory (in health care)	Berg (1999), Berg et al. (2003), Bostrom and Heinen (1977), Coiera (2007), Trist (1981)	Socially developed aspects of using a system need to be balanced with the technical aspects (and vice versa). Subsequently, both social and technical (sociotechnical) elements of a given situation need to be accounted for and respected when expecting humans and technology to coexist.	QI aspects have historically suffered because of deterministic lenses applied to the situation. Sociotechnical theory attempts to balance the importance of social and technical factors in the development, implementation, and use of ICT. Subsequently, any potential for QI stems from respecting that social and technical forces (and their interplay) need to be considered in metrics/definitions of success.	Ash et al. (2007), M. I. Harrison et al. (2007), Koppel et al. (2005), Koppel, Wetterneck, Telles, and Karsh (2008), Meeks, Takian, Sittig, Singh, and Barber (2014), Sittig and Singh (2010)

| STS | MacKenzie and Wajcman (1999), Pinch and Bijker (1984), Woolgar (1991) | Structure and politics have important roles in shaping technology. Technology determinism or focus concerned merely with the *impact* generated by technology does not recognize the numerous complex and dynamic interactions of technology and society.

Social agents or actors are essential in the construction, organization, and labeling of technology. | A larger focus is placed on social actors within the generation of quality. Although STS lenses have been critiqued as potentially affording too much emphasis on social actors, QI within the STS spectrum could be viewed as manipulating technology through a complex process of (re)interpretation, eventually leading to the technology's use and value espoused by its respective social actors. | De Rouck, Jacobs, and Leys (2008), Timmons (2003), M. Wilson (2002) |

ANT, actor–network theory; ICT, information and communication technology; QI, quality improvement; STS, science and technology studies.

action (Lower, 2006; Walsham, 1997). Regardless, the ability of an *actor* to perform action is not located within the entity itself; rather, action is stimulated and derived from the actor's location within larger *networks* of actors. Therefore, when individual actors come together, networks of actors (i.e., actor-network) can form, align, and stimulate action through a process called *translation.* For instance, in isolation, the nonhuman actor, a pencil, is unable to perform the action of making notations on a piece of paper by itself. If the pencil actor is introduced into a larger collection of other actors, including a human, a piece of paper, and a writing surface like a table, the pencil actor may be used by the human to generate notations in the form of writing on the piece of paper. That said, if the pencil actor is not available within the evolving network of actors (e.g., human, piece of paper, writing surface in form of a table), the human may not be able to generate the action of writing on the piece of paper.

Although seemingly logical and commonsensical, when exploring reality in which both human and nonhuman actors are granted privilege in potentially symmetric fashions, a number of new analytical considerations can be posed. For instance, introspective questions may be generated around which an actor possesses more *agency* or *importance* in the evolving network of a pencil, human, piece of paper, and writing surface. From one perspective, the human actor is the most important actor within this evolving network. If needed, the human could potentially seek a multitude of other writing-apparatus actors (e.g., pen, marker, chalk, etc.) to complete the action of writing on a piece of paper. On the other hand, an equally strong argument could also be made that the pencil actor is the most important actor in the evolving network of a human wishing to write on a piece of paper. The action of writing by a human is fully contingent and mediated on the pencil actor being accessible and available in the evolving network. Without the immediacy of the pencil actor, the larger network of actors working together in synergy (to generate the action of a human writing on paper) is unable to materialize. Although the translation of various actors—a pencil, human, piece of paper, and writing surface—may be a simplistic representation of ANT's deconstructive power, the lens can provide some uniquely interesting analysis when used to explore deeper elements of the translation processes of actor-networks.

A final key element of ANT's conceptualization is the idea of Black Box Network. A Black Box Network is a stabilized actor-network in which all the translation elements that were undertaken during the inscription–translation process described earlier become formalized and appear as "a single actor from the perspective of other actors" (Lower, 2006, p. 98). When Black Box Networks stabilize, all the actors comprised within the network are hidden, and do not represent as single entities; rather, the action generated by the network is viewed as a unified force from the perspective of other actors in the system. For instance, when an intravenous (IV) pump works normally during the medical care of a patient, this activity could be conceptualized as a Black Box Network, along with its other peripheral actors (e.g., patients, nurses, IV solutions, etc.). If the intravenous pump were to fail during the delivery of intravenous fluid to a patient, a larger cascade of action and retranslation of what was once an established Black Box Network might occur, including (a) the dissolution of processes that were commonplace when the intravenous pump operated normally (e.g., a patient receiving intravenous fluid); (b) the establishment of backup processes, with new or modified actors in place of the intravenous pump (e.g., the requirement of a nurse to use a gravity-feed intravenous system); and (c) the stabilization of a new actor-network in which not all the important actors in the situation are not overly satisfied with the outcome or result (e.g., disgruntled clinicians who have to continuously adjust the drip rate of the gravity-fed intravenous system).

How Users of ANT View Reality

Proponents of ANT do not see differences between human and nonhuman actors from an analytical stance, and are also encouraged to avoid fixing actors to predefined scales or levels of analysis. As part of an encompassing ANT perspective, levels of observation or analysis of phenomena should not be a priori constrained or outlined. As stated by Latour (1991), "[t]he socio-technical world does not have a fixed, unchanging scale, and it is not the observer's job to remedy this state of affairs" (p. 119). Because all actors possess potential agency and power to facilitate action with larger networks, constraints should not be applied by the researcher to the environment in which analysis is taking place. Actors should be allowed to move through and between levels and structures, "induced by the actors themselves" (p. 119). As a departure from traditional perspectives that demand *fixing* to a preassigned level of analysis (e.g., individual level, organizational level, etc.), users of ANT must appreciate that actors are dynamic entities that may possess agency well beyond their immediate contexts or environments. Being receptive "to follow the actors themselves" (Latour, 2005, p. 22) through various contexts, environments, and structures is a central tenet within all work underpinned by ANT. In essence, a practitioner/researcher using ANT as a theoretical lens is far more concerned with following actors of emergent importance through their actions, rather than deduced subscription to actors they *think* will be of future importance. However, although the "follow the actors" mantra of ANT is well meaning, it can generate a situation that leads a practitioner/researcher on a never-ending quest for new actors and networks for consideration. It has been suggested by other proponents of ANT (Cresswell, Worth, & Sheikh, 2010; Cresswell et al., 2011) that a pragmatic approach to using ANT may assist in normalizing this inherent weakness of the lens to the extent that a practitioner/researcher using ANT will need to draw conceptual and pragmatic boundaries to satisfy the purposes of his or her research project. Although it may be an interesting analytical exercise to follow actors through various distant structures and networks, determinations will need to be made as to the extent to which these leads are followed, and if they are significant enough to have an impact on the immediate research project at hand. Therefore, depending on the perspectives and needs of the practitioner/researcher, ANT can be a self-limiting approach because of the specificity of the questions being asked, and the span of impact of the proposed findings.

Pragmatic Use of ANT for QI Endeavors Within Informatics Activities

Although seemingly complex, ANT yields its most significant value as a sociotechnical perspective when it is used in a pragmatic fashion—and in doing so this approach avoids (or minimizes) the purely theoretical descriptions of situations. For instance, in the preceding sections, the word *actor* was used to describe a variety of *things* (e.g., including humans and technology). To clarify the semantics, this labeling of things as *actors* (or inscriptions) does tend to become cumbersome with repetitive use. A more pragmatic strategy would be to appreciate that humans and technology are different, and not dwell on their "differentness"; but rather focus on providing accurate and detailed descriptions of how various actors (whether they be humans or nonhumans) interact with each other and the environment they occupy. When ANT's language is distanced from overt discussion of actors, networks, translation, and inscriptions, the value of the lens to assist in the deconstruction of situations is made more salient. Similarly, the interpretability of analysis and findings can be increased, especially because a practitioner/ researcher does not feel obligated to define all elements as an actor, or inscription, or some other element of purist ANT vernacular.

This pragmatic approach to describe human–technology relationships is further outlined in two case scenarios, which demonstrates the operational power of the lens to stimulate rarely posed questions to better frame and address important QI activities involving informatics. Similarly, through the presentation of the following two case scenarios (i.e., acute care computer provider order entry [CPOE] implementation, and, social media usage within a public health unit), the deconstructive power of ANT as a sociotechnical lens through which to view the composition of reality will also be demonstrated.

Using ANT in Conjunction With QI Activities: Evolved Approaches and Tools

ANT is a perspective that possesses the most functional power when it is used within a geographically bound context in which all actors of immediate importance are located within the larger environmental network. Historically, users of ANT have enjoyed success with this lens by using it in conjunction with ethnographic approaches or other naturalistic methods that endorse exploring situated phenomena. By using a pragmatic interpretation of ANT (as described earlier), the hybridization of the lens with a wider range of established methods and approaches can be considered. For instance, the AHRQ (2005) currently supports the use of a modified Donabedian model of patient safety to QI (Coyle & Battles, 1999; Donabedian, 1980), in that the model allows a practitioner/ researcher to perform an "examination of how risks and hazards embedded within the structure of care have the potential to cause injury or harm to patients . . . [including whether] . . . individual or team failures in a health care delivery setting are consistently identified as a leading cause of negative patient outcomes" (AHRQ, 2005, p. 2). Although Coyle and Battles's (1999) modified Donabedian model outlined a number of antecedents, structure, process, and outcome variables important to evaluating the quality of medical care, the model is also inherently social-centric in its conceptualization (Carayon et al., 2006) to the extent that nonhuman artifacts and actors (like health technology) are largely minimized or missing from the model's predefined *environment, structural, process,* and *outcome* variables. Therefore, the authors of this chapter believe that the Coyle and Battles (1999) model might benefit from inclusion of both technically and sociotechnically generated variables, which would assist in refining the functionality of the established model and increase sensitivity toward complex health care environments that involve technology.

To do this, ANT-inspired perspectives can be used to help retrofit previously established QI models, such as Coyle and Battles's (1999), into a more sociotechnically receptive heuristic for practitioner/researcher use. For instance, if, hypothetically, the original Coyle and Battles (1999) framework is used to evaluate medication administration safety within a health care context underpinned by a CPOE system, then the CPOE actor (and its role) may be minimized. Because all Donabedian-inspired models (like Coyle and Battles's) afford conceptual privilege to clinicians and providers, the humanistic lens of the model's focus reduces the potential for technical and structural actors to possess agency or importance within the evaluation. Further, because CPOE systems are typically implemented with the mentality that they improve safety (Koppel et al., 2005), a priori assumptions about their value and role within the larger environment may further add to the CPOE's minimization as an important actor within the larger environment.

Although models, such as Donabedian's (1988), favor socially constructed ideals of reality, this is not to suggest that these models are averse to evolution or improvement. For instance, the structural elements of the Coyle and Battles (1999) model could be made more sensitive to the importance of technical actors, and the fluidity of all actors within the context. As a key element of ANT, the ability of actors to move freely between levels and structures should be entertained as a reality of sociotechnical environments (Latour, 2005), and not artificially controlled by a practitioner/researcher. This evolution could also be viewed as a strength in that it fulfills the authors' desire to develop future models that help practitioners "determine whether [study] outcomes were due to the [study] interventions or to patient factors" (Coyle & Battles, 1999, p. 6).

Therefore, although Coyle and Battles's (1999) model offers a usable logic model from which to conceptualize patient safety, it is recommended that a practitioner/researcher wishing to use their model *add* new variables (or actors and their related networks) to the existing model in an iterative process, dependent on the environment, that are relevant to their QI activity. Instead of relying only on the variables described in the established model to predict some element of the QI pathway, it is suggested that practitioners/researchers use pragmatic interpretations of ANT to help identify sociotechnically constructed variables (e.g., how clinicians interact with the CPOE; how patients' outcomes are related to usage behaviors of the CPOE by nurses; etc.), which will be likely more important to the evaluation at hand as a result of their specificity and emergence from the QI environment. Subsequently, by combining the Coyle and Battles (1999) model with the reactivity provided by ANT, variables of interest will not be static or overly a priori deduced. Rather, the established QI models like Coyle and Battles (1999) provide the initial inspiration and conceptual grounding for an evaluation; after the grounding is established within the QI environment, ANT becomes the dominant lens that drives a practitioner/researcher to seek out other important actors and networks for study and examination (and subsequent revision of the operational QI model being used to assist in the endeavor). In this fashion, blurring traditional models of QI with reactive sociotechnical lenses like ANT assists in generating a pragmatic methodology that appreciates the structure of the established QI model (i.e., Coyle and Battles), but is immensely more dynamic due to its subscription to ANT principles, which allow for the discovery of other important mediating actors that are sometimes buried within the complex environment.

ANT AND QI METHODS COMBINED: CASE STUDY EXAMPLES

Case Study 1: Medication Administration With Closed-Loop CPOE

Background

A practitioner/researcher seeks to evaluate the effectiveness of a newly implemented closed-loop CPOE system that is linked with a patient-medication barcoding identification system. The CPOE and related automated dispensing processes have been in place for roughly 1 month on the acute care pilot unit, and a QI analysis is scheduled to determine clinician adoption of the new medication administration practices.

Clinical Context

Nurses on this pilot implementation unit have historically administered medications using a manual paper-based process, with unit dosing available for most medications supplied by the pharmacy. Over the past month, there has been a significant amount of trepidation voiced by the nurses, clinicians, and some administrative staff in regard to the CPOE implementation. Although clinicians have been supported by clinician superusers, mixed perceptions regarding the value of the CPOE and its usability to the nursing role are commonly voiced as complaints of the newly implemented system. Possible QI topics for evaluation within this case, resulting from sociotechnical dimensions, are as follows:

▶ Nurse-specific quality aspects in regard to the new CPOE and automated medication dispensing protocols
▶ Workflow and work-process evolution with the presence of the new CPOE and medication system
▶ Unintended consequences and outcomes of process evolution in regard to the introduction of the new CPOE and medication processes
▶ Frequency or prevalence of medication or sentinel events, pre- and post-implementation
▶ Efficiency and work-time sampling of new CPOE processes versus previous paper-based methodologies

Various dimensions resulting from the sociotechnical perspective can be derived based on the scenario described. Table 3.2 reflects some potential approaches that use a sociotechnical perspective to approach improvement. The case continues discussing how a sociotechnical theoretical framework can be combined with traditional PDSA approaches to achieve a focused approach to improving the CPOE and medication barcoding process described earlier.

QI Context

A practitioner/researcher decided to explore the *safety elements* of the CPOE and related medication administration technology and the first important QI activity to be addressed was to optimize the electronic health record in her institution. To do this, she elected Langley et al.'s (2009) approach to improvement strategies

(continued)

ANT AND QI METHODS COMBINED: CASE STUDY EXAMPLES (*continued*)

TABLE 3.2 Resulting Sociotechnical Dimensions for Consideration in QI

End User	Workflow and Processes	Patient Safety	Measures of Impact
User attitudes, perceptions, and satisfaction of system	Larger workflow redevelopments, including all clinician and administrative staff	Generation of new types of medication errors or potential for latent errors	Work-time sampling pre- and postimplemen-tation
Comments on system functionality, system quality, impacts on care-provider role	Impacts on patients, family, and visitors in terms of new medication administration processes	Number/severity of medication errors pre–post implementation	Comparison of efficiency on similar unit that has not undergone CPOE implementation
User adoption, acceptance, and compliance with new processes	Impacts with other previously developed work patterns or other related HIT systems	Reporting of errors	Impacts on client care, both perceived and measurable
	New workarounds developed by all types of human actors (e.g., housing, physical services, clinicians, pharmacy, dietary, etc.)		
	Workarounds and other end-user-specific developed processes		

CPOE, computerized physcician order entry; HIT, health information technology; QI, quality improvement.

as a suitable framework to drive the quality endeavor. Langley et al. suggest three important steps prior to moving into the PDSA cycle: (a) determine what you want to accomplish, (b) determine how you will measurably know you made a difference with the improvement, and (c) determine what changes can be made to the

ANT AND QI METHODS COMBINED: CASE STUDY EXAMPLES (*continued*)

process that will be considered an improvement from a quality, safety, or efficiency standpoint.

Because it was the researcher's goal to help improve the immediate process to benefit longer term outcomes, selection of the PDSA model was congruent with the larger overall purpose of the QI initiative. In this model, the focus is on what is to be accomplished with improvement strategies. Additionally, the model stresses a measureable difference based on the improvement strategy. This approach offers a way of designing a comprehensive approach to patient safety and quality focused on the process to be improved. In this case, it is the medication administration process. The Langley et al. approach capitalizes on Deming's fundamental improvement process within the PDSA improvement model noted in Figure 3.2. To explicitly address medication administration safety, emphasis is on medication errors and focusing on the identification of processes that lead to error to redesign the process using the PDSA cycle for improvement.

After selecting her theoretical lens to help inform the QI activity, the practitioner/researcher narrowed her focus of patient safety on *medication errors and near misses generated pre- and postimplementation of the CPOE and related medication system*. Given the researcher's knowledge of sociotechnical perspectives (and ANT), she was cognizant that only exploring the medication errors noted in the incident and error reporting system pre- and postimplementation would likely fail to provide her an encompassing perspective of the true frequency or mechanism of medication-related errors/near misses. Subsequently, the researcher decided to

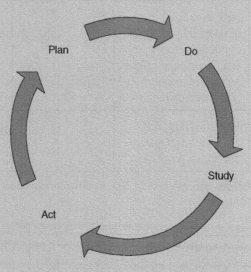

FIGURE 3.2. PDSA improvement model.

(*continued*)

ANT AND QI METHODS COMBINED: CASE STUDY EXAMPLES (*continued*)

approach this situation using mixed research methods, first commencing with qualitative interviews with key staff and clinicians about their experiences using the CPOE system. By doing key interviews with staff, the researcher hoped to generate new perspectives and variables that could be valuable for further exploration and analysis.

After conducting interviews with staff nurses, physicians, clerical staff, clinical informatics, and pharmacy department actors, a deeper level of understanding regarding the current state of CPOE use was generated. Two major workflow issues arose from the data generated in the interviews: (a) scanning of medication barcodes and patient ID bands was found to be a cumbersome process. Similarly, it was found that patient ID bands were often removed from the patient and affixed to the IV poles or other medical equipment beside the respective patient; (b) the barcode scanners were immensely frustrating to use if the barcode on the medication was bent or slightly damaged. This resulted in nurses generating an override (i.e., the nurse does not validate the patient's ID and/or medication as outlined by the new medication administration guidelines) of the new medication administration process.

Quantitative data drawn from traditional reporting sources demonstrated that nurses had been utilizing the override features of the barcode scanning technology on a regular basis, over each shift. Trending over time demonstrated that the use of the override functionality has retained a consistent baseline frequency per shift, which was noted to be increasing in prevalence over the month. Reassuringly, medication errors and near misses did not change significantly over the month, as per the formal reporting data.

Further qualitative workflow shadowing of clinicians also confirmed some of the less than ideal practice actions outlined by participants in the key informant interviews (e.g., the taping of patient ID bands to either the bedside or an IV pole in close proximity to the patient). Direct observation of nurses demonstrated to the practitioner/researcher that nurses had an increasing propensity to use the scanning override if the barcode scanner should become temperamental, or not work "the first time." Subsequently, instead of seeking assistance or trouble shooting use of the barcode scanner, its function and importance in the medication administration process were circumvented if the scanner presented a slight usability issue (or a barcode on the medication could not be read on the first scanning attempt). Similarly, it was noted by the researcher that nurses spent a significant amount of time "worrying about scanning" their medication instead of "thinking about" various medication administration best practices. It was also noted through direct observation that some nurses diminished their clinical judgment during the medication process because "the computer and barcode scanners say it is okay to give the medication."

(*continued*)

ANT AND QI METHODS COMBINED: CASE STUDY EXAMPLES (*continued*)

Although reported medication errors had not increased (or decreased) with the implementation of the CPOE, a number of new potential latent errors and compromises to medication administration best practices of nurses were likely facilitated by the introduction of the CPOE actor. Similarly, the technology had an unintended consequence of (at times) facilitating the dilution of a clinician's judgment surrounding the administration of medication.

Subsequently, through the mixed-methods QI analysis, a new range of sociotechnically based variables and constructs was uncovered that would be of importance when conducting future QI initiatives. For instance, the ID badge actors of patients were not static entities and possessed a significant amount of importance within the medication process (i.e., the ability of the ID badge to be removed from the patient and placed near the patient on other transient medical equipment). Nurses also commented and demonstrated that the barcodes on the medication (and the subsequent barcode scanner actor) possessed some unique usability and human factors flaws, which over time exacerbated the workarounds and circumvention of formalized processes. Finally, the frequency of reporting of medication errors did not seem to be directly influenced by the implementation of the CPOE system. Given the aforementioned issues confronted by nurses and other clinicians using the system, the evidence from this stage of the QI endeavor anecdotally suggests that *new* types of medication errors or near misses have unknowingly occurred; in spite of this, recognition and awareness of these new types of errors by clinicians and staff (and metrics from which to codify them) likely would need to be developed through future QI activities. This case study further emphasizes why Langley et al.'s three points are critical to determine prior to beginning a process. The approach taken by the researcher using a sociotechnical perspective (ANT) helped to determine what was needed to improve the process, how to measure the effectiveness of improvement, and what really needed to be improved prior to launching into improvement cycles of PDSA.

Case Study 1: Conclusion

Subsequently, in following the Langley et al. (2009) PDSA model, the "Act" element should seek to further explore and address the new perspectives outlined earlier through future and ongoing QI activities (i.e., latent medication errors/near misses, usability aspects of the barcode scanner, education surrounding patient ID bands). Further discussion of QI methods is fully covered in subsequent chapters.

Case Study 2: Social Media and Public Health

Background

A practitioner/researcher sought to evaluate the effectiveness of a social media campaign operated by a local public health unit in the health-promotion area of

(*continued*)

ANT AND QI METHODS COMBINED: CASE STUDY EXAMPLES (*continued*)

family and parenting health. The health unit generated its own corporate Facebook page, and has been using the page to discuss with other Facebook users (principally serving, but not limited to, their geographic catchment region) concerns about a number of parenting topics, including breastfeeding, postpartum care, and other infant/child health concerns.

After a prolonged pilot and feasibility test, the use of Facebook was in place for nearly 6 months. The health unit currently staffs the Facebook page during working hours, Monday through Friday, and responds to *all* comments and questions left by users. Nurses supporting the Facebook page have been trained in social media engagement, and follow a flexible engagement rubric to prevent inadvertent public discussion of personal health issues on the public page. For concerns and discussions that become "too personal," users of the page are directed to a call the center operated by the public health unit, where more confidential consultation can be delivered by public health nurses. If users attempt to troll or postinflammatory/inappropriate comments on the page, the nurses follow a detailed response protocol to determine their course of action.

Clinical Context

Nurses and leadership at the public health unit were interested in conducting a QI analysis regarding the use of Facebook to connect and address health questions posed by users. Since Facebook was never originally conceptualized as a health-promotion tool, a number of legal, ethical, and privacy considerations had to be vetted well in advance of the pilot testing and implementation. In this public health-program, the nurses supporting the Facebook page possess autonomy in regard to the content they post, and strategize information that they believe to be relevant to their followers online.

Anecdotally, the nurses and health unit leadership were confident that the Facebook page was successfully engaging Internet users regarding parenting health issues. However, nurses and leadership were less clear about how to continue to maximize the success they have generated, and continue to improve quality in their service delivery via the Facebook platform. The team focused on the following areas: attitudes of users, perceptions and satisfaction, consumer engagement, workflow and processes, and impact on health-promotion.

As with the prior case, the team examined the different dimensions resulting from the technical perspective based on this public health unit's use of technology to impact health outcomes. Table 3.3 reflects some potential options that use a sociotechnical perspective to approach improvement combined with the Donabedian model. The case continues discussing how a sociotechnical theoretical framework can be combined with Donabedian's model to achieve a focused approach to evaluating this public health initiative using technology (Facebook) as an intervention to engage health consumers.

(*continued*)

ANT AND QI METHODS COMBINED: CASE STUDY EXAMPLES (*continued*)

TABLE 3.3 Sociotechnical Dimensions for Consideration of Health Outcomes

End User	Processes/ Interventions	Structure	Outcome Measuring Engagement
User attitudes, perceptions, and satisfaction of system	Evolving communication for a social space	Policy evolution using social media within health unit	Analytic tools (e.g., Facebook analytics) to determine the approximate geographic location of users, linger time on page, and search terms utilized to arrive on the Facebook page
Comments on system functionality, system quality, impacts on care-provider role	Developing engaging messaging	Nursing staff requirements to man social media presence	Generation of metrics related to content sharing, *liking*, and number of emergent conversations stimulated by users and nurses
User adoption, acceptance, and compliance with new processes	Building an online community of health-promotion practice	Staff training utilization	Frequency of posts and other engagement activities from high-, medium-, and low-volume users
	Response time to message posted by users	Development time required by clinicians to repackage health information for social media environment	Search engine optimization statistics of online presence
	Sentiment analysis of posts		

(*continued*)

ANT AND QI METHODS COMBINED: CASE STUDY EXAMPLES (*continued*)

QI Context

A team decision to explore *user engagement* with the public health Facebook page was an important first QI activity; this exploration established a baseline for future comparison. To conduct this analysis, the practitioner/researcher elected to use an approach inspired by Donabedian (1988), which underscored the important role of the nurse in this social communication modality. Donabedian's classical framework identifies three overriding dimensions of health care evaluation: structure, process, and outcomes (Donabedian, 1988).

After selecting the Donabedian (1988) theoretical lens from which to drive the QI activity, the practitioner/researcher narrowed *the assessment to engagement activities generated within the parenting Facebook page*. Of particular interest was how nurses engaged with Internet users by shaping health-promotion messages. Subsequently, the practitioner/researcher was also interested in the reactivity of users to these forms of engagement.

Because of the nontraditional nature of social media evaluations, the practitioner/researcher was cognizant that only reviewing basic Facebook website metrics (e.g., number of unique visitors or page views) was not an overly informative methodology from which to generate deeper insights into user engagement characteristics. Subsequently, using the Donabedian (1988) approach with a sociotechnical-framed lens (drawn from a pragmatic understanding of ANT), a number of other considerations related to the Facebook page were theorized even before collecting and reviewing engagement data. The following are questions considered by the researcher and the team evaluating the public health initiative:

▶ Will this QI endeavor be focused specifically on nurses, Internet users, or the relationship between the nurses and users of the Facebook page?

▶ What theoretical model will be used to best approach the QI question(s)—will this model be reactive to the two-way engagement ideals of a socially generated online space?

▶ Will the QI endeavor be conceptualized as an approach (process), or, as a tool to acquire some deeper level knowledge regarding a process?

▶ What evaluation methods will be used? How will quantitative and qualitative data be triangulated to assist generating the larger and more comprehensive QI analysis?

▶ What is the purpose of this QI assessment? To provide justification to continue diverting resources to support the use of the Facebook page? To generate empirical evidence as to the effectiveness and usefulness of a Facebook page for a health unit? To develop new engagement strategies/methodologies for public health that are mediated through social media technologies? To better understand the population being served by the public health unit, and generate more targeted health-promotion activities?

(*continued*)

ANT AND QI METHODS COMBINED: CASE STUDY EXAMPLES (*continued*)

First, it was recognized that social media platforms, such as Facebook, are extremely two-way communication tools, using which Internet users and nurses alike come together to form an online community where discussion and information sharing happens. Given this dynamic environment, only exploring the actor of the nurse in the generation and facilitation of engagement would not provide a holistic assessment of engagement. For example, users are able to share posts to their Facebook friends, comment on users posts, and also interact with nurses who pose questions and share health-related content. Because of this two-way (and potentially exponential) dynamic, the construct of *engagement* was conceptualized as a sociotechnical relationship between a multitude of human (e.g., nurses, users, etc.) and technical (e.g., Internet, Facebook, interface devices, etc.) actors.

Given the quantitative and qualitative elements of the QI endeavor at hand, the practitioner/researcher decided to use a mixed-methods approach to best qualify and quantify how the nurses facilitated engagement (and correspondingly, how Internet users also shaped engagement). To explore this construct of engagement, the practitioner/researcher first sought to understand how the nurses organized and operated their Facebook page during working hours. Through observation online, the practitioner/researcher recorded the responsiveness of clinicians to questions posed on the Facebook thread, how many posts were generated by nurses per day, and the reactivity of Internet users to the posted threads (e.g., number and sentiment of comments, likes, shares, etc.). Through observing an emergent day's worth of engagement (and review of previous day's message threads), the practitioner/researcher decided he had a reasonable understanding of the workflow of the clinicians using the Facebook page. Upon summarizing his findings, he sought key informant interviews with staff and nurses who were responsible for the Facebook page's operation. The nurses interviewed confirmed the credibility of the observed data collected by the practitioner/researcher, and offered insights and reflections related to their decision making regarding responding to users' messages and the posting of health-promotion material.

Although impressed with the qualitative findings, the practitioner/researcher and team also wished to triangulate these findings with representative quantitative data of nurse and users engagement within the Facebook page. To do so, quantitative data provided by the analytic program (Facebook Insights) operating in the background of the Facebook page was queried for relevant information (i.e., frequency/number of likes to the main page, number of views to each message thread, and the mechanism through which the user navigated to the site). Through a thorough review of the analytic data, it was found that a significant majority of the traffic to the Facebook page came from habitual users, who frequented the site regularly throughout the week. A smaller percentage (around 20%) were new users who typically arrived at the site through Google search terms, such as "parenting," "breastfeeding," "baby health," "public health," and "help."

(*continued*)

ANT AND QI METHODS COMBINED: CASE STUDY EXAMPLES (*continued*)

With this baseline qualitative and quantitative assessment completed, the practitioner/research and the public health team decided to further refine the focus of the assessment by explicitly using the Donabedian *structure–process–outcome* framework. Using the new insights gained by exploring the Facebook- page use from a sociotechnical perspective, the researcher/practitioner was able to generate more refined considerations to operationalize within the Donabedian framework.

QI Aim: Determine how engagement occurs between nurse-users on the Facebook page, with the secondary aim of sustaining or improving engagement.

Structure: Nurses seek to encourage and endorse engagement of Internet users by posting interesting health-promotion material, responding to questions, and directing users to appropriate health care resources on their Facebook page. Users respond to posts generated by nurses, and also submit their own content and ideas for consideration. Currently, the Facebook page is a two-way dynamic in which engagement in the health content is a mutually synergetic dynamic.

Other potential sociotechnically inspired *structural* aspects that the team considered included the following:

▶ The types of interface devices used by nurses and users to connect to the Facebook page
▶ Evolving usage and privacy settings operated by Facebook
▶ Evolving policy and government legislation in terms of health information
▶ How the Facebook page is conceptualized by its users (e.g., novelty or important resource for health information)
▶ How the Facebook platform encourages or diminishes collaboration between users and nurses

Process: Nurses need to continue to appreciate and (re)learn how to shape health-promotion messages for social spaces that are funny, engaging, and that minimize paternalism. Similarly, various nonstatic policies need to be in place in order to generate appropriate usage guidelines for nurses to avoid crossing ethical or legal boundaries regarding the distribution of health care advice or information to users.

Using social network analysis techniques and data mining, sentiment analyses can be conducted to determine whether users of the Facebook page are receiving information they perceive to be important and relevant to their situation. Similarly, engagement of users in the form of sharing and commenting on postings generated by the nurse (or other users) should also be seen as a behavior change, encompassing health-promotion ideals.

Technical: Nurses should generate best practice guidelines for reshaping clinical and health-promotion information for Facebook audiences. Similarly, nurses should continue to use other related social technologies that help to reinforce Facebook as a main actor in the delivery of health-promotion services related to parenting and family health.

(*continued*)

ANT AND QI METHODS COMBINED: CASE STUDY EXAMPLES (*continued*)

Interpersonal: Nurses should reflect on the value that connecting with users on Facebook has generated, and what new areas of growth have arisen. Because communication with Facebook offers a different community modality from which to connect with health-professionals, exploring users' satisfaction or receptivity to new forms of engagement is warranted to fulfill a baseline quality assessment.

Other potential sociotechnically inspired *process* aspects considered by the team included the following:

▶ Further refine nurses' abilities to generate messaging that is engaging and relevant to a potentially heterogeneous population of users with a variety of needs.

▶ Continue to evolve and refine engagement actions in lieu of new and emergent social technologies (e.g., mash-up of other social platforms alongside Facebook, like Twitter and Instagram).

▶ Proactively evaluate how users evolve over time, in terms of their engagement styles, frequencies of use, and purposes for using the Facebook site.

▶ Continue to revisit the workload requirements to maintain an active and responsive Facebook page, especially one that is potentially synergized with other social platforms or other traditional communication technology (e.g., call center, face-to-face clinic days).

Outcomes: Both nurses and users should possess positive perceptions toward the use of Facebook and the translation of health-promotion knowledge. In the case of the nurses, engagement could be evaluated as the way users translate and evolve posted health information. Similarly, nurses would benefit from knowing how many users frequent, access, and engage with the content in a social format (e.g., liking and sharing). From the perspective of the users, an engagement outcome could qualitatively be shaped in the form of a positive sentiment analysis. Similarly, quantitative engagement metrics could also be combined with qualitative data to generate better ideas of behavior change with the user population, and whether the material presented on the Facebook page continues to attract new users, via different entry mechanisms on the Internet (e.g., Facebook ads, Google search, shared link from a current user, etc.)

Other potential sociotechnically inspired *outcomes* aspects considered by the team included the following:

▶ Increased engagement from Internet-user populations who are hard to locate or reach

▶ A stabilized level of usage and engagement by users on a daily and weekly basis

▶ An increase in engagement after the introduction of other social tools that build the presence and reputation of the Facebook page as an authoritative source of parenting health information

(*continued*)

ANT AND QI METHODS COMBINED: CASE STUDY EXAMPLES (*continued*)

> ▶ An increase in the trend of sharing, distributing, and modifying (in a positive or negative fashion) material generated and shared by nurses on the Facebook page with other Internet users.
>
> ### Case Study 2: Conclusion
>
> From this modification of a Donabedian process, deeper insights into the engagement activities of both nurses and users may be ascertained. The *structure–process–outcome* approach offers a usable logic model from which to drive a QI activity, and can be modified to endorse relationships between actors (e.g., like social technology and nurse-users) in meaningful ways to help stimulate deeper inquiry.

SUMMARY

Overall, this chapter has introduced a range of topics and concepts, including the building blocks of science, sociotechnical perspectives, ANT, and QI approaches for use within nursing informatics endeavors. Similarly, the authors of this chapter have advocated using the reactive sociotechnical lens of ANT as a heuristic from which to help inform and evolve traditional QI models for use within health informatics projects. It is hoped that through this marriage of methods and methodologies, deeper insights into how HIT can be both used and evaluated within patient and consumer populations to improve care quality will be generated for the profession.

Finally, this chapter has advocated the reconceptualization of the evaluation of QI activities within the informatics specialty involving HIT. To do this, mixed research methods, utilizing both quantitative and qualitative sources of data, are advocated in order to generate better and more nuanced triangulated evidence in terms of the quality and effectiveness of various HIT. Through this iterative approach, it is hoped that future QI activities will continue to use theoretical and conceptual frameworks from which to drive evaluation, and will remain cognizant of the various context and sociotechnical forces at play in all evaluation research.

EXERCISES AND QUESTIONS FOR CONSIDERATION

Consider a QI opportunity in your clinical setting related to sociotechnical interactions. Using the case studies discussed and the information provided in this chapter, consider the theoretical approaches described and the Langley et al. approach to improvement strategies. Reflect on the following questions related to the QI opportunity identified:

1. Will this QI endeavor be a prospective, retrospective, or cross-sectional activity?

2. What theoretical model will be used to best approach the question(s)?

3. Will my theoretical model need to be evolved to capture subtle sociotechnical considerations of the environment?

4. Will I be conceptualizing this QI endeavor as an *approach* (process), or as a *tool* to acquire some deeper level of knowledge regarding a process or quality indicator?

5. What evaluation method(s) will I use (e.g., quantitative, qualitative, mixed methods)?

6. What is the purpose of this QI—safety improvement, accreditation, gauge the effectiveness of the new HIT within practice, and so forth?

REFERENCES

Agency for Healthcare Research and Quality. (2005). *Chapter 4: Medical team training: Medical teamwork and patient safety: The evidence-based relation.* (No. AHRQ2005). Rockville, MD: Author. Retrieved from http://www.ahrq.gov/research/findings/final-reports/medteam/chapter4.html

Ash, J. S., Sittig, D. F., Dykstra, R. H., Guappone, K., Carpenter, J. D., & Seshadri, V. (2007). Categorizing the unintended sociotechnical consequences of computerized provider order entry. *International Journal of Medical Informatics, 76* Suppl 1, S21–S27. doi:10.1016/j.ijmedinf.2006.05.017

Bagozzi, R. P. (2007). The legacy of the technology acceptance model and a proposal for a paradigm shift. *Journal of the Association for Information Systems, 8*(4), 244–254.

Bakken, S., Stone, P. W., & Larson, E. L. (2008). A nursing informatics research agenda for 2008–18: Contextual influences and key components. *Nursing Outlook, 56*(5), 206–214.e3. doi:10.1016/j.outlook.2008.06.007

Batalden, P., Davidoff, F., Marshall, M., Bibby, J., & Pink, C. (2011). So what? Now what? Exploring, understanding and using the epistemologies that inform the improvement of healthcare. *Quality and Safety, 20*(1), i99–i105. doi:10.1136/bmjqs.2011.051698

Benbya, H., & McKelvey, B. (2006). Toward a complexity theory of information systems development. *Information Technology & People, 19*(1), 12–34. doi:10.1108/09593840610649952

Berg, M. (1999). Patient care information systems and health care work: A sociotechnical approach. *International Journal of Medical Informatics, 55*(2), 87–101. doi:http://dx.doi.org/10.1016/S1386-5056(99)00011-8

Berg, M., Aarts, J., & van Der Lei, J. (2003). ICT in health care: Sociotechnical approaches. *Methods of Information in Medicine, 42*(4), 297–301. doi:10.1267/METH03040297

Berwick, D. M. (1989). Continuous improvement as an ideal in healthcare. *New England Journal of Medicine, 320*(1), 53–56.

Berwick, D. M. (2003). Improvement, trust, and the healthcare workforce. *Quality and Safety in Health Care, 6*(6), 2–7. doi:10.1136/qhc.12.suppl_1.i2

Berwick, D. M. (2008). The science of improvement. *Journal of the American Medical Association, 299*(10), 1182–1184. doi:10.1001/jama.299.10.1182

Berwick, D. M., Nolan, T. W., & Whittington, J. (2008). The triple aim: Care, health, and cost. *Health Affairs (Project Hope), 27*(3), 759–769. doi:10.1377/hlthaff.27.3.759

Boaden, R., Harvey, G., Moxham, C., & Proudlove, N. (2008). *Quality improvement: Theory and practice in healthcare.* (No. NHS-III2008). Coventry, UK: NHS Institute for Innovation and Improvement.

Bostrom, B. R. P., & Heinen, J. S. (1977). STS perspective MIS problems and failures : A socio-technical perspective part I: The causes. *MIS Quarterly, 1*(3), 17–32.

Brown, S. J., Cioffi, M. A., Schinella, P., & Shaw, A. (1995). Evaluation of the impact of a bedside terminal system in a rapidly changing community hospital. *Computers in Nursing, 13*(6), 280–284. doi:PMID: 8529141

Callon, M. (1986). Some elements of a sociology of translation: Domestication of the scallops and the fishermen of St Brieuc Bay. In J. Law (Ed.), *Power, action and belief: A new sociology of knowledge* (pp. 196–223). London, UK: Routledge.

Carayon, P., Schoofs Hundt, A., Karsh, B. T., Gurses, A. P., Alvarado, C. J., Smith, M., & Flatley Brennan, P. (2006). Work system design for patient safety: The SEIPS model. *Quality and Safety in Health Care, 15*(Suppl. 1), i50–i58. doi:10.1136/qshc.2005.015842

Carrington, J. M. (2012). Development of a conceptual framework to guide a program of research exploring nurse-to-nurse communication. *Computers, Informatics, Nursing, 30*(6), 293–299. doi:10.1097/NXN.0b013e31824af809

Chang, I., Hwang, H., Hung, W., & Li, Y. (2007). Physicians' acceptance of pharmacokinetics-based clinical decision support systems. *Expert Systems with Applications, 33*(2), 296–303. doi:10.1016/j.eswa.2006.05.001

Chinn, P. L., & Jacobs, M. K. (1983). *Theory and nursing: A systematic approach.* St. Louis, MO: Mosby.

Codman, E. A. (1916). The classic: A study in hospital efficiency: As demonstrated by the case report of first five years of private hospital. *Clinical Orthoapedics and Related Research, 471*(6), 1778–1783. doi:10.1007/s11999-012-2751-3

Coiera, E. (2004). Four rules for the reinvention of health care. *British Medical Journal, 328,* 1197–1199. doi:10.1136/bmj.328.7449.1197

Coiera, E. (2007). Putting the technical back into socio-technical systems research. *International Journal of Medical Informatics, 76* Suppl 1, S98–S103. doi:10.1016/j.ijmedinf.2006.05.026

Coyle, Y. M., & Battles, J. B. (1999). Using antecedents of medical care to develop valid quality of care measures. *Journal of the International Society for Quality in Health Care/ISQua, 11*(1), 5–12.

Cresswell, K. M., Worth, A., & Sheikh, A. (2010). Actor-network theory and its role in understanding the implementation of information technology developments in healthcare. *BMC Medical Informatics and Decision Making, 10*(1), 67. doi:10.1186/1472-6947-10-67

Cresswell, K. M., Worth, A., & Sheikh, A. (2011). Implementing and adopting electronic health record systems: How actor-network theory can support evaluation. *Clinical Governance, 16*(4), 320–336. doi:10.1108/14777271111175369

Davis, F. D. (1989). Perceived usefulness, perceived ease of use, and user acceptance of information technology. *Management Information Systems Quarterly, 13*(3), 319–340. doi:10.2307/249008

Davis, F. D., Bagozzi, R. P., & Warshaw, P. R. (1989). User acceptance of computer technology: A comparison of two theoretical models. *Journal of Management Sciences, 35*(8), 982–1003. doi:http://dx.doi.org/10.1287/mnsc.35.8.982

DeLone, W. H. (2003). The DeLone and McLean model of information systems success: A ten-year update. *Journal of Management Information Systems, 19*(4), 9–30.

DeLone, W. H., & McLean, E. R. (1992). Information systems success: The quest for the dependent variable. *Information Systems Research, 3*(1), 60–95. doi:10.1287/isre.3.1.60

Deming, E. W. (1986). *Out of the crisis.* Cambridge, MA: Massachusetts Institute of Technology, Center for Advanced Engineering Study.

De Rouck, S., Jacobs, A., & Leys, M. (2008). A methodology for shifting the focus of e-health support design onto user needs: A case in the homecare field. *International Journal of Medical Informatics*, 77(9), 589–601. doi:10.1016/j.ijmedinf.2007.11.004

Donabedian, A. (1980). *Explorations in quality assessment and monitoring volume 1: The definition of quality and approaches to its assessment*. Ann Arbor, MI: Health Administration Press.

Donabedian, A. (1988). The quality of care: How can it be assessed? *Journal of the American Medical Association*, 260(12), 1743–1748.

Donabedian, A. (1989). The quality of care: How can it be assessed? *Journal of the American Medical Association*, 260(12), 1743–1748. doi:10.1001/jama.1988.03410120089033

Drucker, P. F. (1971). What we can learn from Japanese management. *Harvard Business Review*, 49(2), 110–122.

Edwards, P. J. (2006). *Electronic medical records and computerized physician order entry: Examining factors and methods that foster clinician it acceptance in pediatric hospitals* (Doctoral dissertation). Retrieved from https://smartech.gatech.edu/handle/1853/11591

Effken, J. A. (2003). An organizing framework for nursing informatics research. *Computers, Informatics, Nursing*, 21(6), 316–323; 324–325.

Ellis, B. (2010). Complexity in practice: Understanding primary care as a complex adaptive system. *Informatics in Primary Care*, 18, 135–140.

Engeström, Y. (1987). *Learning by expanding: an activity-theoretical approach to developmental research*. Helsinki, Finland: Orienta-Konsultit.

Engeström, Y. (2001). Expansive learning at work: Toward an activity theoretical reconceptualization. *Journal of Education and Work*, 14, 133–156. doi:10.1080/13639080123238

Englebardt, S. P., & Nelson, R. (2002). *Healthcare informatics: An interdisciplinary approach*. Independence, KY: Gale, Cengage Learning.

Fawcett, J. (1984). *Analysis and evaluation of conceptual models of nursing*. Philadelphia, PA: F. A. Davis.

Geels, F. W. (2007). Feelings of discontent and the promise of middle range theory for STS: Examples from technology dynamics. *Science, Technology & Human Values*, 32(6), 627–651. doi:10.1177/016224 3907303597

Goossen, W. (2000). Nursing informatics research. *Nurse Researcher*, 8(2), 42–54.

Graves, J. R., & Corcoran, S. (1989). The study of nursing informatics. *Journal of Nursing Scholarship*, 21(4), 227–231.

Greenhalgh, T., & Stones, R. (2010). Theorising big IT programmes in healthcare: Strong structuration theory meets actor-network theory. *Social Science & Medicine*, 70(9), 1285–1294. doi:10.1016/j .socscimed.2009.12.034

Grinspun, D., Virani, T., & Bajnok, I. (2001). Nursing best practice guidelines: The RNAO (Registered Nurses Association of Ontario) project. *Hospital Quarterly*, 5(2), 56–60.

Guyatt, G., & Drummond, R. (2002). *Users' guides to the medical literature: A manual for evidence-based clinical practice* (1st ed.). Chicago, IL: American Medical Association.

Harrison, M. I., Koppel, R., & Bar-Lev, S. (2007). Unintended consequences of information technologies in health care: An interactive sociotechnical analysis. *Journal of the American Medical Informatics Association*, 14(5), 542–549. doi:10.1197/jamia.M2384

Harrison, R. L., & Lyerla, F. (2012). Using nursing clinical decision support systems to achieve meaningful use. *Computers, Informatics, Nursing, 30*(7), 380–385. doi:10.1097/NCN.0b013e31823eb813

Hasu, M. (2000). Constructing clinical use: An activity-theoretical perspective on implementing new technology. *Technology Analysis & Strategic Management, 12*(3), 369–382. doi:10.1080/09537320050130606

Holden, R. J., & Karsh, B. (2010). The technology acceptance model: Its past and its future in health care. *Journal of Biomedical Informatics, 43*(1), 159–172. doi:10.1016/j.jbi.2009.07.002

Hurtado, M. P., Swift, E. K., & Corrigan, J. M. (2001). *Crossing the quality chasm: A new health system for the 21st century.* (No. IOM2001). Washington, DC: Institute of Medicine.

Kannampallil, T. G., Schauer, G. F., Cohen, T., & Patel, V. L. (2011). Considering complexity in healthcare systems. *Journal of Biomedical Informatics, 44*(6), 943–947. doi:10.1016/j.jbi.2011.06.006

Koppel, R., Metlay, J. P., Cohen, A., Abaluck, B., Localio, R. A., Kimmel, S. E., & Strom, B. L. (2005). Role of computerized physician order entry systems in facilitating medication errors. *Journal of the American Medical Association, 293*(10), 1197–1203. doi:10.1001/jama.293.10.1197

Koppel, R., Wetterneck, T., Telles, J. L., & Karsh, B.-T. (2008). Workarounds to barcode medication administration systems: Their occurrences, causes, and threats to patient safety. *Journal of the American Medical Informatics Association, 15*(4), 408–423. doi:10.1197/jamia.M2616

Korpelainen, E., & Kira, M. (2013). Systems approach for analysing problems in IT system adoption at work. *Behaviour & Information Technology, 32*(3), 247–262. doi:10.1080/0144929X.2011.624638

Langley, G. J., Moen, R., Nolan, K. M., Nolan, T. W., Norman, L., & Provost, L. P. (2009). *The improvement guide: A practical approach to enhancing organizational performance* (2nd ed.). San Francisco, CA: Jossey-Bass.

Latour, B. (1991). Technology is society made durable. In J. Law (Ed.), *A sociology of monsters: Essays on power, technology and domination* (pp. 103–131). London, UK: Routledge.

Latour, B. (2005). *Reassembling the social: An introduction to actor-network-theory.* London, UK: Oxford. doi:10.1234/12345678

Law, J., & Hassard, J. (Eds.). (1999). *Actor network theory and after.* London, UK: Blackwell.

Lewin, R. (1992). *Complexity: Life at the Edge of Chaos.* Toronto, ON: Maxwell Macmillan Canada.

Lomov, B. (1981). The problem of activity in psychology. *Psikhologicheskii Zhurnal, 2*(5), 3–22.

Lorenz, E. N. (1972, December). *Predictability: Does the flap of a butterfly's wings in Brazil set off a tornado in Texas?* Address presented at the meeting of the American Association for the Advancement of Science, Boston, MA.

Lower, U. (2006). Standards development. *Interorganisational standards: Managing web services specifications for flexible supply chains* (pp. 69–111). New York, NY: Springer.

MacKenzie, D., & Wajcman, J. (1999). *The social shaping of technology.* New York, NY: Open University Press.

Matney, S., Brewster, P. J., Sward, K. A., Cloyes, K. G., & Staggers, N. (2011). Philosophical approaches to the nursing informatics data-information-knowledge-wisdom framework. *Advances in Nursing Science, 34*(1), 6–18. doi:10.1097/ANS.0b013e3182071813

Meeks, D. W., Takian, A., Sittig, D. F., Singh, H., & Barber, N. (2014). Exploring the sociotechnical intersection of patient safety and electronic health record implementation. *Journal of the American Medical Informatics Association, 21*(e1), e28–e34. doi:10.1136/amiajnl-2013-001762

Murphy, J. I. (2013). Using plan-do-study-act to transform a simulation center. *Clinical Simulation in Nursing, 9*(7), e257–e264. doi:10.1016/j.ecns.2012.03.002

Nardi, B. (1996). Activity theory and human-computer interaction. In B. Nardi (Ed.), *Context and consciousness: Activity theory and human-computer interaction* (pp. 7–16). Cambridge, MA: MIT Press.

Pabst, M. K., Scherubel, J. C., & Minnick, A. F. (1996). The impact of computerized documentation on nurses' use of time. *Computers in Nursing, 14*(1), 25–30. doi:PMID: 8605657

Paley, J. (2007). Complex adaptive systems and nursing. *Nursing Inquiry, 14*(3), 233–242. doi:10.1111/j.1440-1800.2007.00359.x

Pinch, T. J., & Bijker, W. E. (1984). The social construction of facts and artefacts: Or How the sociology of science and the sociology of technology might benefit each other. *Social Studies of Science, 14*, 399–441. doi:10.1177/030631284014003004

Plsek, P. E., & Greenhalgh, T. (2001). Complexity science: The challenge of complexity in health care. *British Medical Journal (Clinical Research Ed.), 323*(7313), 625–628.

Rahimi, B., Timpka, T., Vimarlund, V., Uppugunduri, S., & Svensson, M. (2009). Organization-wide adoption of computerized provider order entry systems: A study based on diffusion of innovations theory. *BioMedicalCentral: Medical Informatics and Decision Making, 9*(52). doi:10.1186/1472-6947-9-52

Samuels-Dennis, J., & Cameron, C. (2013). Theoretical framework. In G. LoBiondo-Wood, J. Haber, C. Cameron, & M. Singh (Eds.), *Nursing research in Canada: Methods, critical appraisal, and utilization* (pp. 27–47). Toronto, ON: Elsevier.

Sittig, D. F., & Singh, H. (2010). A new sociotechnical model for studying health information technology in complex adaptive healthcare systems. *Quality and Safety in Health Care, 19*(Suppl. 3), i68–i74. doi:10.1136/qshc.2010.042085

Sleutel, M., & Guinn, M. (1999). As good as it gets? Going online with a clinical information system. *Computers in Nursing, 17*(4), 181–185. doi:PMID: 10425817

Staggers, N., Gassert, C. A., & Curran, C. (2001). Informatics competencies for nurses at four levels of practice. *Journal of Nursing Education, 40*(7), 303–316.

Staggers, N., & Parks, P. L. (1993). Description and initial applications of the Staggers & Parks Nurse-Computer Interaction Framework. *Computers in Nursing, 11*(6), 282–290.

Sugimori, Y., Kusunoki, K., Cho, F., & Uchikawa, S. (1977). Toyota production system and Kanban system: Materialization of just-in-time and respect-for-human system. *International Journal of Production Research, 15*(6), 553–564. doi:10.1080/00207547708943149

Thompson, C., Snyder-Halpern, R., & Staggers, N. (1999). Analysis, processes, and techniques: Case study. *Computers in Nursing, 17*(3), 203–206.

Timmons, S. (2003). Nurses resisting information technology. *Nursing Inquiry, 10*(4), 257–269.

Trist, E. (1981). *The evolution of socio-technical systems: A conceptual framework and an action research program.* Toronto: Occasional paper 2. Ontario Ministry of Labour/Ontario Quality of Working Life Centre.

Turley, J. P. (1996). Toward a model for nursing informatics. *Image, 28*(4), 309–313. doi:10.1111/j.1547-5069.1996.tb00379.x

Van Onzenoort, H. A., Van De Plas, A., Kessels, A. G., Veldhorst-Janssen, N. M., Van Der Kuy, P. H. M., & Neef, C. (2008). Factors influencing bar-code verification by nurses during medication administration in a Dutch hospital. *American Journal of Health-System Pharmacy, 65*(7), 644–648. doi:10.2146/ajhp070368

Varpio, L., Hall, P., Lingard, L., & Schryer, C. F. (2008). Interprofessional communication and medical error: A reframing of research questions and approaches. *Academic Medicine: Journal of the Association of American Medical Colleges, 83*(10 Suppl), S76–S81. doi:10.1097/ACM.0b013e318183e67b

Venkatesh, V., Morris, M. G., Davis, G. B., & Davis, F. D. (2003). User acceptance of information technology: Toward a unified view. *Management Information Systems Quarterly, 27*(3), 425–478. doi:10.2307/30036540

Walsham, G. (1997). Actor-network theory and IS research: Current status and future prospects. In A. Lee, J. Liebenau, & J. DeGross (Eds.), *Information systems and qualitative research* (pp. 466–495). Great Britain: Springer.

Wilson, M. (2002). Making nursing visible? Gender, technology and the care plan as script. *Information Technology & People, 15*(2), 139–158. doi:10.1108/09593840210430570

Wilson, T., & Holt, T. (1996). Complexity science and clinical complexity. *British Medical Journal, 323*(7314), 685–688. doi:10.1136/bmj

Woolgar, S. (1991). The turn to technology in social studies of science. *Science, Technology & Human Values, 16*(1), 20–50. doi:10.1177/016224399101600102

Zhang, H., Cocosila, M., & Archer, N. (2010). Factors of adoption of mobile information technology by homecare nurses: A technology acceptance model 2 approach. *Computers, Informatics, Nursing, 28*(1), 49–56. doi:10.1097/NCN.0b013e3181c0474a

CHAPTER 4

National Health Care Transformation and Information Technology

David M. Bergman, Susan McBride, and Mari Tietze

OBJECTIVES

1. Review recent efforts to expand access and use of health information technology (HIT) in the United States.

2. Discuss how various programs are designed to be layered to support one another, particularly with regard to HIT adoption and use.

3. Demonstrate the link between HIT usage and ways to capitalize on payment reform.

4. Describe the important roles that advanced practice nurses play in interprofessional teams within many of these national HIT initiatives.

5. Review best practices used in the nation to examine case studies on how organizations can successfully implement strategies to fully realize the national aims.

KEY WORDS

EHR incentive program, health information exchange, Beacon project, National Quality Strategy, accountable care organizations

CONTENTS

INTRODUCTION

Electronic health records (EHRs) have been around in some form since the 1970s, but prior to the passage of the Health Information Technology for Economic and Clinical Health (HITECH) Act in 2009, their penetration rate has been relatively modest. As late as 2009, fewer than 15% of nonfederal acute care hospitals had implemented even basic EHRs (Charles, Gabriel, & Furukawa, 2014; Jha et al., 2009). In the past several years, the nationwide EHR penetration rate improved substantially. By 2013, 78.4% of primary care providers had adopted an EHR system, with 48.1% using an EHR with more advanced features (Hsiao & Hing, 2014). In the same year, 94% of hospitals were using some form of EHR, with 59.4% using more advanced EHRs (Charles et al., 2014). In particular, the EHR penetration rate has markedly increased since 2010, when the implementation of the HITECH Act began. Although impressive, these improvements in EHR adoption cannot be sustained without the full integration of EHR technology into all aspects of hospital and practice management. The adoption of EHR technology is only one step toward the effective use of HIT for which advanced practice nurses will have to play a major role.

The many programs created through the HITECH Act were each designed to address discrete challenges related to EHR adoption and use. When considered as a whole, these various efforts were not merely a hodgepodge of interventions, but a sophisticated, coordinated effort designed to address major shortcomings in the HIT ecosystem. Some interventions targeted adoption challenges, others workforce needs, and still others were intended to bolster exchange capabilities. By addressing each of these major shortcomings, the HITECH Act's primary goal was to build a nationwide HIT infrastructure that was capable of supporting other changes to the health care sector, particularly those concerning improvements in quality of care and reductions in overall cost.

Four years into building the HIT infrastructure, there is evidence to support the assertion that HIT adoption has been successful (Jha, 2013). However, HIT adoption for adoption's sake was never the goal. As the Affordable Care Act (ACA) has been rolled out over the past several years, a subtle but significant shift has taken place: with payment model changes, incentive payments, and coverage expansion, the emphasis is now on *using* the infrastructure, not just building it.

Of course, there are still major challenges concerning the HIT infrastructure. Interoperability standards for some aspects of care are still under discussion, technology platforms like EHRs and health information exchanges (HIEs) continue to lack plug-and-play functionality that would lower implementation costs and encourage data exchange, and many HIEs are based on limited datasets. Nonetheless, with nationwide adoption of HIT at current levels, enough infrastructure exists in enough communities such that significant improvements in care are now possible.

Advanced practice nurses—particularly those trained in informatics—are extremely well positioned to help realize the potential of HIT to improve care and lower costs. This chapter serves to review the major programmatic initiatives created through the HITECH Act—from the EHR incentive program to the Regional Extension Center (REC) program—and to describe how each component was intended to address key shortcomings within the HIT ecosystem. A major focus also includes how these policies are aligned, and how they are driving substantial changes in the coordination, delivery, and funding of health care. Additionally, this chapter describes ways that the HIT ecosystem is and can be leveraged to support quality outcomes with the explicit engagement of advanced practice nurses.

Recognizing the need to promote HIT, President George W. Bush, in 2004, created the Office of the National Coordinator for Health Information Technology (ONC-HIT) by executive order. Until the passage of the HITECH Act in 2009, ONC served primarily as a convener, and sought to build consensus on the development of standards that the HIT sector could deploy. When created, the goal of ONC was to promote full adoption of EHRs for the entire country by 2014. The task was substantial in that in 2004, just 20% of office-based physicians were using even a rudimentary EHR system, and fewer than 10% of hospitals were using even computer provider order entry (CPOE; Ash & Bates, 2005).

By 2009, some progress had been made regarding adoption. At that time, approximately 48% of primary care practices were using some form of EHR, but fewer than half of those used an EHR with functions that today would be considered basic (Hsiao & Hing, 2014). Furthermore, just 12% of hospitals reported using EHR systems (Charles et al., 2014). If ONC was going to help realize the promise of HIT, something would need to change.

In the midst of the economic turmoil that occurred at the end of 2008 and into 2009, Congress passed and President Barack Obama signed into law the American Reinvestment and Recovery Act, or "ARRA." Approximately 50 of the 400 pages comprising ARRA were dedicated to a separately named Act, called the HITECH Act. As early as March of 2009, the HITECH Act was described as reflecting the conviction that "electronic information systems are essential to improving the health and health care of Americans" (Blumenthal, 2009, p. 1477). In this way, the HITECH Act was strategically linked to efforts that reached fruition a year later in March 2010 with the passage of the ACA. As shown later in this chapter, the two laws are inextricably linked in critical operational ways. As noted by Dr. David Blumenthal shortly after he became the third national coordinator for HIT, the HITECH Act was a "substantial down payment on the financial and human resources needed to wire the U.S. healthcare system" (Merrill, 2009, p. 1)— activities that would prove crucial to health care reform.

RAPIDLY EXPANDING HIT

The HITECH Act included funding provisions for both mandatory spending through Centers for Medicare & Medicaid Services (CMS), and for programmatic spending for HIT adoption support through the ONC-HIT for a total of six major initiatives. The mandatory spending initiative—the EHR Incentive Program—was administered by CMS, whereas the programmatic spending largely went through ONC (see Figure 4.1). Individually, each of these initiatives was designed to address different ways of supporting widespread adoption and use of HIT. Additionally, these different initiatives were intended to build on and support one another. The six initiatives were:

▶ *The EHR incentive program*: A 5-year program of increasing complexity to encourage providers and hospitals to adopt and meaningfully use EHRs

▶ *The EHR certification program*: A national standard of functionalities that providers and hospitals could reference to ensure that their EHR was capable of supporting meaningful use (MU)

▶ *The State HIE program*: A program for states to build a nationwide technological infrastructure that supports the secure exchange of clinical content between relevant care providers

▶ *Regional Extension Center (REC) program*: A program to provide technical assistance to primary care providers in small and safety-net practices to facilitate selection, adoption, and use of EHRs; the REC program was explicitly intended to help providers qualify for the EHR incentive program

▶ *Beacon community program*: Beacon grants went to communities already relatively advanced in terms of adoption and use of EHRs. These large grants of approximately $17 million were designed to help communities more explicitly connect the use of HIT—EHRs, HIEs, and other emerging forms of technology like Short Message Service (SMS) messaging—to improvements in community health outcomes as demonstrated by standardized quality measures.

▶ *Workforce development*:

  • *Community-college curriculum*: These programs provided funding to four specific cohorts of communities around the country to develop and deploy a curriculum that provided certification to individuals.

  • *University-based training*: Funding provided to nine colleges and universities (HealthIT Buzz, 2011–2013) to develop a training curriculum for college students.

▶ *Strategic Health IT Advanced Research Projects (SHARP)*: SHARP projects were awarded to four university centers to spur technological innovation regarding the development of EHR technology. Areas of research include:

  • Security and technology

  • Usability and alignment of technology to physician cognition and decision making

  • EHR information architecture

  • Integration and utilization of EHR data for quality-improvement purposes

Ultimately, ONC was allocated just over $2 billion for programs (HealthIT Dashboard, 2013), the EHR incentive program, a mandatory program administered by CMS, was estimated to require funding of $26.8 billion by the end of FFY2014 (Rangel, 2009) (see Figure 4.2). For a breakdown of the allocation to ONC, see Figure 4.3.

As these programs developed, it also became clear that there were crucial ways of leveraging this burgeoning infrastructure to achieve additional health-related goals and objectives. Program initiatives, such as the accountable care organizations (ACOs) that were embedded in the ACA, required more robust technological infrastructure and subsequent policy documents. One key policy document was the National Quality Strategy (NQS), which laid out plans to link these separate initiatives in ways that were explicitly tied to improvements in community health, quality of care, and reduced cost. To see how these programs were designed to mutually support one another, and how they related to each other, see Figure 4.4.

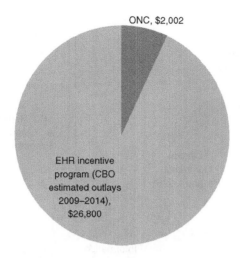

FIGURE 4.1. Health IT-related funding through the HITECH Act (in $ millions).

Note: The Health Information Technology for Economic and Clinical Health Act created a mandatory spending program—the electronic health record incentive program—through the Centers for Medicare & Medicaid Services. Based on Centers for Disease Control estimates, the EHR incentive program was expected to result in direct outlays of $26.8 billion through 2014. The HITECH Act also provided the statutory authority to create key programs, administered by the Office of the National Coordinator for Health Information Technology, to support HIT expansion. These programs include the Regional Extension Center program, the state health information exchange program, and the Beacon Program, among others.

CBO, Congressional Budget Office; ONC, Office of the National Coordinator for Health Information Technology.

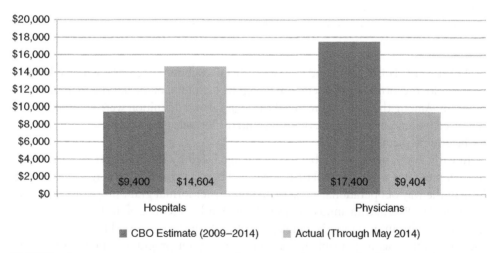

FIGURE 4.2. EHR incentive program estimated versus actual payments (2009–2014; in $ millions).

Note: Through 2014, the Congressional Budget Office estimated that the electronic health record incentive program would result in direct outlays of $26,800 million, with roughly $9,400 million to hospitals, and $17,400 million to physicians. Through May 2014—4 months shy of the close of the 2014 fiscal year—the EHR incentive program had distributed a total of $24,008 million, with $14,604 million in payments to hospitals, and $9,404 million in payments to physicians. CBO, Congressional Budget Office.

Of these six programs, only one—the EHR incentive program—was not housed completely within the ONC. Even so, ONC's policy committee, a group of stakeholders meeting under the Federal Advisory Committee Act (FACA), was charged with developing the initial framework and recommendations defining what it meant to achieve "meaningful

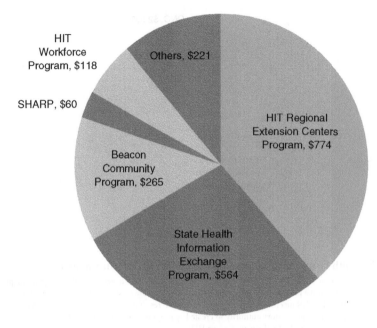

FIGURE 4.3. HITECH Act allocation for ONC by program (in $ millions).

Note: The Health Information Technology for Economic and Clinical Health Act allocated $2.002 million for programs in the Office of the National Coordinator related to HIT adoption. The three largest programs were the Regional Extension Center program, the state Health Information Exchange program, and the Beacon community program, which together accounted for more than 75% of ONC's HITECH Act allocation.

HIT, health information technology; SHARP, Strategic Health IT Advanced Research Projects.

use" of an EHR. This recommendation was officially submitted to CMS, where it became the basis for the formal rules operationalizing the definition of MU for the EHR incentive program. Among the concepts realized through further definition were eligibility criteria, incentive amounts, program duration, and the formal attestation process, in addition to the criteria themselves.

In early 2009, perhaps the biggest challenge faced by the HITECH Act and all its nascent programs was that, until then, ONC had been a policy-focused organization with little in the way of operational capacity to administer formal grant programs. In 2008, for example, ONC had an annual budget of $60.5 million (Office of the National Coordinator for Health Information Technology, 2010). With the passage of the HITECH Act, suddenly ONC was responsible for administering grant programs totaling $2 billion, more than a 33-fold increase.

In addition to this challenge, many of these programs were explicitly designed to build off of other programs. This was perhaps no more evident than in the REC program. The REC program, as an example, was designed to get small practices to adopt and meaningfully use "certified" EHRs. Yet, at the time the initial REC funding-opportunity announcement (FOA) was released in 2009, there were no ONC-published certification criteria for EHRs, no certifying body, and certainly no certified EHRs. Furthermore, CMS published the notice of proposed rulemaking defining the "meaningful use" in late December 2009, a rule that didn't become final until June of 2010, 2 to 4 months *after*

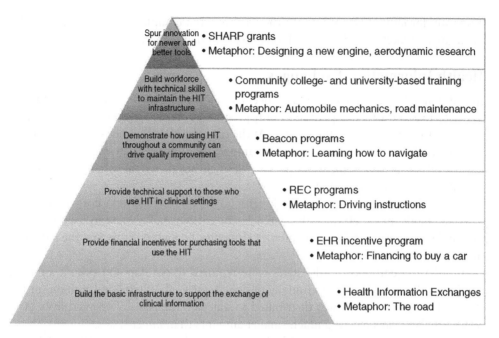

FIGURE 4.4. HITECH Act initiatives.

Note: The Health Information Technology for Economic and Clinical Health (HITECH) Act initiatives were explicitly designed to build off of and support one another. They were designed to provide both foundational support for health information technology (HIT), and to develop new and innovative approaches to guide long-term development.

EHR, electronic health record; HIT, health information technology; REC, Regional Extension Center.

60 of the 62 REC program awards had been announced. These RECs were therefore "on the clock" to deliver their 4-year goals before the operational definitions had even been published.

EHR Incentive Program

The EHR incentive program became the framework for promoting EHR adoption. This initiative provided funds to eligible providers and eligible hospitals for the adoption and "meaningful use" of certified EHR technology. In order to understand the magnitude of this program, each component first needs to be examined.

Although the EHR incentive program is broadly administered by the CMS, it is also partially implemented through state Medicaid offices. "Eligible providers"—health care practitioners in various categories—can qualify for these funds, so long as they meet a billing threshold for Medicare or Medicaid claims. Eligible Medicaid providers—those with a total number of billings greater than 30% in most cases—can qualify for up to a total of $63,750 per provider over 5 years. Meanwhile, eligible Medicare providers can qualify for $44,750 per provider over the same period. In this way, the amount providers can qualify for is dependent on which program they qualify under. However, providers meeting both billing thresholds can claim incentives only through one program. In addition, nurse practitioners (NPs) are eligible for Medicaid incentives, and under specific circumstances physician assistants may also qualify. Hospitals, meanwhile, are eligible to qualify for *both* Medicare and Medicaid through a complex formula that includes Medicare and Medicaid billings and total inpatient days, among other elements.

Health Information Exchanges

In addition to the creation of the EHR incentive program, the HITECH Act also funded the ONC to administer an application-only program to states or their designated entities to build HIE capabilities in their states. At the time the HITECH Act was passed, there were a handful of exchanges in operation around the country, each operating with different levels of success. Some were specific to a single health system, whereas others were broadly supported in a community.

HIEs typically fall into three major designs: (a) the central data repository model, (b) a federated model in which the HIE references the existence of content in local repositories, and (c) a hybrid model that combines elements of data repository and the federated models.

In order to qualify for funds, states were required to develop and submit a formal application for these funds. As initially designed, ONC allocated $564 million for the state HIE program, which was distributed to states on the basis of covered lives. As a result, smaller states received much smaller amounts than larger states.

At the same time, states had a wide degree of latitude to implement HIE models that could leverage local infrastructure and address local needs. ONC's primary concern was with the development of a functional, sustainable infrastructure that was capable of supporting MU. As originally conceived, ONC intended to create the capability for all local HIEs to roll up to a nationwide HIE that was capable of referencing the existence of local clinical content. However, early in 2011, this goal was delayed in favor of the use of what became known as the Nationwide Health Information Network Direct (NwHIN Direct), or simply Direct. The Direct protocol functions much like a secure e-mail system that enables clinical content to be transmitted electronically in a way that is consistent with privacy obligations enforced under the Health Information Portability and Privacy Act (HIPAA). In order to encourage the development of the Direct capability, ONC required states to support the Direct protocol. Additionally, ONC required EHRs to support the Direct functionality in order to become certified.

Beacon Programs Leading the Way

If the REC program was designed to help small practices with the basic adoption and use of EHRs, the Beacon program was designed to demonstrate the kinds of clinical quality improvements that are possible in communities with more robust EHR adoption. In early 2010, ONC made available $250 million for the Beacon communities program, a cooperative agreement program for communities with at least 30% EHR adoption among ambulatory care providers.

Ultimately, 17 communities were designated Beacon communities and were awarded between $12 and $16 million each. Communities were charged with a three-part aim:

1. Improve population health
2. Test innovative approaches
3. Build HIT infrastructure and capacity to exchange clinical information

Functionally, over the 3 years of the cooperative agreement, Beacon communities were put in the position of demonstrating how HIT can be used to drive measureable improvements in health. According to the Funding Opportunity Announcement (FOA) "the Beacon community grants program will provide funding to communities to demonstrate the vision of the future where hospitals, clinicians, and patients are meaningful users of HIT, and together the community achieves *measurable improvements in health care quality, safety and efficiency*" (ONC-HIT, 2009, p. 8). In pursuit of that fundamental goal, they were asked to support, where possible, broader HIT initiatives like their local REC program(s) and/or development of an HIE.

The Beacon communities were broadly representative of the country and were expected to develop findings, processes, and approaches that could be leveraged to support ways of leveraging HIT in other communities around the country. Among the Beacon communities were health systems centered in large urban areas (Detroit, MI; San Diego, CA; and Cincinnati, OH), substantially rural communities (eastern Maine [Bangor], Mississippi Delta [Greenville], and Inland Northwest [Spokane, WA], and all areas in between (Rein, 2012).

Each community was required to identify a set of validated clinical quality measures against which they would evaluate their performance. Some chose measures related to vaccination rates, whereas others looked at diabetes management. The programs were given substantial latitude to identify measures that were germane to their community, and to use the federal dollars to address barriers or technological innovations that would enable achievement of the goals. Although there were some similarities among communities, as a general rule, each Beacon community was a unique program with unique goals, addressing challenges that were specific to each community.

The experience of the Beacon communities collectively informed a series of "learning guides" that are designed to inform communities seeking ways to improve population health. There are six guides:

1. Improving hospital transitions and care management using automated admission, discharge, and transfer alerts

2. Strengthening care management with HIT

3. Capturing high-quality EHRs data to support performance improvement

4. Enabling HIE to support community goals

5. Using HIT capabilities to support clinical transformation in a practice setting

6. Building technology capabilities for population health measurement at the community level

Each of these guides provides valuable insight into both the challenges that communities face in the adoption of HIT and how to overcome some of those obstacles. As additional communities around the country begin to leverage their HIT infrastructure, these findings can help them avoid mistakes and follow successful strategies.

REC Programs

If the HIEs and EHRs were the technological backbone of the HITECH Act, the REC program created the "boots on the ground" to support EHR adoption. Based on the extension programs in agriculture and manufacturing, the REC program was explicitly laid out in the HITECH Act. By late 2009, just a few months after HITECH was passed in February 2009, ONC released the initial FOA for the REC program. This FOA allocated $774 million to support primary care providers in small practices with the adoption and MU of EHR technology.

As originally conceived, the REC program had a collective goal of supporting 100,000 primary care providers around the country in achieving Stage 1 of Meaningful Use of EHRs. By September 2010, every area of the United States, including Puerto Rico and Guam, was covered by one of the 62 RECs, each of which was responsible for supporting a defined number of primary care providers (see Figure 4.5). Although nominally a target agreed on between the REC itself and ONC, the target number was loosely based on the total estimated number of primary care providers in the REC's region, with the minimum being 1,000 priority primary care providers (PPCPs). Although there were a few RECs targeting as many as 8,000 PPCPs, the average PPCP target size was approximately 1,350.

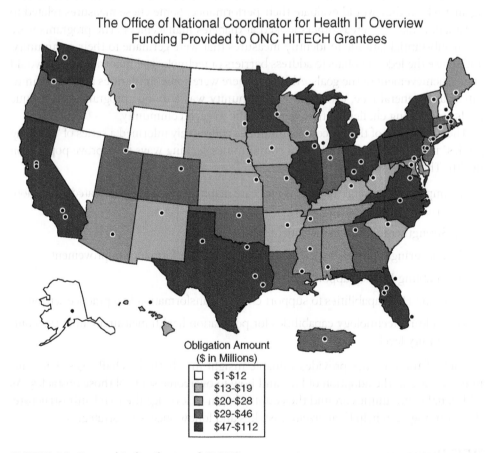

The Office of National Coordinator for Health IT Overview
Funding Provided to ONC HITECH Grantees

Obligation Amount
($ in Millions)
- $1-$12
- $13-$19
- $20-$28
- $29-$46
- $47-$112

FIGURE 4.5. Geographic distribution of 62 RECs.

Note: There were 62 Regional Extension Center programs around the country, covering every state and territory. Some populous states—California, Florida, New York, and Texas—were served by multiple RECs. Less populous states (MN and ND, MT, and WY) were sometimes combined and served by a single REC.

Funding for RECs was divided between "core" funding, and "direct" funding. RECs could use between $500,000 and $750,000 of their allocation for "core" funding for a 2-year period. Core funding was intended to support building the operational infrastructure for the REC services—hardware and software purchases, initial hiring of staff, partnership agreements, and so on. The long-term plan for the RECs was to design business units to support the regions that can sustain post-HITECH funding to provide HIT services and support for the region. The infrastructure in the United States would need long-term support that did not exist at the launch of HITECH; the RECs were created to provide that support.

Direct funding, meanwhile, was tied to the achievement of specific operational milestones with PPCPs:

▶ Enrollment with the REC

▶ Go-live on an EHR

▶ Attestation that the provider had achieved MU

RECs were eligible for a total of $5,000 in direct support and, with ONC approval, could choose different amounts for each milestone. With few exceptions, RECs elected earn $1,666.67 per milestone, simply dividing the total amount across the three milestones. For an REC with a target of 1,000 PPCPs and 2-year core support of $750,000, this meant a budget of $6.5 million ($1.5 million for core, $5 million for direct).

Originally, the REC program was designed to be a 4-year cooperative agreement. In the first 2 years, local programs were required to provide a 10% match to be eligible for the remaining federal 90% of funding. In the last 2 years, this was supposed to be reversed, with local programs providing 90% of the funding to obtain the 10% federal match. As the first 2 years drew to a close, however, it became clear that there was not yet enough local support to sustain the REC programs. To address this, Secretary Sebelius exercised her authority to modify the program to maintain federal support at the 90% level, without altering the total amount available to the program (Blumenthal, 2011).

From the beginning, the REC program faced a number of significant challenges over and above the operational challenge of getting providers to purchase EHRs. Many of these had to do with emerging specificity coming from other programs. Until ONC defined certification criteria and a certifying body, there could be no "certified" EHR technology; until CMS published final rules for "meaningful use" there could be no "meaningful use" of EHRs; however, other challenges were a function of having 62 very different programs with differing business strategies to deploy the regional support services.

The newly created REC programs began with significant differences in size, scope, and initial challenges. Significantly, about 80% of REC programs were housed in three major types of parent organizations: Quality Improvement Organizations (QIOs), universities, and Health Center Controlled Networks (HCCNs). The remaining 20% of organizations housing REC programs represented a wide range of parent organizations. These differences, in turn, meant that REC programs started with different levels of native expertise and with various levels of operational capacity.

ONC approached these challenges with both personnel and technology. First and foremost, each REC program was assigned an ONC project officer who had primary responsibility for communicating program requirements and ensuring that programs were meeting milestones. Additionally, ONC created a number of affinity groups, known as Communities of Practice (COPs), with regular conference calls that were supported by a combination of project officers and contractors with unique expertise in the area.

Project officers facilitated regular calls with the leadership of each REC program. Calls tended to focus on the completion and updating of detailed operations plans, or "ops plans." The ops plans contained detailed work plans on different components of program activities as they related to program goals. Importantly, these ops plans also contained detailed forecasts regarding when and how milestones were expected to be achieved. The ops plans also contained detailed descriptions of operational threats, which were mined to identify broader threats across multiple programs.

The nature of the project officer calls changed as the program evolved—early calls focused on getting grantees up and running; later calls focused on efforts to ensure timely achievement of milestones and to address barriers for providers and small hospitals getting to MU of their EHRs. However, the major purpose of the calls was to provide information to programs and obtain information about programs. Both roles were critical. Because these were new programs in a new agency, there were no established practices to fall back on and many aspects of the programs required additional explanation. For example, REC programs needed guidance on how to define a milestone that was achieved for direct service purposes, what the implications were for their ability to draw down funds, and how to request the release of additional federal dollars.

In addition to the project officer support, ONC also created a series of COPs, each of which was focused on unique challenges. Some of these were designed to bolster the operational capabilities of the RECs. One COP focused on practice and workflow redesign. This COP discussed the implication of EHR adoption on practice workflows, and ended up producing a series of workflow templates that REC grantees used to further conversations with practices they were supporting and to kick-start the workflow redesign process. These templates were also used to teach practices how to do their own workflow redesign (see Chapter 9 for more detail on use of templates). Another COP discussed implementation issues related to the evolving operational definition of MU and some of the clinical quality measures that were affiliated with it. Other COPs focused on issues that were specific to a subset of REC grantees. For example, there was a COP for RECs serving rural communities, and another for RECs that were also QIOs, and still another for RECs serving critical access hospitals (CAHs).

ONC also implemented two web-based platforms—a community portal with a message board type platform known as the Health Information Technology Resource Center (HITRC), and a customer relationship management (CRM) platform. The HITRC evolved from a general platform for posting content to one that was closely linked to specific COPs, and back again to a general platform. It functioned both as an asynchronous platform where individual RECs could post internally developed materials they found effective for use by other RECs, and as a place to obtain content that other RECs had posted. This community of RECs presented a unique opportunity to culminate best practices for fast-track deployment of EHRs and to help providers and hospitals interpret the regulations and achieve MU.

Early in the REC initiative, the HITRC was designed to be a clearinghouse of information on supporting the REC programs and EHR implementations particularly for those REC grantees that lacked specific operational expertise. An explicit component of the cooperative agreement approach was to have REC programs learn from each other. The HITRC and the COP were the main two vehicles through which ONC facilitated this learning environment.

ONC also supported RECs through a CRM platform, which became the primary reporting platform for each of the REC programs. Individual REC programs had the option to have the CRM prepopulated with provider content from a source they identified or from Medicare and Medicaid data. In any event, each REC program was expected to track its outreach efforts on a practice-by-practice basis, and to do some of its EHR implementation project management through the CRM tool. This helped grantees by providing a ready-to-go tool, and enabled ONC to monitor activity and progress.

Despite some early challenges, the REC program has been a striking success. As of the end of January 2014, RECs had enrolled nearly 150,000 providers, had supported more than 130,000 in achieving go-live status, and supported nearly 90,000 providers in attesting to MU (HealthIT.gov, 2014).

Research and Technology Development SHARP Grants

In addition to programs building the HIT infrastructure through HIEs and EHR implementations, ONC also funded a grant program that supported innovations to advance existing technology. The SHARP grants were awarded to universities or research institutions and were designed to support innovative research that would address critical areas of EHR functionality. "SHARP" is an acronym for Strategic Health IT Advanced Research (HealthIT.gov, 2013). Under this program, four grants were awarded to address target issues: privacy and security, physician cognition and decision making, health application design, and use of EHR data.

There were four target areas for the SHARP grants, and each awardee was responsible for a single area of innovation and research. Unlike other ONC grants and cooperative agreements, the SHARP grants were not expected to have an immediate impact on HIT deployment. Rather, they inform the broader milieu of HIT, and their impact is felt more obliquely in the application of their conceptual findings. These grants have directly and indirectly produced scores of academic papers and presentations on topics that are both narrow and broad.

SHARP-S Privacy and Security

The University of Illinois at Urbana—Champaign (UIUC) was awarded the SHARP-S grant in order to advance the privacy and security associated with HIT. Specifically, the grant focused on privacy and security for EHRs, HIEs, and telemedicine. Additionally, through the course of the grant, UIUC began to focus on the connectivity between health-related sensors and devices, particularly implants like insulin pumps.

In addition to exploring the governance around accessing health data—for example, the process through which an identity becomes authenticated for access purposes—this SHARP-S grant explores some of the technological aspects of identity authentication.

SHARP-C Physician Cognition

The University of Texas at Houston (UTHouston) was awarded the SHARP-C grant to explore the relationship between the presentation of information in an EHR user interface and the impact of that presentation on physician decision making. This project defined four focus areas:

▶ Work-centered design-of-care process improvements in HIT, which focus on EHR usability and workflows

▶ Cognitive foundations for decision making: implications for decision support

▶ Automated model-based clinical summarization of key patient data

▶ Cognitive information design and visualization: enhancing accessibility and understanding of patient data (HealthIT.Gov, 2013)

SMART Application

Harvard University was awarded a SHARP grant in order to develop and deploy a modular, interoperable health data infrastructure known as the "SMART" platform. The SMART platform—substitutable medical apps and reusable technology—represents an effort to apply an iPhone "app" store functionality to EHRs. As currently designed, it is primarily a tool used to view data contained in another EHR, with limited capability to write information into a patient record; however, this is intended to evolve over time. The SMART tool sits conceptually on top of the EHR, where it reads and presents patient record data in ways that are significant to the provider. The SMART platform application list is still relatively limited.

SHARP: Secondary Use of EHR Data

The SHARP grant, awarded to the Mayo Clinic College of Medicine of Rochester, MN, is designed to address the uses of data that are now available via EHRs. There are six target areas for this grant:

▶ Two (clinical data normalization and natural language processing) are focused on preparing data to support deeper analysis of content

▶ The remaining four focus on ways of applying data in different situations. For example, one target area—phenotyping—is designed to support identification of patients with a host of clinical characteristics. This is particularly important for streamlining the process of identifying candidates for clinical trials and involves reviewing or summarizing a potentially wide range of clinical information. Another target area is focused more broadly on data quality when looking for patients with specific criteria. Still another explored ways of calculating clinical quality measures associated with MU Stage 2.

In addition to the SHARP grantees named earlier, a grantee of the National Institutes of Health (NIH) was designed as an affiliate program, given that it has made use of the same goals. This program, called MD SHARP, was designed to develop further plug-and-play functionality for medical devices. This grant award was made to the Medical Device Plug-and-Play (MD PnP) interoperability program based at the Center for Integration of Medicine & Innovative Technology (CIMIT) and Massachusetts General Hospital (part of the Partners HealthCare System). This program was intended to support development of standards that can be adopted by industry, as well as a supportive ecosystem of tools that were ready for deployment.

Although the SHARP grants together consisted of only $60 million of the ARRA funding, they provided important funding to further our conceptual and practical understand of how HIT can be used and applied in various settings.

Workforce Development

Passed during the worst financial crisis since the Great Depression, the HITECH Act also contained programs to support workforce development, making explicit the connection between advancing the HIT infrastructure and the development of new jobs. There were a total of four grants for workforce development collectively worth $116 million. Together, these four programs were designed to create a mini-ecosystem that was intended to support the workforce needs of the HIT sector.

The largest award—of $68 million—went to five consortia of community colleges to implement short, nondegree training programs. These programs were intended to serve 10,500 individuals in all 50 states with training in six different areas of HIT. And yet, as of October 2013, these programs had served more than 19,000 individuals (National Opinion Research Center [NORC], 2014). The curriculum for the community college program was part of a separate but related award for $10 million, and included a component related to the dissemination of curriculum materials to community colleges outside of the participating consortia.

ONC also made substantial awards of $38 million for a university-based training program. These awards went to nine colleges or universities to expand or create training programs requiring more substantial technical skills, including those related to health information management, public health, and privacy and security. More than 1,600 individuals had received a master's degree or certificate of advanced study as of October 2013.

The final component of this initiative was awarded to the Northern Virginia Community College to develop a competency exam. Although this certification was available to anyone, it was primarily geared toward those individuals who had completed the community college training programs.

As a microcosm of the broader HITECH Act, these programs clearly demonstrate how the separate initiatives were intended to support broader development of the HIT ecosystem. Collectively, these programs were intended to train both higher skill and lower skill individuals and to deliver them and their skills to a population—clinics, hospitals, and private-sector companies in HIT—rapidly ramping up to deploy services.

The certification for nondegree individuals was particularly important both for those who attained the certificate and to potential employers. The certificate for graduates became a differentiator and, for employers, it became a way to identify individuals with more advanced skills, creating a virtuous cycle.

INTERLOCKING RELATIONSHIPS AMONG PROGRAMS WITHIN THE NATIONAL STRATEGY

When looking at this collection of programs funded through the HITECH Act, it is tempting to see them as separate and distinct programs, each of which serves a separate constituency. However, these are best thought of as a cohort of interlocking programs, each of which is designed to support the others. Broadly speaking, each program is designed to compensate for different challenges, any one of which could derail or slow broad adoption efforts. See Table 4.1 for side-by-side comparison of the challenges related to the program.

Seen like this, it is clearer how these programs are interrelated and how each builds on the others. In this way, it is also clear that the three most critical programs are the EHR incentive program, the REC program, and the state HIE program, because without them most of the subsequent work would have been fruitless.

Prior to the HITECH Act, the HIT sector was largely stuck in a chicken-and-egg scenario: providers were reluctant to adopt EHRs because there were few providers with whom to exchange clinical content, and there was little clinical content to exchange because few providers were using EHRs. To address this problem, the HITECH Act first provided a massive infusion of funding to build the HIT infrastructure (the HIEs) and finance the purchasing of EHRs (EHR incentive program), and second, provided the technical assistance to connect EHRs to the HIE infrastructure. All three programs were closely linked to each other, and depended on the availability of the others to be truly effective.

Looking specifically at the exchange of clinical content, these different programs each address a discrete but linked challenge. The HIEs enable the capacity to exchange clinical content. They both provide the mechanisms and administer the interoperability criteria that are used in a specific community. Meanwhile, the EHR incentive program

TABLE 4.1 Comparison of the ONC Programs and Challenges	
Challenge	Program
Lack of broadly available technological infrastructure	EHR certification program and state HIE program
Lack of providers using technological infrastructure	EHR incentive program
Lack of technical support resources for critical or vulnerable providers	REC program
Lack of skilled employees to support EHR adoption and use	Community college certification program and university-based training
Lack of support for linking HIT adoption to improvements in community health	Beacon programs
Slow pace of technological innovation for EHRs	SHARP grants
Lack of alignment strategies leveraging HIT adoption and use	NQS/Million hearts

EHR, electronic health record; HIE, health information exchange; HIT, health information technology; NQS, National Quality Strategy; ONC, Office of the National Coordinator; REC, Regional Extension Center; SHARP, Strategic Health IT Advanced Research Projects.

provides both funding and progressively more challenging MU criteria. The funding helps providers purchase an EHR capable of exchanging clinical content. However, the MU criteria link the availability of funding to specific exchange milestones. In this way, too, the progressively more challenging stages of MU—going from Stage 1's testing of the capability to exchange clinical content, to Stage 2's limited requirement for some exchange, to Stage 3's proposal for more robust exchange—mirror the development and expansion of the exchange capacity in communities around the country. And finally, the REC program provides critical technical assistance to providers to help them purchase an EHR, connect to an HIE, and meet the progressively more challenging MU criteria. Of course, in meeting the MU criteria, the providers then qualify for the EHR incentives, completing the circuit.

Link to the ACA

Although there are many ways the Patient Protection and Affordable Care Act is linked to the HITECH Act, our discussion here focuses on two provisions of the ACA outside of coverage expansion that have important implications for the HITECH Act. The first area concerns a broad-based, consensus document—the NQS—intended to guide the development of health policy and implementation; the second area—payment reform—concerns the implementation of ACOs. In different but crucial ways, these two provisions of the ACA begin the process of routinizing how a robust HIT environment can work in practice, and work effectively to better care for all Americans.

Beginning in 2011 and annually thereafter, the secretary of Health and Human Services (HHS) is required to deliver a report to Congress known as the NQS. It was created through a consensus-based process that brought together leadership from many health-related divisions within HHS, and sought input from many external stakeholders and organizations supporting improvements in health quality (Department of Health and Human Services, 2011). At a high level, the NQS lays out three broad aims—better care, healthy people/healthy communities, and affordable care—which are intended to serve as a framework for each of the different health-related agencies within the HHS. Additionally, the NQS identifies six priority areas:

▶ Making care safer by reducing harm caused in the delivery of care

▶ Ensuring that each person and family are engaged as partners in their care

▶ Promoting effective communication and coordination of care

▶ Promoting the most effective prevention and treatment practices for the leading causes of mortality, starting with cardiovascular disease

▶ Working with communities to promote wide use of best practices to enable healthy living

▶ Making quality care more affordable for individuals, families, employers, and governments by developing and spreading new health care delivery models

Since its initial publication in 2011, the NQS has served as a guidepost and framework for different divisions within HHS and other federal agencies.

Shortly after the 2011 NQS was released, HHS began a robust effort to identify ways of operationalizing the strategy, specifically among 24 key health-related agencies.

Programmatically, this was an opportunity to identify ways in which individual agency programs could align existing efforts with broader strategies and to coordinate with synergistic programs in other agencies. For example, shortly after the publication of the 2011 NQS, the Substance Abuse and Mental Health Services Administration (SAMHSA) began an effort to categorize all their programs in ways consistent with the NQS. This facilitated alignment with other agencies, for example, the ONC-HIT on issues concerning the privacy and security of substance abuse treatment information in an electronic setting.

Additionally, 2011 and 2012 saw federal agencies begin the process of harmonizing the use of quality measures. As described in the 2012 NQS, "the proliferation and use of quality measures across settings and by numerous programs has created an increasingly complex environment for health care providers with an often burdensome volume of measurement" (Department of Health and Human Services, 2012, p. 13). Not only was it burdensome administratively for providers, but also the measurement variations made it difficult for consumers and others to make true comparisons.

But perhaps most important, the NQS gave stakeholders at a variety of levels ways of thinking about how to leverage the existing infrastructure to support broader health and public policy goals. Because the health care sector in the United States is so complex, achieving measureable population health improvements requires coordination and alignment at multiple levels. Rarely does a single stakeholder own the responsibility in its entirety. Rather, every stakeholder can play a role, sometimes with little effort, which collectively can produce outcomes far greater than the sum of the efforts. See Figure 4.6 to better understand the requirement alignment of different domains that can affect care quality.

When the Million Hearts® initiative was announced in September of 2011 by the Centers for Disease Control (CDC), this quickly became a central theme in the NQS and a way to focus alignment across different stakeholders and sectors. Broadly speaking, the Million Hearts initiative is a coordinated effort to prevent a million heart attacks and strokes between 2012 and 2017. Yet each stakeholder—federal agencies, providers,

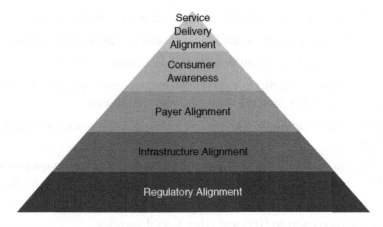

FIGURE 4.6. HIT domains.

Note: Ultimately, health information technology is a component of a larger set of initiatives used to transform the delivery of health care in the United States. Effecting this transformation requires the right kind of alignment across all these domains.

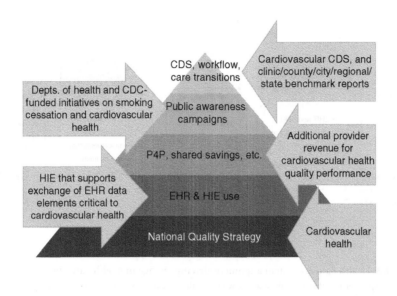

FIGURE 4.7. Alignment and interaction with the delivery system.

Note: This is an example of how the right kind of alignment within different domains can encourage the right kind of interaction at the level of individual care delivery.

CDC, Centers for Disease Control and Prevention; CDS, clinical decision support; EHR, electronic health record; HIE, health information exchange; P4P, Partnership 4 Patients.

payers, consumers, and others—can play a substantial role in helping to achieve this change. This is illustrated in Figure 4.7.

Important Link Between HIT Usage and Payment Reform

In addition to the NQS, the ACA also began a large experiment with an emerging model of health care delivery and financing, known as an ACO. In this model, providers or groups of providers agree to assume some level of risk with regard to the treatment of a large cohort of individuals. Using a hypothetical example, General Hospital enters into a contract with a health insurance company to manage all health care for 5,000 people. In exchange, the health insurance company will pay General Hospital $10,000 per member per year. If General Hospital spends less than $9,000 per member per year and demonstrably maintains clinical quality for all 5,000 members enrolled in its ACO, General Hospital will keep $500, and the health insurance company will keep $500.

Even though this is a crude illustration, it is clear that the onus is on General Hospital to effectively coordinate and manage care and to continually monitor clinical quality measures to ensure that effective care is being delivered. This is only possible with a robust HIT infrastructure. Figure 4.8 shows the linked chain of activities.

SUMMARY

This chapter has reviewed the federal initiatives under the HITECH Act of 2009 and the complementary programs within CMS to incentivize providers to rapidly adopt and implement EHRs and HIE. The research and development strategies under the SHARP-C federal initiatives were reviewed, as were as the workforce development initiatives.

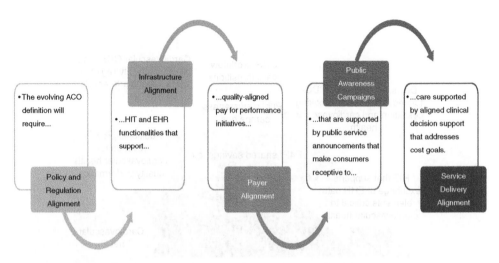

FIGURE 4.8. Health care ecosystem alignment driving change in health care outcomes.

Note: Using a single sentence, this figure illustrates how to align the various aspects of the health care ecosystem in order to drive changes in health care outcomes.

ACO, accountable care organization; EHR, electronic health record; HIT, health information technology.

This chapter reflects what occurred in the United States to reinforce, incentivize, and press forward for a nation connected with health initiatives. The picture reflected in this chapter is a significant design strategy implemented by these interconnected federal plans to support the nation in this effort.

EXERCISES AND QUESTIONS FOR CONSIDERATION

Consider content covered with respect to how technology has been deployed and supported throughout the nation by the federal regulation within the HITECH Act:

1. Do you believe this was a good strategy for the United States with respect to improving patient safety, quality, population health, and cost? Support your response with the evidence.

2. What are the critical components under the HITECH Act, and how do these programs interrelate?

3. What are the programs of the HITECH Act? Do you believe these programs have been successful? Support this response with evidence.

REFERENCES

Ash, J. S., & Bates, D. W. (2005). Factors and forces affecting EHR system adoption: Report of a 2004 ACMI discussion. *Journal of the American Medical Informatics Association, 12*(1), 8–12. doi:10.1197/jamia.M1684

Blumenthal, D. (2009). Stimulating the adoption of health information technology. *New England Journal of Medicine, 360,* 1477–1479. doi:10.1056/NEJMp0901592

Blumenthal, D. (2011). *DHHS health information technology extension program.* (Notice No. FR Doc. 2011–1447). Washington, DC: GPO.Gov.

Charles, D., Gabriel, M., & Furukawa, M. F. (2014). *Adoption of electronic health record systems among U.S. non-federal acute care hospitals: 2008–2013.* (ONC Data Brief No. 16). Washington, DC: HealthIT.Gov.

Department of Health and Human Services. (2011). *National strategy for quality improvement in health care.* (Congressional Report No. DHHS-2011). Washington, DC: Agency for Healthcare Research and Quality.

Department of Health and Human Services. (2012). *National strategy for quality improvement in health care.* (Congressional Report No. DHHS-2012). Washington, DC: Agency for Healthcare Research and Quality.

HealthIT Buzz. (2011–2013). *University-based training.* Retrieved from http://www.healthit.gov/buzz-blog/category/university-based-training/

HealthIT Dashboard. (2013, January). *Office of the National Coordinator for HealthIT overview: Funding provided to ONC-HITECH grantees.* Retrieved from http://dashboard.healthit.gov/onc/

HealthIT.Gov. (2013). *Strategic health IT advanced research projects (SHARP).* Retrieved from https://www.healthit.gov/policy-researchers-implementers/strategic-health-it-advanced-research-projects-sharp

HealthIT.Gov. (2014). *HealthIT Dashboard.* Retrieved from http://dashboard.healthit.gov/rec/

Hsiao, C., & Hing, E. (2014). *Use and characteristics of electronic health record systems among office-based physician practices: United States, 2001–2013.* (National Center for Health Statistics, Data Brief No. 143). Washington, DC: U.S. Department of Health and Human Services, Centers for Disease Control and Prevention.

Jha, A. K. (2013). *As the debate over Obamacare implementation rages, a success on the IT front.* Retrieved from http://thehealthcareblog.com/blog/2013/07/12/as-the-debate-over-obamacare-implementation-rages-a-success-on-the-it-front/

Jha, A. K., DesRoches, C. M., Campbell, E. G., Donelan, K., Rao, S. R., Ferris, T. G., . . . Blumenthal, D. (2009). Use of electronic health records in U.S. hospitals. *New England Journal of Medicine, 360,* 1628–1638. doi:10.1056/NEJMsa0900592

Merrill, M. (2009). *Blumenthal says HITECH faces challenges.* Retrieved from http://www.healthcareitnews.com/news/blumenthal-says-hitech-faces-challenges

National Opinion Research Center. (2014). *Evaluation of the information technology professionals in health care ("Workforce") program.* (Summative Report No. March 2014). Bethesda, MD: NORC, University of Chicago (Health IT).

Office of the National Coordinator for Health Information Technology. (2009). *Beacon community cooperative agreement program: Funding opportunity announcement and application instructions.* (No. BCCAP-2009). Washington, DC: Department of Health and Human Services.

Office of the National Coordinator for Health Information Technology. (2010). *Justification of estimates for appropriations committees.* (No. ONC-HIT-2010). Washington, DC: HealthIT.Gov.

Rangel, C. B. (2009). Congressional Budget Office, U.S. Congress, *HITECH Act letter.* Washington, DC: Recipient.

Rein, A. (2012). *Beacon policy brief 1.0: The Beacon community program—Three pillars of pursuit.* (Report Brief No. BPB-2012). Washington, DC: HealthIT.Gov.

CHAPTER 5

Consumer Engagement/Activation Enhanced by Technology

Mari Tietze, Patricia Hinton Walker, and Elaine Ayres

OBJECTIVES

1. Compare national initiatives in support of patient engagement.
2. Identify patient care-related engagement approaches.
3. Describe key patient-engaging provider competencies.
4. Discuss technology available to support patient engagement.
5. Summarize how patient engagement, cost, and technology relate to ideal patient care delivery.

KEY WORDS

Accountable Care Act, HITECH Act, National Strategy for Quality, interprofessional education/collaborative, patient engagement, patient activation, technology, costs

---

CONTENTS

INTRODUCTION

In the book *A Sea of Broken Hearts: Patient Rights in a Dangerous, Profit-Driven Health Care System* by James (2007) details events in which failure of integrated care ended in the death of a 19-year-old, his son. James wrote the book in an effort to change the health care system to a patient-centered and truly engaged approach. Foundational to engagement is the claim in the 2001 Institute of Medicine (IOM) report (Committee on Quality of Healthcare in America, 2001) of 10 minimal expectations in any patient bill of rights document. Given James's experience in the death of his son, he prioritized the following list as (James, 2007, p. 143):

1. *Science and education*: Patients should have care based on the best scientific evidence available with recognized standards and guidelines. Your provider and specialists will be allowed to provide care only if they have the proper education/ certifications.

2. *Transparency*: Care will be kept confidential but nothing should be kept a secret from the patients.

3. *Anticipation*: Patients shall receive preventive care that reduces their risk of illness; their provider has a "duty to warn" the patient of lifestyle choices that pose health risks and how to manage those risks.

4. *Information*: Patients should know what they want to know when they want to know it, having full access to their medical record in a timely way.

5. *Safety and accountability*: Patients shall not be harmed by errors of omission or commission in care; however, mistakes will occur. When they do, the patient or survivors have the right to unbiased assessment of treatment by a jury of peers.

Patient rights and the delivery of safe care are expected to be facilitated by information technologies such as the electronic health record (EHR). This chapter focuses on the key elements needed for that to happen and the associated role of patient engagement/ activation.

BACKGROUND AND PERSPECTIVE

Patient Engagement by Definition

More than half (51%) of U.S. consumers with chronic conditions believe the benefits of being able to access medical information through electronic medical records (EMR) outweigh the perceived risk of privacy invasion, according to the Accenture 2014 Patient Engagement Survey of more than 2,000 U.S. consumers. Interestingly, the differences among consumers with chronic conditions are notable. The highest percentage of individuals who believed that the benefits of EMR outweighed the privacy risk was among those with cancer (57%), whereas those with asthma and arthritis showed the lowest percentage (48%; Ratliff, Webb, & Safavi, 2014). In terms of this consumer-perceived risk of privacy invasion, organizations, such as the Aligning Forces for Quality (AF4Q) and Partnership 4 Patients (P4P), are working to place the patient at the center of health care decision making and in more control of his or her data, thereby mitigating the trend toward perceived risk of privacy invasion (Aligning Forces for Quality, National Program Office, 2015; Centers for Medicare & Medicaid Services [CMS], 2014).

A 2012 report provides sound evidence that communicating with patients about their health care decisions yields optimal outcomes (Alston et al., 2012). The aim of such a report was to increase the use of the available evidence for medical decision making. The approach was intended to instill awareness and demand for medical evidence among patients, providers, health care organizations, and policy makers. This had the potential to yield better care, better health, and lower costs. The authors of this report were participants drawn from the Evidence Communication Innovation Collaborative (ECIC) of the IOM Roundtable on Value & Science-Driven Health Care, which sought to "improve public understanding, appreciation, and evidence-based discussion of the nature and use of evidence to guide clinical choices" (Alston et al., 2012, p. 3).

ECIC participants, such as communication experts, decision scientists, patient advocates, health system leaders, and health care providers, have indicated that "shared decision making is the process of integrating patients' goals and concerns with medical evidence to achieve high-quality medical decisions" (Alston et al., 2012, p. 3). In support of this, they cite a 2011 Cochrane systematic review of 86 clinical trials in which patients' use of evidence-based decision aids led to (a) improved knowledge of options; (b) more accurate expectations of possible benefits and harms; (c) choices more consistent with informed values; and (d) greater participation in decision making (A. M. O'Connor, Llewellyn-Thomas, & Flood, 2004; Schoen et al., 2007; Stacey et al., 2014). Other studies on patient engagement (Schoen et al., 2007) suggested that providing patients with clearly presented evidence has been shown to impact choices, resulting in better understanding of treatment options and screening recommendations, higher satisfaction, and choices resulting in lower costs (Kennedy et al., 2002). Several studies stated that engaging patients in their own medical decisions leads to better health outcomes (A. M. O'Connor et al., 2004; K. O'Connor, 2007; Schoen et al., 2007).

National Initiatives

One of the first widely known definitions of "patient engagement" was introduced by the Centers for Medicare & Medicaid Services (CMS) in the standard requirements for meaningful use (MU) of the EHR. CMS packaged patient engagement as a quality metric via the Health Information Technology for Economic Clinical Health (HITECH) Act. The HITECH Act indicated that increased patient and consumer engagement in their own care should be a major focal point of Stage 2 MU of an EHR and that patients must begin to access online digital data. The Office of the National Coordinator for Health Information Technology (ONC-HIT) has established a website (www.healthit.gov) to promote consumer engagement in gaining access to his or her own health information. Additionally, since it was noted that evidence from Stage 1 data for MU of an EHR indicated that most patients did not realize they could request digital data, the following requirements were included in the Stage 2 standards:

▶ More than 5% of patients must send secure messages to their provider and more than 5% must have access to their online health data.

▶ Electronic exchange providers must send a summary of care record for transitions of care and referrals, 10% of which must be sent electronically (CMS, 2014).

This addition increases the involvement of information technology in the effort to meet MU requirements for patient engagement/activation.

As part of its efforts to improve the health of U.S. citizens, the federal government has provided reports that define the status of health and the associated evidence-based approaches to prevent poor health outcomes. One such report is the National Quality Strategy (Department of Health and Human Services, 2012). This report is provided each year to the U.S. Congress as a means to define the status of health improvement efforts throughout the country. Of interest to consumers/patients is that one of the six major components of the strategy is "engaging individuals and families in their care" (p. 1). An example is the Flex Medicare Beneficiary Quality Improvement Program, which is based on the assertion that high-quality care is not only safe but also timely, accessible, and consistent with individual and family preferences and values. Individuals are said to stay healthier when they and their families actively engage in their care, understand their options, and make choices that work for their lifestyles. This program provides technical assistance and national benchmarks to participating hospitals to improve health care outcomes in person-centered care (Federal Office of Rural Health Policy, 2014). The three-phase project emphasizes person-centered care by focusing on improving health care services, processes, and administration.

National Prevention Strategy (National Prevention Council, 2014) is a companion report to the National Quality Strategy report that focuses on endorsing preventive health care tactics aimed at the top U.S. health concerns. As noted in Chapter 2, there are four major components of the strategy; "empowered people" is one of the components.

Decision making is a complex process, influenced by personal, cultural, social, economic, and environmental factors, including individuals' ability to meet their daily needs, the opinions and behaviors of their peers, and their own knowledge and motivation. The goal of having a nation of empowered people is guided by four key recommendations, all of which can be facilitated by information technology (National Prevention Council, 2014). They are as follows:

▶ Provide people with tools and information to make healthy choices.

▶ Promote positive social interactions and support healthy decision making.

▶ Engage and empower people and communities to plan and implement prevention policies and programs.

▶ Improve education and employment opportunities.

These recommendations (National Prevention Council, 2014) are supported by descriptions of specific activities that can be accomplished by numerous stakeholders in this process of preventive health improvement for our nation. Those listed for health care systems, insurers, and clinicians are as follows:

▶ Use proven methods of checking and confirming patient understanding of health promotion and disease prevention (e.g., teach-back method).

▶ Involve consumers in planning, developing, implementing, disseminating, and evaluating health and safety information.

▶ Use alternative communication methods and tools (e.g., mobile phone applications, personal health records [PHRs], and credible health websites) to support more traditional written and oral communication.

▸ Refer patients to adult education and English-language instruction programs to help enhance understanding of health promotion and disease prevention messages (p. 2).

As a result of the recently enacted Patient Protection and Affordable Care Act (ACA), thousands of additional U.S. citizens and their family members are expected to enter the U.S. health care system, the environment in which the National Quality Strategy and the National Prevention Strategy initiatives exist (ACA; Berwick & Hackbarth, 2012; Keehan et al., 2011). The ACA expands health insurance coverage in three ways: (a) by subsidizing private plans offered through the health insurance marketplaces, (b) by substantially increasing eligibility for Medicaid, and (c) by banning insurance practices that penalized people with even minor health problems (Collins, Rasmussen, & Doty, 2014). Preliminary findings indicated that the uninsured rate for the 19 to 64 age group declined from 20% in the period July to September 2013 to 15% in the period April to June 2014, which means that there were an estimated 9.5 million fewer uninsured adults and that the uninsured rate fell significantly for people with low and moderate incomes and for Latinos (Collins et al., 2014).

The ACA, by itself, includes provisions for cutting payments and raising revenues that will achieve about $670 billion of gross savings for CMS according to Berwick and Hackbarth (2012). It is suggested that patient engagement/activation has the potential to mitigate some of the waste related to failures of care delivery, failures of care coordination, and overtreatment (Berwick & Hackbarth, 2012; O'Kane et al., 2012). However, according to the Institute for Healthcare Improvement (IHI), accountable care organizations (ACOs) are also a "step in the right direction" (Torres & Loehrer, 2014, p. 62). Broadly speaking, ACOs (led by hospitals, health systems, physician groups, or other entities) are charged with providing coordinated, high-quality care to assigned beneficiaries while also meeting quality metrics and financial targets. By doing this, the ACO is able to contribute to the savings generated by the program (Torres & Loehrer, 2014), thereby serving as a motivator for optimal health care delivery. Commonly, the use of information technology to support such improvement efforts is key to their success (Appleby, 2014; Hibbard & Greene, 2013).

Aligning Forces for Quality (AF4Q) is the Robert Wood Johnson Foundation's signature effort to lift the overall quality of health care in 16 targeted communities across America (Robert Wood Johnson Foundation, 2014). Summary reports distill some of the key lessons learned by these regional alliances of providers, patients, and payers, indicating that programs that are most successful have encouraged collaboration among patients, have made physician practices transparent, involved patients in quality-improvement efforts, and have begun engaging patients to influence health care systems or policy formation (Robert Wood Johnson Foundation, 2014).

PATIENT CARE-RELATED ENGAGEMENT APPROACHES

Organizing Frameworks

Although several organizing frameworks exist to guide the engagement of patients in their health care delivery, those associated with the major U.S. payer, the federal government, have the most at stake. As such, studies supporting frameworks by the Agency for Healthcare Research and Quality (AHRQ) of the National Institutes of Health (NIH) from the U.S. Department of Health and Human Services (DHHS) tend to be grounded in rigorous research such as randomized controlled trials (see James, 2013 for a summary). One such framework is that created by Carman et al. (2013), titled the Patient Engagement in Health and Health Care Framework.

According to the research studies supporting the Patient Engagement in Health and Health Care Framework (see Figure 5.1), patient and family engagement offers a promising pathway toward better quality health care, more efficient care, and improved population health. Because definitions of patient engagement and conceptions of how it works vary, the framework first presents the different forms of engagement, ranging from consultation to partnership. Next, it presents the levels at which patient engagement can

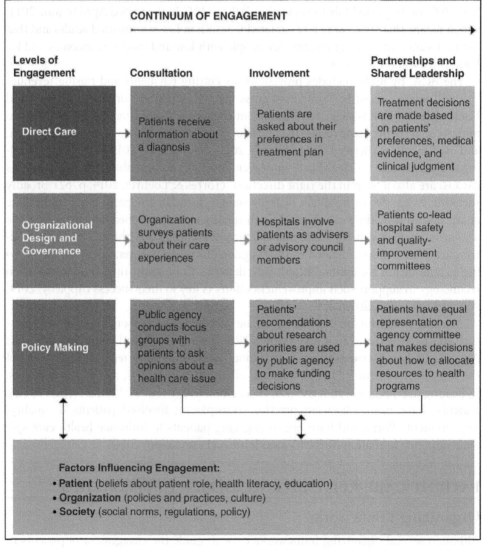

FIGURE 5.1. Patient and family engagement framework.
Source: Carman et al. (2013).

occur across the health care system, from the direct care setting to incorporating patient engagement into organizational design, governance, and policy making. The factors that influence whether and to what extent engagement occurs are included. The framework explores the implications for the development of interventions and policies that support patient and family engagement, and offers a research agenda to investigate how such engagement leads to improved outcomes (Carman et al., 2013).

An expansion on the Carmen et al. framework for patient engagement is the model published by the Healthcare Information Management Systems Society (HIMSS) Center for Patient- and Family-Centered Care (Healthcare Information and Management Systems Society, 2014). The HIMSS model includes meaningful-use categories that support provider efforts to meet the EHR federal requirements for patient engagement (see Appendix 5.1 for details of the diagram). It guides health care organizations in developing and strengthening their patient engagement strategies through the use of eHealth tools and resources and assists health care organizations of all sizes and in all stages of implementation of their patient engagement strategies. This framework can help organizations navigate the path toward more efficient and effective models of care that treat patients as partners instead of just customers (Healthcare Information and Management Systems Society, 2014).

Patient and Family Needs

As per the National Prevention Strategy, people's basic health care needs should be met regardless of age, gender, race, or socioeconomic status (National Prevention Council, 2014). Evidence-based needs were prioritized in the National Prevention Strategy report in 2014. The report indicated that people should live free of tobacco, prevent drug abuse and excessive alcohol use, eat healthfully, be physically active, avoid injury and violence, be proactive about their reproductive and sexual health, and pursue mental and emotional well-being. The report goes on to explain the roles of government and other stakeholders in achieving each of these aforementioned parameters and in realizing the importance of patient and family engagement.

Language clarity and health literacy are important to patient and family health care needs. Some groups are more likely than others to have limited health literacy. Certain populations are most likely to experience limited health literacy:

- Adults older than 65 years
- Racial and ethnic groups other than Caucasians
- Recent refugees and immigrants
- People with less than a high school degree or the general equivalency diploma (GED)
- People with incomes at or below the poverty level
- Nonnative speakers of English (Office of Disease Prevention and Health Promotion, 2010)

The report calls for health literacy to be a national priority effort and sets guidelines and standards for improvement.

Use of DNA analysis (especially in Scandinavian countries) is becoming more common in guiding health care decisions. This comprises efforts to educate patients and prevent adverse health conditions. DNA analysis has been embraced by consumers/patients to better manage their future health care decisions. A company called 23andMe provides a reading of 23 chromosomes for an individual (23andMe, 2014). This and other such organizations are covered in more detail in Chapter 24.

Websites, such as blogs, have evolved for the sharing of health care experiences, including information about health conditions and associated providers (medical professionals and health care facilities). Patients like Me (www.patientslikeme.com) and Invisible Disabilities Association (www.invisibledisabilities.org/) are two such sites that have proven popular and helpful to consumer/patients. A site dedicated to the use of technology that supports self-management of health is Health Tech and You (www.healthtechandyou.com).

PROVIDER APPROACHES/COMPETENCIES

Interprofessionalism for Patient Engagement

In support of efforts for patient engagement, studies have indicated that interprofessional approaches to care delivery are most successful. Interprofessional education (IPE) collaboratives have convened where the definition and associated competencies for health care professionals are outlined (Interprofessional Collaborative Expert Panel, 2011; World Health Organization, 2010). A key component of interprofessional education/collaboration is that professionals are all focused on the same goals for the patient and are acutely aware of each other's roles. According to the expert panel report, in addition to the understanding of professional roles, information technology is an equally important component of this approach. As noted in Chapter 2, the depiction of interprofessional teamwork as defined by the IOM IPE core competencies expert panel illustrates the interdependencies of the core interprofessional team competencies such as utilizing informatics, providing patient-centered care, applying quality improvement, and employing evidence-based practices (Figure 5.2; Interprofessional Collaborative Expert Panel, 2011).

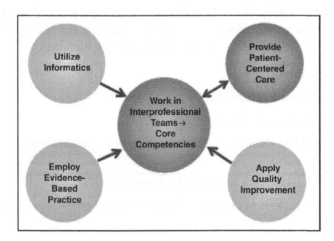

FIGURE 5.2. Pat Interprofessional teamwork and IOM CORE COMPETENCIES.
Source: International Collaborative Expert Panel (2011).

Patient engagement, also known as patient activation, is said to improve patient outcomes and decrease the cost of care delivery (Hibbard & Greene, 2013). Patients make many choices in their day-to-day lives that have major implications for their health and their need for care. Chronic disease patients must often follow complex treatment regimens, monitor their conditions, make lifestyle changes, and make decisions about when they need to seek professional care and when they can handle a problem on their own. Patient activation is:

- ► Understanding that one must take charge of one's health *and* that actions determine health outcomes
- ► A process of gaining skills, knowledge, and behaviors to manage health
- ► Having confidence to *make* needed changes (Hibbard & Greene, 2013)

Hibbard and colleagues have developed a 13-item self-report survey that measures patient activation levels. Based on results, patients fall into one of four categories, indicating a low to high level of patient activation. Each level has an associated health care coaching approach and content. Together these two components of patient care delivery have resulted in overall medical costs that were 5.3% lower than fees charged for those receiving only the usual support. They also had 12.5% fewer hospital admissions and 20.9% fewer preference-sensitive heart surgeries (Carman et al., 2013).

Provider-Based Models

Several provider-based models exist that can guide patient engagement efforts by their focus on patients and their families. One such model is described by Denham in the Family Health Model (Denham, 2003) in which the social construction of family health has contextual, functional, and structural dimensions. Examples of contextual aspects of the Family Health Model are the *family members, member traits, community context, resources, and threats*, for example (p. 9). Similarly, examples of functional aspects of the model are *developing persons, developing family, member relationships*, and *core processes*, for example (p. 9). Finally, examples of structure aspects of the model are routine type, routine characteristics, routine meaning, and routine participants (p. 9). Collectively, these aspects of the model provide for the overall perspective of a family and suggestions for considering the family when dealing with a given patient.

The Betty Neuman Model of health is closely aligned with family-centered care (www.nursingtheories.weebly.com/betty-neuman.html). The Neuman Systems Model views the client as an open system that responds to stressors in the environment. The client variables are physiological, psychological, sociocultural, developmental, and spiritual. The client system consists of a basic or core structure that is protected by lines of resistance. Subsequently, the human being is viewed as an open system that interacts with both internal and external environmental forces or stressors. The human is in constant change, moving toward a dynamic state of system stability or toward illness of varying degrees within a given environment that includes the family.

Family systems theory (FST) is derived from the broader framework of general systems theory (Bowen, 1978, p. 153). According to systems theory, a system is defined as a whole with interrelated parts in which the whole is more than the sum of its parts.

People are viewed as part of their environment rather than separate from it and characterized by patterns of emotional interactions carried from generation to generation.

The Institute for Patient and Family Centered Care (IPFCC; www.ipfcc.org/about/index.html), a nonprofit organization founded in 1992, represents an approach to the planning, delivery, and evaluation of health care that is grounded in mutually beneficial partnerships among health care providers, patients, and families. It redefines the relationships in health care in that it recognizes the vital role that families play in ensuring the health and well-being of infants, children, adolescents, and family members of all ages. They acknowledge that emotional, social, and developmental support are integral components of health care. They promote the health and well-being of individuals and families and restore dignity and control to them.

Patient- and family-centered care is an approach to health care that shapes policies, programs, facility design, and staff day-to-day interactions. It leads to better health outcomes and wiser allocation of resources, and greater patient and family satisfaction. One popular tool from the IPFCC is the hospital readiness assessment document (www.ipfcc.org/tools/downloads-tools.html). The 24-page document, which was created in partnership with the American Hospital Association (AHA) includes an extensive survey of questions to rate a given hospital's patient and family centeredness characteristics. Based on these results, the document includes guidelines for beginning an IPFCC project.

Patient-Engaging Provider Competencies

The ability to engage patients and their families in effective health care delivery practices is a matter of growing concern for those involved in outcomes management and financing of such care delivery, for example, as noted in CMS meaningful-use standards 2, where metrics for provider reimbursement are based on patient engagement levels. This notion was initially introduced in the 2003 IOM report titled *Health Professions Education: A Bridge to Quality* (National Research Council, 2003) in which educators and accreditation, licensing, and certification organizations were charged with the mandate that students and working professionals develop and maintain proficiency in core areas of patient-centered interprofessional competencies.

One example of a profession that has embraced the notion of interprofessional competencies is nutrition and dietetics. Ayres and colleagues (Ayres, Greer-Carney, Fatzinger McShane, Miller, & Turner, 2012) have in fact described a process through which multiple disciplines harmonize on defined interprofessional collaborative competencies with a focus on information technology application. As background, the authors indicated that, as a result of HITECH and meaningful use, health care has entered the digital age. The 2011 Dietetics Workforce Demand Study conducted a future scan of trends and issues that will shape dietetics practice in the future (Rhea & Bettles, 2012). A consistent theme of this study was technology driving change for all areas of practice, as well as the potential for practitioners to embrace technology and new forms of information management to remain competitive in the marketplace. In support of this trend, a three-round online Delphi study was conducted among nutrition and dietetics professionals. In round three, there were almost 100 participants, all comprising educators, clinical/community, informatics, or food service professionals. Using the Nancy Staggers model of information technology (Staggers, Gassert, & Curran, 2002), competencies by level of practice were categorized. The study provided a summary of the 216 competencies by category and by level of practice and indicated that a range from "novice" to "informatics expert" could be identified. This range of competencies was explored and quantified in regard to computer skills, informatics knowledge, and informatics skill. This master list of competencies by level of practice is available at www.eatright.org/NIDelphi2012. It is assumed that competencies at the lower levels of practice apply to higher levels of practice.

The rigorous work depicted through this study has provided a list of interprofessional informatics competencies on which health care professionals could potentially align. The categories, terminologies, and associated nomenclature should be adopted by multiple health professions as a way to enhance health care delivery collaboration.

TECHNOLOGY SUPPORT FOR PATIENT ENGAGEMENT

The Health Research Institute (HRI) 2014 report estimated that the $2.8 trillion U.S. health care industry is being upended by companies attuned to the needs and desires of empowered consumers (PricewaterhouseCoopers, 2014a). These new entrants from the retail, technology, telecommunications, consumer products, and automotive industries are centered on consumer transparency, convenience, and prevention. For example, $267 billion is estimated for their fitness and wellness market. Using a device attached to a phone, 46.9% of customers surveyed have checked for an ear infection at home and 38.6% have had a live visit with a physician via their smartphone and a webcam (PricewaterhouseCoopers, 2014a). Another HRI study indicated that 43% of consumers surveyed prefer an online health care website with different options and different prices so they can optimally compare the overall value (PricewaterhouseCoopers, 2014b).

Patients also have made contributions to the empowered consumer movement. They may contribute through patient generated health information (PGHI). As part of a national eHealth collaborative, PGHI was evaluated by technical experts and summarized in a December 2013 report (National eHealth Collaborative, 2013). The general approach would be to have the PGHI entered into the health system electronically. Examples of medication-related PGHI items are medication (history, current), medication adherence (including over-the-counter medication), medication reactions/symptom reporting, and so on. Although concerns existed on both the patient and the provider side, the main emphasis for success is that expectations be managed well. Providers and patients must have a shared understanding about what information would be most valuable, how data should be shared, and what will happen after they share the data (National eHealth Collaborative, 2013).

Based on these findings for consumer spending and potential PGHI, the use of information technology has been identified as a means to enhance, expedite, and optimally support the patient information content for patient health care decision making. Patient engagement starts with giving patients the tools they need to understand what makes them sick, how to stay healthy, and what to do if their conditions get worse. It means motivating and empowering patients to work with clinicians—to be active participants in their care by asking questions, knowing their medications and medical history, bringing friends or relatives to appointments for support, and learning about care that may be unnecessary. It can also mean giving them a seat at the table to improve the care that hospitals and doctors' offices provide (Robert Wood Johnson Foundation, 2014).

The technology-based PHR (Agarwal, Anderson, Zarate, & Ward, 2013; Lau et al., 2013) and mobile health care are important components of the consumer/patient engagement effort. Because of their complexity, these are addressed in other chapters.

HEALTH CARE COSTS AND TECHNOLOGY

Some suggest that the current approach to health care reform and, ultimately, health care cost reduction, is not on the right track because of financial misalignment (Mechanic, 2008). However, others indicate that with a robust focus on infrastructure and technology, the needed transitions can be achieved (Feldman, Murtaugh, Pezzin, McDonald, & Peng, 2005; Murtaugh, Pezzin, McDonald, Feldman, & Peng, 2005).

In the fall of 2013, a group from the Consumers Union and from the Robert Wood Johnson Foundation met to explore potential solutions to the rising cost of health care (Consumers Union, 2014). It was noted that health care spending consumes more than $1 of every $6 we earn, but many consumers are often unaware of the real cost of health care. The impact is felt by individuals, families, employers, and those crafting state and federal budgets in that rising health care costs undermine wage growth. Between 1999 and 2009, almost all increases in compensation have taken the form of paying rising health premiums and almost none have been allocated to increasing the take-home paycheck. Rising health care costs force trade-offs in our national and local government budget priorities, reducing the money available for education and other important programs. The report indicated that our current path is unsustainable, and it is evident that good, quality health care can be delivered for less money (Consumers Union, 2014).

An extensive effort by the IOM to determine how our nation can provide high-quality care at low cost was described in a 450-page report (Smith, Saunders, Stuckhardt, & McGinnis, 2012). Essentially, the committee members from the payer and provider organizations across the nation believed that achieving a learning health care system that is aligned to promote continuous improvement in care is necessary. Four fundamental characteristics of such a system were identified (p. S-11):

▶ *Science and informatics*: (a) real-time access to knowledge and (b) digital capture of the care experience

▶ *Patient–clinician partnerships*: engaged, empowered patients

▶ *Incentives*: (a) incentives aligned for value and (b) full transparency

▶ *Culture*: (a) leadership-instilled culture of learning and (b) supportive system competencies

Recommendations, followed by specific strategies for stakeholders, are described in the full report (Smith et al., 2012). There are three major categories of the committee's recommendations: (a) fundamental elements, (b) care improvement targets, and (c) supportive policy environment. Of significance to information technology professionals is the fact that "digital infrastructure" and "data utility" (p. S-20) are *the* two components of the fundamental elements category.

SUMMARY

Characteristics of patient engagement/activation are becoming more well-known to patients and providers. Much of this is fueled by the government initiatives in which value-based reimbursement focuses on patient engagement/activation. The use of organizational frameworks, coupled with family involvement, help to foster a patient's involvement in his or her care. On the other hand, providers should have the interprofessional skills and knowledge necessary to support patient engagement. Technology support for patient engagement and for cost reduction is discussed in detail in Chapter 15, as well. Advanced practice RNs and other advanced interprofessionals would benefit from these skills.

EXERCISES AND QUESTIONS FOR CONSIDERATION

1. As an information technology professional, your role in support of patient engagement is guided by the five components of interprofessional teamwork and IOM core competencies described in Chapter 2. Using these components, describe how you and your colleagues reflect each component.

2. There are four specific activities identified as supportive of preventive health care (National Prevention Council, 2014). Select one of these four activities and describe a situation in which you have conducted such an activity.

   a. Use proven methods of checking and confirming patient understanding of health promotion and disease prevention (e.g., teach-back method).

   b. Involve consumers in planning, developing, implementing, disseminating, and evaluating health and safety information.

   c. Use alternative communication methods and tools (e.g., mobile phone applications, PHRs, and credible health websites) to support more traditional written and oral communication.

   d. Refer patients to adult education and English-language instruction programs to help enhance understanding of health promotion and disease prevention messages.

3. Ayres et al. (2012) used a Delphi technique to gain consensus among a variety of health care professionals. Review this master list of competencies provided by the level of practice that is available at www.eatright.org/NIDelphi2012.

   a. Identify where you would categorize your informatics competencies.

   b. Identify other competencies that could be added to address consumer engagement and self-reported health data.

4. According to Hibbard and Greene (2013), patient activation is:

   a. understanding that one must take charge of one's health *and* that actions determine health outcomes.

   b. a process of gaining skills, knowledge, and behaviors to manage health.

   c. having confidence to *make* needed changes (Hibbard & Greene, 2013).

   Explain which of these three characteristics would be the most difficult for you to implement and why.

5. Consider content covered with respect to policy changes in the United States and the strategic plan needed to improve care and drive down cost through use of health information technology. Give one example of an information technology policy change that has supported patient engagement.

CASE STUDY EXAMPLE

Consider the following case study example.

Aims and objectives: To evaluate the outcome of a coherent nursing practice in the form of a partnership that addresses the complexity of living with chronic obstructive pulmonary disease.

Background: Chronic obstructive pulmonary disease is a wide-ranging and progressive chronic disease that not only requires the relentless attention of the persons having the disease but also requires family involvement (Ingadottir & Jonsdottir, 2010). Particular consideration is required in health care for those with an advanced and complicated stage of the disease.

Please respond to the following questions:

1. How would you use the Patient Engagement in Health and Health Care Framework to plan a patient engagement approach for the patient and family?
2. What type of information technology would you advise to support the care delivery?

REFERENCES

Agarwal, R., Anderson, C., Zarate, J., & Ward, C. (2013). If we offer it, will they accept? Factors affecting patient use intentions of personal health records and secure messaging. *Journal of Medical Internet Research, 15*(2), e43.

Alston, C., Paget, L., Halvorson, G., Novelli, B., Guest, J., McCabe, P., . . . Von Kohorn, I. (2012). *Communicating with patients on health care evidence.* (Discussion paper). Washington, DC: Institute of Medicine.

Aligning Forces for Quality, National Program Office. (2015). *Aligning forces for quality: Improving health and healthcare in communities across America.* Retrieved from http://forces4quality.org/about-us

Appleby, C. (2014). *Want to improve patient satisfaction? Try integrating technology* (No. Satis2014). InsightON. Retrieved from http://www.insight.com/insighton/healthcare/want-improve-patient-satisfaction-try-integrating-technology/

Ayres, E. J., Greer-Carney, J., Fatzinger McShane, P. E., Miller, A., & Turner, P. (2012). Nutrition informatics competencies across all levels of practice: A national Delphi study. *Journal of the Academy of Nutrition and Dietetics, 112*(12), 2042–2053. doi:10.1016/j.jand.2012.09.025

Berwick, D. M., & Hackbarth, A. D. (2012). Eliminating waste in US health care. *Journal of the American Medical Association, 307*(14), 1513–1516. doi:10.1001/jama.2012.362

Bowen, M. (1978). *Family therapy in clinical practice.* New York, NY: Jason Aronson.

Carman, K. L., Dardess, P., Maurer, M., Sofaer, S., Adams, K., Bechtel, C., & Sweeney, J. (2013). Patient and family engagement: A framework for understanding the elements and developing interventions and policies. *Health Affairs, 32*(2), 223–231. Retrieved from http://content.healthaffairs.org/content/32/2/223.full

Collins, S. R., Rasmussen, P. W., & Doty, M. M. (2014). *Tracking trends in health system performance: Gaining ground: Americans' health insurance coverage and access to care after the Affordable Care Act's first open enrollment period.* (Brief). New York, NY: The Commonwealth Fund.

Centers for Medicare & Medicaid Services. (2014, November). *Stage 2: Meaningful use.* Retrieved from http://www.cms.gov/Regulations-and-Guidance/Legislation/EHRIncentivePrograms/Stage_2.html

Committee on Quality of Healthcare in America. (2001). *Crossing the quality chasm: A new health system for the 21st century.* Washington, DC: National Academies Press. Retrieved from http://www.nap.edu/catalog.php?record_id=10027

Consumers Union. (2014). *Addressing rising health care costs workshop summary: A pioneering meeting of advocates seeking to address health care costs.* (No. RWJF410914). Princeton, NJ: Consumer Union–Robert Wood John Foundation.

Denham, S. (2003). *Family health: A framework for nursing.* Philadelphia, PA: F. A. Davis.

Department of Health and Human Services. (2012). *National strategy for quality improvement in health care.* (Congressional Report No. DHHS-2012). Rockville, MD: Agency for Healthcare Research and Quality.

Federal Office of Rural Health Policy. (2014). *FLEX Medicare beneficiary quality improvement project* (No. FLEX2014). Retrieved from http://www.ruralcenter.org/sites/default/files/MBQIP%20Overview%20for%20CAHs.pdf

Feldman, P. H., Murtaugh, C. M., Pezzin, L. E., McDonald, M. V., & Peng, T. R. (2005). Just-in-time evidence-based e-mail "reminders" in home health care: Impact on patient outcomes. *Health Services Research, 40*(3), 865–885.

Healthcare Information and Management Systems Society. (2014). *HIMSS center for patient- and family-centered care.* Retrieved from http://www.himss.org/library/NEHC

Hibbard, J. H., & Greene, J. (2013). What the evidence shows about patient activation: Better health outcomes and care experiences; fewer data on costs. *Health Affairs* (Project Hope) 32(2), 207–214. doi:10.1377/hlthaff.2012.1061

Ingadottir, T. S., & Jonsdottir, H. (2010). Partnership-based nursing practice for people with chronic obstructive pulmonary disease and their families: Influences on health-related quality of life and hospital admissions. *Journal of Clinical Nursing, 19*(19), 2795–2805. doi:10.1111/j.1365-2702.2010.03303.x

Interprofessional Collaborative Expert Panel. (2011). *Core competencies for interprofessional collaborative practice: Report of an expert panel* (No. ICEP-2011). Interprofessional Education Collaborative. Retrieved from https://ipecollaborative.org/uploads/IPEC-Core-Competencies.pdf

James, J. T. (2007). *A sea of broken hearts: Patient rights in a dangerous, profit-driven health care system.* Bloomington, IN: AuthorHouse.

James, J. T. (2013). A new, evidence-based estimate of patient harms associated with hospital care. *Journal of Patient Safety, 9*(3), 122–128. doi:10.1097/PTS.0b013e3182948a69

Keehan, S. P., Sisko, A. M., Truffer, C. J., Poisal, J. A., Cuckler, G. A., Madison, A. J., . . . Smith, S. D. (2011). National health spending projections through 2020: Economic recovery and reform drive faster spending growth. *Health Affairs, 30*(8), 1594–1605. doi:10.1377/hlthaff.2011.0662

Kennedy, A. D., Sculpher, M. J., Coulter, A., Dwyer, N., Rees, M., Abrams, K. R., . . . Stirrat, G. (2002). Effects of decision aids for menorrhagia on treatment choices, health outcomes, and costs: A randomized controlled trial. *Journal of the American Medical Association*, *288*(21), 2701–2708. doi:joc20530 [pii]

Lau, A. Y. S., Dunn, A. G., Mortimer, N., Gallagher, A., Proudfoot, J., Andrews, A., . . . Coiera, E. (2013). Social and self-reflective use of a web-based personally controlled health management system. *Journal of Medical Internet Research*, *15*(9), e211. doi:10.2196/jmir.2682

Mechanic, D. (2008). Barriers to eliminating waste in US health care. *Journal of Health Services Research & Policy*, *13*(2), 57–58. doi:10.1258/jhsrp.2008.007165

Murtaugh, C. M., Pezzin, L. E., McDonald, M. V., Feldman, P. H., & Peng, T. R. (2005). Just-in-time evidence-based e-mail "reminders" in home health care: Impact on nurse practices. *Health Services Research*, *40*(3), 849–864.

National eHealth Collaborative. (2013). *Patient generated health information: Technical expert panel final report December 2013*. (No. Grant#7U24AE000006-02). Washington, DC: Author. Retrieved from http://himss.files.cms-plus.com/FileDownloads/pghi_tep_finalreport121713_1394215078393_9.pdf

National Prevention Council. (2014). *2014 annual status report*. (No. NPC2014). Washington, DC: U.S. Department of Health and Human Services, Office of the Surgeon General. Retrieved from http://www.surgeongeneral.gov/initiatives/prevention/2014-npc-status-report.pdf

National Research Council. (2003). In A. C. Greiner & Knebel, E. (Eds.), *Health professions education: A bridge to quality*. Washington, DC: The National Academies.

O'Connor, A. M., Llewellyn-Thomas, H. A., & Flood, A. B. (2004). Modifying unwarranted variations in health care: Shared decision making using patient decision aids. *Health Affairs* (Project Hope), (Suppl. Variation), VAR63–72. doi:hlthaff.var.63 [pii]

O'Connor, K. (2007). Toward the "tipping point": A new coalition of groups is working quietly to reform U.S. health care. *Health Progress*, *88*(3), 32–34.

Office of Disease Prevention and Health Promotion. (2010). *National action plan to improve health literacy*. (No. USDHHS2010). Washington, DC: Department of Health and Human Services. Retrieved from http://www.health.gov/communication/hlactionplan/

O'Kane, M., Buto, K., Alteras, T., Baicker, K., Fifield, J., Giffin, R., . . . Saunders, R. (2012). *Demanding value from our health care: Motivating patient action to reduce waste in health care*. (No. Demand2012). Washington, DC: Institute of Medicine. Retrieved from http://www.iom.edu/Global/Perspectives/2012/DemandingValue.aspx

PricewaterhouseCoopers. (2014a). *Healthcare's new entrants: Who will be the industry's amazon.com?* (No. PwC-HRI2014). Dallas, TX: Author.

Pricewaterhouse Coopers. (2014b). *Medical cost trend: Behind the numbers 2015*. (No. PwC-2014). Dallas, TX: Author.

Ratliff, R., Webb, K., & Safavi, K. (2014). *Insight driven health: Consumers with chronic conditions believe the ability to access electronic medical records outweighs concern of privacy invasion* (Survey No. 1). Albany, NY: Accenture. Retrieved from http://www.accenture.com/SiteCollectionDocuments/PDF/Accenture-Consumers-with-Chronic-Conditions-Electronic-Medical-Records.pdf

Rhea, M., & Bettles, C. (2012). Future changes driving dietetics workforce supply and demand: Future scan 2012–2022. *Journal of the Academy of Nutrition and Dietetics*, *112*(3 Suppl.), S10–S24. doi:10.1016/j.jand.2011.12.008

Robert Wood Johnson Foundation. (2014). *What we're learning: Engaging patients improves health and health care* (No. RWJF411217). Princeton, NJ: Author.

Schoen, C., Guterman, S., Shih, A., Lau, J., Kasimow, S., Gauthier, A., & Davis, K. (2007). *Bending the curve: Options for achieving savings and improving value in U.S. health spending* (No. CWF2007). Washington, DC: Commonwealth Fund. Retrieved from http://www.commonwealthfund.org/publi cations/fund-reports/2007/dec/bending-the-curve--options-for-achieving-savings-and-improving-value-in-u-s-health-spending

Smith, M., Saunders, R., Stuckhardt, L., & McGinnis, M. J. (2012). *Best care at lower cost: The path to continuously learning health care in America* (1st ed.). Washington, DC: National Academies Press.

Stacey, D., Legare, F., Col, N. F., Bennett, C. L., Barry, M. J., Eden, K. B., . . . Wu, J. H. (2014). Decision aids for people facing health treatment or screening decisions. *Cochrane Database of Systematic Reviews, 1*, CD001431. doi:10.1002/14651858.CD001431.pub4

Staggers, N., Gassert, C. A., & Curran, C. (2002). A Delphi study to determine informatics competencies for nurses at four levels of practice. *Nursing Research, 51*(6), 383–390.

Torres, T., & Loehrer, S. (2014). ACOs: A step in the right direction. *Healthcare Executive, 29*(4), 62–65. Retrieved from http://www.ihi.org/resources/Pages/Publications/ACOsStepinRightDirection.aspx

23andMe. (2014). *Find out what your DNA says about you and your family*. Retrieved from http://www.23adnMe.com

World Health Organization. (2010). *Framework for action on interprofessional education & collaborative practice*. (No. WHO/HRH/HPN/10.3). Geneva, Switzerland: Author.

APPENDIX 5.1. HIMSS PATIENT ENGAGEMENT FRAMEWORK WITH MEANINGFUL USE CATEGORIES

HIMSS FOUNDATION · National eHealth Collaborative

PATIENT ENGAGEMENT FRAMEWORK

Bands: **INFORM AND ATTRACT** · **RETAIN AND INTERACT** · **PARTNER EFFICIENTLY** · **CREATE SYNERGY AND EXTEND REACH**

Inform Me

Information and Way-Finding
- Maps and directions
- Services directory
- Physician directory

e-Tools
- Health encyclopedia
- Wellness guidance
- Prevention

Forms: Printable
- HIPAA
- Insurance
- Advance directives
- Informed consent

Patient-Specific Education
- Care plan
- Tests
- Prescribed medication
- Procedure/treatment

Engage Me

Information and Way-Finding
- Mobile
  - Nearest healthcare services
  - Symptom checker

e-Tools
- Pregnancy tracking
- Fitness tracking
- Healthy eating tracking
- Option to share progress and health milestones on social media

Interactive Forms: Online
- Patient profile
- Register or pay a bill
- Email customer service
- Schedule a clinic appointment
- Refill a prescription

Patient-Specific Education
- Care Instructions
- Reminders
- Medication
- Preventive services
- Follow-up appointments

Patient Access: Records
- View electronic health record
- Download electronic health record

Empower Me

Information, Way-Finding, and Quality
- Quality and safety reports on providers and healthcare organizations
- Patient ratings of providers, hospitals and other healthcare organizations

e-Tools
- Care plan management
- Virtual coaching
- Online nurse
- Secure messaging

Integrated Forms: EHR
- Record correction requests
- Advance directives (scanned)

Patient-Specific Education
- Materials in Spanish
- Guides to understanding accountable care

Patient Access: Records
- Transmit patient record electronically
- Copy the patient or a healthcare designee when sharing electronic record
- EHR integrated with patient PHR

Patient-Generated Data
- Care experience surveys
- Symptom assessments
- Self-management diaries
- Patient-generated data in EHR
  - Questionnaires
  - Pre-visit
  - Health history
  - Demographics

Interoperable Records
- Integrated with health information exchange (HIE)
- E-referral coordination between providers
- Ambulatory and hospital records integration
- Images and video in EHR
- Commercial labs, radiology, medications

Partner With Me

Information, Way-Finding, and Analytics/Quality
- Patient-specific predictive modeling
- Patient-specific quality indicators
- Patient accountability scores

e-Tools
- Wellness plan
- Advance care planning
- Coordination of care across systems

Integrated Forms: EHR
- Clinical trial records
- Immunization (public health)

Patient-Specific Education
- Materials in Spanish and the top 5 national languages
- Condition-specific self-management tools

Patient Access
- Publish and subscribe
  - Summary of care

Patient-Generated Data
- Shared decision making
- Preference-sensitive care
- Informed choice/consent
- Adherence reporting
  - Medications
  - Self-care
  - Wellness
- Home monitoring
  - Devices
  - Tele-medicine
- Directives
  - Advance
  - Physician orders for life-sustaining treatment
  - Intolerances
  - Allergies
  - Values
  - Preferences

Interoperable Records
- Integrated with clinical trial records
- Integrated with public health reporting
- Integrated with claims and administrative data

Collaborative Care
- Acute
- Long-term post-acute care
- Primary care
- Specialty

Support My e-Community

Information, Way-Finding, and Analytics/Quality
- Care comparison for providers, treatments, and medications
  - Costs
  - Convenience
  - Quality

e-Visits and e-Tools
- e-Visits as part of ongoing care

Integrated Forms: EHR
- (replaced by interoperable collaborative care records)

Patient-Specific Education
- Care planning
- Chronic care self-management
- Reminders for daily care

Patient Access and Use
- Publish/subscribe for complete record
- Distribution of record among care team
- Patient-granted permissions
- Patient-set privacy controls

Care Team-Generated Data
- Shared care plans
  - Episodic
  - Chronic
  - End of life
- Team outcomes
  - Adherence
  - Costs
  - Quality

Interoperable Records
- Integrated with long-term post-acute care records

Collaborative Care
- Chiropractic
- Dentistry
- Alternative medicine
- Home

Community Support
- Online community support forums and resources for all care team members
  - Caregivers
  - Family
  - Friends
  - Clergy
  - Counseling
  - Services

Aligned: Emerging Meaningful Use	Aligned: Meaningful Use 1	Aligned: Meaningful Use 2	Aligned: Meaningful Use 3	Aligned: Meaningful Use 4+

SECTION II

Point-of-Care Technology
(NEHI Model Component #1)

CHAPTER 6

Computers in Health Care

Susan McBride, Richard Gilder, and Deb McCullough

OBJECTIVES

1. Discuss the basics of computer technology related to hardware, software, and networking.

2. Describe hardware specifications and criteria that should be taken into account as a health care system considers purchases of hardware to implement technology.

3. Examine the ergonomics requirements needed when implementing health information technology (HIT) for nursing and other health care professionals.

4. Identify and describe various programming languages utilized in the health care setting.

5. Analyze various types of software utilized in health care settings relevant to HIT, including functionality, usability, human factors considerations, configuration languages, modules versus full platforms, and other important considerations when purchasing software applications.

6. Discuss databases and how a database is configured utilizing Microsoft Access as an example for configuring the basics of a database.

7. Compare and contrast report writing versus raising queries, and provide examples of types of reports versus queries commonly used in the health care setting for quality and patient safety initiatives.

KEY WORDS

hardware, software, human factors, ergonomics, database, query, reports, usability, programming languages, system software, application software, hardware configuration, network typology

CONTENTS

INTRODUCTION

The technology underlying health information systems is an important aspect that advanced practice nurses have to understand, as they are the ones who are to lead teams to adopt and implement HIT systems. This chapter focuses on the "bits and bytes" underlying the systems that we commonly use in the clinical setting. Software selection, configuration, hardware specifications, programming languages, databases, queries, report writing, and other technology specifics important to selection of systems are discussed at length. Additionally, we cover the ergonomics and usability of systems and how to configure systems that work well for clinicians.

BACKGROUND

In health care, we are currently in the very early stages of experimentation with many different concepts in the search for an engine that will enable the powered flight of a fully automated electronic health record. As with the high mortality rates associated with early experiments in aerospace technology, vast portions of the general body of scientific knowledge have been discovered relating to technological advancements in aerospace while we balance safety with innovative technological advancement. The internal engines in the computer are electronic in nature, and similar to an automobile, the automated electronic health care machine has vast potential for good or bad outcomes, depending on how it is designed and used. The cumulative effect of that outcome can be determined by how well we engineer safety into its fundamental designs, and how well we educate, train, and license operators of the electronic health care record "machine." How well we regulate, mandate, and support the interactive behavior of the operators and what the operators do with the machine will determine profitability and viability of the electronic health record.

Historical Perspective

Computers in health care have already solved, and have great potential to solve, some of the most complex and difficult problems that have always challenged health care providers. Health care providers over time have discovered that documentation and archiving of their personal observations of the health care delivery process at the point of care, in a manner that was valid, accurate, immediately retrievable, and accurately reproducible, was a critical advancement in health care. Standardization of common terms used to describe and articulate observations related to health care facilitated the storage, retrieval, and communication of health care experience, knowledge, wisdom, and skills, spanning time, cultures, and geography. Nevertheless, if transferred through oral tradition, inscribed on clay tablets, woven into intricate tapestries of knots, or written in glyphs, the intentional collection, archive, and transfer of knowledge was identified as a critical function of health care for centuries. The intrinsic value of discovered knowledge, and especially knowledge of things that ease suffering, promote health, and significantly assist healing from disease and injury is not new. It became an expected professional behavior that contribution to that shared understanding, through continuous maintenance of this pooled reservoir of information, was also a hallmark of the scientific culture of health care, and that the ability to share information beyond the immediate point-of-care delivery enabled great discovery and widespread implementation and adoption of successful health care interventions. The peer-reviewed publication process present in general science likewise forms an integral part of the structure of modern health care.

The Role of Computers in Health Care

Communication of information is the essence of the role of computers in health care and the primary function of any electronic health care record machine or machine intelligence. In the following sections on hardware, software, and ergonomics, the role that the computer as a health care machine plays in communicating health care information among health care providers, and how that role impacts the delivery of health care at the point of care and beyond, is explored. This impact is growing and accelerating perfectly in line with Moore's Law and is perhaps as significant as the impact that Guttenberg's printing press had on communication of information. Moore's Law, originating in the 1970s, postulates that computing power will double every 2 years (Moore, n.d).

Fundamentals of Communication

Successful communication requires that a minimum amount of understandable signal be present in the communication. Discrimination of the correct information in the signal, even when embedded and surrounded by noise, is a minimum characteristic of the true and accurate transfer of knowledge that occurs when communication takes place. Every medium that has ever been used by one human to communicate with another human, from hand gesture, eye contact, facial expression, spoken words, symbols scribed in sand or on rock, or even written by hand on parchment, is subject to noise. Ink can become smudged, symbols chiseled into rock can become eroded, even facial expressions and nonverbal gestures can be completely misinterpreted; these examples illustrate the concept of signal versus noise. With every communication medium, successful communication of the intended signal is always at risk of misinterpretation, or outright loss, due to noise. When the ratio of signal to noise is very high, successful communication is very high; when the ratio of signal to noise is very low, successful communication is very low. The accurate transfer of a streaming flow of information from a health care provider at the point of care to an electronic health care record in a handoff to the machine, and a return handoff from the machine to the health care provider engaged in providing point-of-contact health care, requires an optimal signal-to-noise ratio. The computer, as "a machine," has great potential to deliver even larger and more complex streams of flowing information in packets routed to wide area networks (WANs) that potentially encompass the entire world. The potential to do that far more rapidly than the human recipient can assimilate and process, in order to stay afloat on the stream (rather than drown in it), poses problems that are addressed by the cognitive sciences that form part of the fundamental foundation of informatics science. Anyone who has experienced the difficulty of carrying on two telephone conversations with two different people simultaneously, by holding two telephone handsets to each ear on the right and left, and talking to both parties at the same time by rotating the mouthpiece up over the head while talking on the left phone or the right phone, yet listens to the feedback in both earpieces of the handsets at the same time, understands this overwhelming complexity. Sounds confusing? Now try it with two conference calls, each with 20 to 30 people, and the potential of all 60 people talking to you (the person in the middle of this stream of signal flowing in from two places at once) at the same time. What would be the potential for misunderstanding or mishandling critical pieces of information? Yet, to the trained ear, even a fairly quiet beep tone of a repeating SOS in Morse code would be crystal clear, even when embedded in the midst of such a chaotic stream of data flow. This is an example of just one characteristic behavior of the electronic health care record machine.

A military aircraft is quite capable of operating in a manner that is very different from what the human body is capable of interpreting and processing. It can execute turns so rapidly and at such high speeds, that even though the aircraft remains intact and the wings do not tear themselves off during the maneuver, the human pilot would be exposed to a lethal level of artificial gravitational forces from centrifugal motion, and would not live through the maneuver even though the aircraft would. Of course, safeguards are built into the aircraft to prevent this from happening accidentally. In contrast, the electronic health care record machine is still at an early stage of development like the first flight at Kitty Hawk in comparison to the current mission to colonize Mars.

We have a very long way to go in order to make the electronic health care record machine as safe and effective as even the common aspirin tablet is today. Aspirin is perhaps one of the most deadly poisons commonly found in any home, yet it is one of the most beneficial medications to keep in store as a critical item in every home. In the future, beyond doubt, there *will* be an electronic health care record machine that enjoys a similar long historic record of being safe and effective when used as directed, but the exact date of that future day and time remains elusive at present.

It has been observed that if one were to automate a bad process, then one would have a bad process that runs automatically. This speaks to the importance of quality-improvement tools, such as workflow redesign, and a focus on improved process being so important to the refinement of computers in health care. We cannot simply automate a paper-based process that had potential flaws in the process, but we must redesign, rethink, and improve processes as we automate the process with computers in health care. This is perhaps the most important cautionary aspect of computers in health care. No doubt the technological advances that made air travel possible have changed the world in ways that none of the first aviators or aircraft inventors could have ever imagined. On the other hand, traveling at such great speed has also resulted in huge disasters and loss of life and property, and has led to the potential spread of global pandemics in a much faster and irreversible manner than would have ever been possible if we had to simply walk from one place to another, or pull a cart behind an animal, or even sail the high seas across continents. Through trial and error, experiment and observation, air travel has become progressively safe and highly reliable. Many versions of electronic health care records and the machines used to manufacture and distribute them are currently being subjected to the same scientific methods that eventually resulted in the modern commercial air travel becoming a common universally available service. The same classic method of posing research questions and formulating hypotheses designed to objectively and mathematically test the hypotheses through trial and error is being employed. Studies are being conducted that evaluate electronic health care records in terms of their effects on mortality rates, readmission rates, and quality of life of the patient populations. Reporting of the findings to a jury of peers through professional journals and publications is no different in informatics science than any other branch of science. What the aerospace sciences have done for air travel, health care informatics sciences are in the process of doing for health care delivery; right now, health care informatics is in the very early stages of scientific discovery.

Health Care Informatics—An Evolving Science

Health care informatics science bridges the highly technical computer, data, mathematical, and communication sciences with the human aspects of cognitive, biological, medicine, and nursing, and other supporting health care sciences. Like a United Nations translator who listens to a person addressing the assembly in his or her native foreign language and immediately relays the correct and accurate interpretation of what is being said into the headphones of the ambassadors and representatives present, capturing even subtle nuances and idiomatic meanings between the lines, health care informatics data scientists serve to facilitate understanding and clear communication among all of the health care delivery team members. Health care informatics science plays a critical role wherever computers are involved in the process of delivering health care.

Health care informatics has evolved and is now rapidly expanding into many specialized roles required by various health care service lines. Medical and surgical doctors have developed expertise as medical and surgical informatics scientists, as have nurses, pharmacists, and other health care professionals. Perioperative surgical nursing was one of the first among the nursing profession to invent, develop, and adopt a standardized codified vocabulary with the intent of incorporating it into the electronic health record as a method of standardized documentation that would have meaningful use for research, patient safety, and health care improvement (Kleinbeck, 1999).

In the background of this discussion of computers in health care, consider that if communication is the essential function of the electronic health care record machine, then the machine plays a very strong hand in the game of automated clinical decision support (ACDS). The logic modules and computational algorithms that operationalize health care logic into a cascade of triggers, warnings, messages, and alarms, are the nature of most of that communication. The differentiation of clinical informatics science is being driven by the health care service line-specific needs that require that the communication input and output that are mediated by the machine are clinically meaningful and useful to the health care provider who must act upon it. Messages that are clinically meaningful and useful to nurses may not be as useful to pathologists, radiologists, or pharmacists. On the other hand, some of the information that is clinically meaningful to nursing may be of critical value to other service lines, and vice versa. How to build the internal mapping between critical data elements that are of universal use to every end user (including the patient) of the electronic medical record (EMR) machine's output is a major challenge for clinical health care informatics science. The map must be wide enough to account for rare and isolated expressions of data elements as a unique field having only one value in the database, and yet must be sufficiently deep enough to accommodate multiple expressions of the same data element value no matter how many records deep it recurs. The resulting map is what makes it possible for programmatic algorithms, logic, and rules to be developed that apply to all health care delivery regardless of point of care. This ideal type of map is also sufficiently flexible to provide automated decision support in a context of care that occurs very rarely, but that may result in catastrophic failure if no supplemental support is provided at all to move the clinician's tacit knowledge into action. The ideal ACDS system will enable anyone who interacts with it to make competent decisions, but will never replace the tacit "expert" knowledge, wisdom, and insight that require many long years of experience in professional practice to attain. As a final thought to consider, how do we resolve what can best be described as the "Ansatz conflict"?

The Ansatz, as used in physics and mathematics, is the initial hunch, educated guess, guesstimate, or "best bet, given the odds," that precedes the research question. It is an assumption or a guess that works well to support a given conclusion, with the given facts available at the time the conclusion is drawn. It is a conclusion, not a theory. It is the precursor to legitimate research questions. The human cognitive ability to accurately form vague hunches rapidly from intuitive insights based on an internal body of implicit knowledge that has been neurologically stored over a lifetime of active and passive learning is clearly a definitive aspect of humanity. That those hasty hunches are more often enough than not valid to the point of saving the lives of the human's acting on such "decision support" is a matter of colorful historical record.

Formalization of human intuition and insight and codification of logic in mathematical systems of reasoning have resulted in the ability to document and reproduce the steps required to navigate the problem space. In the process of exhaustively enumerating and analyzing the many paths that lead to a definitive solution set, it has become clear that some of the solution sets are paths that are unique, are rare, and are much shorter, and just as accurate and valid as those that are much longer. Testing hunches prior to acting on hunches in life or death decisions with uncertain outcomes through the proxy of hypothesis testing became less of a gamble on pure chance when the outcomes of the hypothesis tests were collectively applied to the decision as a weight on the hunch. Methods of assigning numerical value to uncertainty, as a way to predict the otherwise unknowable outcomes of high stakes games, was the first stirrings of the concept of probability in the formal mathematical sense of definition as hypothesis tests, with numerical thresholds of acceptance or rejection, that would yield a simple "yes" (or "no") decision. The advent of electronic computing that can take advantage of the same codified logic involved in exhaustively assigning probability to uncertainty in a manner that far exceeds the human man hours that would have been required to render the same decision is having an impact that is still unfolding in human history. One of the areas being influenced by the advent of this new automated decision support is health care.

It is very well understood that ACDS is mechanically providing a "best guess" that the clinician takes into consideration when making a decision. The "Ansatz conflict" arises when the suggested action from the ACDS "best guess—Ansatz" is in conflict with the Anzatz arising from the experienced clinician's gestalt tacit knowledge. There is a very real risk that the experienced clinician, whose Ansatz is actually orders of magnitude more accurate and appropriate than the computer ACDS Ansatz, will suppress and censor his or her own best "conclusion" (which results in a clinical decision), in favor of an automated decision, which often turns out to be only second best when examined in retrospect (not always, but often) by a jury of experienced peers. Until ACDS is capable of exceeding the judgment rendered by a jury of experienced peers in retrospect, widespread use and implementation of ACDS in any point-of-care technology must necessarily proceed with great caution in order to assure the highest standards of safety for patient and provider alike. The true test of how well any given ACDS system or algorithm actually works is found in the false-positive rate and false-negative rate (sensitivity and specificity) of its performance after the fact. We examine, in more detail in Chapter 19, the best practices for implementing and designing clinical decision support systems to best address some of these challenges. Yet, before we fully redesign processes related to the use of computers in health care, it is important to understand the fundamentals on which these machines actually process and communicate information. In the following section we review those basics.

REVIEW OF THE BASICS

The basics of computer technology encompass fundamental building blocks. We will examine some of the basic definitions of how computers function and the origin of some of the terms we use in computer science to describe technology, including the terms "bits," "bytes," "hardware," "software," and conclude with connectivity considerations.

Bits, Bytes, and How They All Fit Together

In the early 1980s, there was a new technical jargon, a new and special language that was an anthropological consequence of the human–machine interaction around computers. The term "computerese" appears in the title of an article written at that time by Lietzke, (1982), to provide a glossary of the new words and terms that were being used to conceptually define unique attributes of computer hardware, software, human–computer interactions, and the common usage of these terms in a ubiquitous jargon. Lietzke clarified and stabilized the modern primary definition, whereas Tukey coined the first use of the term as "professional slang" (jargon). Tukey's usage was an idiomatic and linguistic drift at the time of first use, to describe two distinct concepts of "binary" and "digit," "bit-digit" or "bit." Tukey's concept of "binary digit" (Bit) was indeed the root concept, but Lietzke, in the process of clarifying a term that had been in use for 38 years, finalized the whole concept that data can be "counted" representationally by the number of "binary digits" in the data; hence, Lietzke added the concept of "unit of measure" to Tukey's existing "binary digit." After that clarification in 1984 (Dickey, 1984), the use of "bit" to accurately describe computational architecture as a standard unit of measure (8 bit, 16 bit, 32 bit, 64 bit, 128 bit, 256 bit, chip sets, etc.) cemented the definition as a unit of measure in place.

The bit has only two possible values and the two values it is allowed to have are the "digits" zero (0) or one (1), hence the term "binary" in the phrase "binary digit." A bit is a binary digit and always has a value of either 0 or 1. If 1 is always taken to mean "on" (as opposed to "off"), and if 0 is always taken to mean "off" (as opposed to "on"), then the bit is universally understood to represent mutually exclusive values. The switch is either in the "on position," or is in the "off position." Although in human experience, it is quite possible to be completely drenched from a water hose when the valve is "half open," any such behavior of bits in a computer would have prevented the next phase of growth and development of computational algorithms based on the ability to form bits into special aggregations of eight bits, which form the set of 256 unique combinations of bits, each known as a "byte."

Although Lietzke actually clarified many of the terms, the jargon word "bit" was actually used for the first time in 1946 by mathematician John Wilder Tukey, as an abbreviated contraction of the term "binary digit." Twelve years later, in a 1958 article published in the *American Mathematical Monthly*, Tukey is also attributed as the first to define the programs that electronic calculators ran on, describing them as "software," differentiating the code from "the hardware," including the tubes, transistors, wires, tapes, and the like (Leonhardt, 2000). The intentionally misspelled term "byte" was invented by Werner Buchholz in 1956, spelled with a "y" to prevent confusion of "bite" with "bit" (Buchholz & Bemer, 1962). The byte is the basic whole unit of information roughly corresponding with letters and symbols in an alphabet that can be used to form the written codex of a phonetic language with unique codes that can be assigned to retrievable computer data archives known as "the memory." With its 256 possible unique symbolic alphabetic values formed by the natural frequency of 2 to the 8th power (2^8) possible combinations of zeros or ones in any of the eight allowed positions, the byte forms the computational alphabet of machine language. The difference between the base 10 system of measurement and the base 2 system of measurement has historically always been a source of confusion because of the similarity between the two. The byte also serves as a scale measure of data size, often classified by orders of magnitude in units of exponential power. The binary (base 2) prefix terms (kilo, mega, giga, etc.) form the basic unit of measure for data file size and are exactly the same as the decimal (base 10) prefix names already in use for labeling decimal quanta. Binary has its own special quanta names based on the fundamental radix (base) of 1,024 bytes of data information. The byte, therefore, represents alphanumeric symbols and text characters, the smallest standard unit of data information that can be archived, transmitted, or manipulated, and that can be reliably retrieved from memory, regardless of the media used for memory archive. At the smallest level, it only takes one bit of data to discriminate true (1) and false (0). In the world of data storage and retrieval, it requires 2 bytes (16 bits) to define one word composed of alphanumeric text symbols. At that rate of exchange, one kilobyte of data (1,024 Bytes) can contain 512 words (Yuri, n.d.). The comparisons of decimal to binary prefix terms are illustrated in Table 6.1.

The Joint Electron Device Engineering Council (JEDEC) and the International Electrotechnical Commission (IEC) set standard definitions that are shown alongside the decimal definitions by their order of exponential magnitude in Table 6.1. The IEC is one of the organizations that are recognized and entrusted by the World Trade Organization (WTO) for monitoring the national and regional organizations that agree to use the IEC's international standards (International Electrotechnical Commision [IEC], 2014). The JEDEC is an independent semiconductor engineering trade association that sets standards for terms, definitions, letter symbols for microcomputers, microprocessors, and memory-integrated circuits. The purpose of the standard is to promote the uniform

TABLE 6.1 Comparison of Decimal to Binary Prefix Terms

Exponential Order of Magnitude	Decimal					Binary						
	Radix Base	Bytes	Scientific Notation	Symbol	Name	Radix Base	Bytes	Scientific Notation	JEDEC* Symbol	JEDEC Name	IEC* Symbol	IEC Name
1	1000	1,000	1.000E+03	kB	kilobyte	1024	1,024	1.024E+03	KB	kilobyte	KiB	kibibyte
2	1000	1,000,000	1.000E+06	MB	megabyte	1024	1,048,576	1.049E+06	MB	megabyte	MiB	mebibyte
3	1000	1,000,000,000	1.000E+09	GB	gigabyte	1024	1,073,741,824	1.074E+09	GB	gigabyte	GiB	gibibyte
4	1000	1,000,000,000,000	1.000E+12	TB	terabyte	1024	1,099,511,627,776	1.100E+12	–	–	TiB	tebibyte
5	1000	1,000,000,000,000,000	1.000E+15	PB	petabyte	1024	1,125,899,906,842,620	1.126E+15	–	–	PiB	pebibyte
6	1000	1,000,000,000,000,000,000	1.000E+18	EB	exabyte	1024	1,152,921,504,606,850,000	1.153E+18	–	–	EiB	exbibyte
7	1000	1,000,000,000,000,000,000,000	1.000E+21	ZB	zettabyte	1024	1,180,591,620,717,410,000,000	1.181E+21	–	–	ZiB	zebibyte
8	1000	1,000,000,000,000,000,000,000,000	1.000E+24	YB	yottabyte	1024	1,208,925,819,614,630,000,000,000	1.209E+24	–	–	YiB	yobibyte

*JEDEC, Joint Electron Device Engineering Council is an independent semiconductor engineering trade organization and standardization body.

*IEC, International Electrotechnical Commission is an international standards organization that prepares and publishes international standards for all "electrotechnology."

use of symbols, abbreviations, terms, and definitions throughout the semiconductor industry (JEDEC, 2002). Table 6.1 illustrates the dramatic difference in maximum-size increase in bytes at each stepwise order of magnitude increase, due to the difference in the radix (base) size being acted on by the order (exponent) of magnitude. The standard radix for binary data is 1024.

Hardware Considerations

Hardware includes many devices in the health care industry, including system peripherals and aspects of the computer that make up the physical components of the system. Figure 6.1 reflects a visual of a typical hardware setup for a personal computing (PC) system. Within the computer, in the actual case, are important elements, including the motherboard, central processing unit (CPU), random access memory (RAM), power supply, video card, hard disk drive (HDD), solid-state drive (SSD), optical drive (e.g., BD [Blu-ray disc]/DVD/CD drive) and the card reader (SD/SDHC, CF, etc.). Table 6.2 defines each of these elements and describes its basic function. When we purchase any PC for use in health care, we have to pay special attention to the components of the system, particularly with respect to the processing speed, storage size, and the type of graphic interfaces you would need based on the requirement of the system. We also have to consider aspects of how and when that piece of equipment will be used with respect to patient care.

Hardware Selection and Specifications

Decision making regarding the right hardware for implementation involves the interprofessional team and should include management, users, and systems analysts in the information technology (IT) sector. The vendors will provide information on their specific hardware components, but the systems analyst within the IT department frequently recommends hardware options for the team to consider and provides information based

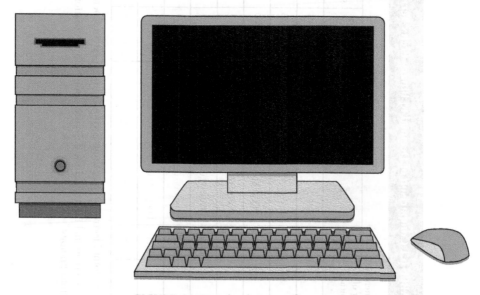

FIGURE 6.1. Basic hardware configurations.

TABLE 6.2 Internal Components of the Computer

Component	Definition	Function
Motherboard	The mother board is the backbone of the computer	Connects all of the parts of the computer together
CPU	Often thought of as "the brains" of the computer	Responsible for interpreting and executing most of the commands from the computer's hardware and software
RAM	The working memory of the computer	Allows a computer to work with more information at the same time in active memory processing
Power supply	A converter that supplies the power to the machine	Used to convert the power provided from the outlet into usable power for the many parts inside the computer case
Video card	Graphics adapter or expansion card	Allows the computer to send graphical information to a video display device such as a monitor, TV, or projector
HDD	Data storage device and an electromechanical magnetic disk drive	The hard disk drive is the main, and usually largest, data storage hardware device in a computer where the operating system, software and most files are stored
SSD	Data storage device; no moving (mechanical) components	Storage device that is typically more resistant to physical shock, runs silently, has lower access time, and less latency, but more expensive than hard disk drive
Optical drive (e.g., BD/DVD/CD drive)	Optical storage devices	Optical drives retrieve and/or store data on optical discs like CDs, DVDs, and BDs

BD, Blu-ray disc; CPU, central processing unit; HDD, hard drive; RAM, random access memory; SSD, solid-state drive.

on which the team can make an informed purchasing decision. Depending on the varied options, hardware will typically have disadvantages and advantages, which should be considered prior to purchase. The workload for the system, purpose of the hardware, and end-user interface needs are criteria to be considered and, most important in the clinical setting, the answer to the question "how and where will that hardware be used with respect to patient care?" is very crucial. The end-user and workflow considerations

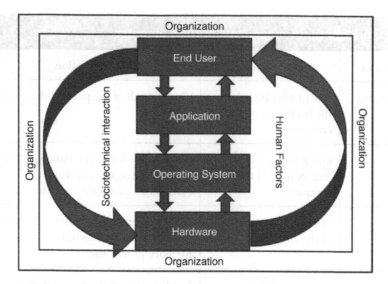

FIGURE 6.2. Sociotechnical interaction: hardware, software, and human factors.

for the hardware components are critical considerations as well. We cover workflow redesign in Chapter 9. Figure 6.2 is a schematic that reflects the interaction points for the sociotechnical interaction of the end user, application layer, operating system, and the hardware. In this chapter, we focus on some of the issues and considerations that are relevant to health care with respect to these interaction points. Human computer interaction (HCI) is considered a subcategory within the larger field of human factors science.

Human Factors and System Ergonomics

Human factors is defined as "the field of study focused on understanding human elements of systems, in which 'systems' may be defined as software, medical devices, computer technology, and organizations" (McCormick & Gugerty, 2013). Figure 6.2 reflects these interaction points of the end user (human) and the software and hardware within the health care organization. *Ergonomics* is defined by Wilson (2013) using a systematic approach, which the authors believe is particularly relevant to health care and HCI. Wilson defines ergonomics in terms of human factors as follows: "Ergonomics/human factors is, above anything else, a systems discipline and profession, applying a systems philosophy and systems approach" (Wilson, 2013, p. 5). Other aspects that also apply to the field of human factors include the field of cognitive science and how the end user interfaces and interacts with the software, equipment, and the graphic user interface (GUI). In addition, the field of ergonomics and human factors science involves a workflow within the system, which is covered in Chapter 9.

Hardware and Infection-Control Issues

One crucial factor that is unique to health care relates to infection control and the possible transmission of microbes via the hardware within the clinical setting. This specific concern is an excellent example of how HCI, human factors, and the environment impact patient safety and quality. As the number of devices increase, the possibility for infection to be transmitted through direct patient contact and use of the hardware for patient care compounds. Neel and Sittig (2002) reviewed the literature to determine possible links to nosocomial infections transmitted through colonization of microbes on hardware acting as a vector for the infections. These findings indicate how health care professionals can be cognizant of the mode of transmission to design interventions to potentially prevent infection when viewing the computer hardware as a potential vector for infection. The review of the literature indicates that there is significant opportunity for some serious transmission of infection, and of particular concern are the findings relating to methicillin-resistant *Staphylococcus aureus* (MRSA). MRSA was directly correlated to the keyboard MRSA colonization and MRSA infection in at least two intensive care unit (ICU) patients using pulse-field gel electrophoresis to determine that the isolates were of the same genus and species. Neel and Sittig indicate that there are steps that can be taken to prevent the transmission of infection by keeping in mind the route of transmission. They recommend knowing the risk factors that predispose a patient to serious infection, following strict hand-washing protocols, using gloves as appropriate, and working with infection control professionals to develop and adhere to policies for cleaning and decontamination of all hardware. Finally, these two researchers advise us to think in terms of the interaction among the patient, hardware, and clinician, and how that piece of equipment is used within the workflow to identify instances that might transmit infection given the sociotechnical interaction reflected in Figure 6.2 and the chain of infection depicted in Figure 6.3.

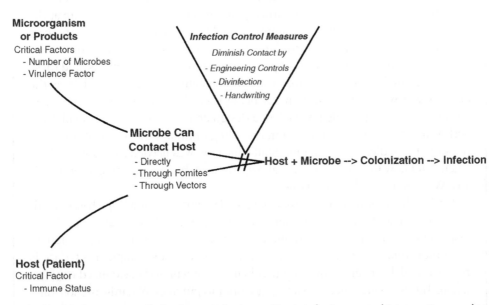

FIGURE 6.3. Steps potentially leading to infection and basic infection-control interventions used to decrease the risk of infection.

Source: Neel and Sittig (2002).

CASE STUDY LESSONS LEARNED: CASE STUDY OF ERGONOMIC–HUMAN FACTORS IN BARCODE SCANNING

Recently, a health care system evaluated its knowledge-based medication administration process, which utilized barcode scanning. The process was implemented with the goal of providing support for a higher standard of nursing care, with inherently fewer medication errors. Incorporation of computer-assisted ACDS in real time and at the point-of-care delivery required barcode scanning of the patient's armband and each individual unit-dose medication that was labeled with a barcode.

During the process of performing the actual nursing care tasks of medication administration to multiple patients on a medical–surgical hospital floor, several distinct human factor and ergonomic problems were identified. The type of computer hardware "Workstations on Wheels" (WOWs), or "Computers on Wheels" (COWs) exhibited limited mobility when pushed on carpets, because of the selection of smaller wheels on the cart that the workstation was mounted on. Network issues of crowding around Wi-Fi hotspots resulted in significant reduction of access speeds. With no external and extra batteries that could be charged separately, batteries of WOWs required frequent recharging; they were anchored to stationary charging locations, essentially removing them from service until charged. Lack of standardized maintenance and internal cleaning of cooling fan and airflow vents led to overheated/broken computers and WOWs. Log-in configurations added many time-consuming layers with excessive logon–logoff interruptions required to navigate among multiple secure systems and data silos during the process of assembling and transporting the medications that had to be administered from the satellite pharmacy storage bins to the point of care at the patient bedside, where barcode scanning would be carried out during the process of administering routine meds to the patient. It was discovered that some computer workstations were capable of performing at much higher speeds, and these became favored workstations that were in constant crowded use, whereas the other slower workstations were never being used. Reporting of slow or broken hardware was compounded by lack of a designated technical support field agent with primary job responsibility of maintaining optimal function of all workstations on the medical–surgical unit. Staff education was needed to establish when, where, and how to report suboptimal performance, broken equipment, or unreliable Wi-Fi or network access issues.

During the implementation phase of barcode scanning knowledge-based medication administration, it became apparent that having a global strategy for device installation configuration is extremely important for successful implementation. Each individual point-of-care location where any human–computer interface is required to deliver care, requires individual assessment and customized configuration. The assessment needs to take place prior to purchase of hardware, software,

(continued)

CASE STUDY LESSONS LEARNED: CASE STUDY OF ERGONOMIC-HUMAN FACTORS IN BARCODE SCANNING (*continued*)

and peripherals (scanners, sensors, etc.), and must necessarily include testing of all reasonably anticipated human–computer end-user workflows and tasks that are expected to be performed in the context of actual point of care. Identification, classification, and categorization of different tasks and workflows associated with different user groups and service lines were critical factors for success and were found to be best determined largely by the workflow and task being performed in the context of the actual point-of-care delivery. Anticipation of utilization barriers and consideration of time of day as a barrier resulting from peak network bandwidth congestion was also an important success strategy. Careful observation of unit layout and workflow that incorporated frontline staff and rehearsal of dry-run scenarios based on proposed ACDS workflows were of key importance.

Time, motion, and efficiency videography studies of the entire stepwise ACDS process involving frontline staff acting as patients and caregivers were performed over several weeks. Analyses of the videographic journals in time-lapse compression, transforming hours of observations into a few intense minutes revealed numerous barriers, bottlenecks, and inefficiencies present in the actual ACDS process. Issues identified were hardware placement given the physical layout of the actual point-of-care delivery room. The computer workstation and the barcodes being scanned were placed in physically separate locations that were convenient for the cabling and the barcode, but awkward and inconvenient for the end user nurse. The nurse was required to negotiate barriers in order to deliver care in the room. Workstation behavior required nurse–console interactions with keyboard and mouse at almost every step in the ACDS barcode scanning workflow procedure. The resulting human–computer interface behavior required the nurse to physically walk back and forth along the three sides of the room. The patient's bed and armband with the barcode to be scanned was located on one side of the room, the console with keyboard and mouse was located on the opposite side of the room, and the unit-dosed barcoded medications were located on a third side of the room on the only available shelf workspace at the foot of the patient bed. The walk-around distance among the three sides of the room, plus having to walk back and forth between the computer console and the barcode on the packaged medications arrayed side by side (they were checked off of a hand-written pick list with the hand-held laser scanner), added significant time to the administration of all patient medications on the unit. The significant time added during time-and-motion efficiency recordings did not include interruptions to the process from overhead pages, telephone calls, family members, or requests for immediate attention and help from fellow staff or physician demands. The time-compression analyses performed were therefore conservative underestimations of normal variations in the actual workflow.

(*continued*)

CASE STUDY LESSONS LEARNED: CASE STUDY OF ERGONOMIC-HUMAN FACTORS IN BARCODE SCANNING (*continued*)

Questions to consider:

1. What hardware and peripherals might have served the organization better than WOWs, wall-mounted units, kiosks, or desk workstations?
   a. Secure wireless-enabled personal electronic devices (iPad, Nook, Surface, etc.) with optical, near-field, Q-code or barcode scanning capabilities
   b. Secure voice-recognition "speech to text" interface and wearable augmented reality interface (i.e., "Google Glass," Virtual Reality 3 sight–sound–touch input/output) wearables; smart-vests, and smart-shells

2. How might they have configured the hardware differently?
   a. Incorporating frontline staff and end-user feedback to guide device selection
   b. Identifying end-user group service line-specific tasks and their unique work-flow dynamic requirements

3. What are the implications to patient safety and quality?

There are many important objective lessons to be learned from this case study, including hardware placement, human factors considerations, and implications for ACDS. Points to consider related to the case are as follows:

▶ Successful implementation of ACDS is associated with dramatic reduction in adverse events due to accidental human factor errors.

▶ Poor implementation of ACDS is associated with an increase in accidental adverse events because of staff frustration and resorting to "work-around," "cutting corners," and abandonment of automation all together, just to deliver actual care.

▶ Poor implementation of ACDS is a financially unsustainable and risky business model. Damages and punitive damages awarded in settlements related to actual or perceived accidental injuries attributable to ACDS implementation require mitigation of risk strategies to avoid loss. Accelerated turnover of frustrated, highly mobile nursing and physician staff to competitor health care provider organizations is also a low-quality outcome of poor ACDS implementation.

▶ The quality of ACDS implementation is a direct reflection of workplace environment health, and this in turn synergistically affects patient safety culture as well as the overall quality of care ultimately provided.

The issues reflected in this short case relate largely to the ergonomic issues involved with comfort, ease of use, and practical functionality when it comes to the effects of hardware, software, and peripherals on workplace health. Detrimental workplace ergonomic designs characteristically exhibit an absence of the comfortable and healthy attributes of the high-quality ergonomic designs that take human factors into account. The assessment of ergonomic quality surrounding the human–computer interface is therefore a core clinical health care informatics skill, and especially so in the modern clinical workplace environment that relies on the computer-enabled clinical informatics world of ACDS.

Hardware Specifications

Performance of the system and configuration of hardware are also important points for consideration, including factors such as time required per transaction as well as data input and output by the end user; how the hardware should be configured given its purpose is yet another point for consideration. The volume of information that will be managed, how much data can be processed before the system has reached maximum capacity, and its use in the current state with anticipation of future growth should be taken into consideration. These types of decision points are discussed in more depth in Chapter 8 with respect to hardware (Kendall & Kendall, 2014).

The considerations noted here take into account hardware specifications—specifications that typically include parameters such as processing speeds, memory requirements (RAM and HDD requirements), necessary interface equipment, operating system requirements for running the clinical software. Table 6.3 presents a sample of what a technical specification for a clinical information system setup might look like for a clinical environment application server.

Software Considerations

Software is a vast topic that has many options available, and the number of available options depends on the category. Those considerations may also take into account proprietary software or open source options in the form of free ware. In this section we discuss the different types of software and considerations for selecting the right type of software.

TABLE 6.3 Sample Recommended Specifications for a Clinical Information Server

Processor	2 × Six Core Xeon E5-2620 or higher
Memory	8 GB RAM
Network interface card	1 Gbit
Primary hard drive(s)	2 × 300 GB SAS in RAID 1
Repository hard drives	6 × 300 GB SAS or more in RAID 5
Operating system	Microsoft Windows 2008 R2 (64-bit) Standard Edition SP1
Database software	Microsoft SQL 2008

SQL, structured query language.

Source: Philips (2014).

Programming Language Classifications

Programming is a mechanism for transforming information into a computer in the form of machine code, which instructs the computer to do some type of task. Programming language can be classified into different levels. A program that resides in the memory of a computer executes codes or commands to complete a function or task, telling the computer how to perform some operation relevant to the program's function. Machine code is the primary language for the computer and consists of binary 0s, and 1s, and it is considered "first-generation" machine language; it is also referred to as "low language." The second-generation level (2GL) is a step higher and constitutes assembly languages that use reserved words and symbols that have special and unique meaning. It is considered a low-level language similar to machine language, but uses symbolic operation code to represent the machine operation code. The assembly code is specific to the machines, including the computer and CPU (Janssen, 2014c). Third-generation languages (3GL) were intended to be easier to use, and higher level languages provided a programmer-friendly language. Some examples of this type of code include FORTRAN, BASIC, Pascal, and the C-family (C, C+, and C++; Janssen, 2014d). Fourth-generation programming languages (4GL) are more in line with the "human language" and therefore easier to work with than 3GL. 4GL are considered domain-specific and high-productivity languages and include aspects such as database queries and report generators, as well as GUI creators, database programming, and scripts. Many of the 4GL are data oriented and use structured query language (SQL) developed by IBM and also adopted by the American National Standards Institute (ANSI; see Chapter 7 on data standards; Janssen, 2014b). Fifth-generation languages (5GL) utilize visual tools to support programming. One such frequently used language is Visual Basic. Further, some consider 5GL to be types of constraint logic or problem-solving-based programming. PROLOG is a programming language that fits into this description (Janssen, 2014a).

Types of Software

Software can be categorized as (a) system software that is used to start and run the computer, (b) application software that generally has a purpose or function specific to its use (e.g., accounting/financial applications), or (c) programming tools that are used to compile programs and link or translate computer program source code and libraries that belong to either the system software or the application. Figure 6.2 demonstrates how the software relates to the end user and to the various types of software. Table 6.4 features the types of system software used across industries. Systems software is related to what the software does within the computer system to support the use of the computer. For example, the device-driver software operates and manages all devices attached to the computer. Table 6.5 lists the application software typically categorized by intended use, such as business software that is used for managing admissions, discharge, and transactions for patients in hospitals and health care systems. This is not an exhaustive list but instead gives the reader an idea of how software fits within the categories for either systems or applications. Review the table and see whether you can think of other software that might fit into some of these categories, given the definitions and descriptions.

TABLE 6.4 Types of Internal Components of Computer Software	
Type	**Description**
Operating system	The software that is responsible for the direct control and management of the hardware and running application software
Open source software	Free source code access licensed for use by an open community of developers and end users; proprietary software is owned and distributed for commercial use
Boot loader or bootstrap	The small program that loads and executes the command to "boot up" the computer; the program is stored in the RAM
Device drivers	A program that operates the various devices on the computer, such as printers and peripherals; the driver provides software interface to the hardware device
Firm ware	Controls the devices typically seen in items such as mobile phones and digital cameras
GUI	A graphics display with user-friendly point-and-click capability that allows the end user to interact with the computer through the mouse and touch pad
Middle ware	Software that resides as an interface between the operating system and the applications that allows developers to control input/output devices, also referred to as "software glue"
Utility software	Software that helps analyze, configure, optimize, or maintain the computer

GUI, graphical user interface; RAM, random access memory.

Software Selection of an EHR

EHR is perhaps the most important criterion for software selection in the current setup of health care organizations, particularly given the emphasis in the United States on creating a national health information network across the country with full interoperability between care settings. The selection of EHR software emphasizes the importance of strategic decisions that align with the organizations' overall improvement and business plans.

The basis on which EHRs are selected for a hospital or provider is very specific to that organization, and as such should be both a cost and quality decision based on the needs of the organization and the end users within the organization. Involving the end user in the selection of EHR software is critical to the success of adoption, implementation, and effective "meaningful" use of the EHR software. An entire chapter is dedicated to this topic; however, we note a few important considerations on EHRs here. Hartley

TABLE 6.5 Types of Application Software	
Type	**Description**
Business software	Used by and for specific business functions in health care; e.g., this would be admission, discharge, and transactions software components frequently imbedded in the EHR as a module component seamlessly interfaced in the background so that data is passively collected as fast as it is entered or becomes available
Communications or messaging software	Used to exchange files and messages between systems remotely; health care systems require encryption of data to meet HIPAA regulatory requirements when using communications or messaging-type software
Data-management software	Source software with the primary function of managing a database in a particular structure, usually relational or object oriented
Graphics software	A type of software that allows the end user to manipulate graphic images on the computer; usually has the capability to import and export graphics file formats
Simulation software	Software that allows the end user to model real phenomenon with a set of mathematical formulas used in health care professional training to simulate events rather than have students practice on patients
Gaming or video software	Software that uses interaction with a user interface to generate visual feedback on a video device
Spreadsheet software	Software that allows data to be analyzed in a tabular format with data organized in rows and columns that can be manipulated by formulas
Word processors	Software that performs processing of text (words) to compose, edit, format, or print written material
Workflow software	Software used to reflect a process or steps within a process that provides functionality to create workflows with a diagram-based graphical designer approach
Presentation software	Software used to create slide presentations that allow typesetting and graphical design to create a professional looking presentation quickly

EHR, electronic health record; HIPAA, Health Information Portability and Accountability Act.

and Jones (2005) outline 12 essential steps that should be completed prior to the purchase of an EHR. These steps are as follows:

Step 1: Establish the budget

Step 2: Establish the right team

Step 3: Engage the team, but be clear on the decision-making lead

Step 4: Prioritize requirements

Step 5: Assign fact-finding duties and responsibilities to the team members

Step 6: Develop the request for proposal (RFP)

Step 7: Develop a scorecard to rate the products

Step 8: Schedule on-site demonstrations

Step 9: Determine return on investment (ROI)

Step 10: Negotiate the contract

Step 11: Agree on the purchase plan

Step 12: Ask for help if needed (Hartley & Jones 2005)

The Office of the National Coordinator (ONC) provides excellent resources to providers, including various tools used to help make software selection easier for organizations with minimal resources. These tools highlight the steps, noted by Hartley and Jones (2005), that providers should follow when selecting and purchasing an EHR. These elements include the following:

1. Contracting templates
2. Demonstration of the software and scenario-based evaluation of the product, complete with scenarios for hospitals, clinics, and federally qualified health care clinics
3. Reference checks on the software with other providers with instructions on how and what to ask
4. RFP templates
5. Evaluation tools based on measureable criteria important to the organization (score card templates)
6. Meaningful use comparisons between product tools
7. Pricing and ROI calculators (Hartley & Jones 2005)

HealthIT.gov (2014) provides tools on its website to guide a provider through the process of EHR selection and considerations. In addition, elements, such as the RFP, are discussed in full in Chapter 8.

When selecting software for any purpose, attention should be paid to important criteria such as price, function, and end-user requirements; it is also crucial to include a very structured methodical approach to decision making by involving the entire team in the decision-making process. The ONC, through tools developed primarily by the Regional Extension Centers (RECs), provides organizations with many of these types of tools to help follow this structured approach. The following case study demonstrates how these steps and tools were put to use by a rural health clinic.

CASE STUDY: EFFECTIVE SELECTION AND DEPLOYMENT OF AN EHR IN A RURAL LOCAL PUBLIC HEALTH DEPARTMENT

Contributed by Deb McCullough, DNP, RN, FNP
Andrews County Health Department

Issues: A small rural local health department (LHD) implemented an EHR using a step-by-step implementation guide (Hartley & Jones, 2005). The project incorporated national standards and requirements to meet Stage 1 Meaningful Use criteria under the HITECH Act (2009).

Description: The LHD formed a seven-member interprofessional team with defined roles and responsibilities to prepare for EHR implementation. The team collaborated with the West Texas HIT Regional Extension Center; attended a regional conference on EHR meaningful use, clinical decision making (CDS), quality, and safety; reviewed the LHD's services, payor and funding sources, current charting and billing systems, perceived benefits of EHR implementation; and developed the vision, goals, and criteria for the project's success. After EHR vendor training, the LHD went live in September 2011 employing a big-bang approach.

Step-by-Step Implementation Process: The LHD followed a step-by-step guide for medical practice EHR implementation. Step 1 consisted of learning the basics of EHRs with support of the REC. During Step 2, the staff conducted workflow analyses, compared paper administrative and patient care workflows to EHR workflows, participated in vendor demonstrations, and identified EHR champions. Additional considerations were rural connectivity issues and whether to host the server on site or in an Internet cloud-based service offered by EHR vendors. Rural providers have specific issues related to Internet connectivity that must be taken into account. During Step 3, the LHD determined the appropriate EHR based on the budget and workflow needs and connectivity requirements and purchased the EHR. The LHD selected eClinicalWorks as its vendor because of the vaccine inventory-and-management component and the ability to meet the LHD's clinical needs; they elected to host it on site due to connectivity constraints within the rural community. The fourth step addressed the EHR implementation phase: changing from paper medical records to an EHR.

Pre- and Post-Implementation Workflow Analyses and Redesign: The staff reviewed multiple processes and conducted workflow analyses and redesign. In July 2011, stakeholders from the LHD and Texas Department of State Health Services (DSHS) met to review Texas Health Steps (THS) Medicaid forms and documentation requirements. Prior to the EHR, the LHD staff completed 20 forms during an initial THS visit. The LHD seized the opportunity to redesign and streamline THS documentation to avoid transitioning a dysfunctional paper process to an electronic format. After EHR implementation, the staff struggled with the cumbersome and difficult-to-navigate THS documentation structure within the EHR. To improve the workflow

(continued)

CASE STUDY: EFFECTIVE SELECTION AND DEPLOYMENT OF AN EHR IN A RURAL LOCAL PUBLIC HEALTH DEPARTMENT (*continued*)

processes, decrease staff frustration, increase consistency, and meet the documentation requirements, the LHD director/system administrator built the streamlined DSHS forms into the EHR. The forms included the history of children younger than 5 years, history of children of all ages, interval history, tuberculosis questionnaire, physical exam, and health education/anticipatory guidance. The director added age-specific immunization and THS order sets and clinical decision support alerts.

Lessons Learned: A proactive multidisciplinary team approach is essential for implementing an EHR in a small LHD. A hosted EHR has advantages for a small LHD. Collaboration and consultation with a regional REC, local public health, and state funding sources are essential to provide expertise and implement a meaningful EHR applicable to the setting. The EHR can impact prevention and wellness across the life span by providing accessible preventive health services documentation and CDS; paper charting was reduced by 98%.

Recommendations: Successful EHR implementation and use includes strong leadership and visions, policies on key issues, goal setting, planning, and communication. Critical factors, particularly when rural facilities are resource constrained, involve utilizing the support of the REC to provide a step-by-step process, selecting a vendor by matching the capabilities of the EHR to the staffs' requirements, as well as perceived benefits. Also critical was redesigning workflow with an improvement focus and ensuring flexibility and capacity for creating documentation components within the EHR.

Consider the following questions:

▶ Which tools do you believe the clinic used to help with this process?
▶ How do you see that the REC might have helped with this process, given what you read in earlier chapters and the current chapter on software selection considerations?
▶ What hardware considerations do you think this organization considered?
▶ Why would cost be a critical issue for this organization, and what other considerations might they have given their public health purpose?
▶ How do you think rural providers and clinics present unique challenges when implementing EHRs?

Networking, Connectivity, and Configuration of Hardware

Networking and connectivity of systems in health care comprises diverse areas ranging from radiology medical imaging departments to specialty care units, business administration, and information services. Networking expanded in the 1990s, as the cost of data storage (hardware) and communications technologies became available at lower costs. Health care is also diverse in terms of size and scope of the organizations and communities served from small rural facilities to major networks of health care systems distributed across the United States and in some cases internationally. As such, we have a vast array of requirements within the industry to address connecting, networking, and configuring the connectivity of technology to support the health care industry. Additionally, there are emerging trends in cloud computer and mobile technology that create expanded capacity; yet, we also need to incorporate older architecture as we move into the future. In the following section, we cover older technologies as well as some of the newer configurations for connectivity and remote access.

Networking and Communications

Typical networking relates to connections between and among two or more computers. Local area networks (LANs) involve computers and printers connected by wire or radio frequency, whereas a WAN is a network that uses high-speed, long-distance communication networks or satellites to connect computers over greater distances than LANs. Ethernet connections are a means of communicating using an architecture that relies on a detection and avoidance protocol for routing data that permits larger networks and faster data transmission. The *Internet* is defined as "the single worldwide computer network that interconnects other computer networks, on which end-user services, such as World Wide Websites or data archives, are located, enabling data and other information to be exchanged" (William, 2012). The Internet was originally created in 1969 during the Cold War and used by the department of defense. Today, the Internet is used worldwide by networks of computers now maintained primarily by service providers. Some important Internet terms are listed here:

- ► FTP is an abbreviation for "file transfer protocol," and is a common means for transferring files within the Internet from one computer to the other.

- ► TCP/IP is an acronym for transmission control protocol/Internet protocol. TCP and IP are two protocols developed by the U.S. military for the purpose of allowing computers to communicate over long-distance networks. TCP is a verification mechanism for the packets of data, whereas IP relates to the actual data packets between the given nodes of the Internet.

- ► HTML, or hyper-text markup language, is the programming language that most webpages are based on that control display of information via the web browser.

- ► HTTP is an acronym for hyper-text transfer protocol and is the means by which data is transferred via the web.

- ► HTTPS indicates that the website uses a secure socket layer (SSL) for security purposes. This is an important consideration for the protection of health care information, or other information such as your personal banking or credit card information. You can determine whether a website is secure by viewing the URL (uniform resource locator) in the address field of your web browser. If the web address starts with "https://" you can be assured that the website has been secured using SSL (TechTerms.com, 2014).

Network typologies have several different types of physical layout or "typology." These configurations include tree network, star network, ring network, and bus network (Figure 6.4). Network typologies have pros and cons depending on the configuration. Bus configurations are dependent on the total length of the network and the distance

Star Network Typology

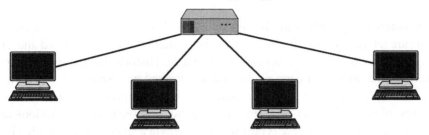

Bus Network Typology

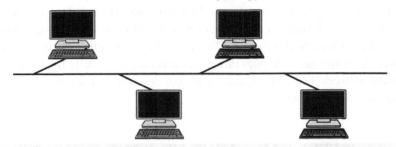

Tree Network Typology

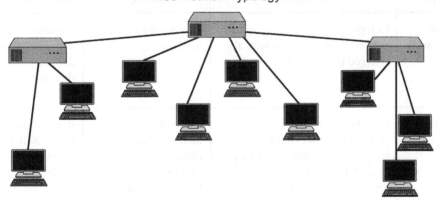

Ring Network Typology

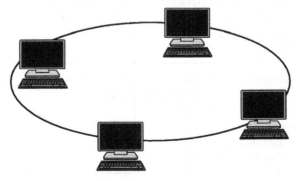

FIGURE 6.4. Network typologies.

the computers are spaced within the network. Total distance, number of computers, and spacing are relevant to the efficiency with a bus configuration. It is confined and cannot be expanded as fully as the other options available. Historically, this was the type of network used mainly on a copper wire and was limited by distance or size of the network, or length of the cable between computers, which impacts timing and efficiency. This type of network is an inexpensive setup but obviously has limitations and is seldom used. Star networks are typically connected via a switch or hub, with a limited number of computers on the network. With the tree, one builds off the switch and connect a switch to switch, and this configuration works using the Internet. Expansion is available with the tree network typology. Ring networks are set up in a circular configuration with the signals transmitting around the ring until the envelope containing the data, or package of information, finds the designated address. This configuration is set up in a circular fashion and it can be difficult to add a computer; when one computer goes down, the entire network goes down, but it is easy to identify the location of the failure in the network. (Zanbergen, n.d.) Table 6.6 describes these topologies and their advantages and disadvantages.

TABLE 6.6 Network Typologies Advantages and Disadvantages			
Type	**Description**	**Advantages**	**Disadvantages**
Star network	Computers or other devices are connected to a central hub, also referred to as a switch	Easy to install and manage	Bottlenecks can occur because data passes through the hub
Ring network	Computers or other devices are connected to one another in the shape of a circular closed loop such that devices connect directly to two other units (one on either side)	Offers high bandwidth and span distances, relatively easy to install, easy to locate points of failure	If one computer goes down, the entire network is down
Bus network	Computers or other devices are connected to a central cable referred to as a bus or backbone	Inexpensive and easy to install	Not as stable as other configurations
Tree network	A tree typology combines characteristics of linear bus and star topologies consisting of groups of star-configured workstations connected to a linear bus backbone cable	Improves network scalability	Expensive to configure and maintain

Source: Mitchell (2014).

Communication Protocols

Communication protocols include TCP/IP, FTP, and simple mail transfer protocol. An FTP is a standard network protocol used to transfer computer files over a network, such as the Internet, and was defined earlier in the Network and Communications section. This communication protocol has become the industry standard for interconnecting computer hosts, networks, and the Internet. One of the most widespread communication protocols today is the use of wireless Internet. Protocols, such as Bluetooth, IEEE802.11, and wireless application protocols, are expanding the growth along with the availability of mobile devices such as our cell phones. Mobile computing is expanding in the health care industry and thus is a very important computing protocol for consideration, which is discussed in more detail in Chapter 16.

Cloud Computing

Cloud computing is also referred to as "software as a service," and although we could have classified this under the software subheading, we elected to place the discussion in the hardware section, as cloud computing is often selected because organizations do not want to host their own servers, invest in the infrastructure (hardware), and deal with the security requirements that are becoming very significant (see Chapter 14 for further details). Cloud computing is a solution hosted typically by a company providing its software on a server that can be accessed from the Internet; it is considered a new way of accessing services but not necessarily a new technology (Kuo, 2011). The service model of cloud computing and software as a service is noted as one of the top emerging trends in the Gartner 2014 report *The Top 10 Strategic Technology Trends for 2014* (Cearley, 2013/2014).

Client Server Architecture

A client server setup involves different configuration considerations as well, including whether the client is a thin client with no software loaded to the desktop versus a thick client with software and perhaps some processing applications on the desktop. "Thin" indicates there is very little computing power on the desktop, whereas "thick" indicates software and computing power to drive the software are loaded on the desktop. Many software applications that we purchase in health care have configurations similar to this. Many of our EHRs run on thin client configurations, whereas many of our analytic tools have processing and software running off of the desktop, but we access data off of a server hosted by the organization in a data warehouse setup.

Key Terms in HIT

This section discusses key terms relevant to today's HIT revolution under the HITECH Act, including terms defined in Table 6.7. Common terms frequently used in the health care setting are often confused by the average clinician. There are differences in definitions of an EHR versus and EMR that are often mistaken. According to the ONC, the EMR is defined as an electronic record of health-related information on an individual that can be created, gathered, managed, and consulted by authorized clinicians and staff *within one health care organization*. However, an EHR is defined as an electronic record of health-related information on an individual that conforms to nationally recognized interoperability standards and that can be created, managed, and consulted by

TABLE 6.7 Definitions of Key HIT Terms		
EMR	EHR	PHR
An electronic record of health-related information on an individual that can be created, gathered, managed, and consulted by authorized clinicians and staff within one health care organization	An electronic record of health-related information on an individual that conforms to nationally recognized interoperability standards and that can be created, managed, and consulted by authorized clinicians and staff across more than one health care organization	An electronic record of health-related information on an individual that conforms to nationally recognized interoperability standards and that can be drawn from multiple sources while being managed, shared, and controlled by the individual

Reproduced from the National Alliance for Health Information Technology (2008).

authorized clinicians and staff *across more than one health care organization*. A third type of record important to and controlled by the health care consumer is the personal health record (PHR). The PHR is defined as an electronic record of health-related information on an individual that conforms to nationally recognized interoperability standards and that can be drawn from multiple sources while being managed, shared, and controlled *by the individual*.

SUMMARY

We have discussed background information, including the history of computers in health care and the important role that computers have and will play in the future. Health care informatics is an evolving science that involves the overlap between computer science and use of clinical information to inform patient care, quality, patient safety, and population health. In addition, we have discussed hardware and software configuration considerations, examined a case study relating to ergonomics and human factors that impact patient care when not addressed strategically, and related additional information concerning software selection in rural settings. We have also discussed programming languages, types of software, EHR selection, as well as the importance of understanding hardware, software, networking, and the specifications of technical requirements that impact the EHR selection decision.

EXERCISES AND QUESTIONS FOR CONSIDERATION

Evaluate the physical environment of IT in a hospital or clinic setting. Consider the HCI as you observe clinicians using the EHR in the clinical setting. Your assessment should include the following tasks:

1. Identify the location of the EHR on the unit and observe clinicians using the system.

2. Obtain input from the nursing staff who use the technology in the chosen setting.

3. Assess the site for the following:

   - The layout of the nursing unit

   - Location of technology in relation to patient care areas

   - The type of equipment available

   - The structure, size, and function of existing furniture, flooring, equipment, and so forth

   - Nursing staff input on functionality and challenges

4. Analyze the impact of the existing ergonomic design on nursing work, patient safety, and quality of care.

5. Describe the challenges in ergonomic design.

6. Develop a plan to solve identified challenges.

7. Create an electronic visual representation of the layout of the area and document issues noted and a plan of action.

REFERENCES

Buchholz, W., & Bemer, R. W. (1962). Natural data units. In W. Buchholz (Ed.), *Planning a computer system: Project stretch* (1st ed., pp. 33–40). New York, NY: McGraw-Hill.

Cearley, D. W. (2014). Gartner report: The top 10 strategic technology trends for 2014. *Forbes.* Retrieved from http://www.scribd.com/doc/220080178/Gartner-The-Top-10-Strategic-Technology-Trends-for-2014 (Original work published 2013)

Dickey, J. P. (1984). Custom CMOS architecture for a handheld computer. *Hewlett-Packard Journal: Technical Information from the Laboratories of the Hewlett-Packard Company, 35*(7), 14–17.

Hartley, C. P., & Jones, E. D. (2005). *EHR implementation: A step by step guide for the medical practice.* Chicago, IL: AMA Press.

HealthIT.gov. (2014). *How to implement EHRs: Step 3—Select or upgrade to a certified EHR.* Retrieved from http://www.healthit.gov/providers-professionals/ehr-implementation-steps/step-3-select-or-upgrade-certified-ehr#resource_table

International Electrotechnical Commision (IEC). (2014). *International standards (IS).* Retrieved from http://www.iec.ch/standardsdev/publications/is.htm

Janssen, C. (2014a). *Fifth generation (programming) language—5GL.* Retrieved from http://www.techopedia.com/definition/24309/fifth-generation-programming-language-5gl

Janssen, C. (2014b). *Fourth generation (programming) language—4GL.* Retrieved from http://www.techopedia.com/definition/24308/fourth-generation-programming-language-4gl

Janssen, C. (2014c). *Second generation (programming) language (2GL).* Retrieved from http://www.techopedia.com/definition/24305/second-generation-programming-language-2gl

Janssen, C. (2014d). *Third generation (programming) language—3GL.* Retrieved from http://www.techopedia.com/definition/24307/third-generation-programming-language-3gl

JEDEC. (2002). *Terms, definitions, and letter symbols for microcomputers, microprocessors, and memory integrated circuits.* (No. JESD100B.01). Arlington, VA: JEDEC Solid State Technology Association.

Kendall, K., & Kendall, J. (2014). Project management. *Systems analysis and design* (9th ed., p. 57). Boston, MA: Pearson.

Kleinbeck, S. V. M. (1999). Development of the perioperative nursing data set. *AORN Journal, 70*(1), 15–28. doi:http://dx.doi.org.ezproxy.ttuhsc.edu/10.1016/S0001-2092(06)61851-6

Kuo, A. M. (2011). Opportunities and challenges of cloud computing to improve health care services. *Journal of Medical Internet Research, 13*(3), e67. doi:10.2196/jmir.1867

Leonhardt, D. (2000, July 28). John Tukey, 85, statistician; coined the word "software." *New York Times.* Retrieved from http://www.nytimes.com/2000/07/28/us/john-tukey-85-statistician-coined-the-word-software.html

McCormick, K. M., & Gugerty, B. (2013). Human factors in healthcare IT. In *Healthcare information technology exam guide* (p. 368). New York, NY: McGraw-Hill.

Mitchell, B. (2014). *Computer network topologies.* Retrieved from http://compnetworking.about.com/od/networkdesign/ig/Computer-Network-Topologies/

Moore, G. E. (n.d). *Moore's law.* Retrieved from http://www.mooreslaw.org/

The National Alliance for Health Information Technology. (2008). *Defining key health information technology terms.* (No. NAHIT-2008). Washington, DC: Department of Human and Health Services. Retrieved from https://www.nachc.com/client/Key%20HIT%20Terms%20Definitions%20Final_April_2008.pdf

Neel, A. N., & Sittig, D. F. (2002). Basic microbiologic and infection control information to reduce the potential transmission of pathogens to patients via computer hardware. *Journal of American Medical Informatics Association, 9*(5), 500–508. doi:10.1197/jamia.M1082

Philips. (2014). *Hardware specifications.* Retrieved from http://www.healthcare.philips.com/main/products/healthcare_informatics/products/cardiology_informatics/hardware_specifications/

TechTerms.com. (2014). *Definition: Secure sockets layer (SSL).* Retrieved from http://www.techterms.com/definition/ssl

William, C. (2012). *Collins English dictionary—Complete & unabridged: Internet* (10th ed.). London, UK: HarperCollins. Retrieved from http://dictionary.reference.com/browse/internet

Wilson, J. R. (2013). Fundamentals of systems ergonomics/human factors. *Applied Ergonomics, 45*(1), 5–13. doi:10.1016/j.apergo.2013.03.021

Yuri, K. (n.d.). *Units of information and data storage.* Retrieved from http://www.translatorscafe.com/cafe/EN/units-converter/data-storage/10-5/kilobyte-word/

Zanbergen, P. (n.d.). *How star, bus, ring & mesh topology connect computer networks in organizations.* Retrieved from http://education-portal.com/academy/lesson/how-star-topology-connects-computer-networks-in-organizations.html#lesson

CHAPTER 7

Electronic Health Records and Point-of-Care Technology

Mary Beth Mitchell and Susan McBride

OBJECTIVES

1. Discuss the evolution of the electronic health record (EHR) within hospitals, including federal initiatives, health care system impact, and clinical rationale.

2. Describe the process for implementing EHRs in hospitals, focusing on project life cycle and nursing's role in ensuring a successful go-live.

3. Explain the impact of integration on the EHR, including managing disparate systems, point-of care devices, and device integration.

4. Explore the role of governance in EHR optimization to increase nursing adoption and utilization and understand how nursing informatics supports the sustainability of the EHR.

5. Discuss EHR recognition programs and how they promote value, utilization, and outcomes associated with the EHR.

KEY WORDS

electronic health record, point-of-care technology, barcode medication administration, Rogers's Diffusion of Innovation model, innovators, early adopters, laggards, adoption, implementation, evaluation, interoperability

---

CONTENTS

INTRODUCTION

Since the 1960s, the promise of an electronic health record (EHR) that would bring together all aspects of a person's health in a collective and cohesive way to provide a systematic longitudinal record of his or her health and health care encounters across the life span, regardless of location, intervention, behaviors, and lifestyle has been on the horizon. The desire to provide access to health care resources, continuity of care for all individuals, and holistic management of a person's quality of life have influenced the rapid development of health information technology (HIT) over the past two decades in ways never imagined. This chapter describes the impact of the EHR on the health care community, including consumers of health care, the government and other regulatory bodies, and vendors of goods and services. Most important, it explains what this means for clinicians and the patient experience.

To fully understand this development of HIT over the past three decades, one only has to start with the present. In the health care environment of 2014, an idealized state of health care starts with an individual engaging in healthy behaviors. The person accesses his or her health information via a web-based portal on a mobile device that manages and reports all relevant health information. Information from wearable devices that provide vital signs and activity routinely download and aggregate data; lab data, such as blood sugars, urine tests, and so forth, are monitored and results provided. Health history data are available and continually updated as situations change and health problems are added and resolved. Every encounter with the health care system results in information within a patient record, whether it be an office visit to a provider, a hospital encounter, or interaction with other community services, including emergency medical services, health centers, and long-term care facilities. This information is now accessible by patients, families, and health care providers. In addition, this information is organized and defined within a framework of rules and tools that provide reports, reminders, alerts of potential or real problems, treatment options, interventions, and outcomes. Patient education is given to the patient, is auto-assigned, or sought out by the patient based on documented activities, and the patient's response to education, to treatment, his or her compliance, and other patient activities are recorded and considered in the total health picture. Over time, a longitudinal picture of a person's health emerges and this information can be compared with that of other patients in other places and systems to provide information about populations with similar health patterns that can guide future research, best practices, as well as manage the health of the single patient across his or her life span.

HISTORY OF EHRs IN HOSPITALS

EHRs have become increasingly prevalent since the 1990s because of the national initiatives taken to drive EHR adoption. However, as far back as the mid-1960s, it is believed that around 73 hospitals had some type of health record in an electronic format. Often, universities and corporations worked together to develop these early EHRs, such as University of Utah working with 3M or Harvard working with Mass General, to create their own version of various health record components. These were not full EHRs, but rather specific programs that provided functionality in limited ways (Atherton, 2011).

However, in the 1970s, the federal government implemented an EHR system within the Department of Veteran Affairs called the De-Centralized Hospital Computer Program, which was used nationwide. In addition, the Department of Defense also implemented the composite health care system (CHCS) to serve as the patient record for all military personnel worldwide (National Center for Research Resources [NCRR], 2006).

By the 1980s, there was more work done to develop and increase the use of EHRs in the field of medicine, as its use became better defined and a greater potential for improving health was recognized. The Institute of Medicine (IOM) launched a study in the mid-1980s on the potential of EHRs to improve patient clinical care (Dick & Steen, 1991). This study, The Computer-Based Patient Record, originally published in 1991 and again in 1997 with revisions, was the first to call for the widespread implementation of EHRs to provide timely, accurate health data and to improve the quality of care while reducing costs (Dick, Steen, & Detmer, 1997).

In 1987, an EHR standards-developing organization called Health Level Seven International (HL7) was formed to develop standardization around EHRs, thus recognizing the growing industry of health records and the need for integration and communication across platforms, systems, and organizations. Today, HL7 has become the standard in 55 countries for the exchange, integration, sharing, and retrieval of health information.

With the increasing awareness of the potential of EHRs, along with development of standards, and the increase in companies developing clinical applications, organizations started moving toward some type of electronic systems within hospitals. Certainly, lab systems were often early clinical systems used within hospitals, as were patient registration systems, but wide adoption of full, integrated EHRs did not occur until the 2000s.

In 1999, the IOM issued the landmark report *To Err Is Human: Building a Safer Health System*, in which the IOM ascertained that tens of thousands of Americans die every year as a result of potentially preventable medical errors. In 2001, the IOM issued another report, *Crossing the Quality Chasm: A New Health System for the 21st Century*, in which the need for high-quality, evidence-based, standardized health care for all was emphasized. These reports explained that part of the reason for the schisms in care across the country was lack of a technological infrastructure, uncoordinated care, and lack of organization in a system that is often difficult to navigate and manage across multiple encounters and interactions with health care providers. The IOM believed that a fundamental component needed to address the problems plaguing the health care system in America was to advance technology, indicating that technology, including the Internet, "holds enormous potential for transforming the health care delivery system, which today remains relatively untouched by the revolution that has swept nearly every other aspect of society" (Institute of Medicine [IOM] Report, 2001, p. 15). In addition, the report emphasized the need for a "national commitment" to building an information infrastructure to support health care delivery, consumer health, quality measurement and improvement, public accountability, clinical and health services research, and clinical education. The goal was to eliminate most handwritten clinical data by 2010. Thus, began the drive to improve quality of care through the adoption of EHRs and implementation of national initiatives to promote the use of EHRs (IOM, 2001).

CURRENT DRIVERS BEHIND AN EHR NATIONAL INITIATIVE IN THE UNITED STATES

Even though the two landmark IOM reports promoted the use of EHRs to improve patient quality and safety, and even though there were more sophisticated and developed systems, adoption of fully integrated EHRs remained low through the first part of the 21st century. Hospitals were starting to purchase and implement pieces of EHRs, such as radiology systems, operating room (OR) systems, or even barcoding of supplies or medications; but a fully integrated EHR was still not implemented in most hospital systems. In 2009, a study found that only 9% of hospitals surveyed had basic or comprehensive EHR systems, and only 17% of hospitals had computer provider order entry (CPOE) implemented for medications (Jha et al., 2009); thus, the Health Information Technology for Economic and Clinical Health (HITECH) Act was born.

As early as 2004, President George W. Bush highlighted the need for hospitals and health care providers to implement and adopt the use of EHRs over the next 10 years by stating in his State of the Union Address: "By computerizing health records, we can avoid dangerous medical mistakes, reduce costs, and improve care" (The White House, 2004). To support this effort, he created the Office of the National Coordinator (ONC) within the Department of Health and Human Services to oversee and manage the adoption of EHRs through development of standards for interoperability, provide for certification of EHRs that met these standards, and develop a national infrastructure to support health information exchanges (HIE). As the advancement of EHRs continued within hospital and physician practices, there came an ever-growing focus on the use of technology in health care.

Government Initiatives and Mandates for EHR Use

In 2009, President Barack Obama made an unprecedented move and mandated the use of EHRs by all health care providers and hospitals. The economic stimulus bill of 2009, the American Recovery and Reinvestment Act (ARRA), also allowed up to $29 billion for the adoption and utilization of EHRs. The ONC and the Centers for Medicare & Medicaid Services (CMS) would support and manage the HITECH Act through the administration of financial incentives for organizations that demonstrated "meaningful use" (MU) of EHRs to improve patient care and clinical outcomes. The HITECH Act represents one of the largest federal investments ever in health technology, demonstrating a broad consensus and commitment to fully realizing the potential of EHRs to transform the health care system (Blumenthal, 2011).

The "MU program," as it has become known, is overseen by the ONC and administered by CMS. There are guidelines for providers and hospitals that define the criteria that demonstrate meaningful use of a certified EHR. These criteria define thresholds that must be met, ranging from recording patient information as structured data to exchanging summary care records. CMS has established these thresholds for eligible professionals, eligible hospitals, and critical access hospitals (CAHs). The MU program includes three stages, with increasing requirements for participation. All providers begin participating by meeting the Stage 1 requirements for a 90-day period in their first year of meaningful use and a full year in their second year of meaningful use. After meeting the Stage 1 requirements, providers will then have to meet Stage 2 requirements. Eligible professionals participate in the program on the calendar years, whereas eligible hospitals and CAHs participate according to the federal fiscal year. These requirements are outlined in a statutory rule-making process with the stages outlined in the HITECH Act (2009).

By law, to meet the requirements of the MU program, the user must:

▶ Use a certified EHR

▶ Exchange health information

▶ Report quality measures

Figure 7.1 reflects these key areas under the meaningful use measures, including both core and menu-set measures (also see Appendix 1.1 on Meaningful Use Stage 1 and Stage 2 comparisons).

BENEFITS OF THE EHR FOR IMPROVING SAFETY AND QUALITY

Although MU has been a key driver of EHR adoption, the benefits of the EHR are well known, and volumes of research have been published to support these benefits. As organizations deploy these systems and they are fully integrated and adopted throughout an organization, the benefits are realized by providers, nurses, and other clinicians, and even patients and families

EHRs are known to do the following:

▶ Improve quality of patient care

▶ Increase patient participation in care

▶ Improve accuracy of diagnoses and health outcomes

▶ Improve care coordination

▶ Increase efficiencies and provide cost savings

Quality of patient care is positively impacted through the use of clinical decision support (CDS) consisting of rules and alerts to manage the breadth of information within the EHR. This may be drug-allergy checking or advisories for management of certain conditions. Certainly, legibility of the record, real-time access from virtually any location, and integration of data from other systems promote quality initiatives within the organization. Reporting is also enhanced as more robust patient information is more readily available through a variety of reporting tools. Also, provider order entry and barcode

MU Stage 1 - Core and Menu Items

Legend by domain:

D1 Improve Quality, Safety, Efficiency	D2 Engage Patients & Families	D3 Improve Care Coordination	D4 Improve Public & Population Health	D5 Ensure Privacy & Security for Personal Health Information

Core Objectives

Computerized Provider Order Entry (CPOE) for Medication Orders	Medication Allergy List	Clinical Decision Support Rule
D1 - Improve Quality, Safety, Efficiency	**D1 - Improve Quality, Safety, Efficiency**	**D1 - Improve Quality, Safety, Efficiency**
Drug Interaction Checks	Record Demographics	Electronic Copy of Health Information
D1 - Improve Quality, Safety, Efficiency	**D1 - Improve Quality, Safety, Efficiency**	**D2 - Engage Patients & Families**
Maintain Problem List	Record Vital Signs	Clinical Summaries
D1 - Improve Quality, Safety, Efficiency	**D1 - Improve Quality, Safety, Efficiency**	**D2 - Engage Patients & Families**
e-Prescribing	Record Smoking Status	Electronic Exchange of Clinical Information
D1 - Improve Quality, Safety, Efficiency	**D1 - Improve Quality, Safety, Efficiency**	**D3 - Improve Care Coordination**
Active Medication List	Clinical Quality Measures (CQMs)	Protect Electronic Health Information
D1 - Improve Quality, Safety, Efficiency	**D1 - Improve Quality, Safety, Efficiency**	**D5 - Ensure Privacy and Security for Personal Health Information**

Menu Objectives

Drug Formulary Checks	Patient Electronic Access	Immunization Registries Data Submission
D1 - Improve Quality, Safety, Efficiency	**D2 - Engage Patients & Families**	**D4 - Improve Public and Population Health**
Clinical Lab Test Results	Patient-specific Education Resources	Syndromic Surveillance Data Submission
D1 - Improve Quality, Safety, Efficiency	**D2 - Engage Patients & Families**	**D4 - Improve Public and Population Health**
Patient List	Medication Reconciliation	
D1 - Improve Quality, Safety, Efficiency	**D3 - Improve Care Coordination**	
Patient Reminders	Transition of Care Summary	
D1 - Improve Quality, Safety, Efficiency	**D3 - Improve Care Coordination**	

FIGURE 7.1. HealthIT.gov tables of meaningful use.

Adapted from HealthIT.gov (n.d.).

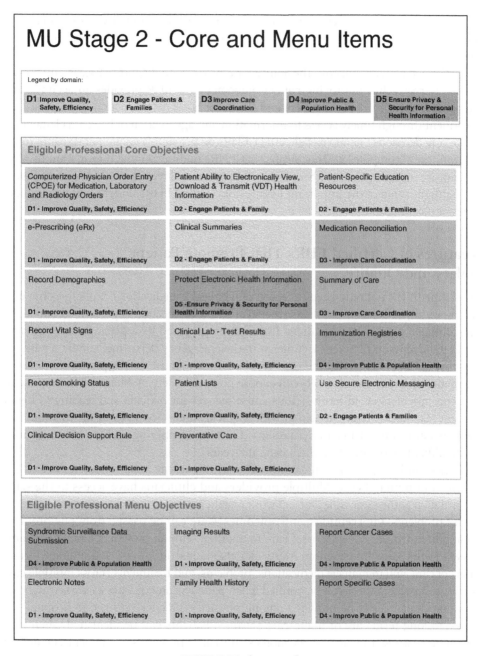

MU Stage 2 - Core and Menu Items

Legend by domain:

| **D1** Improve Quality, Safety, Efficiency | **D2** Engage Patients & Families | **D3** Improve Care Coordination | **D4** Improve Public & Population Health | **D5** Ensure Privacy & Security for Personal Health Information |

Eligible Professional Core Objectives

Computerized Physician Order Entry (CPOE) for Medication, Laboratory and Radiology Orders	Patient Ability to Electronically View, Download & Transmit (VDT) Health Information	Patient-Specific Education Resources
D1 - Improve Quality, Safety, Efficiency	D2 - Engage Patients & Family	D2 - Engage Patients & Families
e-Prescribing (eRx)	Clinical Summaries	Medication Reconciliation
D1 - Improve Quality, Safety, Efficiency	D2 - Engage Patients & Family	D3 - Improve Care Coordination
Record Demographics	Protect Electronic Health Information	Summary of Care
D1 - Improve Quality, Safety, Efficiency	D5 -Ensure Privacy & Security for Personal Health Information	D3 - Improve Care Coordination
Record Vital Signs	Clinical Lab - Test Results	Immunization Registries
D1 - Improve Quality, Safety, Efficiency	D1 - Improve Quality, Safety, Efficiency	D4 - Improve Public & Population Health
Record Smoking Status	Patient Lists	Use Secure Electronic Messaging
D1 - Improve Quality, Safety, Efficiency	D1 - Improve Quality, Safety, Efficiency	D2 - Engage Patients & Families
Clinical Decision Support Rule	Preventative Care	
D1 - Improve Quality, Safety, Efficiency	D1 - Improve Quality, Safety, Efficiency	

Eligible Professional Menu Objectives

Syndromic Surveillance Data Submission	Imaging Results	Report Cancer Cases
D4 - Improve Public & Population Health	D1 - Improve Quality, Safety, Efficiency	D4 - Improve Public & Population Health
Electronic Notes	Family Health History	Report Specific Cases
D1 - Improve Quality, Safety, Efficiency	D1 - Improve Quality, Safety, Efficiency	D4 - Improve Public & Population Health

FIGURE 7.1. (*continued*)

medication administration (BCMA) have removed many of the process and human factor effects of patient care, leading to a reduction in errors and improved quality (HealthIT.gov, n.d.).

The use of EHRs has also increased patient and family participation in care. Through online tools and portals, patients now have access to their patient information and can message providers and other members of the health care team, request medication refills, schedule appointments, and view education. All these initiatives result in a more positive patient experience as well as a patient informed in his or her health management process.

EHRs can actually improve the ability for a provider to diagnose disease and reduce medical errors, thus improving patient outcomes. The EHR provides an accurate and comprehensive picture of the patient and allows for faster determination of diagnosis and treatment through timely access to information and aggregation of key data elements to drive care decisions (Jamoom et al., 2011). EHRs do not simply contain or transmit information, they "compute" it. This means that EHRs manipulate the information in ways to improve outcomes in a number of important functional requirements. We review them to highlight some of the important features of certified EHRs under the federal guidelines of meaningful use.

Features of Certified EHRs That Promote Patient Safety and Quality

A qualified EHR not only keeps a record of a patient's medications or allergies but also automatically checks for problems whenever a new medication is prescribed and alerts the clinician to potential conflicts. Information gathered by a primary care provider and recorded in an EHR tells a clinician in the emergency department about a patient's life-threatening allergy and the emergency staff can adjust care appropriately, even if the patient is unconscious. EHRs can expose potential safety problems when they occur, helping providers avoid more serious consequences for patients and leading to better patient outcomes. EHRs can help providers quickly and systematically identify and correct operational problems. In a paper-based setting, identifying such problems is much more difficult and correcting them can take years.

EHRs can help provide care coordination across an encounter of care or across the entire continuum of care. Multiple providers and clinicians have access to the same information at the same time and can work together, providing documentation on a variety of problems, interventions, and outcomes. Care can be passed from one provider to another or from one episode of care to another, with all providers having the same access to the same information. Alerts can also be used to notify and manage transitions of care, and to manage medications, problems, and treatments across multiple care settings. Provider offices can be notified when patients enter or leave a care setting; care summaries can easily be provided among physician practice settings, to hospital settings, to long-term care or home-care settings. Patients can be identified when they return to a care setting and notifications sent to alert providers of a patient's change in status. The possibilities for care management of patients across the entire continuum of care is changing the face of health care and improving patient outcomes as well as reducing costs (Bell & Thornton, 2011).

Other efficiencies and cost savings are recognized from EHR adoption within an organization. Certainly form reduction and timely access to information can reduce operation costs. In addition, the quality and safety impact can result in significant cost avoidance of care related to delays in care or medical errors. Table 7.1 highlights some important findings from a national study of physicians' perspectives of their EHRs offering insight into the benefits of an EHR (Jamoom et al., 2011).

TABLE 7.1 National Study Reflecting Benefits of the EHR

► 79% of providers report that with an EHR their practice functions more efficiently
► 82% report that sending prescriptions electronically (ePrescribing) saves time
► 68% of providers see their EHR as an asset with recruiting physicians and other staff
► 75% receive lab results faster
► 70% report enhanced data confidentiality

EHR, electronic health record.

Finally, the incentives from MU have a direct cost impact. Millions of dollars have been paid to providers and health care organizations, with a projected $19 billion being paid over 5 years. Cost avoidance from a decrease in errors will also provide additional savings; it is estimated that within a large organization it is possible to save between $37 million and $59 million over 5 years (Bell & Thornton, 2011). Figure 7.2 is an infographic created by HealthIT.gov to emphasize the progress made on moving from paper-based records to the EHR and looks to the future of what is next when considering new and emerging technology. The ONC created these resources for use by organizations to help emphasize the importance of adoption and implementation of EHRs to the health care industry, as well as to emphasize the value proposition.

EHR IMPLEMENTATION AND ADOPTION

When deciding to adopt and purchase an EHR, many factors impact an organization's decision. There are basically three different ways to approach an EHR decision: a single-vendor solution, best of breed, or a combination of both.

In a single-vendor decision, typically one vendor provides all the clinical applications needed. This could include everything from patient registration, to all the clinical systems, to the financial and charging systems. Clinical applications include all the patient and ancillary systems, such as clinical documentation, order entry, obstetrics (OB), perioperative, as well as ancillary systems such as lab, radiology, pharmacy, cardiac catheterization lab, gastrointestinal lab, and more. In a best-of-breed approach, organizations look for the best system for each function, such as a separate OB system, or separate laboratory system, with potentially different vendors for multiple applications within a single hospital or organization. There are many considerations for each of these approaches. In a single-vendor approach, there is clear integration of applications among departments; often these applications work together to provide a cohesive user experience, and rules and alerts work across the applications. In a best-of-breed approach, departmental systems are selected and implemented based on the specific and unique workflows within that department, often with advanced functionality for specifically defined clinical needs. Examples of these systems are an OB system, or lab system, or radiology system. Following a best-of-breed approach requires a very strong network infrastructure to integrate these systems and standardize processes as much as possible. Users may need to switch between systems or access multiple systems to manage their work. Often organizations have a combination of a single EHR vendor, with a general platform for many of the clinical systems, but use some best-of-breed systems to supplement specific departmental systems

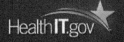

Electronic Health Records:
How they connect **you** and **your** doctors

You and your doctor can share your data more effectively and quickly with other health care providers. There are multiple benefits to YOU. For example, you can eliminate the time and hassle of taking multiple tests or exams.

Where We Were

There was a lot of paper.

Most medical data was not electronic, so the exchange of information between the following health care providers may not have been possible:

- Your doctor and a pharmacy
- Your doctor and another trusted health care provider
- Your doctor and a hospital

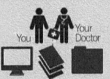

You   Your Doctor

pharmacy   trusted provider   hospital

Physicians' use of
EMR/EHR systems
increased from
18% ➡ **57%**
in 2001   in 2011[1]

Where We Are Now

Many doctors are using electronic health records.

Doctors, labs, pharmacies, and hospitals can store patients' health data electronically. This will help:

- Make your doctor visits faster
- Seamlessly coordinate your care among all your doctors
- Allow you to be in full control of all your medical data

You   Your Doctor

pharmacy   trusted provider   hospital

2 out of 3 people
would consider
switching
to a physician who offers access to medical records through a
secure
Internet connection[2]

What can you do with access to your health record?

Check to make sure your information is correct and complete

Keep track of important health information (e.g. vaccination records and test results)

Have your medical history available if you are changing doctors or visiting a specialist

Keep track of all your medicines and dosages

Having electronic access to your medical record can help you better manage your health.

80%
Americans who **have access to** their health information in electronic health records use it[3]

65%
Americans who **don't have electronic access** to their health information say it's **important to have it**[4]

E-health tools and mobile devices can help you better manage your personal health and wellness.

17 million
Number of consumers using **mobile devices to access health information** in 2011[5]

27%
Adults who use the internet have tracked the following:[6]

weight   diet   exercise routines   health indicators   symptoms

 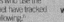 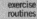
People who are **more engaged** in their health actually get **better health care**[7]

FIGURE 7.2. HealthIT.gov infographic on electronic health records.

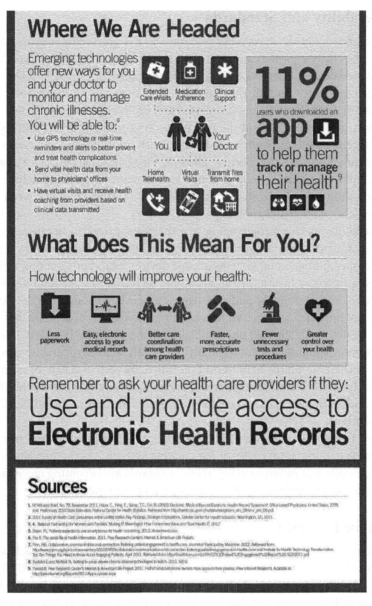

FIGURE 7.2. (*continued*)

based on their needs. Finally, some organizations may even develop or build their own systems; however, with the increasing numbers of vendor systems that cover a wide range of functionalities and workflows, this approach is no longer used within most organizations, except in large organizations that can provide the build-and-support expertise to commit to this approach. Ultimately, the culture of the organization, the resources available to support the EHR, as well as the priorities for use of the EHR will provide the basis for which type of system best meets the needs of the organization.

Interoperability and Standards

Another component of the decision to purchase an EHR is interoperability. Interoperability describes the extent to which systems and devices can exchange data, and interpret that shared data. For two systems to be interoperable, they must be able to exchange data and subsequently present those data so that they can be understood by a user (HIMSS, 2013). This allows data to be shared and exchanged across systems, within an organization, and also outside of the organization. Through interoperability, systems can work together synergistically to enhance health information management, as well as reduce redundancy or data collection, allowing for aggregation of data for analytics and reporting. Interoperability among systems is what makes it possible to have different applications within an organization, and also allows sharing of data between organizations, providers, or other stakeholders.

Interoperability has been challenging over the years, primarily because of the lack of health care standards. Standards provide a common language and set of expectations that enable interoperability among systems and/or devices. Standards are now being developed across a variety of health care applications, such as device standards, system standards, terminology standards, and reporting standards. Through the development of standards, not only are systems able to communication and transfer data, but organizations both locally, nationally, and internationally, are beginning to be able to transfer data. Some of the more common system standards for health care interoperability are reflected in Table 7.2. These standards have important functions with oversight of essential components of the EHR as well as supporting exchange of clinical data. Table 7.2 briefly defines several of these standards. Chapter 12 covers the evolution and details relating to these standards.

Certified EHRs must comply with standards of interoperability and provide various standards to allow for transfer of data among systems. As the prevalence of EHRs expand nationally and internationally, these standards are becoming more mature and detailed in scope and definition, allowing for greater interoperability.

Request for Proposal

Because there are so many options for types of EHRs, and varying approaches based on organizational priorities, culture, and resources, a request for proposal (RFP) is often a first step in determining which EHR solution best meets the needs of an organization or hospital. An RFP is a document that provides a structured approach to obtaining criteria that are relevant to an organization's needs in defining an EHR. An RFP can help narrow down the options for selecting an EHR solution by requesting specific information from several key vendors. Each vendor responds and the responses are evaluated by the organization and two to three vendors are then selected to pursue in greater detail. This allows an organization to get specific information about a vendor, and then compare several vendors using the same criteria. These are sent to the vendors with a completion date, and then the vendor sends back the completed RFP. Table 7.3 highlights a minimum set of information that organizations should consider in an RFP. We discuss this further in Chapter 8 on the systems development life cycle (SDLC).

RFPs provide the due diligence for an organization seeking multiple vendors/solutions to select an EHR. Through the RFP process, they can better define the approach to an

TABLE 7.2 Common System Standards Important to EHRs	
Common System Standards	Importance to EHR
HL7	Health Level 7 is a standards oversight organization that has developed an EHR Records Management and Evidentiary Support Functional Profile (RM-ES FP). The RM-ES FP provides functions in an EHR system that can help an organization maintain a legal record for business and disclosure purposes, help reduce a provider's administrative burden, and reduce costs and inefficiencies caused by redundant paper and electronic record keeping (see www.hl7.org/).
ANSI	American National Standards Institute (ANSI), a private, not-for-profit member-based organization that oversees the U.S.'s voluntary standards and conformity assessment system. HL7 is one of several ANSI-accredited standards developing organizations. ANSI is relevant to health care technology, including pharmacy, medical devices, imaging, or insurance (claims processing) transactions (see www.ansi.org/).
SNOMED	Systematized Nomenclature of Medicine (SNOMED) Clinical Terms is a comprehensive clinical terminology originating in pathology. SNOMED provides the core general terminology for the EHR and contains 311,000 active concepts. Maintained by International Health Terminology Standards Development Organization in Denmark (see www.ihtsdo.org/).
LOINC	Logical Observation Identifiers Names and Codes (LOINC) is a standardized database providing a set of universal names and ID codes used for identifying laboratory and clinical test results used primarily to facilitate exchange of clinical data (see https://loinc.org/).
ISO	International Standards Organization (ISO) defines the set of requirements for the architecture of a system that processes, manages, and communicates information (see www.iso.org/iso/home.html).
RxNorm	RxNorm provides normalized names for clinical drugs and links names to drug vocabularies commonly used in pharmacy management and drug interaction software (see www.nlm.nih.gov/research/umls/rxnorm/).
UMLS	Unified Medical Language System (UMLS) is collection of controlled vocabularies that provide specialized vocabularies, code sets, and classification systems for many health care domains (see www.nlm.nih.gov/research/umls/).

TABLE 7.3 RFP Basic Elements

▶ Organization's name and description
▶ Contact information for questions about the RFP from the vendors
▶ Background and demographics of the organization, including financial stability
▶ Services requested; what the organization is looking for in a product or service
▶ Criteria, information, and guidelines for completing the RFP
▶ Evaluation criteria as to how the information will be used in the RFP process
▶ Selection process as to how and when vendor selection will be determined and next steps for the vendor
▶ Specific criteria about the vendor with a detailed questionnaire of the requested information; may be in survey format or case study format, but the intent is to garner the specific functionality of the system being evaluated

---

RFP, request for proposal.

EHR and select a smaller group of vendors that meet their requirements. The next steps beyond the RFP include live or virtual demonstrations of the system, site visits to see the system in use in other organizations, and a budgetary review. The selection process for an EHR may take several months to over a year. The selection of an EHR is often one of the largest investments a health care organization makes and involves the input from and review by multiple levels of staff, including clinicians and how they use the system.

Implementation of the EHR

The implementation of an EHR follows a very specific process called system development life cycle (SDLC). SDLC is used by engineers and developers in creating systems, but it is also the accepted process for managing a project, such as an EHR implementation, from decision making to beginning a project, to completion of the project. An SDLC approach has a definite time frame—a beginning or initiation point, and an end or closure point. This section reviews the SDLC approach to EHR implementation. There are several different constructs for managing projects of the magnitude and scope of an EHR implementation, but SDLC follows a very specific group of activities defined within each phase, thus further defining the project steps and requirements.

Initiate the Project

The initiation phase of the project is one of the most important stages of an EHR implementation process because this is where the organization's culture, leadership goals, and purpose of the project are defined. It is necessary that the strategic goals of the organization are aligned with the scope of the project in terms of time, resources, and financial impact. The project scope and charter are clarified, and documents are created that define every aspect of the project. It is critical that organizational leaders understand the impact of this project and are able to fully support it throughout the entire project life cycle. In addition, this is where project teams may be defined, resources identified, key deliverables identified, and the entire project scope defined. In the initiation phase, there are often "roadshows" to provide demonstrations of the system and get staff feedback and buy-in of the impending project. Also, during this time, clinical staff may be requested to leave their units and become part of the project's build-and-design team for an extended period of time. The project team is defined and the resources needed for EHR implementation are obtained.

Analysis Phase for EHR Implementation

In the analysis phase, the requirements of the project are further defined. The types and extent of hardware required are determined and interfaces needed for interoperability are defined. How the "roll-out" of implementation will be managed and the types of training and support that will be required are also identified in this phase. All the aspects that make a project implementation successful are analyzed and defined, including how the organization will migrate from the old system or workflow to the new system. Part of the analysis is determining the roll-out plan, such as whether all areas will go live at the same time, often referred to as a "big-bang" approach, or whether there will be a more phased implementation approach, going unit by unit, or only putting in specific functionality at a time. Also, the following questions have to be answered:

▶ What type of devices will be used?

▶ How many of such devices are required?

▶ Will fixed devices be used? If so, what will be their size and configuration?

▶ How will the infrastructure support additional hardware and computers?

▶ Where will the additional hardware and computers be located?

The device management aspect of the project is critical to the success of the implementation and needs to be managed as a key component of the overall project.

Design Phase of the EHR Implementation

In the design phase of the project, gap analysis is done to evaluate the old workflows and define the new workflows. In this process, end-user clinicians define every step of the tasks that are part of their work and those tasks are mapped as an existing state. Then, the new workflows are defined by the staff using the functionality of the EHR being implemented as the future state. Gaps between the existing state and future state are identified, as well as key components of the workflow that are required. Organizational culture and approach to care have an important role in this design analysis in terms of getting the system adopted. The EHR provides only functionality; through the design phase, it is up to the organization to determine how the tools will be operationalized and used to facilitate the desired workflows. This step should involve nurses and clinicians at all levels to provide input and support of both the existing workflows as well as the new, desired workflows. Additionally, in the design state, data dictionaries are established, nomenclature is standardized within the EHR, and expectations for use and compliance are established.

Implementation Phase of the EHR Implementation

During the implementation phase, policies and procedures are written to define the workflows, training materials are developed, and testing is completed. There are several types of testing done within the project, starting with unit testing to ensure that the system performs correctly within the build. Then there is integrated testing, in which the workflows are tested, and testing among various systems is done to ensure data are interoperable and are moving through the system. Finally, there is end-user testing, or user-acceptance testing, in which the staff using the system test the workflows and approve the functionality and the support of the workflows. Testing is ongoing throughout the entire project build, but the final user-acceptance testing ensures that the system meets the requirements originally defined by the organization. Training of staff occurs usually within the 4 to 6 weeks preceding the actual "go-live" of the system, superusers are defined, and schedules are created for the implementation time period. The actual implementation, or "go-live," occurs at a point and time that is usually supported by the builders, developers, and superusers for a specific time period. During the actual implementation, additional staff may be needed to manage the clinical activities while everyone is learning the systems. It is critical that everything possible be done to minimize impact on patient care during the EHR implementation and that quality and patient safety are maintained during the go-live time frame. There should be adequate support and resources available to help the staff adjust to the new system without affecting patient care.

Support and Maintenance Phase

Once the system goes live and is stabilized, the postimplementation phase begins. There should be an evaluation of the implementation by all members of the project team, as well as by the staff using the system. Lessons learned are considered and a long-term, sustainability plan is put into place. In the support that occurs after the system goes live, there should be ways to make requests for enhancements, ways to report breaks or problems with the system, and ways to train and communicate ongoing changes to the users. The initial project will close at this point, but the project management of an EHR never really ends. Governance needs to be defined for how ongoing requests, optimization opportunities, enhancements, and upgrades will be managed. Communication is critical to the post implementation support plan, and there should be a structure in place within the organization to report to all staff impacted by the system. Business recovery plans or downtime plans detailing how staff will manage if there is a failure of the system, or if the system has to be taken offline at defined times for upgrades or maintenance, also need to be put in place.

One thing to note about a systems life-cycle approach is its similarity to nursing process. Nursing informaticists can use their knowledge of nursing process to facilitate an SDLC methodology. Figure 7.3 shows how SDLC aligns with the nursing process.

Workflow Analysis

In order to have a successful EHR implementation, it is important not to just look at the functionality of the system in terms of how the system responds or the features of the system, but rather to develop the EHR around the workflows of the clinicians who will be using the EHR. Workflows are critical in the overall adoption of the EHR by the clinicians who will use it. The workflows will guide the steps in system performance. Most systems can support a variety of steps or functions within a specific workflow, such as medication administration or a patient history, but the culture of the organization and existing workflows should be considered when designing and building the EHR. On

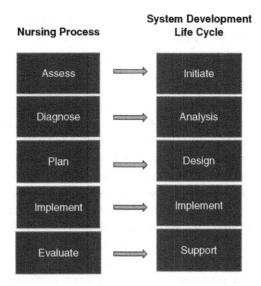

FIGURE 7.3. Nursing process and SDLC alignment.

the other hand, it is critical not to take existing workflows that are used in a manual system (or even with another EHR), and try to recreate those same workflows. Many organizations tried to replicate their paper forms electronically only to discover that the workflows did not flow smoothly from one function to another. Therefore, although these clinical workflows are critical to the success of the system, reimplementing existing paper-based workflows for an EHR leads to further problems. So, how do these workflows get defined? How do the analysts know the workflows? What is the best workflow to use to build in the EHR?

Current State Analysis

One way to look at workflow management is to define existing workflows and create diagrams or maps to evaluate and document the "current state." The current state analysis helps define all the critical workflows used by the clinicians. What is frequently discovered in the current state analysis is inconsistency of practices, demonstrating that not everyone follows the same workflow for the same process. To implement a successful EHR, these variances among caregivers, units, and shifts are critical to examine, document, and address in a workflow redesign effort. Questions that need to be addressed with respect to medication management are as follows:

▶ How are patients properly identified?

▶ How is medication reconciliation done?

▶ Where does the responsibility lie for all steps in the process, and when is it started and when is it actually completed?

A current state analysis takes the end user who performs the functions and lays out the process for each workflow he or she performs. Additional areas that are critical to examine include admission history, managing orders, medication administration, care planning, dressing changes, daily care, vital signs, and patient education. Each workflow is completely diagramed with all steps defined and then agreed on by the staff to verify each workflow. This current state analysis is the basis for the next phase of workflow management, which is the workflow redesign phase.

Future State Analysis

The workflow redesign phase is focused on designing the workflows for the same functions in the new electronic environment. This is the "future state" workflow design process. In the future state workflow design, the staff, often with the EHR analysts, will review the functionality of the system and create new workflows that take both key and important elements from the current state but also account for the functionality of the EHR to optimize and streamline these workflows. One would expect these new workflows would have any redundancy removed, be cleaner, and easier to follow with fewer steps, and this is most often the case. If the EHR provides efficiency and safety, then many of the redundant steps and inefficiencies of paper systems are removed and the new workflows are much easier to follow and adopt by the staff. An example of a current state and future state workflow for one organization implementation of the EHR is provided later in this chapter. Note the reduced number of steps and the increased efficiency of the future state workflow based on the EHR functionality. It is important to note that these are new workflows, and not existing workflows, placed in the EHR environment. However, it is possible to retain the overall culture of the organization in the development of the future state workflows.

There are several advantages to working through this workflow management exercise. First, the staff using the actual workflows, particularly the clinicians, should be an integral part of workflow development. Second, this presents a perfect opportunity to establish consistency for a specific process, thus providing an opportunity to increase standardization and update and reeducate policies and procedures to ensure all staff know and follow the new workflows. Finally, workflow management decreases variability while increasing efficiencies. Therefore, the effort placed on workflow management will standardize processes and involve the clinical staff, thereby increasing accountability, while decreasing variability.

The Build Process Using "Use Cases"

On completion of workflow design, the build occurs based on the specifications of the workflow design. An approach that builds the design for end users, based on workflows, is the object-oriented approach, which is based on "use cases." Use cases establish a foundation for evaluating information design in an EHR that categorizes and describes discrete functional scenarios and determines how computer interactions are carried out. A use case describes a system's behavior and how it responds to a stimulus (or activity) and can be used to define activities. Use cases serve as a framework demonstrating and establishing the relationship between high-level clinical functions and related standards in information design and usability. Through combining use cases with basic principles of system usability and design, an effective and practical framework for the evaluation of EHRs can be established (Armijo, McDonnell, & Werner, 2009). Basically, there is an actor and a process, or function, and the process for building the functionality is based on how the actor interacts or "uses" the system. This situation is an excellent example of the actor–network theory described in Chapter 3 in an applied practical use (see Chapter 3 for more details).

There are basically use cases for every workflow, and these use cases help the analysts understand what the needs of the users are and allow them to adapt the functionality to meet the workflow. Use cases are an excellent way of designing specifications when there are end users of the system who are not the technical developers, and the developers may not understand the workflows they are designing. Nursing informaticists are key, however, to helping in the design of both the use cases and the technical specs of how the system performs to provide the functionality desired to accommodate the workflows the clinicians developed. The use-case approach is an efficient way to build the system because it is a systematic approach designed to ensure that technology meets the needs as described by the individuals using the system. Figure 7.4 shows a schematic based on a use case in a clinical setting. In this diagram, we see the patient presenting for treatment and interacting with the provider (clinician); the EHR boundary represents information that is captured and managed within the system. Stakeholders who interact with the EHR are the patient, clinician, staff support, and those who manage data that are internal and external to the system.

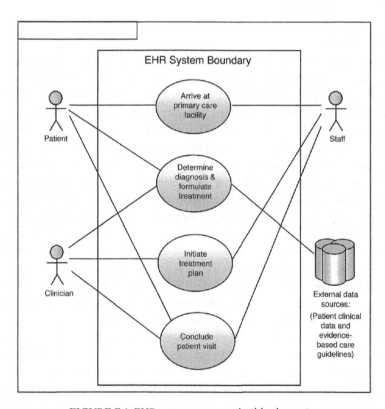

FIGURE 7.4. EHR system use-case build schematic.

EHR, electronic health record.

Source: Armijo et al. (2009).

Support Phase: Superusers and Nursing Informaticists' Role

Once an EHR is fully implemented, there is a tendency to think, "Well the EHR is now implemented, and the project is over." Although a project has a defined start and end time, and projects do close, the EHR remains a dynamic, ever-changing process within the organization. It is critical that all staff in a health care system or clinical practice understand that the EHR is never "done," and the ongoing support and optimization of the system needs to continue. One of the most standard ways to maintain support both during and after an EHR go-live is through the use of superusers and nursing informaticists.

Nursing Informatics' Role

The nursing informatics (NI) role is critical to success because the NI content expert understands both the clinical aspects of how the EHR affects the clinicians and the patients, and can assess and monitor the impact of the technology on patient care and the clinician's experience. The NI content expert understands both the workflows and the system functionality, and is uniquely positioned to provide the expertise on solving problems, establishing best practices, and adapting policies and procedures to support the defined workflows of the EHR. These functions are critical to optimization of the EHR in the clinical setting and align with the nursing informatics role and competencies discussed in Chapter 2.

Superusers' Role

Superusers are staff who are designated to be a resource to assist end users within their units or departments. Superusers are critical to the success of an EHR implementation in that they provide staff support and are the first-line resource to assist end users with basic questions about workflow and functionality. Superusers usually volunteer to be a superuser, or are asked by their managers, but are usually someone with a strong interest in the EHR and often in technology. It is important, during a go-live, that superusers are given time away from their patient care responsibilities to learn the system very well and to be available to staff to answer their questions and help support them during go-live. Superusers usually provide support to a group of staff or users, either within a department or unit, and serve as the first line of support or the "go-to" person for all staff. In addition, it is important for superusers meet as a group routinely and to stay abreast of issues or concerns that are raised so they can address them. They also are usually the first ones to get information on fixes, approved work-arounds, and policy changes, so they can communicate them back to their staff. The superuser is the pivotal, point person during the go-live and should have no other responsibilities than to provide support and to keep staff up to date with information on key changes needed to move forward.

Once the go-live is complete, superusers should stay engaged and committed to the EHR, as well as get used to thinking in terms of expanded use of technology, such as incorporating devices such as intravenous (IV) pump integration into the EHR platform. Superusers continue to grow in their expertise of the system and remain in the support role for the unit or department for all matters concerning the EHR. Often, superusers are responsible for communicating changes and ongoing reinforcement of workflows, policies, and EHR functionality. Superusers, along with the nursing informaticists, can ensure the ongoing adoption, optimization, and support of the EHR. Because superusers stay

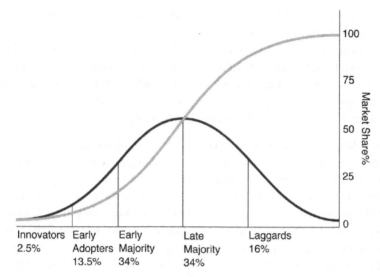

FIGURE 7.5. Rogers's innovations theory. Based on Rogers (1962).
Source: Sahin (2006).

engaged even after the implementation of the EHR and continue to support both the staff
and the efforts of EHR optimization and changes with growth in expertise of the EHR,
many superusers may move on to pursue work in NI, or other information technology-
related positions.

EHR Adoption

Adoption refers to how well the staff and users actually use and embrace the system as part
of their routine daily activities. Adoption of the EHR by stakeholders, including leadership, clinicians, support staff, and patients, align with more mature stages in accordance
with the diffusion of innovation theoretical framework (Rogers, 2003). Rogers (2003)
depicts the spread or diffusion of innovation as a bell-shaped curve. Rogers describes
this model as "the classifications of members of a social system on the basis of innovativeness" (Rogers, 1995, p. 22). This classification includes innovators, early adopters, early
majority, late majority, and laggards (Figure 7.5). In each adopter category, individuals
are similar in terms of their innovativeness: "An *innovation* is an idea, practice, or project
that is perceived as new by an individual or other unit of adoption" (Rogers, 2003, p. 12).
Innovativeness has been described as a socially constructed process that is aligned with
an individual's willingness to change what is familiar (Braak, 2001). For Rogers, innovativeness helps to understand the desired and main behavior required in the innovation–
decision process.

When looking at adoption of an EHR, this same pattern emerges and users can be
identified within each category of the diffusion of innovations curve.

▶ *Innovators*: Innovators on average account for about 2.5% of the organization's
population and may include the nursing informaticists, champions, and superusers. They embrace the technology and understand the potential of the EHR in
improving the safety and quality of patient care, as well as the clinician experience.

They seek to help define the system and are often testers involved in the design of the workflows. Innovators often are innovators in other areas of their lives, not just with an EHR implementation; they may have the latest mobile device or the newest gadget, and generally are on the cutting edge with regard to how they interact with technology. Innovators constantly push for advanced functionality of the system, pushing the limits of the system and creatively thinking of ways to improve existing workflows and functionality.

▶ *Early Adopters*: Early adopters may also be champions, nursing informaticists, or superusers, and represent about 13.5% of the organization's population. They may also be users who are engaged and ready to start using the system to its fullest potential and offer a positive response on the implementation. Early adopters look for the bugs in the system and seek to find solutions. They are willing to support the system with their peers and other staff, and to promote use of the system. They follow the defined workflows and ask questions in areas of uncertainty. Early adopters may look for better ways to perform specific workflows, if they feel the workflows are not optimized or could work better. They are supportive of the system but are also realistic in their approach, yet they remain positive while looking for solutions to problems or issues. An example of an early adopter's contribution is spending extra time to complete a workflow in the EHR, such as medication reconciliation, or completing a nursing history that may have been done quickly in the old environment but now is taking longer to complete as the adopter tries to understand the correct workflow.

▶ *Early and Late Majority*: These adopters represent the largest number of the staff, approximately 68%, and consist primarily of the staff using the system on a regular basis. They understand the need to use the system and that they are required to use the system, but they may not be looking for ways to improve on its use or ways to use it better. Early-majority staff often use a portion of the system well but may have forgotten or not adopted certain workflows well and need to be supported and reminded of key features. Over time, they improve in their use and may speak favorably of the system, but only to the extent that it meets their needs and provides efficiencies for them in the course of the day. They are not interested in technology for technology's sake and will adopt based on how well the system meets their needs in providing safer or better patient care, or in providing for organizational efficiencies. Late adopters may be somewhat resistant to the new system and have to be shown how it will improve their work. They often use workarounds and may even continue to use old workflows, trying to use as little of the new system as they can. As the system begins to work for them, they are willing to adopt and incorporate the new workflows. They need a lot of support from superusers and nursing informaticists, and need to see the evidence that the EHR improves patient safety and quality or improves their own efficiency. The early and later majority may use the system for those areas that are required but may also utilize paper to make notes, such as printing the Medication Administration Record (MAR) or writing on a piece of paper the days when all medications are due, but use the barcoded medication administration when giving meds. Over time, they give up their old workflows in favor of the new workflows. Eventually, this group will also adapt to the system and become supporters.

▶ *Laggards*: Laggards represent the final 16% of the staff; they are the most resistant to the use of anything new, resisting change of any type. They are often fearful of change or feel they do not have the technological knowledge to change. They express concern about patient safety, may talk about changing jobs, or leaving the workforce all together rather than adjust to the new methods. They complain about the system and try to use the old workflows. An example may be a physician continuing to write paper orders, when all the other physicians are entering orders via CPOE. Another example could be a nurse not using the barcoded medication administration and continuing to manually check the five rights of medication administration. They are concerned about their own ability to use the EHR, as well as experience a feeling of loss of control in the many changes that are occurring. Laggards need a lot of support from superusers as well as direction from management to use the system. In their use of the EHR, they often do not know the designed workflow, and create inefficient ways to access information, thus confirming that the EHR does not improve care or efficiencies. With support, laggards can be brought along to gain the same level of adoption as other staff. However, they need a lot of reinforcement of the correct workflow as well as providing the laggards with real-world examples that demonstrate the value of the system. Examples might include providing the laggard with information related to how the new technology has addressed near misses and medication errors through use of electronic barcode administration. Once laggards adopt the EHR, they are very supportive. In fact, a recommendation aligned with the DI model is to include the laggards in the design team from the beginning or employ them as superusers to help gauge and understand the concerns likely to be expressed by staff.

Adoption of an EHR can be measured through qualitative studies, such as surveys, questionnaires, or interviews. There are standardized evidence-based surveys that measure adoption of the EHR and are relatively easy to administer. Organizations often conduct surveys of their workforce at regular intervals before and after the EHR implementation to evaluate the adoption over time. Other ways to measure adoption or success of the EHR may be through calls to the help or service desk, rounds performed by the nursing informaticist, and by having general discussions within various committees and meetings.

Case Scenario of Early Adopters and Laggards

A federally qualified health center (FQHC) serving a large indigent population within a rural community is staffed with two nurse practitioners (NPs), a licensed vocational nurse (LVN), and two administrative support staff. The clinic has early adopters in one of the NPs and the LVN, whereas the second NP and LVN are clearly laggards, refusing to document in the EHR and continuing to do everything on paper. The administrator for the clinic is very frustrated with barriers to adoption of the EHR and is beginning to think the clinic may have wasted dollars investing in the system. The FQHC administrator has solicited the help of the Regional Extension Center (REC) to assist their efforts.

The REC sends a nursing informaticist to assist in the clinic. One of the first things the NI does is to examine the workflows and discuss with staff why the EHR is not working for them. One of the main things the NI assesses in the interview process with the staff is to determine the adoption status using Rogers' diffusion of innovation model as a guide to determine where the adoption resistance is and to develop solutions to help the clinic overcome the resistance. Consider the following questions:

1. How can the NI determine the level of adoption of each staff person?
2. Why do you believe it is important to identify which are the early adopters and which are the laggards?
3. How might the NI utilize that information to address barriers to adoption?
4. What could the clinic have done differently when it initiated the EHR that might have prevented the resistance to adoption that the clinic is experiencing?

EHR Evaluation

Evaluation of how effective the adoption of an EHR has been can be measured through qualitative studies, such as surveys, questionnaires, focus groups or ethnographic observational methods, staff interviews, and workflow analysis before and after implementation of the system. There are standardized evidence-based surveys that measure adoption of the EHR that are relatively easy to administer. Two surveys that examine clinicians' experience with their clinical information system (CIS) or EHR are the ISET and the CISES. The *Information Systems Evaluation Tool*, 2nd edition (Smith et al., 2012), developed by Children's Mercy Hospital, was designed to measure the nurse's satisfaction with a CIS and includes a brief demographic survey of the participant and of the participating hospital. The CISIES survey—the Clinical Information Systems Implementation Evaluation Scale—was developed by Dr. Brian Gugerty to measure the nurse's satisfaction with a CIS (Gugerty, Maranda, & Rook, 2006).

Organizations often conduct surveys of their workforce at regular intervals, before and after the EHR implementation, to evaluate adoption over time. The ISET was developed by Children's Mercy Hospital and expanded for use under a Robert Wood Johnson Foundation research study that funded expansion of the effort to include other hospitals throughout the nation with benchmarking reports to compare one's hospital's experiences to others of similar size (Smith et al., 2012).

Other ways to measure adoption or success of the EHR may be through calls to the help or service desk, rounds performed by a nursing informaticist, and general discussion within various committees and meetings. Quantitative measures of quality defining success are recommended by the authors to track and monitor improvement over time using methods described in Chapter 20.

POINT-OF-CARE TECHNOLOGY AND THE EHR

Within the full scope of patient care, there are systems and functions that interact between the patient and the EHR, such as medication administration or glucose testing. These functions are provided at the patient's side, and involve being present with the patient to interact with the technology. Point-of-care (POC) testing allows for testing and diagnosis at the patient's side and can be conducted anywhere the patient is, such as the home, physician office, ambulance, or hospital bedside (National Institutes of Health, 2010). This technology allows for quick, on-the-spot testing, with immediately available results. Additionally, these results can be downloaded directly into the EHR through interface engines. This decreases the risk of error in manually entered results, and the results are immediately available to caregivers for making treatment decisions. There are many innovative devices emerging, particularly those that engage the patient in his or her own care to monitor and maintain health and well-being, including such things as fitness measuring devices, scales, biometric devices, as well as FDA-approved medical devices, such as insulin pumps, pacemakers, defibrillators, and so forth, which can be interfaced with EHRs and patient portals. These types of technologies are discussed in Chapter 15, which covers patient portals and personal health records. The potential for advancement in POC devices is one of the most rapidly growing areas in the health care industry with tremendous potential for improvement in patient safety, quality, and population health.

Barcode Administration

In the hospital, one of the most common POC technologies utilized is BCMA. In BCMA, medication is prepared and delivered to the patient by scanning the patient's armband and the medication, after which an electronic process occurs that verifies the five rights of medication administration using a barcode reader. The reader verifies the patient information and the medication information; the system then proceeds to double check for any drug–drug interactions and allergies, and then verifies that this is the right patient and the right time as the patient is scanned with the barcode reader. BCMA has greatly reduced medication errors, anywhere from 20% to 50% (Poon et al., 2010). Barcoded blood administration is also becoming increasingly common within the EHR. This is similar to BCMA, except that with blood administration, the specific unit of blood is associated with the patient, via the product identification, in addition to the blood administration time and type.

POC Testing

POC testing is also common within the EHR environment. One of the most common types is blood glucose monitoring. Integration with the EHR occurs when the clinicians verify the patient by scanning the patient's armband with the glucose reader and then performing the glucose test. The result is then uploaded directly into the EHR for that patient. This is done either through wireless upload, immediately resulting in readings on the glucose levels, or by synching the glucose meter with a docking station that sends the results to the lab and then to the EHR via a secure router. This type of POC testing is expanding to include such things as iStat for various electrolyte tests obtained at bedside, and tests for laboring patients such as protein and glucose. The benefits of POC testing are primarily the immediate availability of the results and decrease in transcription errors of the value through manual entries. In addition, there is less likelihood of documenting the lab result on the wrong patient. On the downside, however, these results need to be verified by the clinician, and often by the lab, and can be problematic if a lab value is accepted into the record that was not obtained accurately, or if an inaccurate result was obtained because of user error in collecting the specimen, or if there was a problem with the device. In addition, the EHR also provides CDS as well as rules and alerts related to the results as they are verified and entered into the record, such as the need for insulin for a high glucose reading. However, these devices are not intended to replace the clinician's clinical judgment but to provide an adjunct to support the clinician in terms of ease of use, manual-error reduction, and efficiency.

Many types of POC systems require Food and Drug Administration (FDA) approval, because the barcode reader interacts with the patient and the FDA regulates all medical devices that interact with patients. EHR vendors are starting to obtain FDA approval for this type of technology (U.S. Food and Drug Administration, 2014). Other examples of patient POC devices that require FDA approval are fetal monitors, blood glucose monitors, blood pressure monitors, and other vital sign monitors, in addition to devices used for barcode blood administration. FDA approval has been a challenge for the EHR vendors because the requirements for FDA approval are specific to the devices that interact with the patient, and these vendors tend to be software developers, not hardware systems manufacturers with expertise in developing for FDA approval. However, as customer demand for POC has increased, the trend now is for the software vendors to seek more and more FDA approval for their POC technology. However, the niche systems that provide a specific device and function, such as a fetal monitor system, are still able to meet the demand of customers to connect the device into the EHR through integration and interfaces with the EHR.

INTEROPERABILITY AND INTEGRATION OF THE EHR

A successful EHR is dependent on its ability to integrate interoperably into a cohesive clinician experience and reflect an accurate patient record. Most EHRs today, under certifications for EHRs under the HITECH Act, have the ability to reveal a patient's journey across the continuum, from various encounters, from a physician office visit, to a hospital encounter, even to the patient's home. Population health and meaningful use have increased the need for interoperability and in stage 2 of meaningful use include opportunities to incorporate the patient's own personal data within the patient portals. This section addresses various types of interoperability often seen within the EHR that impact the user experience of the EHR and the opportunity to decrease redundancy in data entry.

Device Integration

Device integration is expanding in functionality and scope across the EHR platform. Basically, device data integration is the ability to pull in data from source systems, such as cardiac systems, anesthesia machines, ventilators, blood pressure monitors, and pulse oximetry, integrating data from the devices into the EHR. The device data goes through an integration system or engine, where they are formatted for the EHR and seamlessly sent to the patient's record in a pending verification state. The clinician verifies the information and accepts it into the permanent record. Device integration prevents transcription errors, is available in real time, and can be pulled into the record as frequently as 1-minute intervals. Device integration is especially prevalent in intensive care units, surgeries, and other procedural areas where frequent vital signs are obtained. One of the biggest challenges with device integration is the expense associated with implementation because of the requirements of devices to translate the monitoring data into EHR data through interface engines.

Integration of Disparate Systems

Many EHR vendors are making functionality more inclusive to accommodate all aspects of the patient experience. However, it is still difficult for single EHR vendors to have expertise in all types of systems, especially in niche systems specifically designed for a single function, such as OB surgery or cardiology. Specialty departmental systems are often installed and implemented at different times over many years, so the functionality of the EHR is constantly in flux. Therefore, many organizations still have disparate systems in use, often with some systems being more outdated and some systems using newer technology. These systems are often referred to as "legacy systems." The use of multiple legacy systems can create challenges within the overall EHR integration strategy. For example, a hospital may have had an OR system in place for many years (legacy system) when they implement a new EHR. The OR system with older technology may not be able to fully integrate into the new EHR. Another example is a hospital that has an EHR vendor, but chooses to implement a different obstetric (OB) system that is specialized only for OB, and as a result more fully meets the needs of OB documentation and reporting requirements. However, the clinician still has certain functions that have to be documented in the EHR for cohesiveness of the patient record. Procedural areas, such as surgery, lab, radiology, or cardiology, often have very specialized systems that need to be integrated into the overall EHR. Therefore, interoperability and the ability to integrate these disparate systems are key to having a fully integrated EHR. This continues to be a work in progress, and most organizations take a very strategic approach in how to manage the integration of disparate systems and their older legacy systems. Key factors that impact these strategic decisions may include:

▶ *Safety and quality*: Is there a safety or quality benefit of a system that manages only one aspect of care, and is that benefit quantifiable?

▶ *Functionality*: Are there specific functions that are required, which are not met within one system and require a different system?

▶ *Efficiencies*: How well do the data integrate into a seamless system? Is there redundancy of data?

▶ *Ease of use*: How easy and simple is it for the clinician to use and interact with the system because of the specificity of the system's department-specific functionality?

▶ *Costs*: How justified are the replacement costs of legacy systems and costs of management of disparate systems in terms of technical resources?

▶ *Return on investment*: Is there more value in using a separate system and can that value be quantified in either direct cost savings or cost avoidance?

Regardless of the type of system used, most organizations have some component of integration of various systems. As a result, the management of this integration requires resources, technical expertise, and ongoing monitoring to maintain an efficient user experience.

Challenges With POC Technology and Device Integration or With the EHR

Although POC devices and integration of the devices have increased efficiency as well as safety through direct data integration, there are still many challenges that need to be addressed by an organization adopting this technology. We cover here a few of those issues and challenges.

Mobile Access

Many POC or integrated devices are mobile and require local area wireless technology often referred to as "Wi-Fi." These devices access data via the local area wireless network to pull the data from the device to the patient's record. As mobility increases in the organization, Wi-Fi access needs also increase. Management of "dead" spots, where the Wi-Fi is inaccessible, slow, or drops the connection, is often a challenge and frustration for staff and, as a result, decreases efficiency. The infrastructure must be continuously updated, expanded, and maintained to ensure proper connectivity for all mobile devices using wireless integration of POC data.

Data Reliability and Validity

As with POC testing, competence of the clinician to obtain the test and validate the data must be assured. When data are electronically submitted to the EHR, the validity and verification of the data are critical. Validity checks are often built into the systems but, to ensure accuracy, require the clinician to follow the designed workflows using the POC device according to the designed protocol for use. Management of data reliability and validity is often the responsibility of the department that "owns" the data, such as the lab being responsibile for POC blood sugar results, or the blood bank being responsible for quality control of blood bag accuracy. In manual systems, the quality control was part of the workflow between the clinician and the host system. In an electronic environment, it can be challenging to maintain the quality and integrity of the data coming from the POC system, and these electronic systems do not mean that clinicians should not continue to institute clinically responsible validity checks. This is particularly important when older legacy systems are integrated with new technology.

Management of Rules and Alerts

CDS through the use of rules and alerts for data obtained outside the defined parameters is one of the safety advantages of the EHR. However, if rules and alerts are too frequent, or do not require some type of response, it can be easy for the clinician to ignore them, or not process the information in the alert. Defining the rules and alerts so that they are presented only when there is a true safety concern is a challenge with most systems, and nursing informaticists are key in helping to define the parameters for these rules and alerts based on the clinical evidence. For example, a nurse scans the patient and the medication for administration, and receives an alert that it is too early to give the medication. The nurse elects to give the medication despite the alert, overriding the alert. Sometimes these actions may be appropriate based on the nurse's clinical judgment, but they also can be safety concerns. Knowing when to put a required hard-stop in the system is an important consideration. A hard-stop is an alert that the clinician receives that warns him or her against moving forward with a task until certain requirements are met. An example of this might be when a nurse navigates to a medication documentation screen and receives a hard-stop alert that this is the wrong patient for the drug. In certain circumstances, clinicians can select an override for an alert, such as giving a medication early or late, and these are decisions that are best made by clinicians. Ongoing evaluation of rules and alerts to monitor how they are used, how many times they fire, and whether the alerts are acted on correctly or consistently overridden are critical measures for evaluation of the effectiveness of the CDS system. Maintenance of alerts and rules aligned with clinical guidelines are also best managed by clinical informaticists. It is important that pharmacy staff have input into the system and pharmacy leadership is involved in designing alerts and rules that involve medication administration. These efforts are clearly the role of the interprofessional teams designing the CDS systems for organizations.

Over-Reliance on Technology

The safety functions of the EHR are well documented (Sittig & Ash, 2007), and especially within POC and device integration, safety features can be dramatic. It is not uncommon to see reductions in medication errors of over 50% with BCMA. Along with this comes the expectation by clinicians that these systems are fail-safe, and it may be easy for clinicians to miss an alert, or to not follow the correct workflow because they believe the system will prevent them from making an error. Staff education must emphasize that these systems are only a tool, an adjunct to care; it is important to keep this in mind when using POC technology and the EHR, just as with any other piece of equipment.

Manual Association of Devices to the Patient

One of the challenges regarding device integration is identifying the device with the patient. Often, devices, such as ventilators, critical care monitors, blood pressure machines, and anesthesia machines, have to be linked to the right bed or patient. The clinician may have to select the device name to associate it to the patient within the EHR. Challenges arise when patients move, such as a transfer to another level of care or when the patient is discharged. If the device is not removed from that patient or bed, then the data from the device could be downloaded to the wrong patient's EHR. Over time, the technology will automatically associate the device to the patient, but in most systems today, the clinician must perform a step to associate and disassociate the patient to and from the device, and ensure that the data that's coming from the device into the record is being recorded for the correct patient.

Evaluation and Acting on Results

Finally, there is also a challenge regarding awareness of results. Often, unlicensed personnel may obtain the data recorded in the EHR and communication of the values to the nurse may be slow or not occur at all. For example, a nursing technician obtains the reading of a POC blood glucose and the value is directly integrated into the EHR. If the value is high or low, the technician may not notify the nurse directly, assuming that the nurse will see the value in the record. Or, nurses may accept values coming from monitors, such as vital signs or other cardiac devices, and, if not properly reviewed and acted upon, they could potentially accept values that are not true values, such as a high heart rate caused by movement, or they could accept data without noting that action should be taken, such as when a low blood pressure is recorded. It is easy to get the data into the EHR with POC technology and device integration; often data may not be analyzed, communicated, or acted upon.

HIT is not a replacement for critical thinking and for professional nursing practice. These systems can provide increased efficiencies for the clinician, as well as increased patient safety when used correctly, and strong policies and workflows will help guide the clinician to use POC testing and device management correctly, paying attention to rules and alerts, and following the defined best practices. Nursing informaticists are critical in helping define the best practices, providing education and training to staff on their importance, and ensuring nursing policies are adapted to reflect the requirements related to the technology and the most up-to-date evidence.

SUSTAINABILITY AND CHANGE MANAGEMENT

EHRs are typically implemented over a period of years, although we have seen many organizations begin implementation with the big-bang approach, defined as rapidly adopting an implementation strategy into an organization in as few as 3 to 6 months. Additionally, given the multiple POC devices that continue to improve and expand with options to integrate into the EHR, the result is that the "complete" system does not exist. Basically, the implementation of the EHR is never complete. There are always additional projects, new functionality, new technology, changes in regulatory requirements, and user workflows that require ongoing management to sustain the overall patient record. Although projects have definite start and end times, the EHR is really a series of projects that must be assessed and managed through the lifecycle of the EHR (see Chapter 8 for SDLC specifics). This section addresses some of the components of ongoing management of the EHR, or sustainability.

Change management is the process that organizations use to manage the ongoing requirements and development of their systems. In the EHR, change management may consist of the changes to the functionality of the various applications or systems that comprise the EHR. It may also be changes to workflows, or policies and procedures that affect the technology. Organizations develop change management processes to accommodate the ongoing sustainability and future development of their systems; this process may be based on specific models of change management or internally developed. Change management typically follows a basic life-cycle process of assessing the problem, or area to be changed, designing the solution or the change needed, training and implementing the change, and then evaluating the impact and success of the change. However, we cover here four key areas that are often high priority in the field of change management.

Maintenance Requests

Maintenance change requests are a part of the normal organization processes that continue to evolve as part of everyday practice. Maintenance may include adding lab tests to an order panel and changes in medication dosage recommendations from the FDA. Maintenance requests are often the most prevalent but do not take the tremendous resources that the build and training phases of implementation do. They are often considered the day-to-day business of managing the system.

Regulatory Changes

There are also required changes that are governed by regulatory requirements that need to be incorporated into practice, which may have a significant impact on the resources needed to create and manage these changes, as well as to educate and to incorporate these changes into practice. There may be new changes from the Joint Commission that impact the EHR and clinical practice, as well as ongoing recommendations for core measures, Surgical Care Improvement Project (SCIP) measures, MU, and other regulatory requirements. Often, implementation of these changes has time requirements; managing these changes effectively and efficiently creates additional challenges to staff. Examples of regulatory changes might include implementing functionality to accommodate medication reconciliation, managing immunization reporting requirements, or improved ability to provide electronic patient discharge instructions.

Patient Safety Changes

Patient safety is certainly the top priority within the organization and managing the EHR to maintain and support patient safety is a critical function for informaticists. Changes may be needed to help promote patient safety, or to prevent a functionality or workflow that can impact patient safety. Change requests that have a true patient safety impact are often given highest priority in terms of available resources to manage the change. An example of this type of patient safety issue is the removal of drugs from order sets that have been determined to be unsafe. Often safety issues are managed through introduction of alerts, or stops in the system, which require the user to interact with the system in a very specific manner to stop an error from occurring.

User Requests

Requests by users of the system, based on their own unique needs, comprise a significant number of requests. Examples of these types of common requests are additional selection options in a structured list of assessment criteria or interventions, order sets developed, and clinical flowsheets moved, added, or deleted. Users may have very good knowledge of the functionality of the system and present very good ideas, or they may request changes that would negatively impact the system and that are in direct conflict with other requirements or system functionality. Processes should be in place to manage user requests and ensure that they meet the needs of the organization, as well as enhance the workflows and functionality of the system. Often, user requests may actually be in conflict with each other, or may have a downstream impact on some other workflow. Prioritization and use of decision trees as to how the organization makes these decisions are important considerations when managing scarce resources in HIT staff.

Strategic Development

Finally and perhaps most important, changes need to align with the ongoing vision, mission, and future strategic goals of the organization. Strategic plans should include impact on the EHR, and future development and additional implementations should be considered in the ongoing management of the EHR. In addition, planning for regular upgrades and enhancements to the system should be part of the strategic plan budgeted and planned for on an ongoing basis.

Governance

In order to have a successful change management and sustainability plan, a strong governance model is fundamental. Governance consists of the leadership and organizational structures and processes that ensure that the organization's information technology sustains and extends to the organization's strategies and objectives. Governance programs can help define the prioritization of information technology (IT) projects, how changes are identified and managed, and the approval process for requests. Governance programs provide the structure around the change process, including the organizational goals. Important questions for organizations to consider related to governance are: (a) To what extent do the end-user clinical staff provide inputs or contribute to decisions about changes? (b) How are changes communicated to staff? (c) How often are changes put in place? and (d) How are the resources to make the changes allocated?

A governance program defines all these requirements and provides methods for how requests are entered, reviewed, approved (or denied), prioritized, implemented, communicated, and put into production. Although developing a governance program seems straightforward, it is often very difficult to create and manage a governance program. Staff need a way to make requests and have those requests approved in a timely manner. Often, the requests far exceed the available resources to meet the demand, and it is difficult to know which requests should move forward. Also, having end-user input is important to any governance program, but it is often difficult to define user groups and maintain them over time, so getting consensus on requests from users may be difficult or slow.

Nursing informaticists have a key role to play in helping manage the governance process. They are uniquely positioned to facilitate the management of the clinical need for requests, manage end-users expectations, and assist IT with how to translate requests into functional requirements, and manage training and communication to staff who are affected. A governance program generally evolves over time, through many iterations, and nursing informaticists are a key part of any governance discussion and process to achieve success.

Downtime Contingency Planning for the EHR

The unavailability of the EHR can represent a potential patient safety event, disruption of patient care, or negative impact to the work of the clinician. Organizations must have a plan in place to manage both documentation and access to patient information for clinical decision making in the event the system is unavailable, resulting in a system "downtime." An organization's policies and practices for managing continued patient care and business practices when systems are unavailable is the business continuity plan (BCP). Organizations are required to have BCPs in place as a component of the HIPAA security rule and staff should be aware of the practices outlined in the contingency plan to maintain safe patient care should they face a system downtime (Ruano, 2003).

There are several reasons why the EHR may be unavailable. Often systems require downtime for maintenance, upgrades, or other planned events. These planned downtimes are coordinated between the technical and clinical resources to best manage the downtime. This is typically coordinated during night shift when there is the least impact on patient care and busy daytime activities. These types of downtimes are communicated, and staff should be aware of how to maintain ongoing access to information during the downtime. An unplanned downtime may occur when there is any interruption in access to the system. This could be due to an application failure, such as the application itself failing for some reason. In this case, other systems may be operational, but one or more systems are offline. Another type of downtime is due to a network failure, where the systems may be working, but there is no access to the applications by the clinicians due to the network failure. In this type of downtime, many systems may be impacted, including all computers and other applications that run on the hospital network.

Organizational policies should guide staff on how to respond and manage when the system is down. This may include when to transition to "downtime procedures," how to print reports of patient information, how to access paper-based forms for documenting, and downtime recovery. EHRs have functionality that allows the user to either view data during a downtime, or ways to print out reports with patient data up until the time of the downtime. It is up to the organization to define the practices around this functionality. In addition to knowing when to move to downtime procedures, and what is required to be entered into the EHR after the downtime, it is also critical to understand how to manage other procedures that may be impacted by a system downtime. BCMA or other device integration and the transfer of data to other systems need to be acknowledged and managed during a downtime.

Safe HIT has several criteria to help minimize the potential for a system failure or downtime of the EHR resulting in risk to patient safety. The criteria are presented as checklists geared for self-assessment. The recommended practices are outlined in the Contingency Planner Safety Assurance Factors for the EHR Resilience (SAFER) guide. This guide is designed for self-assessment in nine areas to support organizations in safer use of EHRs. One of these nine areas is contingency planning. There are worksheets for each of the nine areas that begin with a checklist for recommended practices. We encourage the reader to visit the ONC's website and walk through all of the SAFER guide principles, which are complete with interactive references and supporting materials, and guide the end user through how to assess an organization (HealthIT.gov, 2014). The SAFER guide breaks assessment into three phases. The first phase relates to hardware, equipment, paper backup, data and software backups, policies, and procedures for patient identification. Phase two of the assessment relates to using HIT safely, including staff training on downtime and recovery procedures, communications strategies, policies, and procedures on continuity of safe patient care; the user interface of the maintained backup or read-only EHR is clearly differentiated. The third phase is focused on the monitoring and testing approach used to prevent and manage EHR downtime. The authors suggest that the reader review the SAFER guide on the HealthIT.gov website for detailed information and tools on how to address patient safety and Health IT through use of this guided process (http://www.healthit.gov/buzz-blog/electronic-health-and-medical-records/safer-guides-optimize-safety).

IMPACT OF NURSING INFORMATICS

NI has a significant impact on all aspects of the EHR. From project planning, to implementation, to sustainability, NI is critical to the success of the organization's ability to manage their EHRs. When looking at the scope and standards of NI, it is easy to align NI with the EHR, from the planning, to communication and training, to implementation, and then governance and optimization. Nursing informaticists are key in understanding and affecting all aspects of the EHR. Nursing informaticists in hospitals have a primary responsibility of working with clinical staff and promoting the use of the EHR in clinical practice, helping ensure proper workflows, adoption, and identification of optimization opportunities. It is imperative that they understand both the clinical side of patient care and the EHR as a tool to promote and support patient care, while also understanding the IT needs and requirements for ensuring a solid EHR development and build, while managing with IT resource availability and change management processes. Over time, NI can establish an identity, not just within nursing and not just within IT, but as a unique profession and contributor to a body of knowledge used to advance technology and the EHR for clinicians and to improve patient outcomes while promoting nursing efficiencies and patient safety.

CASE STUDY: A SUPERUSER AT THE GO-LIVE OF THE EHR IN THE EMERGENCY DEPARTMENT

A hospital within a large integrated delivery system was scheduled to go live with their EHRs. The chief nursing informatics officer had protocols in place to train both the staff and the superusers for all units. Superusers were trained thoroughly on the EHR in advance and dedicated to the exclusive assignment to support the staff on the unit during go-live and thereafter.

The superuser for all units is an experienced clinician working within the unit. In the ED, volume for that particular ED had significantly increased over the past year and there were staffing shortages. Additionally, many of the nurses were older nurses with significant ER experience, but very little computer experience. In contrast, there were also new, young nurses with very little experience in the ER, but computer literates who considered themselves to be advanced PC users.

On the day of go-live, the superuser looked up to see one of her proudest and most efficient ED senior nurses reduced to tears. The nurse was very frustrated, stating, "How am I going to learn something like this new system with a full patient load and be expected to accurately document on all these patients?" The nurses were specifically told: "Do not document later, but document in real time."

The savvy superuser assessed where she was with her EHR documentation, determined what her immediate clinical support needs were, suggested that they delegate certain clinical tasks, and the superuser assumed some of the critical nursing tasks herself so that the nurse could calmly focus on documenting in the

(continued)

CASE STUDY: A SUPERUSER AT THE GO-LIVE OF THE EHR IN THE EMERGENCY DEPARTMENT *(continued)*

EHR. The superuser continued to be available to the nurse and others as a resource for the EHR.

1. What did this superuser do that was important to reinforcing the training of this staff nurse on the EHR?
2. How can we think in terms of training professionals in the future on systems that prepare them for real-time documentation using the EHR?
3. Could we consider using simulation as a means for advance training? If so, how do we consider developing simulation labs that simulate the clinical environment, such as this busy ED?
4. Are there other things this superuser might have considered doing to support her unit? If so, what might she have done?
5. How did this superuser use adult learning theory?

SUMMARY

This chapter has covered important aspects of EHRs in the clinical setting. We have briefly explored the history and current drivers of our HIT push for a fully connected health information infrastructure throughout the United States. Benefits of the EHR for improving patient safety and quality have been discussed, particularly as this relates to certified technology under the HITECH Act. We have paid significant attention to ways to adopt, implement, and maintain an EHR. Special attention has gone into outlining the importance of aligning interprofessional teams through the process of implementation. Roles, such as the informaticists, clinicians, information technology analysts, superusers, and others, have been discussed in terms of supporting adoption, implementation, sustainability, and maintenance. In addition, we have emphasized the importance of POC technology that interfaces with the EHR, and focused on important aspects of adoption, implementation, and maintenance that should be considered by organizations. This chapter aligns with best practices for SDLC and takes into consideration important safety factors such as downtime planning. Finally, we close with the importance of governance and the NI role within the governance infrastructure.

EXERCISES AND QUESTIONS FOR CONSIDERATION

Resource Required: Season 9, *Grey's Anatomy*, "The Perfect Storm"

Download or purchase this episode from *Grey's Anatomy*, Season 9. Watch the disaster that occurs in this fictional film. Although this is, perhaps, an overdramatization of a natural disaster and subsequent events, there are a number of important lessons organizations can learn from this episode when preparing for major downtime issues. This story reflects a number of important components that relate to HIT with respect to disaster preparedness, technology, and business continuity. Watch the episode and reflect on the following questions:

1. With respect to technology, how were the hospital staff, patients, and clinicians impacted by the storm?
2. What business continuity issues compounded the situation?
3. Was this hospital prepared for this event with respect to its business continuity planning?
4. What happened to the EHR and how did they try to prepare in advance for the downtime of the EHR during this natural disaster? Did it work effectively?
5. What about POC devices that support patient care, medication administration, and other supportive devices that critically impact care?
6. What happened with these devices and how might these events have been mitigated?
7. What other issues did you see in this television show that will help organizations think through preparedness for business continuity and downtime of critical POC technology such as what is reflected in this show?
8. Which of the HIPAA regulations does this episode relate to and how?
9. Outline a plan to prepare an organization for such an event, including how you might simulate and prepare staff.

REFERENCES

Armijo, D., McDonnell, C., & Werner, K. (2009). *Electronic health record usability: Evaluation and use case framework* (No. 09(10)-0091-1-EF). Rockville, MD: Agency for Healthcare Research and Quality.

Atherton, J. (2011). Development of the electronic health record. *Virtual Mentor, American Medical Association Journal of Ethics, 13*(3), 186–189.

Bell, B., & Thornton, K. (2011). From promise to reality achieving the value of an EHR. *Healthcare Financial Management, 65*(2), 51–56.

Blumenthal, D. (2011). Wiring the health system: Origins and provisions of a new federal program. *New England Journal of Medicine, 365*(24), 2323–2329. doi:10.1056/NEJMsr1110507

Braak, J. V. (2001). Individual characteristics influencing teachers' class use of computers. *Journal of Educational Computing Research, 25*(2), 141–157.

Dick, R., & Steen, E. B. (1991). *The computer-based patient record*. Washington, DC: National Academies Press.

Dick, R. S., Steen, E. B., & Detmer, D. E. (Eds.). (1997). *The computer-based patient record: An essential technology for health care* (Revised ed.). Washington, DC: The National Academies Press.

Gugerty, B., Maranda, M., & Rook, D. (2006). The clinical information system implementation evaluation scale. *Journal of Studies in Health Technology and Informatics, 122*, 621–625. Retrieved from http://ebooks.iospress.nl/publication/9287

Health Information and Management Systems Society. (2013). *What is interoperability?* Retrieved from http://www.himss.org/library/interoperability-standards/what-is-interoperability

Health Information and Management Systems Society. (n.d.). *Why do we need interoperability standards*? Retrieved from http://www.himss.org/library/interoperability-standards/why-do-we-need-standards

Health Information Technology for Economic Clinical Health Act. (2009). Public Law 111-5 American Recovering and Reinvestment Act of 2009, Title XIII Health Information Technology for Economic and Clinical Health Act.

HealthIT.gov. (2014). *Safety assurance factors for EHR resilience (SAFER): Self assessment contingency planning* (No. SAFER-012014). Office of the National Coordinator for Health Information Technology. Retrieved from https://www.healthit.gov/sites/safer/files/guides/safer_contingencyplanning_sg003_form_0.pdf

HealthIT.gov. (2015). *How to implement EHRs*. Retrieved from www.healthit.gov/providers-professionals/ehr-implementation-steps/step-5-achieve-meaningful-use

Health Level Seven International. (n.d.). *About health level seven international*. Retrieved from http://www.hl7.org/about/index.cfm?ref=nav

Institute of Medicine. (2001). In R. Briere (Ed.), Executive Summary. *Crossing the quality chasm: A new health system for the 21st century* (2001). Washington, DC: National Academy Press. Retrieved from http://www.nap.edu/openbook.php?isbn=0309072808

Jamoom, E., Beatty, P., Bercovitz, A., Woodwell, D., Palso, K., & Rechtsteiner, E. (2011). *Physician adoption of electronic health record systems: United States, 2011*. NCHS data brief, no 98. Hyattsville, MD: National Center for Health Statistics.

Jha, A. K., DesRoches, C. M., Campbell, E. G., Donelan, K., Rao, S. R., Ferris, T. G., . . . Blumenthal, D. (2009). Use of electronic health records in U.S. hospitals. *New England Journal of Medicine, 360*(16), 1628–1638. doi:10.1056/NEJMsa0900592

National Center for Research Resources. (2006). *Electronic health records overview* (No. NCRR-2006). McLean, VA: National Institutes of Health, National Center for Research Resources. Retrieved from http://www.himss.org/ResourceLibrary/ResourceDetail.aspx?ItemNumber=10878

National Institutes of Health. (2010). *Point of care diagnostic testing*. (Fact Sheet No. NIH-2010). Washington, DC: Author.

Poon, E. G., Keohane, C. A., Yoon, C. S., Ditmore, M., Bane, A., Levtzion-Korach, O., . . . Gandhi, T. K. (2010). Effect of bar-code technology on the safety of medication administration. *New England Journal of Medicine, 362*(18), 1698–1707. doi:10.1056/NEJMsa0907115

Rogers, E. M. (1995). *Diffusion of innovations* (4th ed.). New York, NY: The Free Press.

Rogers, E. M. (2003). *Diffusion of innovations* (5th ed.). New York, NY: The Free Press.

Ruano, M. (2003). Understanding HIPAA's role in business continuity, disaster recovery. *Confidence, 11*(10), p. 3. Retrieved from http://library.ahima.org/xpedio/groups/public/documents/ahima/bok3_005209.hcsp?dDocName=bok3_005209

Sahin, I. (2006). Detailed review of Rogers' diffusion of innovations theory and educational technology-related studies based on Rogers' theory. *Turkish Online Journal of Educational Technology, 5*(2), 14–23.

Sittig, D. F., & Ash, J. S. (2007). *Clinical information systems: Overcoming adverse consequences*. Boston, MA: Jones & Barlett.

Smith, J. B., Lacey, S. R., Teasley, S., Hunt, C., Kemper, C. A., Cox, K., & Olney, A. (2012). The Information Systems Evaluation Tool (ISET©), 2nd Edition. Kansas City, MO: Childrens' Mercy Hospitals & Clinics.

U.S. Food and Drug Administration. (2014). *Medical devices: Products and medical procedures*. Retrieved from http://www.fda.gov/MedicalDevices/ProductsandMedicalProcedures/default.htm

The White House. (2004). *Promoting innovation and competitiveness: President Bush's technology agenda*. Retrieved from http://georgewbush-whitehouse.archives.gov/infocus/technology/

CHAPTER **8**

Systems Development Life Cycle for Achieving Meaningful Use

Susan McBride and Susan Newbold

OBJECTIVES

1. Review the systems development life cycle (SDLC) as it relates to product development and system implementation and compare and contrast differences in development versus system implementation.

2. Analyze the SDLC framework and identify each phase and the components of each phase using a four-cycle approach.

3. Understand important tools and competencies necessary for informatics professionals to master SDLC.

4. Examine case studies using SDLC aligning SDLC with meaningful use guidelines, incentives, and the certification program for EHRs.

5. Examine a case study using best practices for SDLC to demonstrate use of the technique.

6. Discuss new methods available to design systems in rapid cycles and to use object-oriented methods for design.

7. Discuss meaningful use in terms of SDLC, comparing and contrasting the roll out of EHRs under meaningful use federal guidelines, product development, and implementation as a case study examining the SDLC framework.

KEY WORDS

meaningful use, systems development life cycle, project management, assessment, implementation, evaluation, request for information, request for proposal, return on investment, cost–benefit analysis, waterfall, rapid application development, agile, commercial off-the-shelf products, unit testing, system testing, integration testing, alpha testing, beta testing, big-bang implementation, command center, core implementation team, superuser

---
| CONTENTS |

INTRODUCTION

The systems development life cycle is a standardized approach used to develop and implement information technology. This framework is often used across industries to structure best practices with regard to information technology development and deployment. It is a phased approach used to analyze and design information systems that is broken into distinct phases (Kendall & Kendall, p. 4). Health information technology (HIT) projects can be deployed in a haphazard manner, or can follow a structured and methodical approach such as with the SDLC. The phases of SDLC are essentially synonymous with the phases of project management with both requiring planning, analysis, design, implementation, and evaluation. This chapter outlines the SDLC framework, discusses each phase, and concludes with a case study that examines the approach used in the United States to deploy electronic health records (EHRs) under the meaningful use requirements.

SYSTEMS DEVELOPMENT LIFE CYCLE

The SDLC is a methodology used to describe the process of building information systems. This approach offers a road map for the development of information systems in a very deliberate, structured and methodological way. The SDLC is also used in software development and is a process of creating or altering information systems. Figure 8.1 reflects the phases within the SDLC. We examine each of these phases and discuss the importance of these steps in deploying information systems. There are some differences in developing products and information systems compared to implementation of new systems or upgrading systems. We discuss those differences within the chapter, and point out the differences in each stage of the SDLC.

Overview of the SDLC

SDLC is a process used by a systems analyst or software engineer to develop an information system that includes extensive planning and analysis that informs the development and evaluation strategies for the information system requirements. One of the most important aspects of SDLC is aligning the needs of the intended customer with the deliverable; if you miss the intended purpose and need of the end user, the project

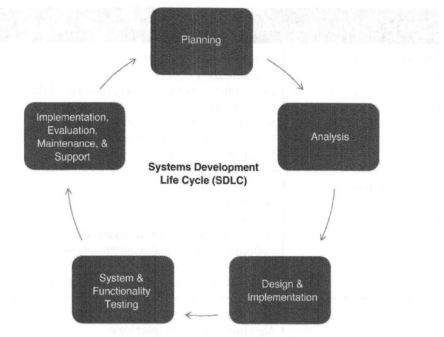

FIGURE 8.1. Phases of the SDLC.

will fail. Successful projects meet or exceed customer expectations. This is the primary goal of SDLC. To accomplish this goal, it is critical that human factors science in the area of human–computer interaction be considered. Zhang, Carey, Te'eni, and Tremaine, (2005, p. 518) define human–computer interaction (HCI) as "an aspect of a computer that enables communications and interactions between humans and the computer. It is the layer of the computer that is between the humans and the computer." Any SDLC should result in a high-quality system that meets or exceeds customer expectations, reaches completion within time and cost estimates, works effectively and efficiently in the current and planned information technology infrastructure, and is inexpensive to maintain and cost-effective to enhance (Newbold, 2014). Although experts disagree on exactly how many phases are found within the SDLC framework, we examine the approach using a five-phase approach noted in Figure 8.1 (Dennis, Wixom, & Roth, 2012, p. 11). We review each of these phases and discuss the importance of completing each phase prior to moving to the next. Table 8.1 reflects important components of each phase.

Planning Phase of SDLC

The first phase of the SDLC is establishing a plan that comprises the overall project goals, including what the project will entail, also called "the scope of the project." It is important to see end-user requirements and to align the scope of the project with clear requirements and understanding of the costs related to the proposed benefits of the new system. The planning phase sets the foundation for a successful project. Key objectives include

TABLE 8.1 SDLC Phases and Important Components of Each Phase	
System planning	System-planning concepts—project management, organization Understand strategic goals and priorities of the organization Vendor, product, and market analysis ROI—Resource considerations and benefit analysis Establishment of the team
System analysis	Needs assessment Feasibility assessment Process analysis Process diagrams—workflows and decision trees Collection of functional requirements—specifications Write an RFP or RFI Participation in system selection and contract issues
System design	Critical success factors Algorithms and principles logic Principles of hardware, software, and interoperability design Process redesign and reengineering concepts Logical database design Physical database design Data and system integrity and security Quality assurance and auditing
System implementation and testing	Implementation strategies System and functional testing Documentation of policies, procedures, and training—user and system Education and training Conversion and "go-live"
System evaluation, maintenance, and support	Operational Technical Financial Social and cultural Enhancements and upgrades User support Backup, recovery, and system monitoring

RFI, request for information; RFP, request for proposal; ROI, return on investment; SDLC, systems development life cycle.

identifying the goals, setting the scope of the project, engaging stakeholders, identifying required functionality, and evaluating costs and benefits.

System-Planning Goals

In the planning stage of system development, selection or deployment of clinical information systems, identification, and assessment are key steps. Important questions to consider are *What do end users or customers need out of the system? Who are the key players in the success of the system? What competencies and tools are needed to effectively function in a systems-analyst role in the planning-goal stage of SDLC?* In order to plan for systems development and implementation, we must have knowledge of the problem, the magnitude of the project, the outcome anticipated, and the finances needed to accomplish the work. We can examine the approach taken with both system development and system selection and implementation; there are some differences to consider. Table 8.2 shows a parallel comparison of the two. Finally, in this section we examine a case study on system selection to determine best practices and tools necessary to be successful in this phase of the SDLC.

In systems development, it is important to fully identify customers' needs and the high-level functionality required by the end users. In commercial industry, it is critical to understand the target market and the market size (market analysis). Key stakeholders should be identified at this stage. For system selection and implementation of a new system, the problem or opportunity for improvement should be clearly examined and understood. The scope of the project is defined with a clear understanding from all stakeholders as to the outcomes expected, as well as all dependencies documented.

TABLE 8.2 Planning Goals for System Development and System Selection and Implementation

System Development	Systems Selection/Implementation
Identify Customer needs High-level functionality Target market and market size Key stakeholders	**Identify** Problem or opportunity Scope Desired outcome Key stakeholders Dependencies
Assess Align with company goals and strategic direction Capabilities of competition Business case	**Assess** ROI Cost: Budget for personnel time, hardware, licensing fees, supplies, and other costs Identify both tangible and intangible benefits

ROI, return on investment.

With respect to assessment when planning goals for system development, it is critical that the project align with company goals and strategic direction. It is also important to identify capabilities of major competitors and to establish the business case for the new product. When assessing the selection and implementation of a new information system, establishing the return on the investment is the major goal. In order to fully accomplish that, an analyst needs a thorough budget, including all personnel's time, hardware, software, licensing fees, supplies, and any other anticipated costs necessary to deploy the system. In addition, both tangible and intangible benefits to the new system should be identified and documented.

System-Planning Tools

Planning tools for product/systems development in this phase include stakeholder analysis, market surveys, and feasibility analysis. Used as system analysis for vendor product development, market surveys include literature reviews, Internet searches, and trade shows. These types of investigations are to be based on the full scope of the competitive market to inform your strategy for product development that will compete in the marketplace and either meet or exceed your market's expectations. Feasibility analysis includes the technical feasibility of developing the system/product and resources required to develop the product for market.

In system implementation, one's most important tool for planning is a customer site visit. Although a systems analyst will thoroughly plan and evaluate products on the market that will meet goals and expectations, seeing the product in place in other institutions is an important way to evaluate how the product will work within your institution. Therefore, some of the most important tools needed for the planning phase include surveys, requests for information (RFIs), requests for proposals (RFPs), analytic tools, gap analyses, and spreadsheets. A proficient systems analyst will master competencies in all of these types of tools.

Informatics Roles in the Planning Phase of SDLC

In addition to a systems analyst role within the planning phase of SDLC, system development and implementation involve interprofessional teams used to accomplish effective planning. Table 8.3 highlights some of the additional roles and skills necessary for both system/product development and system implementation. Many of these roles and skills are discussed later as an output from the process.

System-Planning Outputs

In product development, outputs from the planning phase include a product concept document. This document includes the summary of the customer needs, proposed solution, and potential market for the product. A feasibility assessment is also an output from the process, as well as a product scope document. The product scope document includes the major components the product will and will not contain from a functionality standpoint. In this stage of the SDLC product development, a decision to "go" or "no-go" is made. The organization examines the feasibility and product documentation to determine whether resources necessary to develop the product/system are warranted.

TABLE 8.3 Informatics Roles and Skills Needed for the Planning Phase of SDLC

System Development	Systems Selection/Implementation
Market and user researcher	Project manager
Subject matter expert	Subject matter expert
Systems analyst	Systems analyst
Author of product concepts and scope documents, feasibility assessments, and other artifacts of planning	Author of project charter, gap analysis, system selection plan, RFIs, RFPs, and other artifacts of planning
Respond to RFIs and RFPs	Change manager

RFI, request for information; RFP, request for proposal; SDLC, systems development life cycle.

In system implementation, output also includes a feasibility assessment; product charters are also important output for this stage of SDLC. Project charters clearly outline the goals of the project, measures of success, and define parameters of the project to prevent scope creep. Scope creep occurs when a project expands beyond the project's immediate deliverables and often occurs if a project plan or project charter does not clearly define what is and is not within the deliverable. Another important output for the planning phase involves the team formation.

Implementation Committees and Teams

To begin, an implementation committee is created and a project team that will actually deploy the project is formed. The implementation committee informs "the what and how" and the project team actually accomplishes the "what and how" of the project plan. The committee is responsible for overseeing the project, whereas the project team comprises the technical team that will actually implement the system. Project plans and timelines are also important output that keeps the implementation team on track, and the committee informed of progress. Table 8.4 outlines important committees and teams that are often in place for planning effective information systems.

Feasibility Studies

Feasibility studies are important elements to consider when examining technical, operational, and economic feasibility. Feasibility grids are important tools and a good way to objectively evaluate various product options when selecting a product, or to determine the feasibility of developing a new product or system. Questions to consider in a feasibility study are *Will the technology meet the functionality required of the end users? Will the system work in our environment? Can we afford the system? What are the estimated costs of purchase, maintenance, hardware, software, communications, and human resources?*

TABLE 8.4 Important Structures to Establish in the Planning Phase of SDLC	
Typical Implementation Committees	**Typical Project Teams**
Executive committee	Project core group or build team
Data governance committee	Testing team
Information technology steering committee	Change management/communication team
Physician advisory committee	Training team
	Support team

SDLC, systems development life cycle.

Project Charter

Project charters are important tools used by the informaticist to master system development, deployment, and utilization. Creating project charters is often the first step of project planning. Project charters should include the following basic elements:

▶ *Project champion*: Name of the individual who will "champion" the cause and act as either a formal or informal leader within the organization. Ideally, an executive who can secure the funds for the project is an ideal project champion, or a provider who can harness the support of other providers to adopt and embrace the new system.

▶ *Dates*: This includes the initiation date and the target date for completion.

▶ *Problem or opportunity statement*: An example of an opportunity statement might be: Delay in timely electronic completion of medication orders resulting in higher than expected medication errors caused by tardiness of medication delivery.

▶ *Objective*: An example of an objective relating to the opportunity statement aforementioned might be: To implement a barcode administration system within the nursing department.

▶ *Key stakeholders*: Key stakeholders include clinical leaders, frontline caregivers, information technology (IT) staff, clinical engineering, and other important individuals who might be impacted by change under the project charter.

▶ *Scope*: Scope refers to the parameters of the project and clearly differentiated boundaries as to what the project does and does not entail.

▶ *Target benefits*: Clearly defined benefits that will result when the charter deliverable is accomplished; in the barcode administration project one might expect the target benefit to be a 20% decrease in medication errors relating to timely administration.

▶ *Budget*: The estimated total cost of the project.

CASE STUDY

Obstetricians within Hospital Baby Friendly are threatening to take all of their deliveries to the competitive hospital across the street. The major competitor hospital has the capability for providers to access remotely the EHR of both mom and baby with direct access as well as health information exchange within the region, in addition to maternal and fetal monitoring of all their laboring patients. Your chief executive officer (CEO) has asked you to assess and plan an upgrade of your obstetrical unit within the next 12 months, so that the institution does not lose market share. She wants a cost–benefit analysis done on upgrading the system with an estimated budget, and three vendors to consider in negotiations. She has also indicated that this cannot interfere with plans to meet meaningful use by year end.

As a system analyst, you follow SDLC phases and begin the process of goal planning. Priority setting would include selection, adoption, and implementation of a new system that meets the specifications of the providers and interfaces with the current EHRs in the health care system within the next 12 months. Key stakeholders are nursing staff, providers, and patients.

The first thing you note is that selecting a new system for the obstetrical unit with provider remote-monitoring access of laboring mothers will ultimately improve quality of care for mothers and babies in the institution, improve patient and provider satisfaction, and result in an increased market share for the hospital. This goal clearly aligns with the institution's vision to be the premier hospital for the region, and the mission to promote quality, efficiency, and patient-centered care. The increased quality of care and increased patient and provider satisfaction are intangible benefits, whereas increased market share for the institution equates to tangible dollars. In the planning goals, it is important to identify end-user requirements and, in this case, a clear requirement from the providers was the ability to see the obstetrical and neonatal monitoring information remotely from home or office; to have direct access to the EHR, including mobile technology; and the ability to interface with the regional health information exchange. This goal constitutes a high level of functionality. After you select the team that will include physician, midwifery providers, and obstetrical and neonatal nurses, you elect to have an expectant mother help to inform the decision (one of your nurses who will deliver on the unit in the coming year). You examine goals for the organization of the project and establish priorities, timelines, and your next step is to hear from stakeholder's the specific requirements so that you can distribute an RFI from vendors that you are aware will interface with your existing EHR; the ideal option would be to consider your EHR's obstetrical module, which your institution has not implemented. You know this would be your best option if you are to have your ideal interface to the HIE, mobile computing, and maintaining continuity of care for provider access to mothers and babies' EHRs in the obstetrical unit, nursery, or neonatal intensive care unit. You also know this will impact your cost–benefit analysis and ROI because this is likely your most expensive option. However,

(continued)

CASE STUDY (*continued*)

long-term cost of interfaces to a modular approach will also be an issue and the decision to select a modular approach will have implications for reaching meaningful use requirements. These factors will play into the high-level budget estimates you will prepare and the RFI will specifically ask the vendors how they will address these interface issues, the costs associated with them, and how they will guarantee the product will align with your institution's timeline for reaching meaningful use within the 12-month period. Your budget estimates to your CEO will include these costs on all three options, as well as manpower (personnel) costs, timelines for delivery, consulting, training, hardware, and software.

This case demonstrated how a systems analyst would approach goal planning in the first phase of SDLC. The system analyst identified the goals that would meet high-level functionality required by stakeholders, engaged stakeholders, noted dependencies; prepared an RFI; and examined costs and benefits. The analyst used tools and skills, including conducting the needs assessment, performing the gap analysis between the vendor product options, preparing the RFI and feasibility analysis on all product options, as well as focusing on project management and financial, budget-planning competencies. Project management software and spreadsheets were important software needed to support the goal-planning phase. This systems analyst served not only as the analyst but also as the project manager and change manager, which typically is the case with health care projects in systems planning.

Analysis Phase of SDLC

This section covers in more detail the portion of SDLC related to the analysis phase of systems development and implementation. Analysis is the study of current practices during which end-user requirements for new applications are defined. Key objectives include outlining end-user requirements, data flows, processes and workflows, outlining detailed system specifications, and conducting market analysis.

System-Analysis Goals

System-analysis goals are needed to fully understand and prioritize the gaps in existing products and systems and how the development will address those gaps. In order to effectively analyze, it is important to create a visual depiction of processes and data flows. We cover workflow redesign in Chapter 9 with steps used to accomplish effective planning with adoption, implementation, and evaluation of EHRs and other information systems. Data flow is different in terms of what is mapped and is an important aspect of development and implementation of information systems. Data flow maps answer the question: *How does the data currently flow and how will data to transformed or used within the system?* Data maps are critical to data integrity within new or upgraded systems. As such, data workflow and process maps are fundamental elements of the analysis phase. In addition to these important maps, functional and technical specifications documents are essential. Functional specifications outline the end-user requirements, whereas design specifications define programmer instructions and require technical detail from which coders will develop the product.

When implementing systems in the analysis phase, market surveys are frequently done to assess options for selection and implementation. In addition, tools are developed that provide an objective scoring mechanism for selecting a product. This is a component of the system selection process and is typically developed from the RFP. The RFP is used as a structural guide and from the RFP one determines scores based on functional requirements. What does the end user weigh most heavily, and what might he or she be able to live without? The necessary elements of the RFP are scored more highly than those that are constituted as "nice to have." Other aspects of the analysis phase may also include contract analysis and issues of mitigation or negotiation with prospective vendors. The final component of the analysis phase results in a recommendation and may be in the form of a white paper or report to executive leadership on the decision. Table 8.5 outlines system-analysis goals under both development projects and system selection and implementation projects.

System-Analysis Tools

In the analysis phase of SDLC, analysis tools may include various analytical methods, including both qualitative and quantitative data-analysis methods. Some common qualitative methods include focus groups, observational studies, and artifact analysis. Quantitative tools include RFP and RFI scoring tools to quantify the best product that fits the need of the organization. In addition to these tools, context diagrams, clinical

TABLE 8.5 System-Analysis Goals in SDLC

System Development	System Selection/Implementation
Understand and prioritize gaps and needs	Conduct a detailed assessment of gaps and user needs to understand "must have" functionality of desired system
Understand the diagram-related workflows, data flows, and processes	Conduct market survey
Document functional and technical specifications	Develop RFI and RFP
Outline the anticipated impact of the new system on existing processes and outline future-state workflows, data flows, and processes	Establish a system-selection process, including decision scoring methodology
	Assess organizational readiness for change

RFI, request for information; RFP, request for proposal; SDLC, systems development life cycle.

workflows, and data-flow diagrams are considered "tools of the trade" for the analysis phase of SDLC. Current state assessments and future state assessment are often done in terms of workflow redesign methods and are covered extensively in Chapter 9.

System-Analysis Outputs

Analysis outputs in system development include a report to stakeholders, interviews, and end-user requirements; outputs should also include regulatory requirements. For example, if you are developing products for the cardiac catheterization lab that will connect and interface with cath lab equipment, this may likely constitute a Food and Drug Administration (FDA)-approval process. The output process will also include product scope documents, functional requirements, and technical requirements from which the product can be developed.

In system implementation, common output from the analysis phase of SDLC includes prioritization of end-user requirements, workflows, data flows, and RFI and RFP, product demonstrations, customer reference calls or site visits, product selection scoring documents, final recommendation, and a readiness assessment. This phase of output includes reports, diagrams, and more reports. This output phase requires extensive documentation in both development and implementation types of informatics projects.

Informatics Roles in the SDLC Analysis Phase

Informatics roles for the analysis phase of SDLC include similar roles to the planning phase. These roles are outlined in Table 8.6 with identification of specific roles for system development compared to the roles for system implementation.

Design Phase of SDLC

The design phase of the SDLC is essentially the configuration stage of the SDLC. This is the phase during which the major goal is to convert all the design work into functional and technical requirements software, or in the case of selection and implementation of a new system (example might be an EHR); typically these systems do not come "out of

TABLE 8.6 Informatics Roles for the Analysis Phase of SDLC	
System Development	**Systems Selection/Implementation**
Subject matter expert	Project manager
Systems analyst	Subject matter expert
Author of functional specifications, current and future state diagrams, and other artifacts	Systems analyst
Author of product concepts and scope documents, feasibility assessments, and other artifacts from planning	Author of detailed user requirements, current and future state diagrams, RFIs, RFPs, and other artifacts

RFIs, requests for information; RFPs, requests for proposal; SDLC, systems development life cycle.

the box" ready to use. Commercial off-the-shelf (COT) products require customization. This work is either contracted with the vendor or a service company, or it is done in-house with the design team. This work, regardless of development or implementation of a COT product, requires close alignment with end-user requirements.

System-Design Goals

The goals of systems design in the case of systems development are to convert the functional and technical specifications into software applications in the form of programming code. Prototypes are considered "quick and dirty versions of the system" (Dennis et al., 2012, p. 54). The prototype is tested against the plan, including the vision and scope documents. Hardware and software configurations and interfaces are tested. In addition, with commercial off-the-shelf (COTS) products, system selection, implementation, and template customization are the primary goals. This is the case with our certified EHR products, in which a product is selected and customized for use by an organization. Table 8.7 compares differences in goals for the development approach compared to the system selection and implementation approach. The approaches are similar with development and include a "test run" of the system, but both require that the system, which the team is either building or buying, closely aligns with end-user requirements.

System-Design Tools

Tools for the design phase include software for design and development, different methods for development, and project management tools. The tools for the systems-design phase are similar regardless of build-versus-buy strategies. Table 8.8 compares the types of tools often seen in the development of a system compared to the selection and implementation of a COT product. Note that the output from the analysis phase becomes the development team's blueprint for the system development; likewise, for selection of a system, the analysis drives the configuration activities. With both approaches, project management is an overarching goal and, as a result, tools that support project management are critical to success.

TABLE 8.7 System-Design Goals in SDLC	
System Development	**System Selection/Implementation**
Develop teams and write code to convert functional and technical specifications into software applications	Customization of software, including data elements, documentation templates, and screen design
Usability testing of prototypes and early product versions lead to system enhancements	End-user input and engagement for customization to meet the customers'/clinicians' needs
Stakeholder reviews to ensure that what is built matches the original vision and scope	

SDLC, systems development life cycle.

TABLE 8.8 System-Design Tools in SDLC	
System Development	**System Selection/Implementation**
Software/programming code	Vendor system configuration, including databases, data dictionaries, and documentation forms, flow sheets for screens, security profiles, process redesign maps
Product prototypes	Change management and end-user educational artifacts (e.g., start, stop, continue maps)
Software applications	Project management tracking artifacts
Software development progress-tracking artifacts	Clinical and administrative committee review minutes and approval documents

SDLC, systems development life cycle.

System Configuration in Design Phase

System configuration includes equipment requirements, including computers, processors, and devices necessary for the system either under development or pending implementation. Typically, these specifications are important considerations in the planning and budgeting phases of the project and should be taken into account early in the process. This phase of the SDLC cycle requires creation of the detailed plan on how the configuration that was planned and budgeted will actually be configured in the clinical setting.

Situational Analysis in Design Phase

A situational analysis is also an excellent tool for this stage of SDLC. A situational analysis is a means of scoping and analyzing the broad context or the external environment in which the technology will operate. The following elements or steps have been recommended by the International Union for Conservation of Nature (IUCN). Although not explicit to HIT projects, the process has relevance to this phase of SDLC given the importance of designers fully understanding the context for which they are implementing a system. This is particularly relevant for public HIT projects. The steps for performing a situational analysis are as follows:

1. Define boundaries to be included in the situation awareness that are relevant to the project.

2. Analyze the current state and conditions of people, including identification of trends and pressures requiring attention.

3. Analyze key stakeholders, including groups of people and institutions with a right mandate or interest in resources and their management in the geographic area of the potential project.

4. Design the stakeholders' participation strategy.

5. Perform a current state analysis.

6. Perform gap analyses (International Union for Conservation of Nature, n.d).

Project Management Tools in the Design Phase

Project management is an essential tool of the design phase of the SDLC because it is required to keep implementation and development projects on time, in scope, and within budget. The PMBOK® guide defines project management as: "the application of knowledge, skills, tools and techniques to project activities to meet project requirements" (Project Management Institute, 2013, p. 5). The PMPOK Guide is used by project management professionals as a resource to apply the 47 logically grouped processes categorized into initiating, planning, executing, monitoring and controlling, and closing. We recommend the use of PMBOK as a best practice for project management and refer the reader to the current edition of this guide for more detail on approaches and tools that interprofessional teams can utilize to manage HIT development, selection, and implementation projects (Project Management Institute, 2013, p. 5).

Gantt Charts in SDLC

Gantt charts are an important tool utilized by project managers within the SDLC worthy of focused consideration. The Gantt chart is a specific type of graphic depiction of the project that displays the tasks or activities against a timeline that must be accomplished within the design or implementation project. Karol Adamiecki, a Polish engineer dating back to the 1890s, initially conceptualized the first Gantt chart. The Gantt chart in its more current form was developed from Adamiecki's ideas by an American engineer working in the steel works industry, Henry Gantt. The Gantt chart, according to Gantt.com (2013), allows you to see at a glance:

► What the various activities are

► When each activity begins and ends

► How long each activity is scheduled to last

► Where activities overlap with other activities, and by how much

► The start and end date of the entire project (www.gantt.com/2013)

EHR Project Plan Samples

A typical project plan for an EHR implementation was provided by the American Medical Association (AMA) to members supporting efforts to implement EHRs across the country. Figure 8.2 reflects a sample project plan for EHR implementation. In addition, the Centers for Medicare & Medicaid Services (CMS) had a major initiative to implement EHRs in ambulatory settings that predates the HITECH Act in the form of the doctor's office quality-information technology (DOQ-IT) program, resulting in tools and resources available online (DOQ-IT, n.d.). Quality-improvement organizations across the country were responsible for implementing EHRs in hundreds of clinics. Many of the tools developed out of that program were subsequently used and matured under the HITECH Regional Extension Center program. The basic project plans for implementing EHRs reflect a sample plan developed under DOQ-IT by MassPro under contract to CMS.

Project plan: EHR Implementation			
Task	Duration	Start	Finish
Assessment	5 days	1/8/2006	1/13/2006
Select product selection group	0.5 day	1/9/2006	1/9/2006
Select project development team	0.5 day	1/9/2006	1/9/2006
Complete needs assessments	2 days	1/9/2006	1/10/2006
Develop project charter	5 days	1/9/2006	1/13/2006
Develop preliminary budget	3 days	1/9/2006	1/11/2006
Document current workflows	5 days	1/9/2006	1/13/2006
Patient/provider flow	5 days	1/9/2006	1/13/2006
Filing system for medical records	5 days	1/9/2006	1/13/2006
Telephone triage	5 days	1/9/2006	1/13/2006
Lab results reporting and resolution	5 days	1/9/2006	1/13/2006
Assess office space	5 days	1/9/2006	1/13/2006
Medical records	5 days	1/9/2006	1/13/2006
Exam rooms	5 days	1/9/2006	1/13/2006
Support staff	5 days	1/9/2006	1/13/2006
Patient check-in area	5 days	1/9/2006	1/13/2006
Nursing stations	5 days	1/9/2006	1/13/2006
Share project charter with organization	N/A	1/8/2006	1/8/2006
Planning	10 days	1/9/2006	1/20/2006
Develop general project timeline	1 day	1/9/2006	1/9/2006
Outline key milestones and deliverables	1 day	1/9/2006	1/9/2006
Develop communication plan	2 days	1/9/2006	1/10/2006
Preliminary vendor selection	5 days	1/9/2006	1/13/2006
Educate vendor selection team on EHR requirements	5 days	1/9/2006	1/13/2006
Research potential vendors	5 days	1/9/2006	1/13/2006
Write script for vendor demonstration	1 day	1/9/2006	1/9/2006
Develop and distribute vendor evaluation tool	2 days	1/9/2006	1/10/2006
Contact vendors to set up demonstrations	0.5 day	1/9/2006	1/9/2006
Assess hardware, office configuration options based on assessments	5 days	1/9/2006	1/13/2006
Develop preliminary chart abstraction strategy	10 days	1/9/2006	1/20/2006
Develop preliminary implementation strategy	3 days	1/9/2006	1/11/2006

FIGURE 8.2. Sample EHR implementation project plan from the CMS Doctor's Office Quality-Information Technology (DOQ-IT) program.

EHR, electronic health record.

Source: MassPro (2006).

Selection	15 days	1/8/2006	1/27/2006
Assess practice workflows	2 days	1/9/2006	1/10/2006
Demo products with vendor selection team	10 days	1/9/2006	1/20/2006
Conduct reference checks (site visits or telephone calls)	5 days	1/9/2006	1/13/2006
Meet with vendor selection team to select vendor	N/A	1/8/2006	1/8/2006
Select hardware vendor	5 days	1/9/2006	1/13/2006
Reassess hardware based on selected vendor	5 days	1/9/2006	1/13/2006
Negotiate contract with hardware vendor	15 days	1/9/2006	1/27/2006
Negotiate contract with software vendor	15 days	1/9/2006	1/27/2006
Develop project change control process	2 days	1/9/2006	1/10/2006
Sign contracts	N/A	1/8/2006	1/8/2006
Major update for practice and stakeholders	N/A	1/8/2006	1/8/2006
Implementation	90 days	1/8/2006	5/12/2006
Update project plan with vendor deliverables and dates	5 days	1/9/2006	1/13/2006
Develop pre-training plan based on vendor options	5 days	1/9/2006	1/13/2006
Update implementation strategy	2 days	1/9/2006	1/10/2006
Update chart abstraction strategy	2 days	1/9/2006	1/10/2006
Develop go-live plan	2 days	1/9/2006	1/10/2006
Develop new office workflows	15 days	1/9/2006	1/27/2006
Major update for practice and stakeholders	N/A	1/8/2006	1/8/2006
Install hardware	90 days	1/9/2006	5/12/2006
Install software	90 days	1/9/2006	5/12/2006
Install network and peripherals	90 days	1/9/2006	5/12/2006
Convert data from old system to new system	90 days	1/9/2006	5/12/2006
Test and implement interfaces	90 days	1/9/2006	5/12/2006
Training	5 days	1/9/2006	1/13/2006
Go-Live	N/A		

FIGURE 8.2. (*continued*)

The plan is reflected in Figure 8.2. Additional resources are available to walk a provider through adoption and implementation steps at the following website: http://www.ddcmultimedia.com/doqit/index.html.

In both project plans, you see common components that align with the SDLC selection and implementation goals. Creating a valid and reliable project plan that the team adheres to and one that uses time frames to stay on track and on budget is an important goal for the development stage of SDLC. The DOQ-IT project plan also lists estimated days for each component of the project. This provides an excellent planning guide for organizations to consider when implementing EHRs in the ambulatory setting.

System-Analysis Outputs

Outputs for the design phase of the SDLC are very concrete and structured products of the process. These outputs include such things as system developers' software/programming code, product prototypes, software applications, software development documentation, including tracking of progress and any artifacts. For system implementation, the output includes vendor system configuration documents and a number of elements, which are included in Table 8.8. Change management documentation for the vendor or the design team is an output of the process, as is the end users' education plan and content for deployment. Project management plans are outputs expected in this phase, as well as clinical and administrative committee reviews and approval documents.

Informatics Roles in the SDLC Design Phase

Informatics roles and skills in the design phase require advanced skills and competencies in several areas. In addition to roles that typically align with traditional technology development and implementation projects, there are critical needs in this phase for informatics specialists in several areas. These areas are highlighted in Table 8.9 and discussed in the following section. These roles include significant responsibilities of the development team actually creating a product and content-matter experts informing the design to management overseeing the project.

TABLE 8.9 System-Design Roles and Skills

System Development	System Selection/Implementation
Software/programming code	Vendor system configuration, including databases, data dictionaries, and documentation forms; flow sheets for screens; security profiles; and process redesign maps
Product prototypes	Change management and end-user educational artifacts (e.g., start, stop, continue maps)
Software applications	Project management tracking artifacts
Software development progress-tracking artifacts	Clinical and administrative committee review minutes and approval documents

There are also important functions that are in line with clinical informatics contributions that include designing systems with appropriate display of patient-level data for clinical decision making, design input, database structure, and reports to identify trends to align with quality initiatives, translating end-user requirements into technical specifications. A critical role that nursing informaticists and other clinical informatics specialists frequently play in design teams is to bridge the communication divide between the technical content experts and the clinical end users. In addition, nursing informaticists also customize data elements and forms to meet the clinical needs of the environment where the tool will be utilized, as well as make recommendations for programming changes so that legacy systems fit with the design of the system being developed or implemented. Of particular importance are workflow considerations and interfaces with respect to retrofitting legacy systems with newer technology.

Design Implications Under the Disability Accommodations and Americans With Disabilities Act Requirements

The requirements of the Americans with Disabilities Act (ADA) are an important design consideration for any system within the health care industry. This is not only a consideration for patients who are often disabled, the very reason for interacting with the health care system, but is also a consideration of employees within the health care industry. The ADA was passed into law in the 1990s and its purpose is to protect individuals with disabilities from discrimination in employment and programs offered by state and local governments, and in accessing services that include providers' offices and hospitals (ADA.gov, 2010). As such, during the design phase the developer and the implementer are required by law to take into consideration ADA requirements. When evaluating vendors or assessing the development of a system, a review of the requirements under the ADA is important to consider. Table 8.10 provides resources for developers and implementers to consider relating to the ADA and use of computers and technology.

The AMA advises providers that they need to take into consideration patient access to remote mobile devices and other consumer access portals, including the patient portals, with respect to the ADA. The AMA provides an example of a patient provided with a computer tablet who is asked to register in the clinic with the device. The woman responds that she is unable to do so because she is blind. The woman reports that she had to have the clerk assist her, providing her personal information to someone who otherwise should have had the right to have the information accessible. The AMA provides the following guidance regarding steps to consider for technology in the clinical setting: (a) understand the law, (b) electronic tools or eResources must be useful to patients and employees, (c) conduct self-audits of electronic equipment and software to assure it is compliant with the ADA using consultants if necessary, and (d) utilize available resources to stay well informed (Gallegos, 2013). We provide information to access several of the resources provided by the AMA in Table 8.10.

Methods and Strategies for Designing and Developing Systems

There are a number of design strategies used within software development, including the waterfall method, rapid application development (RAD), and agile techniques; these are highlighted in this section. We conclude by discussing object-oriented design strategies.

TABLE 8.10 Americans With Disabilities Act Design Consideration Resources

Description of the Resource	Website
Americans With Disabilities Act (ADA)	www.ada.gov/
Adapted Computer Technologies is expected to be an industry leader and partner in the field of assistive technologies	www.compuaccess.com/ada_guide.htm
Job Accommodation Networks Accommodations and Compliance series: *Employers' Practical Guide to Reasonable Accommodation Under the American Disabilities Act* (downloadable PDF guide)	http://askjan.org/erguide/ErGuide.pdf
Americans With Disabilities Act design standards	www.ada.gov/2010ADAstandards_index.htm
Web Content Accessibility Guidelines, the World Wide Web Consortium, December 2008	www.w3.org/TR/WCAG/
Federal Information Technology Accessibility Initiative Website	www.section508.gov/
Information Technology and Technical Assistance Training Center	www.ittatc.org/
Center for Applied Special Technology—a nonprofit, educational organization working to expand educational opportunities for all	www.cast.org/
ADA Best Practices Tool Kit for State and Local Governments, Department of Justice, May 7, 2007	www.ada.gov/pcatoolkit/chap5toolkit.htm

Waterfall Development

A waterfall approach to development occurs in a cascade fashion with analysts and users proceeding in a sequenced manner from one phase to the next. The phases are linear in approach and do not cycle back around to inform the former stage. When the phase documentation is complete and the documentation approved, the phase is completed and the next phase begins. See Figure 8.3 for the waterfall approach to development.

Rapid Application Development

The rapid application development (RAD) approach, also referred to as "RAD," resulted from weaknesses inherent in the waterfall approach. RAD deploys software tools and analysis and design strategies to speed up development. The goal is to get systems rapidly into the hands of the end user to test and refine the product to meet the end-user requirements. See Figure 8.3 for examples of two types of RAD development: iterative development and system prototyping. Iterative development is defined (Dennis et al., 2012, pp. 54–55) as a method that "breaks the project into a series of versions that are developed sequentially." The most important components are prioritized and developed initially and deployed in the first version using a "mini-waterfall" approach. Once implemented the end user critiques and provides feedback for incorporation into the next version of the product. The system prototyping method is a design strategy that concurrently addresses the analysis, design, and implementation phases to develop a simplified product, provided to end users to critique and to provide development feedback that is incorporated into the next version of the product (Dennis et al., 2012, p. 54).

Agile Development

Agile development is a technique that is a programmer-driven method that creates a feedback loop with the end users. This technique is based primarily on verbal communication with the end user and does not rely on documentation strategies, as do the waterfall and RAD techniques. The face-to-face interaction with stakeholders is critical to this approach of development. Cycles are typically kept short with feedback loops on small components of the deliverable being turned back to the end user for consideration of how well the product will meet the end user's needs. Cycles can be as short as 1 to 4 weeks in this type of development strategy. There are programming techniques used for this type of development: extreme programming, Scrum, and dynamic systems development. We refer the reader to Dennis et al. (2012) for details on these programming/development techniques.[1]

Testing Phase of SDLC

Prior to implementation of any newly developed system, rigorous testing should occur prior to go-live in order to ensure success. There are a number of tests required of systems prior to implementation. We highlight a number of these techniques and define the various types of testing that should be done prior to implementation of a new system.

Systems Testing Goals and Considerations

Prior to going live with a system that has either been developed or selected for implementation after customization for a clinical setting, a rigorous testing phase should occur. In the testing phase, the goal is to validate that the system works as intended, and to ensure that the components, features, interfaces, devices, reports, screens, and user interfaces are ready for end users in the "live" environment. Factors that are considered are: *Does the system work? Are the interfaces valid? Is it ready for use? Is the system easy to navigate?*

---

[1]Programming strategies are considered beyond the scope of this text.

Waterfall Development

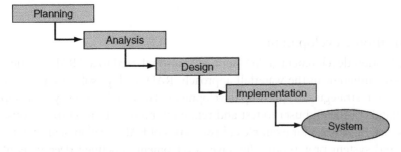

System Prototyping Development

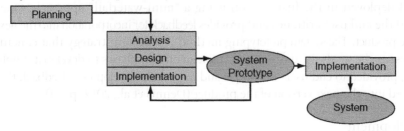

Interactive Development

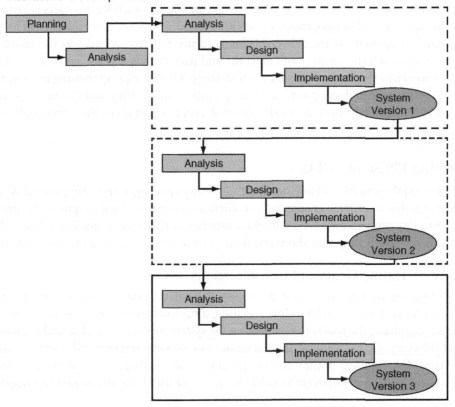

FIGURE 8.3. Design development methods: waterfall, RAD, and agile strategies.
Adapted from Dennis, Wixom, and Roth (2012).

Does the system have appropriate language or reference tables? Is it efficient and intuitive to use?

Testing prior to implementation reduces the probability that the team has missed something.

There are different forms of testing depending on the level of the component of the system. *Unit testing* is one specific component or module that performs a specific task. Integration testing is testing in which one or more modules or components work together (integrate) and function as designed. *System testing* is typically done by the system analyst to make sure the system functions as the designer understood it to be developed. *Integration testing* serves to test how well the different components work together, whereas system testing uses the business requirements to determine whether the system meets end-user specifications given the business it is determined to address. System level also tests the documentation of the product as to whether documentation is accurately reflected. *Acceptance testing* has two levels, alpha and beta testing. *Alpha testing* is done using test data or "made-up" data. *Beta testing* gets a step closer to production with a sample of "real" data to test how the system functions and looks for any errors that might arise.

System-Testing Tools

System-testing tools for development and implementation typically are found multiple system environments, including a build environment, testing environment, training environment, and production or live system. Many different testing types exist, including the tests noted earlier (unit, system, integration, alpha, beta, etc.). In addition to those just mentioned, load and volume testing are critical to confirm that the hardware, software, processing units and servers will handle the anticipated volume, and that response times for the system meet the expectations needed for the clinical environment or business case. Typically, there are test scripts that are used to run the system through the various types of tests. *Automated test scripts* are machine-based execution of the scripts, whereas *load and volume testing* typically employs simulation of simultaneous end users using the system.

System-Testing Outputs

Test results are the primary output of system development and implementation. This includes, at a minimum, the unit, integration, functional, and load/volume testing. The tests should be documented, including any errors or lack of performance and how those issues were rectified and retested for any problem areas prior to going live.

Informatics Roles and Skills in System Testing

Nursing informaticists are frequently used to test the system with scripts to validate data across the system with integration testing, end-user acceptance, system performance; they generally resolve any unanswered problems and questions that might arise in the testing phase. As such fundamental skill needs include the following:

Developing and executing testing plans, including scripts

Validating data integration across disparate systems

Assessing end-user acceptance and system performance (effectiveness)

Identifying and resolving issues with problem-solving and technical skills

System Implementation, Evaluation, and Support Phase

System implementation is the phase in which a system is brought into live use by the end users. When a system is implemented it also requires long-term strategies for ongoing evaluation, maintenance, and support.

Implementation and Support Goals

System implementation is the "go-live" phase of the project and as such requires critical planning prior to implementation of the system, particularly for clinical care. In many respects, implementing a new system is a culture change. An example of significant change is the shift of the paper-based medical record to the electronic record in the form of the EHR. To bring the system into everyday use by clinicians has been and continues to be a major challenge in institutions across the country as organizations press toward fully adopting and meaningfully using EHRs in Stages 1, 2, and soon in Stage 3 of meaningful use. In this phase, focus should be on end-user acceptance, system performance, and the ongoing maintenance and support plan. In routine maintenance, this includes patches and upgrades provided by the vendors. There are also significant concerns related to privacy and security in compliance with Health Insurance Portability and Accountability Act (HIPAA) regulations (see Chapter 14 for details on HIPAA). Supporting end users' needs and problems as they utilize the new system also constitutes a major goal for the implementation and maintenance phases of SDLC. Proper training on the new system is one of the most important components of the implementation phase.

System Implementation, Evaluation, and Support Tools and Strategies

Tools for system implementation, evaluation, maintenance, and support include strategy plans for go-live, data plans for conversion of older data into the new system, a command center and a user-support center. After go-live and moving into the maintenance stages, this function matures into a long-term help desk and clinical units typically have superusers available for help (a role discussed in detail in Chapter 7).

System implementation, evaluation, maintenance, and support include a period during which the system is "pilot tested" by end users prior to go-live. There are two approaches that organizations use with EHR implementation. They are the *phased or incremental approach* and the *big-bang approach*. With the phased approach, units or facilities within a health care system are incrementally brought up on the new system. With the big-bang approach, all units or hospitals in a system go live at once. There is also a third approach, *parallel systems implementation*, in which both the old and new systems are maintained until all units or hospitals transfer over to the new system. In health care, with respect to EHR adoption and implementation, we have seen all three of these approaches used by organizations. An additional tool is found in the form of logs for managing system issues and assessments of end-user needs. Frequently, organizations utilize surveys to assess end-user acceptance and identify areas for improvement planning. An additional critical consideration is contingency plans for both scheduled and unscheduled downtime of the system. Downtime forms, policies, procedures, and reinput data processes need to be addressed prior to implementation. Training materials are also a critical tool for the implementation and support phase of SDLC.

Implementation, Support, and Evaluation Output

Outputs for this phase of SDLC primarily include planning and communication documents. The communication plan is critical to success and requires extensive planning with the implementation team, stakeholders, and executive levels (see Box 8.1).

BOX 8.1 Communication Plan for Go-Live Implementation Phase of SDLC

The communication plan should include:

- ▶ Project communicators and the audience
- ▶ Communication format
- ▶ Communication strategy and change management
- ▶ Channels and elements of communication
- ▶ Stakeholder audiences
- ▶ Communication events
- ▶ Communication instruments and tools
- ▶ Feedback and monitoring effectiveness
- ▶ Communication responsibilities
- ▶ Communication between sites and the vendor project management team
- ▶ Communication to the project team
- ▶ Communications to the executive sponsors and project steering committee
- ▶ Communication log

The planning documents consist of communication plan, training and documentation plan, command center plan, data conversion and go-live plan, and downtime and recovery procedure plan. Current state and future state workflow redesign developed in the analysis phase need to be confirmed and potentially updated post go-live. Policy and procedure revisions are needed to cover the new workflows.

Education and Training Considerations With System Implementation

Educational resources for end users include vendors' sources, system analysts, externally contracted trainers, in-house trainers, other system users with prior experience on the system, and virtual classes. Training on the new system can take on multiple approaches with many organizations using a combination of the training methods that we cover in this chapter. Elbow-to-elbow training is one-on-one training of the end user. Frequently, providers in the ambulatory setting use this method so that patient care in busy clinics is minimally impacted; however, this is an expensive approach. Utilization of superusers described in Chapter 7 is often used by hospitals. This has proven to be a very effective way to bring nursing units onboard with a new EHR or point-of-care device. Staff training is frequently carried out in computer labs that are established for training. It may also occur in a dedicated clinical unit with no patient care occurring. The area is dedicated to training staff on the new system. Computer labs are often used for initial training on EHRs followed by hands-on unit support by the superuser, or elbow-to-elbow support after time spent in the computer lab. Timing of training is critical to success and should be as close to the actual go-live as possible. Large gaps in time from initial training to actual go-live diminish the end users' retention of how to use the new system.

Informatics Roles and Skills in Implementation, Evaluation, and Support Phase of SDLC

Informatics skills and competencies for this phase of SDLC are high-level skills and competencies that align well with graduate-prepared clinicians with expertise in informatics. For example, knowledge of planning, directing, and leading teams is a critical skill set for this phase of the SDLC. In addition, organizational skills for activities, such as assessing the system, logging and maintaining documentation of system issues, and documentation of issue resolution, are required skill sets for this phase. Educational and training support skills include creating and delivering educational training on the new system and supporting the superusers in their roles on the unit. Assessing, analyzing, and planning skills are also required to determine whether the system is meeting the needs of end users and to support planning for changes in the event the system fails to meet the end users' needs or disrupts clinical processes in some manner. Workflow redesign skills continue to be an important skill set combined with fundamentals of quality improvement to optimize the system for end users' needs. We will approach this in detail in Chapter 9 and further in Chapter 22. Frequently, nursing informaticists function in the capacity of an implementation manager. This requires strong leadership, excellent organization, clinical expertise, and the ability to communicate and motivate the end user. The implementation manager should know and understand the current workflows and how they will be redesigned, develop implementation teams that include clinicians, and have a strong working relationship with the project champion. Leadership that empowers clinicians, possesses strong group facilitation skills, provides direction and support for decision making, and enables timely and effective communication among stakeholders are important characteristics that an implementation manager must have.

Implementation teams include interprofessional representation. The members of the implementation team should include clinical experts, match skills with tasks, consider time constraints on the implementation, and have broad representation of all users. Go-live support may take the form of one or more of the following:

▶ *Command Center*: A 24-hour resource center on site for the first 3 days of each rollout.

▶ *Core Implementation Team*: The team is on site the first 24 hours and available by cell or pager for 2 weeks thereafter.

▶ *Superusers*: Coverage is available 24 hours a day, 7 days of the week on all units by a superuser who is familiar with the clinical unit and has been trained as a trainer on the new system. As is noted in Chapter 7, many organizations maintain superusers long term for maintenance and optimization of the EHR. There are two different types of superusers typically seen primarily in the hospital setting. This includes a unit-based RN superuser who is a resource for the staff on the unit. This individual's function is essential for unit buy-in and support. As is discussed in Chapter 7, this individual should not be assigned patients during shifts because she or he provides superuser support to the unit, particularly during go-live. There should be one superuser per unit during go-live covering all shifts. This individual may also perform chart audits to maintain the quality on the unit where he or she is the designated superuser. The other option involves the department RN superuser. This individual may assist with teaching classes and be a part of the support pool during go-live. This option is obviously less resource intensive, but does not maintain the vigil that the unit-based RN superuser provides.

Change management is a critical function of the implementation manager, as well as the implementation team. Change management includes acknowledging opinion leaders who are frequently the early adopters but can also be the resisters. It is important to recognize both, involve users from the beginning of the implementation phase, inform and communicate to users any progress made, respond to concerns in a timely manner, and focus on positive results. Having patience with end-users learning the system and with those resisting adopting the new system is important to the process. And finally, have fun! Activities units can carry out to make it a fun experience include naming the project, designing t-shirts, choosing a mascot, and taking on other similar initiatives. Texas Health Resources had a very creative chief quality officer, Robert Schwab, M.D., who wrote and recorded "The Ballad of Go-Live." The ballad, which was recorded to the tune of Simon & Garfunkel's "Homeward Bound," is a wry chronicle of exasperation and ultimate success in implementing the CareConnect EHR at Texas Health Denton. The CareConnect EHR system is now fully integrated into operations at all 13 wholly owned facilities in the Texas Health Resources family of hospitals. The authors encourage the reader to stop and listen to the following YouTube video as an excellent example of how to make implementation and go-live fun for an organization: www.youtube.com/watch?v= ZEDJku0-hcQ (Courtesy: Schwab & Texas Health Resources, 2012)

Metrics for System Evaluation

Determining what metrics to select for evaluation of the system after implementation is critical to long-term success of an information system. Considerations for metrics should include system stability, evaluation of the system with respect to the strategic plan originally formulated, cost avoidance, risk reduction, and long-range goals for the system.

ROI for electronic information systems and technology in the health care setting is an important consideration, but other success factors include improvements in quality, safety, and population health improvements. *How might the system improve market share, position the organization to participate in at-risk contracts, and better manage data to accomplish that business strategy?* Information systems, when well designed and implemented according to strategic plans for the organization, should better position the organization to succeed in long- and short-terms goals; as a result, the metrics for the system should align with the organization's business strategy.

System Maintenance

System maintenance includes securing the stable, but steady growth of the information system. Upgrades with clinical information systems are expected, particularly with the rapid change underway with EHRs and the stages of meaningful use requirements expanding capability under the HITECH Act. These upgrades are significant with each stage of meaningful use, with workflow redesign considerations, documentation, training, testing, and implementation needed with each major upgrade of the EHR. Budgeting for these types of expected upgrades is a part of the life cycle of a clinical information system.

SDLC: IMPLEMENTATION, ADOPTION, AND ACHIEVING MU: A NATIONAL CASE STUDY ON SDLC

This section discusses the importance of following best practices with respect to SDLC as we think in terms of development and deployment of EHRs in the health care setting. The current federal plan and the manner in which the plan was deployed are examined and discussed as a case study to compare and contrast what and how we deploy EHRs in the United States and to discuss how in many respects we have failed to follow recommendations as outlined by content experts in both the vendor and clinical settings. This section examines steps discussed earlier and recommends ways in which SDLC can be used to help reach meaningful use and address barriers seen in achieving meaningful use.

EHR Development in the United States Under the HITECH Certification Regulations

The federal initiative under the HITECH Act has implemented certification guidelines for all EHRs to lay a platform for the EHRs to be interoperable and to fully meet the intent of the meaningful use guidelines. The certification regulations go through the federal rule-making process and, as a result, are put out for public comment prior to release of the final rules (HealthIT.gov, 2014). CMS and ONC have received comments and responded to those comments in both phase one and phase two release of these guidelines, either indicating they have modified the regulations due to comments or indicating why they are not modifying them and justifying the decision. The response to these comments is also available in the public domain and frequently helps to clarify the intent of the guidelines. When we examine the timing on this feedback loop and the process that has occurred under phase one and phase two of meaningful use, given the SDLC recommended requirements for development of software, we question whether or not this timeline has sufficiently allowed best practice. This is one of the key points made by the Center for Healthcare Information Management Executives (CHIME) as a response to the ONC and CMS in delaying the implementation timeline for Stage 2 meaningful use (Conn, 2014). This presents the challenge we now face in optimizing these systems to work for the end user and to provide vendor feedback to work in partnership with our industry vendors in order to improve the use of these systems for the clinician. Interprofessional teams comprised of HIT professionals, nursing and clinical informaticists, clinicians using the systems for point of care, and other stakeholders are important to the optimization of these systems.

The EHR vendors have had very little time to actually review and interpret the meaningful use certification guidelines and develop products to those specifications. Given those timelines, we might assume that the vendors were using a rapid development and deployment strategies similar to the agile technique discussed earlier, yet the feedback from the market and end users was missing because of timeline constraints imposed by wanting to get the products into the market. EHR vendors had significant pressure to deploy software on rapid development cycles not only because of the certification timing but primarily because their customers or potential customers were looking for EHRs that met the meaningful use guidelines so that they could adopt and implement the certified product and be eligible for the CMS incentive payments under the HITECH Act (CMS, 2013).

Adoption and Implementation of EHRs Under the HITECH Act

The HITECH Act meaningful use guidelines for the providers and hospitals lay out a timeline for adoption and implementation that is incentivized by payments (CMS, 2013). With the incentives for hospitals being millions of dollars, this financial encouragement has created an unprecedented increase in the adoption and implementation of EHRs, which has occurred very rapidly across the industry (Office of the National Coordinator for Health Information Technology [ONC-HIT], 2013). Organizations have approached implementation from essentially one of two ways, either incrementally or through the big-bang approach. Many hospitals have used the big-bang approach to adopt and implement EHRs (Ludwick & Doucette, 2009). As we consider this rapid deployment of EHRs, it is an ideal case study to use to examine how we have either followed practices outlined in SDLC or failed to do so as an industry.

The ONC has emphasized that to achieve meaningful use of EHRs in the true sense of "meaningful use" requires commitment from the entire organization with a team management approach involving leadership, clinicians, and line staff such as front-desk staff, admissions, and unit clerks. ONC promotes meaningful use is a team sport, and has produced an infographic to emphasize that it takes the entire team to get to a full complement of meaningful use measures. The infographic in Figure 8.4 reflects not only the team required to achieve meaningful use but also the workflow redesign required with implementation to meet all of the meaningful use metrics.

SUMMARY

This chapter has covered SDLC and a four-phase approach, including planning, analysis, design, and implementation. Each phase has been examined in detail as to components that should be covered with each phase of implementation and development of health information systems. Strategies for development have been outlined, defined, and discussed, including waterfall, RAD and agile techniques. A clinical case study involving implementation of an obstetrical improvement has been presented in terms of best practices for planning and analysis, and the federal plan for meaningful use has been discussed, noting challenges of development timelines that presented challenges to the health care industry with adoption, implementation, and "meaningful use" of these systems. Finally, the reader is left with questions to consider regarding SDLC best practices and to draw conclusions as to how well we have done as an industry in adhering to these best practices. We must look to the future of evaluation and optimization of the EHRs to fully realize "meaningful use" for our clinicians and patients.

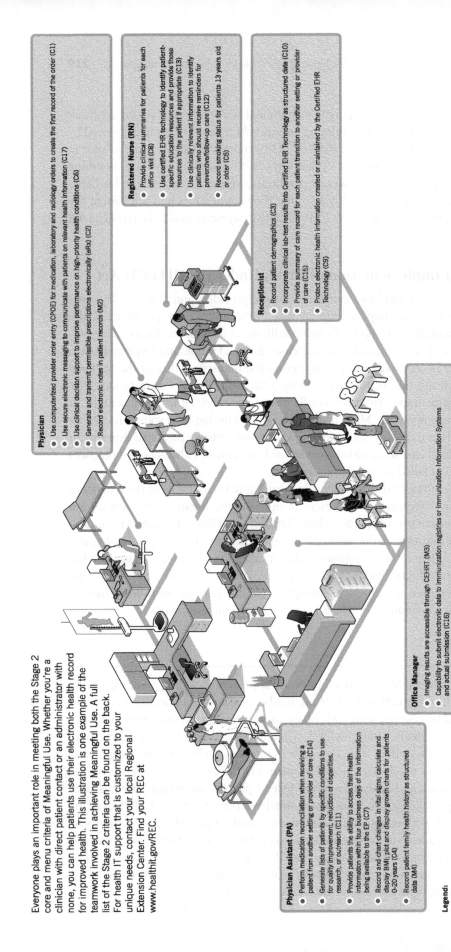

FIGURE 8.4. Meaningful use is a team sport.

Note: Image was provided to Regional Extension Centers working with providers to emphasize how to address barriers in implementation and adoption to successfully achieve meaningful use. The messaging emphasizes the importance of interprofessional teams.

CEHRT, certified electronic health record technology; EHR, electronic health record; EP, expert panel.

Stage 2 Meaningful Use

The Stage 2 definition of meaningful use includes both a core set and a menu set of objectives that are specific for eligible professionals. This gives providers latitude to choose their own path to full EHR implementation and meaningful use. Eligible professionals must meet 17 core objectives and three additional objectives from a menu of six. To learn more about the meaningful use objectives, visit www.healthit.gov.

Core Objectives

C1. Use computerized provider order entry (CPOE) for medication, laboratory and radiology orders directly entered by any licensed healthcare professional who can enter orders into the medical record per state, local and professional guidelines to create the first record of the order.

C2. Generate and transmit permissible prescriptions electronically (eRx).

C3. Record the following demographics: preferred language, gender, race, ethnicity, date of birth.

C4. Record and chart changes in vital signs: height; weight; blood pressure (age 3 and over); calculate and display BMI; plot and display growth charts for patients 0-20 years, including BMI.

C5. Record smoking status for patients 13 years old or older.

C6. Use clinical decision support to improve performance on high-priority health conditions.

C7. Provide patients the ability to view online, download and transmit their health information within four business days of the information being available to the EP.

C8. Provide clinical summaries for patients for each office visit.

C9. Protect electronic health information created or maintained by the Certified EHR Technology through the implementation of appropriate technical capabilities.

C10. Incorporate clinical lab-test results into CEHRT as structured data.

C11. Generate lists of patients by specific conditions to use for quality improvement, reduction of disparities, research, or outreach.

C12. Use clinically relevant information to identify patients who should receive reminders for preventive/follow-up care.

C13. Use CEHRT to identify patient-specific education resources and provide those resources to the patient if appropriate.

C14. The EP who receives a patient from another setting of care or provider of care or believes an encounter is relevant should perform medication reconciliation.

C15. The EP who transitions their patient to another setting of care or provider of care or refers their patient to another provider of care should provide summary of care record for each transition of care or referral.

C16. Capability to submit electronic data to immunization registries or Immunization Information Systems and actual submission except where prohibited and in accordance with applicable law and practice.

C17. Use secure electronic messaging to communicate with patients on relevant health information.

Menu Objectives

M1. Capability to submit electronic syndromic surveillance data to public health agencies and actual submission except where prohibited and in accordance with applicable law and practice.

M2. Record electronic notes in patient records.

M3. Imaging results consisting of the image itself and any explanation or other accompanying information are accessible through CEHRT.

M4. Record patient family health history as structured data.

M5. Capability to identify and report cancer cases to a State cancer registry, except where prohibited, and in accordance with applicable law and practice.

M6. Capability to identify and report specific cases to a specialized registry (other than a cancer registry), except where prohibited, and in accordance with applicable law and practice.

FIGURE 8.4. (*continued*)

EXERCISES AND QUESTIONS FOR CONSIDERATION

Considering the ONC's approach to fostering rapid development of EHRs according to meaningful use stages and vendors' requirements to rapidly develop to those requirements, reflect on the following questions:

1. Do you believe that hospitals and clinics have followed SDLC best practices as outlined in this chapter; if so, how? If not, why do you believe hospitals and clinics have failed to do so?

2. Consider for a moment that you are the executive oversight for an EHR vendor; how would you advise your development team to balance federal requirements and timelines with best practices for SDLC outlined in this chapter?

3. How could the industry have done things differently such that SDLC phases might have been easier to adhere to?

4. What metrics for evaluating EHRs should organizations consider to determine whether patient care is positively or negatively influenced by EHR adoption and implementation driven by the HITECH Act?

REFERENCES

ADA.gov. (2010). The Americans with Disabilities Act of 1990 and Revised ADA Regulations Implementing Title II and Title III: The 2010 regulations. Retrieved from http://www.ada.gov/2010_regs.htm

Centers for Medicare & Medicaid Services. (2013). *The official website for the Medicare and Medicaid electronic health records (EHR) incentive programs*. Retrieved from http://www.cms.gov/Regulations-and-Guidance/Legislation/EHRIncentivePrograms/index.html

Conn, J. (2014). *CMS proposes stage 2 delay*. Retrieved from http://www.modernhealthcare.com/article/20140524/MAGAZINE/305249961

Dennis, A., Wixom, B. H., & Roth, R. M. (2012). In B. L. Golub & Mills, E. (Eds.), *System analysis and design* (5th ed.). Hoboken, NJ: John Wiley & Sons.

DOQ-IT University. (n.d.). *Tools & references*. Retrieved from http://www.ddcmultimedia.com/doqit/ToolsandResources/index.html

Gallegos, A. (2013). Is your EHR ready for the ADA? *American Medical Association*. Retrieved from http://www.amednews.com/article/20130401/profession/130409984/4/

HealthIT.gov. (2014). *EHR incentives & certification: Certification process for EHR technologies*. Retrieved from http://www.healthit.gov/providers-professionals/certification-process-ehr-technologies

International Union for Conservation of Nature. (n.d). *Situational analysis: An approach and method for analyzing the context of projects and programmes*. Retrieved from http://cmsdata.iucn.org/downloads/approach_and_method.pdf

Kendall, K., & Kendall, J. (2014). *Systems analysis and design* (9th ed.). Boston, MA: Pearson.

Ludwick, D. A., & Doucette, J. (2009). Adopting electronic medical records in primary care: Lessons learned from health information systems implementation experience in seven countries. *International Journal of Medical Informatics*, 78(1), 22–31. doi:http://dx.doi.org.ezproxy.ttuhsc.edu/10.1016/j.ijmedinf.2008.06.005

MassPro. (2006). DOQ-IT University Sample Project Plan created by MassPro under contract to CMS. Retrieved from http://www.ddcmultimedia.com/doqit/EHR_Adoption/Planning/L2P9.html

MassPro. (n.d.). Doctor's Office Quality–Information Technology Program (DOQ-IT). *Tools and references.* Retrieved from http://www.ddcmultimedia.com/doqit/ToolsandResources/index.html

Newbold, S. (2014, November). *Systems development life cycle nursing.* Presented at the Nursing Informatics Boot Camp, Austin, TX.

Office of the National Coordinator for Health Information Technology. (2013). *How to implement EHRs.* Retrieved from http://www.healthit.gov/providers-professionals/ehr-implementation-steps

Project Management Institute. (2013). *A guide to project management body of knowledge* (5th ed). Newtown Square, PA: Author.

Schwab, R. (Producer), & Texas Health Resources (Director). (2012). *The ballad of go-live: CareConnect electronic health record implementation with new final verse.* [Video/DVD] Denton, TX.

Zhang, P., Carey, J., Te'eni, D., & Tremaine, M. (2005). Integrating human–computer interaction development into the system development life cycle: A methodology. *Communications of the Association for Information Systems, 15*(29), 512–543.

CHAPTER 9

Workflow Redesign in a Quality-Improvement Modality

Susan McBride, Terri Schreiber, and John Terrell

OBJECTIVES

1. Discuss the fundamentals of workflow redesign and the suggested steps needed to carry out workflow redesign within health information technology (HIT) projects.

2. Examine workflow redesign within a quality-improvement strategy to improve the practice setting using HIT.

3. Outline best practices within the health care industry, including practices established with cooperative work within the Regional Extension Centers across the United States, to use workflow redesign to rapidly deploy electronic health records (EHRs) and to optimize the use of EHRs in clinical settings.

4. Describe some simple steps in using common software available that can support you in designing workflows for your practice setting.

5. Discuss how acute care and ambulatory settings can use workflow redesign to address common barriers.

6. Examine case studies and how to apply the concepts described within the chapter to redesign workflow.

KEY WORDS

workflow, redesign, quality, Regional Extension Centers, meaningful use, barriers, electronic health records, LEAN management, project charter

CONTENTS

INTRODUCTION

Workflow redesign is a fundamental technique used within quality improvement that involves mapping a process to identify areas for improvement or change needed. In the case of implementing electronic health records, this may involve a change in process from paper to electronic records, or it may involve upgrading a system or adding components. In both cases, the focus on workflow is paramount in efforts to avoid the unintended consequences of electronic records use for patient care delivery (Jones et al., 2011).

Regardless of the change process, the techniques for workflow redesign are consistent. Process mapping is a graphic representation of the sequence and actions within a process. Process maps are used to document and learn about the work being performed. They are also used to identify areas of concern and opportunities to improve a process. There are different types of workflows that can be utilized to map a process and the ideal process map often depends on the process involved. Different types of workflow diagrams include the following:

▶ *Simple linear workflow diagrams*: A sequence of steps in a given process with connectors and links within the process depicted in the map.

▶ *Swimlane or cross-functional diagrams or flowcharts*: Flowcharts designed to distinguish a sequence of steps in a given process that show roles and responsibilities for each step.

▶ *Spaghetti diagram*: A layout diagram providing a geographic layout of a work space and how workers or a process move within that space. Each worker or component of a process can be tracked with a different color as the worker or component moves throughout a process.

▶ *Value stream map*: This map is often used in Lean management and documents all the activities within a work area to design, order, produce, and/or deliver a product or service. It is designed to measurably map a process for efficiency and is one of the more advanced process-mapping techniques.

▶ *SIPOC*: SIPOC stands for suppliers, inputs, process, outputs, customer. This type of map provides a high-level view of the process as well as who the suppliers are and what inputs they provide prior to the process and who the customers are and what outputs they receive from the process. Figure 9.1 presents an example of a SIPOC process map for a patient visit to an infusion clinic.

WORKFLOW REDESIGN AND MEANINGFUL USE OF EHRs

The Office of the National Coordinator for Health Information Technology (ONC-HIT) is the principal federal entity charged with nationwide efforts to promote the adoption of EHRs and other health information technology. The Medicare and Medicaid EHR

Suppliers	Inputs	Process	Outputs	Customer
Patient	Vitals results	1. Patient signs in	Completed treatment	Patient
	Lab work	2. Patient called to vital room	Future appointment scheduled	
Scheduling System	Patient appointment template	3. Patient moved to treatment room	Notification of room to be cleaned	Housekeeping
Pharmacy	Chemotherapy	4. Patient receives chemotherapy		
Materials Management	Nursing supplies	5. Patient discharged		

FIGURE 9.1. SIPOC process map example.

Note: A SIPOC map aids the user in showing how the process under investigation fits in with the system around it. This process is an example of a SIPOC for a patient visit to an infusion clinic.

SIPOC, suppliers/inputs/process/outputs/customer.

incentive program offers financial incentives to eligible providers and hospitals who demonstrate the "meaningful use" of certified EHR technology. To be reimbursed for adoption of this new technology, clinicians and other health care support staff must be using the EHR "meaningfully" and in accordance with federal guidelines that define "meaningful use." Criteria set by the ONC and Centers for Medicare & Medicaid Services (CMS) help guide providers in attaining meaningful use as they adopt EHR systems. Yet, providers often struggle with many of the measures within the meaningful use requirements. This often has to do with changes in workflow associated with adopting EHRs and capturing the health information required to meet meaningful use requirements. Additionally, implementation of technology in the clinical settings is an ideal time to stop and rethink processes with the goal of improving clinical quality and efficiency.

WORKFLOW REDESIGN IN A QUALITY-IMPROVEMENT MODALITY

In using workflow redesign within a quality-improvement modality, the goal is to improve patient safety and the overall outcome of care delivered. To accomplish this goal, you need to identify an area or priorities for improvement. We recommend that you start with the end in mind and create a project charter that involves metrics for improvement. For a quality-improvement team, the project charter outlines what the overall goals of the redesigned workflow or quality-improvement initiative are intended to accomplish. The charter becomes the road map for the team to construct and monitor their project. The project charter, coupled with Lean management techniques originally outlined by the Toyota Corporation is a fundamental model for achieving quality and eliminating waste. Lean management techniques compliment workflow redesign and HIT implementation focused on improvement. This chapter discusses best practices with respect to workflow redesign with a focus on quality improvement. The basics of workflow redesign are reviewed and some of the best practices developed from the work of the

TABLE 9.1 HealthIT.gov Tips for Utilizing Workflow Redesign for Quality Improvement	
Tip 1	Identify bottlenecks and inefficiencies in your current workflow. Decide which aspects of your workflow need improvement and prioritize them. Then do the work in stages, creating wins along the way.
Tip 2	Experiment with a new workflow in small ways, or test different ways of doing a task to identify what works best in your practice. Try using the PDSA method.*
Tip 3	Listen to staff. What sounds like resistance is often valuable information about a process issue.
Tip 4	Use standard workflow templates to get started and visualize how the work gets done. Then customize the templates to show the process works in your practice.

*PDSA is discussed in more detail in Chapter 22.

PDSA, Plan-Do-Study-Act.

Source: HealthIT.gov (n.d.).

Regional Extension Centers (RECs) along with case studies to demonstrate applications of steps in workflow redesign are also reviewed. Table 9.1 lists the HealthIT.gov tips for workflow redesign to be considered while developing quality-improvement projects (Office of the National Coordinator for Health Information Technology, n.d.).

Designing a Project Charter

The major issue that should be considered in workflow redesign is to frame the project in a quality-improvement modality. A project charter is an excellent framework to use to establish the plan for improvement and it aligns with LEAN management methods. Figure 9.2 presents a sample project charter with several metrics noted in the center of the charter. To begin the process, it is vital to identify the team that is closest to the process and that understands the components under consideration and goals for improvement. An important consideration is the project champion who is most likely to positively impact the process long term. This is frequently a provider/clinician leader who is willing to take ownership of the process and the improvement goals. Name the process you intend to improve, for example "E-Prescribing Workflow Redesign."

Other considerations in a project charter should include the following elements:

1. What practical problem will be solved?

2. What is the project's main purpose?

3. What metrics will be improved? What is the current performance for those metrics and how much improvement is targeted? Provide specifics on how metrics are computed.

4. Which process steps will be considered in this project? What is the first step and what is the last step?

5. What other scope considerations might exist? Are there constraints on the areas of focus? Are you including or excluding specific populations?

6. Justification for this project: Why is it important? Why is it critical to business success?

7. How will internal or external customers benefit from this project? How does improvement in the metrics that you have selected help them improve their performance?

8. Provide specifics about the project, including names and roles of team members, project timelines, including start and stop dates targeted.

9. Who will approve the project charter? This usually involves an executive champion who may cover any costs of the project, including cost of time spent by staff to accomplish the work.

10. What is the current state workflow map, or the "as is" process?

11. What is the future-state workflow map, or how does your team intend to redesign and improve the process?

12. What resources, people, and departments are required?

Measurement Considerations

Workflow redesign in a quality-improvement modality also involves consideration of the project charter with regard to how you will measure the improvement or impact of the redesign. Outcomes or process measures important to HIT often include financial impact, time, and processing opportunity for improvement, or clinical process or outcomes metrics. The impact of EHRs on financial impact has been a significant concern in many acute care and ambulatory practices, where processes are slowed down by inexperienced end users along with other human factors (Fleming et al., 2014). These areas are particularly relevant to workflow redesign in a quality-improvement modality and are often the target for measurement of a redesigned process relating to HIT.

BEST PRACTICES FOR WORKFLOW REDESIGN

This section discusses how to perform a workflow redesign and highlights best practices, developed from national work under the ONC and the Agency for Healthcare Research and Quality (AHRQ), to refine and recommend processes for workflow redesign. We cover a step-by-step process of how to approach a workflow redesign related to HIT and achieve meaningful use of EHRs as an example of how to effectively design and implement a workflow redesign project. This method for adoption and implementation has been encouraged by both AHRQ and ONC for effective and efficient adoption of EHRs in health care settings in both acute care and ambulatory practice settings.

As discussed earlier in Chapters 1 and 4, the ONC was authorized by the HITECH Act, through the American Recovery and Reinvestment Act (ARRA), and awarded grants for 62 RECs to assist at least 100,000 priority primary care providers in the adoption and meaningful use of EHRs. ONC and AHRQ also established the National Learning Consortium to support and gather best practices from Regional Extension Center (REC)

Team Leader	
Members of the Team	

Element	Description	Specifications				
1. Process	Name of process to be improved.					
2. Project Description	What practical problem will be solved? What is the project's purpose?					
3. Objective	What metrics will be improved, what is the current performance for those metrics and how much improvement is targeted? Provide specifics on how metrics are computed.	Metrics	Current	GOAL	% Improve	units
		Metric 1				
		Metric 2				
		Metric 3				
4. Process Scope	Which process steps will be considered in this project? What is the first step and what is the last step?					
5. Business Case	Justification for this project: Why is it important? Why is it critical to business success?					
6. Benefit to Internal and External Customers	How will internal or external customers benefit from this project? How does improvement in the metrics that you have selected help them improve their performance?					
7. Team Members	Names and roles of team members.					
8. Schedule	Project Start					
	Project Charter Approved					
	Current State Workflow Map					
	Future State Workflow Map					
	Project Completion					
9. Support Required	What resources, people, departments are required?					

FIGURE 9.2. LEAN project charter template.

collaborative efforts as they assisted providers with EHR adoption and meaningful use. One of the collaborative groups was the Practice Workflow and Redesign Community of Practice (PWR CoP). The REC members of the PWR CoP identified a series of priority ambulatory workflows and developed workflow diagrams to be used in assisting providers with workflow redesign, meaningful use, and quality improvement.

Steps to Workflow Redesign

The steps to workflow redesign developed within the Community of Practices (CoPs) and utilized by organizations across the nation follow a series of steps. We highlight and define those steps in the following section.

Identify Process to Be Mapped

Select the process that will be the focus of your improvement work. Start with the workflows that cause a majority of issues or involve the main service that you provide. That will facilitate the fastest workflow improvements and help to build momentum in your organization.

Identify and Involve Individuals Who Perform the Tasks

It is important to assemble the right team members who know the process and are committed to making improvements. It will increase the likelihood of redesigning an optimal process that will be integrated into the day-to-day work of those who are tasked with performing the process.

Map the Current State

Current state, also known as the "as is" process, is the existing workflow for a process. Mapping the current state will allow the team to analyze and identify bottlenecks and opportunities for improvement. Some simple tools that can be used to map the current state include a flip chart or white board, sticky notes, and a marker. Members of the team write the action or task, decisions, and other symbols on a sticky note and place them in order on the flip chart or white board and connect the tasks with arrows. The sticky notes can be rearranged on the board as needed. An advantage of using the sticky-note method is that it requires no special computer software or expertise. Information on how to use common software tools to create workflow diagrams is covered later in this chapter.

Start by walking through the process with the team. The team should observe and capture each task as well as the person who is responsible for completing the task. Also, consider noting the time it takes to accomplish each task. The team will be able to use that information to potentially reassign a certain task to another person if it has the potential for improving efficiency. As the team discusses and maps the current state, keep it focused on the "what" that is actually being done, not the way the policy says it should be. After a draft of the current state is mapped, validate the current state mapping with colleagues who are not on the team but who also perform the tasks.

One of the most frequently asked questions in process mapping is "how detailed should we be?" A process map should show enough detail to provide context for appropriate decision making. On the other hand, if a process is only viewed from a very high level, opportunities to improve may be overlooked. Oftentimes, it may be beneficial to make multiple process maps. One strategy to avoid unnecessary complexity is to start with a high-level process map and break steps identified as needing more understanding into more detail as needed.

Assess Current State Workflow and Identify Opportunities for Improvement

The team should consider any potentially new health information technology the organization has or is planning to adopt when assessing current state workflow. The team should have a solid understanding of the people and tools involved in each step, the number and types of issues encountered in each step, the time it takes to complete each step where the process is taking place, and the total number of steps involved in the process. An understanding of the current state is important for the identification of opportunities for improvement.

Identify Data to Be Collected for Measuring Redesign Outcomes

The purpose of collecting data before, during, and after workflow redesign is to detect whether a change is an improvement. After issues from the current state are analyzed, the team should set specific goals. For example, if the practice would like to improve the capture of smoking status in the EHR, the team should collect data about the number of patients with smoking status entered correctly before and after workflow changes have been implemented.

Map Future "To Be" Processes

Designing the solution for the future state should focus on the efficiency, effectiveness, and quality of care. Ideally, the future state will have fewer steps, faster tasks, and/or less opportunities for failure. Waste should be minimal. After the team has an understanding of the new process, it should map the future process using a diagraming tool so that everyone can visualize who will be doing which task.

Test New Workflows and Processes

Before deploying the new workflows throughout the organization, it is helpful to test the workflows in a controlled environment with as much variability as possible. Try testing the workflows during different times of the day and with a variety of individuals who will be performing the tasks. Adjustments can be made to the new workflows as needed.

Train Individuals on New Workflows and Processes

After the new workflows are field tested, it is important to take the time to properly train all individuals who will be performing the tasks. This important step will enable staff members to complete tasks with high quality, efficiency, and safety.

"Go-Live" With New Workflows

During "go-live" of the new workflows, it may be necessary to lighten the appointment schedule or patient load. It would also be helpful to have extra team members available to help coach individuals through the new workflow and solve any problems that may arise.

Analyze Data and Refine Workflows

At a set frequency, the team should analyze the data and determine whether goals are being achieved. If not, the team will need to investigate any bottlenecks and failure points. Based on the analysis, new workflows should be refined.

USING SOFTWARE TO SUPPORT WORKFLOW REDESIGN

There are several out-of-the-box software tools that allow users to create workflow diagrams by using drag-and-drop interfaces. One commonly used tool utilized in the health care industry for workflow maps will be used to demonstrate how to create a workflow diagram. The tool we utilize is Microsoft Visio Premium 2010 (Microsoft Corporation, 2014). Steps to designing a workflow in Visio are described later. We have also provided a template with standardized shapes used within Visio and other software applications that are common best practices for process mapping. The shapes include such elements

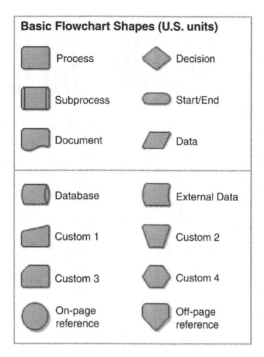

FIGURE 9.3. Common standardized process mapping shapes.
Source: Microsoft Corporation (2014).

as squares for steps in a process and diamonds for decision points (see Figure 9.3 for commonly used shapes in Visio; Microsoft Corporation, 2014).

Steps Needed to Create a Workflow Diagram

The steps used to create a workflow diagram in many of the software applications are similar. In Microsoft Visio 2010, the following steps are used to create a simple workflow diagram:

- ▶ Launch Microsoft Visio.
- ▶ Select a template or blank drawing.
- ▶ Click and drag shapes from the shapes column into the drawing.
- ▶ Double-click on a shape to add or edit text within the shape to describe the step in the process.
- ▶ Click on "Connector," highlight a shape, and drag to another shape to add lines with arrows to indicate the flow of steps or tasks in the process.
- ▶ Shapes and connectors can be resized and moved by clicking a corner and hovering over the object until the cross with arrows or diagonal resizing arrows appear.
- ▶ Shapes and connector can be deleted by clicking on the object and clicking the "delete" button on the keyboard.
- ▶ Save and name the diagram.

OFFICE VISIT WORKFLOW TEMPLATE

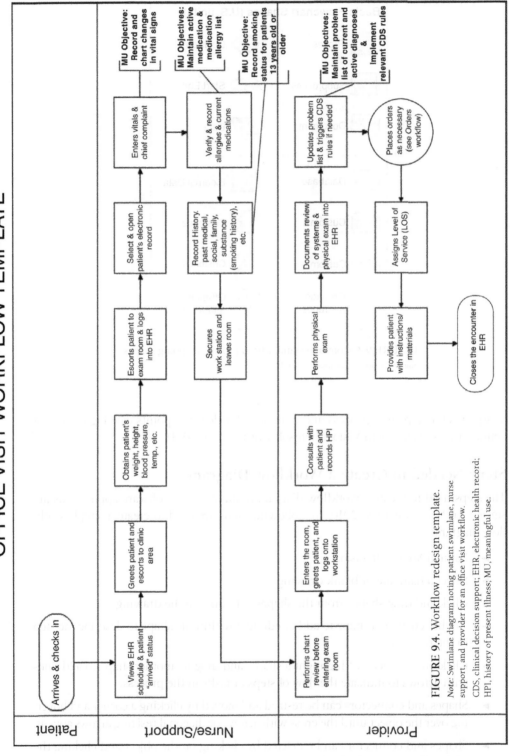

FIGURE 9.4. Workflow redesign template.

Note: Swimlane diagram noting patient swimlane, nurse support, and provider for an office visit workflow.

CDS, clinical decision support; EHR, electronic health record; HPI, history of present illness; MU, meaningful use.

The aforementioned steps reflect a basic workflow, but Visio enables the end user to design swimlane diagrams with roles and responsibilities depicted as well as shapes that reflect decisions, processes, data, documents, and other important functions you may wish to reflect in the diagram. See Appendix 9.1 for screenshots reflecting the steps mentioned here and other functions of Microsoft Visio.

Working With Templates

The RECs across the country focused a great deal of effort in designing support services for providers and small hospitals in workflow redesign of processes, as they adopted an EHR moving from paper to electronic environments, or as they upgraded old systems to certified EHR systems. The RECs participated in CoPs to collaborate and share lessons learned and best practices to help providers meaningfully adopt EHRs. One of these CoPs was focused on practice workflow and redesign (PWR). The PWR CoP identified a series of high-priority workflows in the ambulatory setting and developed templates to help providers kick-start the process of EHR adoption and meaningful use (Health Information Technology Research Center, n.d.). The workflow templates developed by the PWR CoP included "meaningful use" flags on certain steps within a process where meaningful use measures could be collected. Figure 9.4 illustrates a swimlane diagram reflecting the workflows for a routine office visit in the ambulatory practice setting. The full set of workflow templates developed by the PWR CoP is available at www.healthit.gov/node/291. Templates like the ones developed by the PWR CoP can help organizations by using the standardized templates to begin the process. The following are recommended steps for using a template:

1. Identify a template useful to the process you intend to improve.

2. Convene a group of stakeholders involved in the process and have the group examine the template and mark up (pen and paper or electronic approach) the template as to how their process differs from the one reflected in the template. This step frequently identifies additional steps that may equate to potential inefficiencies; often issues are noted by the end users in their notes on their process when comparing it to the template.

3. Use Visio or a similar tool to recreate the workflow based on the organization's notes. Your template may also be a Visio diagram that allows you to take the template into Visio and modify the diagram.

4. Return the modified workflow to your stakeholders and verify that what you have designed in the new workflow diagram is reflective of their process.

5. Finally, observe the process several times in the practice setting to validate that the workflow diagram represents all steps, roles, and responsibilities within the process. Frequently, end users do not always realize what "everyone" does in a process. Observation helps verify what is really occurring and not the perception of what the end user believes is happening. Again, issues in the process and inefficiencies are often identified through observation.

6. If changes are noted by the observer, they should be noted on the diagram and a third version of the diagram prepared.

7. Return to the end user and use the new diagram as an educational opportunity to inform all end users of what is actually happening with respect to the workflow and technology depicted. Use the diagram to identify opportunities for optimizing the technology, improving quality of care, and/or improving efficiencies (eliminating and streamlining process).

Ambulatory Workflows

Ambulatory settings include clinics for specialty and primary care or may also include more complex multispecialty clinics and federally qualified health care clinics. The following is a description of typical workflows in the ambulatory areas that a provider will need to address when attempting to accomplish meaningful use of the EHR.

▶ Patient check-in

▶ Office visit

▶ Appointment scheduling

▶ E-Prescribing

▶ Lab orders and results

▶ Referral generation

▶ Office discharge

Acute Care Workflows

Acute care has a plethora of workflow processes that might benefit from quality-improvement methods and workflow redesign techniques. We highlight a few of the common workflows that present challenges with respect to EHRs and achieving meaningful use. These workflows include admissions processing, medication management, and medication reconciliation, computer provider order entry (CPOE), and patient discharge process.

SUMMARY

This chapter has covered the basics of workflow redesign and has placed this important tool within a framework for quality improvement. The project charter has been discussed as an important mechanism for defining what you intend to do to improve the process, and how you will measure improvement and key components relevant to the redesign. Prior to beginning a workflow redesign project with any major impact to a practice setting, a project charter should be outlined. The chapter has provided an important overview of best practices defined under work done with the REC CoP for workflow redesign, and has identified key areas where workflow maps should be created in order to achieve meaningful use of health information technology in both acute care and ambulatory care settings.

CASE STUDY

The following are case studies highlight the need for workflow redesign. The case can be utilized to think through how you might create a project charter for improvement and construct a workflow redesign.

Case #1: The clinical setting is a small community internal medicine practice that includes eight providers—four physicians, two nurse practitioners (NPs), and two physician assistants (PAs). The practice is pushing hard to get to meaningful use under the Medicare incentive program because the incentive dollars are significant to offset their EHR adoption and implementation expenses. Their largest patient population has Medicare and private insurance. The E-Prescribing rates are very low at less than 10%.

Provider interviews within the assessment process used to examine "as is" workflow status includes the following with respect to findings:

Providers have sent prescriptions that have not been routed to the pharmacy and they do not understand why. Several of the providers refuse to use the EHR for E-Prescribing and would rather handwrite prescriptions and give them to the patient. The senior physician is frustrated by the system and now refuses to use it, stating "I will retire before I will use this system—it doesn't work and I will not use it until you get it fixed!" Other providers are not having as many issues with the system, but believe the system isn't working quite right and do not know whether the problem stems from the pharmacy, EHR, or the way they are using the system. The PAs and the NPs are not having as many issues as the physicians with transmittal of prescriptions.

In addition, you have a serious incident that your team is asked to address related to E-Prescribing by a physician who is inexperienced with the protocols for a particular condition.

Prescribing incident: A new physician who has recently completed residency and joined the clinic is being oriented to the new EHR within the practice. This provider is very computer savvy and takes pride in EHR competency. This provider came from a practice that was highly wired and in one of the areas of the country most advanced in EHRs and health information exchange. The provider is overconfident with the use of the EHR and dismisses any assistance with training, stating, "I fully understand how to use an EHR and don't need your help in training—I've got this covered!"

This physician had an incident that was reported to your team for review:

Dr. Rookie has received a new patient, a Hispanic female post myocardial infarction by 6 months with subsequent congestive heart failure. She is 57 years of age, 225 lbs., and 5'5". Dr. Rookie E-Prescribed metoprolol 100 mg twice a day. After rethinking, the dosage was changed to metoprolol 50 mg twice a day. Dr Rookie assumed the second order would override the original order and, therefore, did not cancel the original prescription. The pharmacy processed and delivered both

(continued)

CASE STUDY (*continued*)

prescriptions to the patient. This resulted in two prescriptions for metoprolol with the patient dosage of 150 mg twice daily. The patient took both prescriptions for the medication for several days before presenting to the ER with severe hypotensive bradycardia.

In the emergency room triage, the nurse received a brown bag of medications and noted two different prescriptions. She asked the patient whether she had been taking both prescriptions; she confirmed she had taken both for several days. The ER physician subsequently accessed the Surescripts network through the hospital EHR and confirmed the medication prescription history from the local retail pharmacy, and called Dr. Rookie about the double prescription.

Dr. Rookie investigated the issue later that week to determine why the system failed expectations. When it was discovered that the system did not have a built-in ability to override the initial order on the same prescription, the physician became defensive and openly critical and reported to your team, "Get this thing fixed—the other system we used in my residency program would have caught this double prescription. This never should have happened!"

EXERCISES AND QUESTIONS FOR CONSIDERATION

1. What are all the major issues noted in the practice setting? Is Dr. Rookies's recent incident and the workflow analysis relevant to successfully achieving a safe and effective meaningful use of an EHR?

2. Prioritize the issues and create a corrective plan of action using the project charter template within the chapter.

3. Define metrics within the project charter that will measure success before and after implementation of the redesign.

4. Within the plan, provide the team's recommended approach as to how to further investigate unexplained issues and how to incorporate community partners in the plan.

5. Discuss how the corrective plan will be monitored and evaluated.

6. What meaningful-use metrics are at play in this scenario in addition to the E-Prescribing metric noted in the case scenario?

7. Describe how a multidisciplinary team approach could improve care within the clinic and further issues with E-Prescribing.

CASE STUDY: E-PRESCRIBING WORKFLOW ANALYSIS

Your multidisciplinary team has requested assistance from your local REC. The Regional Coordinator for the Center (RCC) recommends a process redesign approach to E-Prescribing. The RCC has recently come into the clinic and with your team's help has created a process redesign for E-Prescribing. Outlined here is a workflow template based on E-Prescribing during an office visit (see Figure 9.5). Your team noted the following differences between the recommended workflow and the current practice:

1. When the end user enters a special character into the E-Prescribing field, the EHR does not recognize it. This results in the prescriptions not making it to the pharmacy. This issue frequently occurs when the prescription is written both in English and in Spanish for Hispanic patients.
2. Providers do not always double check protocols or drug benefit information.
3. When a prescription follows an electronic pathway, the Rx is frequently not received at the pharmacy and consequently is not filled.
4. There is not a clinical decision support rule or EHR process to alert providers to block duplicate or revised orders.
5. Your team is not confident that the issue noted in #1, presence of special characters in the E-Prescribing field, is the only reason for lack of receipt by the pharmacy. However, it is the only issue that has been identified thus far. The team suspects other end-user issues, particularly given the various provider behavioral responses to the E-Prescribing process.
6. Your team has preliminarily investigated issues and believes that there may be workflow issues at one large retail pharmacy within a super store. Further investigation reveals that the practice sends a significant amount of business to this pharmacy. The large retail pharmacy has reported potential workflow issues that most likely affect the practice's E-Prescribing process.
7. One of the smaller pharmacies owned by a prominent family within the community only receives electronic faxes. Roughly 30% of the prescriptions are routed to this pharmacy.
8. Using a multidisciplinary approach, your team's overarching goal is to develop a corrective action plan so that the practice achieves a rate of E-Prescribing of 40% or better.

(continued)

CASE STUDY: E-PRESCRIBING WORKFLOW ANALYSIS *(continued)*

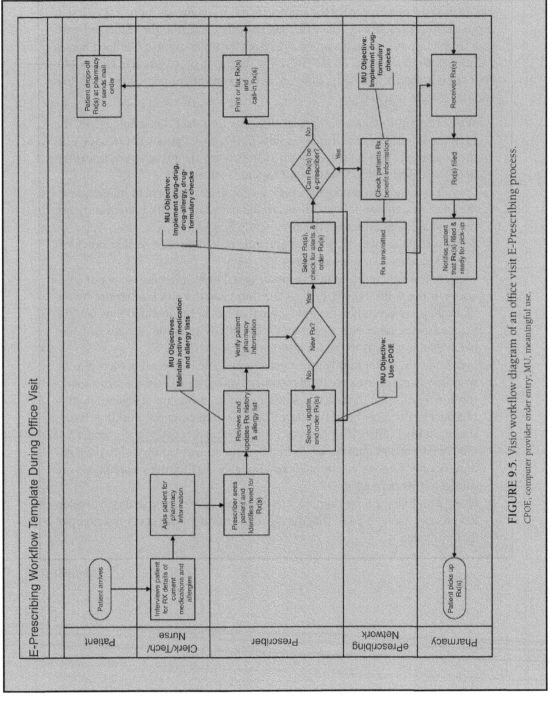

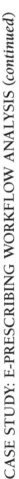

FIGURE 9.5. Visio workflow diagram of an office visit E-Prescribing process.

CPOE, computer provider order entry; MU, meaningful use.

REFERENCES

Fleming, N. S., Becker, E. R., Culler, S. D., Cheng, D., McCorkle, R., Graca, B. D., & Ballard, D. J. (2014). The impact of electronic health records on workflow and financial measures in primary care practices. *Health Services Research*, 49(1pt2), 405–420. doi:10.1111/1475-6773.12133

HealthIT.gov. (n.d.). What are some tips for approaching workflow redesign? Retrieved from https://www.healthit.gov/providers-professionals/faqs/what-are-some-tips-approaching-workflow-redesign

HealthIT.gov. (2011). *Step 2: Plan your approach–Workflow redesign templates*. (No. HITRC-WRDT2). Retrieved from https://www.healthit.gov/node/291.

Jones, S. S., Koppel, R., Ridgely, M. S., Palen, T. E., Wu, S., & Harrison, M. I. (2011). *Guide to reducing unintended consequences of electronic health records* (No. HHSA290200600017I). Rockville, MD: Agency for Healthcare Research and Quality. Retrieved from http://www.healthit.gov/unintended-consequences/

Microsoft Corporation. (2014). *Microsoft Visio Premium* 2010. Retrieved from http://www.digisoftstore.com/Microsoft-Visio-Premium-2010—Retail-Download-_p_40.html

Office of the National Coordinator for Health Information Technology. (n.d.). *HealthIT.gov tips for utilizing workflow redesign for quality improvement* (No. HITgovTips). Washington, DC: Author. Retrieved from http://www.healthit.gov/providers-professionals/faqs/what-are-some-tips-approaching-workflow-redesign

APPENDIX 9.1 MICROSOFT VISIO FUNCTIONS

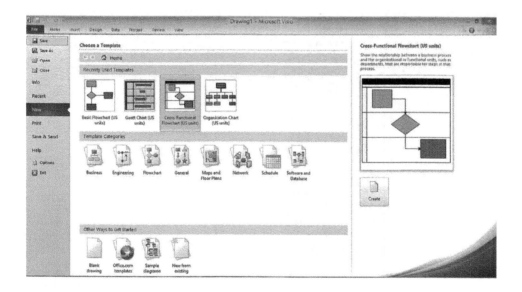

Launch Visio and select the type of swimlane you wish to create, such as the Basic Flowchart or Cross-Functional (also referred to as swimlanes).

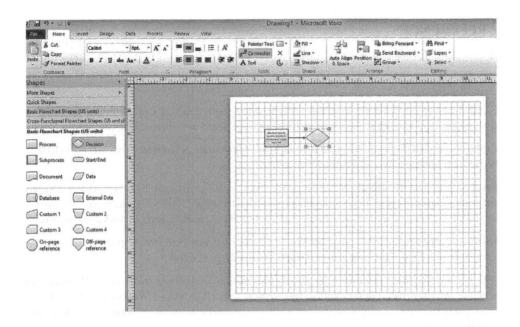

Drag and drop shapes onto the template, click connector, and drag another shape onto the template. Shapes reflected are rectangles for process and diamonds for decisions.

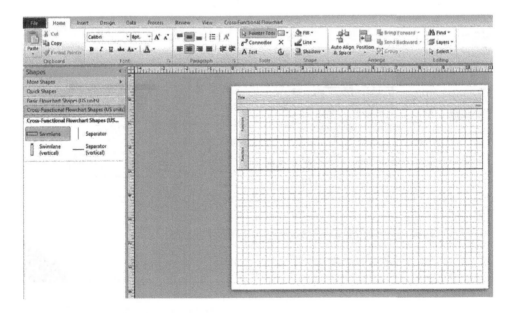

If you wish to create a cross-functional chart with swimlanes, click on "Function" and add roles and responsibilities of the individual and add additional swimlanes by clicking on "swimlane" and dragging it onto the template, where you wish to add the additional lane.

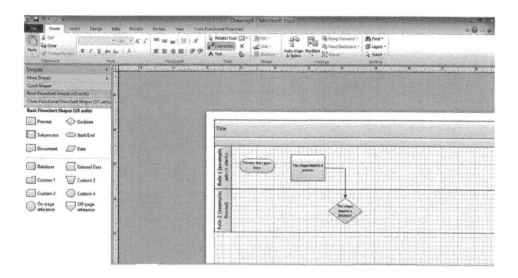

Add shapes and connectors as shown in the figure. This diagram reflects two roles and shapes that indicate start and/or stop of the process, a process (rectangle), and a decision (diamond); note the other shapes shown on the left panel. These are common shapes used in health care settings to reflect different aspects of the process.

CHAPTER 10

Evaluation Methods and Strategies for Electronic Health Records

Susan McBride and Mary Beth Mitchell

OBJECTIVES

1. Discuss and relate evaluation strategies to systems development life cycle (SDLC) fundamentals.

2. Discuss the importance of evaluation strategies for health information technology (HIT) as a fundamental requirement for development and implementation of safe and effective HIT.

3. Discuss evaluation strategies in relation to strategic planning and the significance of such strategies.

4. Describe various methods for designing evaluation programs for HIT.

5. Describe and apply metrics for evaluation of case scenarios relevant to the HITECH Act and maningful use of certified electronic health records.

KEY WORDS

measures, balancing measures, satisfaction, evaluation, strategic planning, return on investment, outcomes, patient safety, end-user acceptance, EMRAM[SM], Davies Award

---

CONTENTS

INTRODUCTION

This chapter reviews methods for evaluating electronic health records (EHRs) from high-level strategic plans for the organization and how well the implementation of the EHR fits that plan versus the actual measures of success. The design and implementation of a program evaluation strategy for EHRs are critical to safe and effective use of technology in the health care setting. Methods for program evaluation lay the foundation for strategies presented, and suggested measures to evaluate EHRs are defined and applied. An approach for EHR implementation involving a strategic focus on continuous quality improvement is emphasized and the evaluation is placed into the context of achieving long-term outcomes for the health care industry using EHRs. Evaluation strategies, including provider acceptance, economic value, quality and safety, consumer engagement, and public health impact, are also discussed. In addition, models of adoption frequently used in the health care industry are examined and compared to broader information systems of evaluation methods described by K. Kendall and J. Kendall (2014). These approaches include determining the value to the end user constituting usefulness or utility. Finally, case studies are presented to consider lessons learned in materials and methods presented.

GENERATING VALUE WITH HEALTH INFORMATION TECHNOLOGY IS STRATEGIC

In order to generate value with the use of any health information technology, an organization must start with strategic thinking. Glaser and Salzberg (2011) state the following: "As an organization develops its IT strategy, it must understand that the acquisition and implementation of an application does not lead to intrinsic value, streamlined processes, improved decision-making capabilities, or reduced medical errors. . . . If value is desired, approaches will have to be developed that manage value into existence" (Glaser & Salzberg, 2011, pp. 12–13). They further outline in an entire text how an organization approaches strategic thinking in order to generate value. So, how does a health care organization design strategy that is aimed at achieving value? This chapter focuses on the evaluation strategies needed in order for organizations to determine whether or not they have achieved value. As with Glaser and Salzberg (2011), text on this topic starting with aligned mission, vision, and objectives are core to any strategic plan.

The EHRs certified under the Centers for Medicare & Medicaid Services (CMS) EHR incentive program are complex systems with tremendous potential for benefits to patient care; however, there are equally as many opportunities for unintended consequences to result from poor implementation. Health care organizations need to establish programs to continually evaluate and improve on the implementation and adoptions of HIT to generate value. Patient safety, quality, and efficiency are key areas to consider when evaluating EHRs and other point-of-care devices. In addition, fundamentals of SDLC that emphasize establishing strategy and goals for all adoption and implementation projects are important considerations prior to implementation of an EHR or supporting point-of-care technologies.

EVALUATION IN THE CONTEXT OF SDLC

SDLC was discussed in Chapter 8, including the importance of establishing clear goals and measureable objectives for any and all HIT projects prior to beginning a development or implementation project. Initiating an HIT project with clear end goals in mind is a method of establishing a baseline for what constitutes "success." Evaluation methods are all about measuring whether or not a project has been successful. So, what constitutes "success" and what are good methods for determining whether or not an EHR implementation has been successful according to plan? Having a framework for evaluation is an important consideration for organizations as they consider implementation of an EHR or consider the status of the EHR they have implemented with respect to overall success. The authors suggest program evaluation methods as an example of one such framework. We also examine several tools and strategies to support strategic thinking aligned with the program evaluation framework.

PROGRAM EVALUATION

Program evaluation is a method used to determine whether an intended HIT solution has met the needs of the organization, end user, or intended purpose. Program evaluation is a systematic way of determining whether the program, in this case an HIT implementation, has been a success. So, how do you determine success? What are the measures that are most important to consider? Do we need balancing measures to determine whether the HIT program has been counterproductive? That is, has it been a benefit in one area but problematic in another? An example of this might be improved patient safety with implementation of computer provider order entry (CPOE), but with negative economic impact caused by poor implementation resulting in inefficiencies, with providers failing to see as many patients on a daily basis as they did prior to CPOE implementation. It is important to consider cost avoidance and risk avoidance as examples of balancing measures. In this case, we would implement measures on medication safety as the target for achieving patient safety, and employ a balancing measure for efficiency, relating to number of patients seen in a day per provider. The goal would be to improve patient safety and, over time (once the learning curve is achieved), maintain or improve efficiencies with respect to provider–patient per day ratios.

The Centers for Disease Control and Prevention (CDC) outlines a methodology to evaluate programs that can be applied to HIT. Figure 10.1 depicts a framework for program evaluation. Within the framework, there are several components to consider, including engagement of the stakeholders, description of the program, focus of the evaluation design, gathering of credible evidence, justification of conclusions, ensuring use, and sharing of lessons learned. According to the CDC framework, "Evaluation involves procedures that are useful, feasible, ethical and accurate" (CDC, 2012).

Engagement of Stakeholders

This section discusses how well the HIT project has engaged the stakeholders within the process and those that the technology was intended to impact. In terms of the EHR and how the Office of the National Coordinator (ONC) and CMS determine that the EHR has been meaningfully used, clearly patient engagement is an important component.

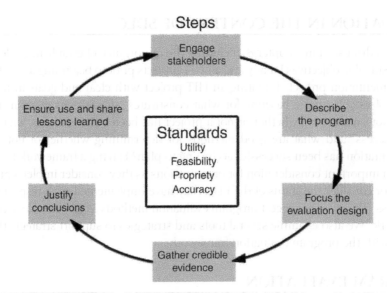

FIGURE 10.1. Framework for program evaluation.
Source: Centers for Disease Control and Prevention (2012).

Patient Engagement as a Factor of Success

An important focus of Stage 2 meaningful use (MU) of the EHR is the engagement of the health care consumer in the EHR. This was one of the most contested and debated component of the Stage 2 MU when the rules were first released. Providers did not want to be held accountable for measuring successful and MU of the EHR by a metric that many felt they had little control over. How could a provider insist on the patient engaging in the EHR? The MU measure in Stage 2 that relates to engagement is in the form of patients viewing and downloading information from their electronic record, or secure messaging between the provider and the patient. For hospitals, MU Stage 2 required that hospitals provide patients with online access to downloadable information from their electronic record and that the hospital track the percentage of patients who actually access that information. Patient engagement has been show to improve health overall. Therefore, one of the key drivers that CMS and ONC were considering to be "MU" of the EHR was this patient engagement component.

Clinician Engagement as a Factor of Success

In terms of SDLC, the engagement of the end user of the technology or "the stakeholders" plays an important role from conceptualization of the project throughout the life cycle of the technology. When considering SDLC methods, it is core to the strategy that the end user is taken into consideration in planning and implementing the technology. When thinking in terms of clinicians' engagement and their satisfaction with the system in regard to SDLC, this should be an important focus of evaluation. We discuss methods for evaluating clinicians' satisfaction and experiences with the clinician information systems they utilize further in the chapter, but for now suffice it to say that clinicians as end users of the EHR are an important consideration when evaluating the overall success of an implementation.

Project Description

In program evaluation, core to success is that the project was well described and thought through in terms of what constitutes success for the program. This too is a fundamental approach described in Chapter 8 that is a basic strategy to any implementation or development project. The project description takes place in the planning phase and includes the scope of the project, timelines, goals, and objectives. In order to effectively evaluate success, an organization must be clear on what the project was designed to accomplish.

Evaluation Design

With program evaluation strategies, evaluation design is built into the program from inception with clear goals on what constitutes success in the project description, followed by a strategy that will evaluate the impact of the program. One method for designing the evaluation methods is the project charter. A well-designed project charter creates discipline in the process, outlining the project in terms of measures of success, timelines, and other parameters important to keeping a team focused on the overall intention of the project or program. In Chapter 9, we described the use of a project charter within the context of improvement of a project using workflow redesign. However, the project charter is also an effective tool for evaluation strategies for the overall HIT projects as described in Chapter 9. Therefore, the authors highly encourage organizations to think in terms of the approach of the EHR evaluation using the charter as a tool to frame the overall intent of the EHR and what the organization wants to effectively accomplish by its use.

Another approach that is frequently used for program evaluation is to establish a logic model structure early in the planning phase that includes data input and output that you expect to achieve with the proposed project. Both the project charter and the logic model are examples of a disciplined approach to program evaluation that rely on well-designed and thoughtful consideration of the plan for improvement, which includes measures of success predetermined by all stakeholders who ultimately validate whether the project has been successful. An example of a logic model is reflected in Figure 10.2 of the book. The model reflected is a results-based logic model for primary health care that provides a conceptual foundation for population-based information systems. This model was designed for use in a primary health care population health strategy that clearly notes inputs as fiscal resources, material resources, and health or human resources. The outputs are noted in terms of what the organizations wish to achieve with products and services (Watson, Broemeling, & Wong, 2009). The logic model is frequently a high-level strategy with the project charter being very explicit and with measureable outcomes. Both tools are useful in EHR program evaluation.

Gathering Credible Evidence

Evidence to suggest that HIT has been successful should be based on reliable and credible information within a health care setting. Data constituting this type of information to evaluate an EHR might include end-user satisfaction, return on investment (ROI), attainment toward MU, or other data outlined in the original project charter and logic model that might include measures of quality related to care delivered using the EHR.

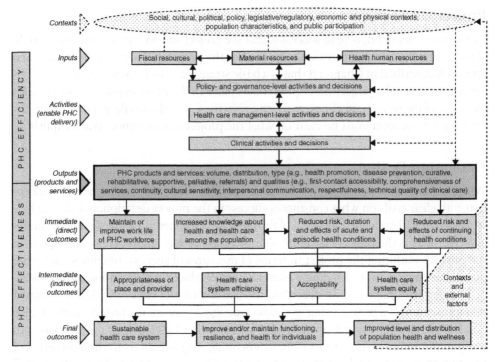

FIGURE 10.2. Results-based logic model for PHC.
Source: Watson, Broemeling, and Wong (2009).

Satisfaction of End Users

There are various methods used to evaluate the satisfaction of the end user in a health care setting. These methods include focus groups and survey approaches to collecting valid information on end-user acceptance and satisfaction. One of the surveys that has been validated for end-user satisfaction is the Clinical Information System Implementation Evaluation Scale (CISIES). The CISIES has been expanded and improved for use across organizations, systems, and types of staff for both formative and summative evaluations of user satisfaction with the various types of clinical information systems implementation (Gugerty, Maranda, & Rook, 2006). Figure 10.3 is a sample of the paper-based survey (pages 1 and 2 of a trifold brochure) that can be deployed in small hospitals and clinics, or expanded as an online survey to include larger hospitals, health care systems, and statewide evaluation of clinical information systems.

Return on Investment

Estimated total costs for the implementation and adoption of an EHR is a primary concern for providers and hospitals. Although EHR CMS financial incentives offset a large portion of total costs for providers and hospitals and motivated many to adopt EHRs, cost continues to be a primary concern for institutions and providers, as they consider adopting an EHR. Fleming, Culler, McCorkle, Becker, and Ballard (2011), in a study conducted across 26 primary care practices in a physician network in north Texas, estimated total costs of the implementation by provider and clinic. The study presented

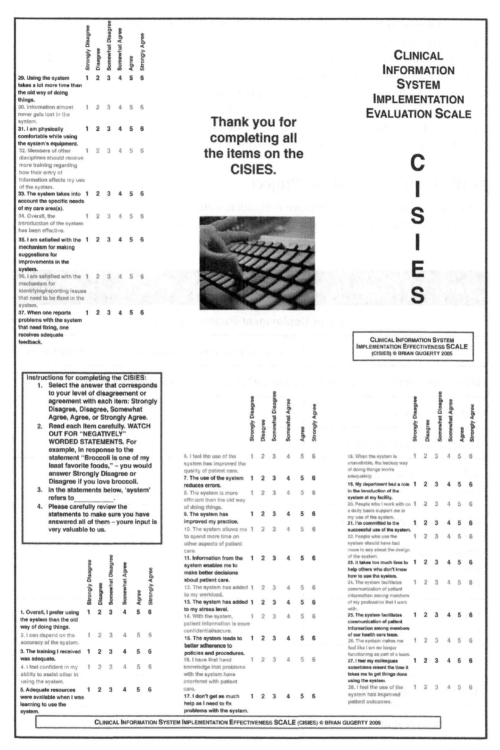

FIGURE 10.3. Trifold paper-based clinical information system implementation evaluation scale.
Source: Gugerty, Maranda, and Rook (2006).

factors that should be included in cost-benefit estimates, including technical expenses for software, hardware, networking, as well as man-hour costs of labor for technical, clinical, and clinician time and effort. Table 10.1 provides a template suggested by Fleming et al. (2011). Although this study was conducted and costs estimated for an ambulatory setting, the authors provide this as a sample template for hospitals to consider as they estimate costs. This research presents practical recommendations on how to examine costs as well as benefits, and can help to guide organizations in thinking about cost-benefit analysis to support return on investment evaluations.

Justify Conclusions of the Project

Justification of the project in program evaluation would address whether or not the program is appropriate, given the expense, and would account for ROI and other important

TABLE 10.1 Estimated Costs for ROI Calculations Template		
Cost of Deployment Factors for EHR		
	Costs per 60 days postlaunch	**1st-Year Costs**
Hardware, Software, Networking, and Other Technical Expenses		
Hardware costs (Fixed)		
Hardware costs (Variable)		
Software licensing and/or hosting (variable)		
Clinical Impact Cost Factors		
Information technology implementation team costs (Fixed)		
Clinical site implementation team costs (Fixed)		
End-user costs (Variable)		
Total Estimated Costs		
Per practice/hospital		
Per physician		

EHR, electronic health record; ROI, return on investment.

Source: Fleming et al. (2011).

factors outlined in the project charter and logic model. Can an organization justify the effort and expense associated with the EHR? Glaser and Salzberg (2011) point to two different types of justifications. One involves smaller components of HIT, such as implementing barcode administration. An organization can more easily justify based on patient safety, quality, and cost that barcode administration is a justified expense. The other type of HIT that Glaser and Salzberg indicate as more difficult to justify is the entire foundation of the EHR platform, which is an ongoing and long-term implementation and maintenance challenge. This is particularly relevant in light of ongoing MU stages that will continue to move the target by achieving "MU" of an EHR according to federal guidelines. Additionally, many organizations are evaluating the EHR and electing to "rip and replace" the system because it is no longer "foundationally" meeting the organization's needs. A "rip and replace" occurs when the EHR that has been implemented no longer meets an organization's needs and it elects to completely replace the system with a new EHR. Glaser and Salzberg indicate that there is likely one of four reasons that an organization will replace an HIT foundation such as the EHR, and that these types of replacements are often difficult to justify. The four areas are as follows:

1. The vendor goes out of business.
2. A new vendor emerges in the marketplace with superior products.
3. There is a serious problem with the EHR, which fails to accommodate new technologies. This is likely to occur in the future with vendors unable or unwilling to continue to invest in older software platforms as MU continues to press vendor development of legacy platforms.
4. Care or the business model shifts and changes dramatically, such as in the case of the risk contracts and requirements of organizations to track cost and quality at higher levels, which result in financial risk to the organization if both quality and cost are not addressed (Glaser & Salzberg, 2011).

Ensure Use

Ensuring use is another factor in a program evaluation approach and is a common method of evaluation seen with EHRs in the health care industry. One of the most well-known approaches has been developed and endorsed by the Healthcare Information and Management Systems Society (HIMSS). The evaluation models developed by HIMSS address the question: "How effectively is the system being used and by whom?" HIMSS has developed two of these types of models. The HIMSS 7 level Electronic Medical Record Adoption Model (EMRAM[SM]) is one of the models, and "the Davies Award" is a more advanced user designation for organizations that have achieved higher levels of innovative use (HIMSS Analytics, 2014a). We describe both of these user-based evaluation models later.

HIMSS EMRAM[SM]

The HIMSS EMR Adoption Model (EMRAM) provides eight progressive levels that define the components organizations are using within the electronic record. This indicates to what extent organizations have implemented the electronic record, as well as how extensively it is being used, which can be considered a measure of EHR adoption by clinicians. According to HIMSS Analytics (2014a), "The EMRAM[SM] identifies and scores hospitals using an 8 step scale that charts the path to a fully paperless environment." Organizations determine their HIMSS EMRAM level based on achieving the defined criteria for each level. Figure 10.4 outlines the key components of each level. We refer the reader to HIMSS for further information constituting the criteria within each level and the method used to determine how an organization works with HIMSS to be identified as a level 0 to 7 organization. We note the model within this evaluation chapter for the purpose of identifying methods currently used and accepted as valid within the industry to evaluate organizations and end-user adoption as one evaluation strategy.

Organizations attest to their level and notify HIMSS so the level can be tracked and monitored over time. The highest level of adoption is HIMSS Stage 7, which demonstrates full utilization of the EHR, including barcode medication administration and medical device integration. In order to achieve EMRAM Stage 7, organizations must demonstrate full adoption of the EHR through a site visit by HIMSS representatives, and provide information demonstrating their use of the EHR. This includes an organizational profile, including how the EHR is used and reports demonstrating compliance with the Stage 7

US EMR Adoption Model[SM]

Stage	Cumulative Capabilites	2014 Q2	2014 Q3
Stage 7	Complete EMR; CCD transactions to share data; Data warehousing; Data continuity with ED, ambulatory, OP	3.2%	3.4%
Stage 6	Physician documentation (structured templates), full CDSS (variance & compliance), full R-PACS	15.0%	16.5%
Stage 5	Closed loop medication administration	27.5%	29.5%
Stage 4	CPOE, Clinical Decision Support (clinical protocols)	15.3%	14.5%
Stage 3	Nursing/clinical documentation (flow sheets), CDSS (error checking), PACS available outside Radiology	25.4%	23.9%
Stage 2	CDR, Controlled Medical Vocabulary, CDS, may have Document Imaging; HIE capable	5.9%	5.3%
Stage 1	Ancillaries - Lab, Rad, Pharmacy - All Installed	2.8%	2.5%
Stage 0	All Three Ancillaries Not Installed	4.9%	4.4%

Data from HIMSS Analytics™ Database © 2014   N = 5,447   N = 5,453

FIGURE 10.4. EMRAM model.

CCD, continuity of care document; CDR, clinical data repository; CDS, clinical decision support; CDSS, clinical decision support system; CPOE, computer provider order entry; ED, emergency department; EMR, electronic medical record; EMRAM, electronic medical record adoption model; OP, outpatient; PACS, picture archiving and communication systems; R-PACS, radiology-PACS.

Source: HIMSS Analytics (2014b).

criteria, such as a CPOE report or a barcode medication compliance report. In addition, a tour of various units and visiting with staff provides information on how the EHR is actually used, and how the staff comply with the various criteria and requirements of Stage 7. Currently, only about 3.4% of hospitals have achieved Stage 7, but the number continues to increase. A complete list of Stage 7 hospitals is available on the HIMSS Analytics website at www.himssanalytics.org/home/index.aspx (HIMSS Analytics, 2014b). The HIMSS EMRAM model provides an indication of evaluation of the EHR through how well organizations are adopting and using the various components within the EHR. There is ongoing discussion at HIMSS about adding additional levels, as more and more functionality becomes available to organizations within the EHR.

Davies Award

The HIMSS Davies Award is another program available through HIMSS Analytics that can help evaluate the EHR in an organization. The Davies Award is an advanced program developed by HIMSS to define how well an organization is using the EHR. According to HIMSS:

> Since 1994, the HIMSS Nicholas E. Davies Award of Excellence has recognized outstanding achievement of organizations who have utilized health information technology to substantially improve patient outcomes while achieving return on investment. The Davies Awards program promotes EHR-enabled improvement in patient outcomes through sharing case studies and lessons learned on implementation strategies, workflow design, best practice adherence, and patient engagement. (HIMSS, 2014a)

Organizations that apply for, and receive the Davies Award are able to demonstrate the value they have received from the EHR. This award is based on the organization submitting five case studies that demonstrate how the EHR is used demonstrating the outcomes achieved. In addition, organizations must be at an HIMSS Stage 6 or Stage 7 on the HIMSS EMRAM scale, thus demonstrating advanced utilization of the EHR. Case studies submitted by organizations for applying for the Davies Award must consist of the following components:

▶ One case study to demonstrate a hard dollar ROI.

▶ One case study showing clinical value or a soft ROI.

▶ Three case studies that demonstrate how the EHR impacted clinical outcomes and improved patient care. These can be anything the organization has done, but should be directly related to patient outcomes, safety, or clinical efficiencies.

The value of applying for the Davies Award comes from allowing an organization to focus on how well the EHR is used and whether it is actually impacting outcomes in a significant way. Just the process of applying for the Davies Award demonstrates the value of the EHR and serves as a mechanism for organizations to reflect on just how effective the EHR is within the organization. The award criteria also require that the evaluation include how the use of the EHR aligns with the organization's strategic goals and key performance indicators (KPIs). Some examples of case studies from Davies Award recipients include the following:

▶ Texas Health Resources reduced the number of cardiac arrests by 62% in 1 year through implementation of modified early-warning systems in their EHR.

▶ Children's Medical Center Dallas has realized a positive ROI of $48.62 million with the implementation of its EHR system, through tying its EHR implementation to its system KPIs.

▶ Lakeland Health System used clinical decision support to reduce incidence of sepsis through early detection. Before the EHR, the mortality rate from sepsis was 16.67% and it dropped to 9.63% within 6 months of implementation of the clinical decision support tools in the EHR.

Further information on this award and the application process for the Davies Award, along with information on all Davies Award winners and accompanying case studies is publically available on the HIMSS Davies website. These cases attest to how the EHR is improving patient care, as evidenced through significant clinical outcomes reported by each of the Davies Award-winning organizations (HIMSS, 2014b). These cases also demonstrate effective methods for organizations to use to evaluate EHRs by examining the alignment of the EHR adoption and implementation strategies and outcomes with the organization's vision, mission, and strategic plans.

Share Lessons Learned

Evaluate the program and discuss lessons learned to inform future projects returning to the stakeholders within an organization to communicate success. This may be in the form of celebrating achievement of MU, or reporting dashboard reports on progress on quality metrics established in the plan. This might also involve dissemination of success stories shared across the industry at conferences, publications, and other vehicles of communication that contribute to colleagues across the nation related to your successes and failures. Learning from failure is as important as successful implementation strategies. The Davies Award winners frequently present at the HIMSS annual conference and share lessons learned, methods for achieving success, and other factors that might be of help to other organizations to support the journey to EMRAM level 6 and 7, as well as their methods for improving outcomes using EHRs (HIMSS, 2014b).

Measures of Success: Useful, Feasible, Ethical, and Accurate

Measures should include utility, feasibility, accurately measure what is intended (reliability and validity) and, above all, be ethical in how evaluation measures are monitored. The primary measures organizations are using in the United States to evaluate EHRs involve attainment of MU measures and reaching thresholds that will provide financial incentives as outlined by the CMS EHR Incentive Program (CMS.gov, 2014). Stage 1 and stage 2 meaningful use measures are noted in Appendix 1.1, comparing phase one and two measures for MU. Phase three MU is in proposal stages and will likely constitute higher achievement of interoperability, patient engagement, and overall value in tracking, trending, and achieving improved patient outcomes (ONC, 2014). These measures structured within the national strategy technically constitute the U.S. framework for evaluating whether EHRs are "meaningfully used."

The importance of accuracy with respect to safe, effective use of the EHR is unquestionably one of the most significant evaluation questions organizations should consider when evaluating the EHR. How accurate is the information documented and how can organizations address issues of inaccuracies and inconsistencies as they develop? We address these important challenges in Chapter 20.

Usefulness can be measured in terms of utility and, according to Kendall and Kendall (2014), provides a very effective way to evaluate the success of information technology projects. In the model outlined by Kendall and Kendall, evaluating utility or usefulness includes possession, form, place, time, actualization, and goal. For each of these categories, the information technology is judged by end users to be poor, fair, or good. If all categories are considered "good," then the project has been a success. If one or more categories are considered "poor," then the organization might want to consider the utility or usefulness of the information system. Definitions of each of the categories are noted in Table 10.2.

There are some important considerations in this model related to end users; note that the possession utility indicates that information has no value if people who use

TABLE 10.2 Categories of Utility/Usefulness	
Category	Definition
Possession utility	Possession utility addresses who should receive the output from the system and make decisions about information from the system, and who has the power to make decisions with information from the system. According to K. Kendall and J. Kendall, information has no value if people who use the system have no power to improve it, or lack the ability to use the system productively.
Form utility	Form utility involves the type of output generated from the system and what "form" the output takes. The output and form should be useful to the end user. The information should also be in an appropriate form to be useful. Form also takes into account too much information to be useful "information overload."
Place utility	Place utility considers the position or location of the information within the system and addresses "the where" or location as a consideration of usefulness.
Time utility	The time utility addresses when the information is delivered and it must be appropriately timed to be useful to the decision maker, if it is too late or too early, then the time utility is not met.

(continued)

TABLE 10.2 Categories of Utility/Usefulness *(continued)*	
Category	Definition
Actualization utility	Actualization utility relates to how the information is used by the decision maker. The system has value if it is implemented, but retains actualization utility if it continues to be of value postimplementation. Actualization relates to long-term value to the decision maker using the system.
Goal utility	The goal utility addresses "the why" and determines whether the system helps the organization achieve long-term success in terms of organizational goals.

Source: Kendall and Kendall (2014).

the system have no power to improve it or lack the ability to use the system productively. The form utility takes into account the output in terms of usefulness to the end user in terms of the quantity of information available. This aspect takes into account human factors and the need to make sure we do not overload the end user with too much information on the EHR screens. In addition, place utility is similar in that it is a factor indicating whether the information is placed in a location that is useful. This too is an aspect of human factors design and whether or not the human–technology interface is designed in a manner intended to best engage the end user and for the information within the system to be cognitively interpreted, processed, and utilized. Actualization is realized when long-term value is determined by the end user. This factor amplifies the importance of determining end-user satisfaction and acceptance of the EHR. Finally, the goal utility once again confirms the importance of strategic alignment with the organization's vision, mission, and goals.

All factors in Table 10.2 are important to consider as they relate to long-term success with EHRs in truly reaching "MU" of EHRs.

ACHIEVING THE "MEANING" IN MU

Classen and Bates (2011, p. 857) state the following: "As the broad adoption of EHRs accelerates, the challenge of ensuring that MU actually leads to meaningful benefits, such as improvements in safety and quality of care, remains a serious concern." These two national leaders in HIT emphasize the need for evaluation tools after implementation of EHRs in order for organizations to reinforce safety and quality along with achieving the MU measures. Classen and Bates (2011) suggest self-assessment tools similar to the Leapfrog Group's assessment tool for EHRs (see http://leapfroggroup.org/). They further recommend ongoing evaluation with an annual review of HIT, including the eight dimensions of the EHR safety model described by D. F. Sittig and Singh (2009). These eight factors are outlined in Table 10.3 and include infrastructure such as hardware and software, as well as content, interfaces, training, communications, policies, procedures, and regulatory requirements.

TABLE 10.3 Eight Dimensions of EHR Safety Model
1. Hardware and software
2. Clinical content
3. User interfaces
4. User training and authorization procedures
5. Clinical workflow and communication
6. Organizations policies and procedures
7. State and federal rules and regulations
8. Periodic measurements of system activity

EHR, electronic health record.

Source: Sittig and Classen (2010).

Classen and Bates (2011) indicate that without a comprehensive evaluation strategy instituted nationally, including the eight facets outlined in Table 10.3, we cannot ensure safe and effective EHR use. The recommended framework includes five essential components:

1. Ability for users to report patient safety events and hazards related to EHR usage.

2. Enhanced certification criteria aligned with best practices in software development and "evidence" that adverse events and hazards have been addressed.

3. Methods to self-assess, attest, test, and report all eight dimensions of safe EHR use outlined in Table 10.3 are in place for clinicians using the EHR.

4. A regulatory oversight mechanism to be put in place at local, state, and federal levels to ensure "in-person accreditation of EHRs."

5. A national board instituted for reporting and investigation of EHR-related adverse events that would receive incident reports (Sittig & Classen, 2010).

SUMMARY

This chapter has discussed the importance of strategies for EHR evaluation that rely on establishing clear goals and objectives based on strategic plans that align an organization's vision and mission with objectives for the HIT program. Additionally, various methods have been explored using a program evaluation outlined by the CDC as a framework for examining aspects of how a program should be evaluated and what components might be important to EHR evaluation. Several methods and tools have been explored in terms of how they fit within the context of program evaluation. The tools included project charters and logic models. MU was discussed as the national framework for evaluation throughout the United States with many organizations determining success by whether or not they achieve MU and draw down the financial incentives from CMS when those outcomes are achieved. This discussion followed with national experts proposing models of evaluation that aligned with safe and effective use of HIT, calling for national models to address safety. Other models have also been discussed, including the HIMSS ENRAM model and HIMSS esteemed Davies Award for advanced EHR users who have achieved nationally recognized health outcomes using their EHRs.

EXERCISES AND QUESTIONS FOR CONSIDERATION

Consider the implementation of the EHR within your clinical setting or a setting you have recently experienced or observed the use of the EHR within. Reflect on Kendall and Kendall's utility model noted within the chapter, and evaluate the system by scoring it with respect to the six categories outlined in Table 10.2. Now, visit the HIMSS website and read the case studies on one of the Davies Award-winning organizations and score the organizations with respect to the six categories of utility or usefulness. Consider the following questions:

1. How does your organization compare to the Davies Award-winning organizations?
2. Do you find the utility model helpful in evaluating the EHRs?
3. How does the approach taken by HIMSS with the Davies Award also address utility and usefulness?
4. What factors noted in the utility model are well aligned with MU, and which are less closely aligned?

Given that the MU measures are the national framework for the United States with respect to EHRs, many organizations are measuring success with respect to adoption and implementation of the EHRs through achieving the financial incentives with CMS on measures reflective of "MU." After reading the chapter and reflecting on the CDC's evaluation model, how well do the MU measures align with usefulness, feasibility, ethics, and accuracy? Compare and contrast MU measures to the concepts of usefulness, feasibility, ethics, and accuracy. Consider the following questions:

1. Are the MU regulations, as outlined in our federal plan, meaningful and useful to the clinicians who use the system and the patients who are impacted by the EHR?
2. Are organizations taking these factors into account in evaluating EHRs in the United States? If yes, how do you believe they are accomplishing these aspects of evaluation, and, if not, what do you believe are the barriers that might be preventing organizations from focusing on these evaluation methods.
3. Are there other methods that might be effective and, if so, what are they? Defend your position with the evidence.

REFERENCES

Centers for Disease Control and Prevention. (2012). *Program Performance and Evaluation Office (PPEO)—Program evaluation.* Retrieved from http://www.cdc.gov/eval/framework/

Classen, D. C., & Bates, D. W. (2011). Finding the meaning in meaningful use. *New England Journal of Medicine, 365*(9), 855–858. doi:10.1056/NEJMsb1103659

CMS.gov. (2014). *EHR incentive programs.* Retrieved from http://www.cms.gov/Regulations-and-Guidance/Legislation/EHRIncentivePrograms/index.html?redirect=/EHRIncentivePrograms

Fleming, N. S., Culler, S. D., McCorkle, R., Becker, E. R., & Ballard, D. J. (2011). The financial and non-financial costs of implementing electronic health records in primary care practices. *Health Affairs, 30*(3), 481–489. doi:10.1377/hlthaff.2010.0768

Glaser, J. P., & Salzberg, C. (2011). *The strategic application of information technology in health care organizations* (3rd ed.). San Francisco, CA: Jossey-Bass.

Gugerty, B., Maranda, M., & Rook, D. (2006). The clinical information system implementation evaluation scale. *Journal of Studies in Health Technology and Informatics, 122*, 621–625. Retrieved from http://ebooks.iospress.nl/publication/9287

Healthcare Information and Management Systems. (2014a). *HIMSS Davies Awards: Awarding IT: Improving healthcare.* Retrieved from http://www.himss.org/library/davies-awards

Healthcare Information and Management Systems. (2014b). *HIMSS enterprise Davies Award recipients.* Retrieved from http://www.himss.org/resourcelibrary/TopicList.aspx?MetaDataID=2803

Healthcare Information and Management Systems Analytics. (2014a). *Maturity models.* Retrieved from http://www.himssanalytics.org/emram/index.aspx

Healthcare Information and Management Systems Analytics. (2014b). *Stage 7 application requests.* Retrieved from http://www.himssanalytics.org/home/index.aspx

Kendall, K. E., & Kendall, J. E. (2014). *Systems analysis and design* (9th ed.). Upper Saddle River, NJ: Pearson.

Office of the National Coordinator for Health Information Technology. (2014). *Federal health IT strategic plan 2015–2020.* Retrieved from http://www.healthit.gov/sites/default/files/federal-healthIT-strategic-plan-2014.pdf

Sittig, D., & Classen, D. (2010). Safe electronic health record use requires a comprehensive monitoring and evaluation framework. *Journal of the American Medical Association, 303*(5), 450–451. doi:10.1001/jama.2010.61

Sittig, D. F., & Singh, H. (2009). Eight rights of safe electronic health record use. *Journal of the American Medical Association, 302*(10), 1111–1113. doi:10.1001/jama.2009.1311

Watson, D. E., Broemeling, A., & Wong, S. T. (2009). A results-based logic model for primary healthcare: A conceptual foundation for population-based information systems. *Healthcare Policy, 5*(Special Issue), 33–46.

Electronic Health Records and Health Information Exchanges Providing Value and Results for Patients, Providers, and Health Care Systems

Susan McBride, Tony Gilman, Anne Kimbol, and George Gooch

OBJECTIVES

1. Define health information exchanges (HIEs) and interoperability in terms of the deployment of the Nationwide Health Information Network (NwHIN) in the United States.

2. Analyze the current and the historical intent of HIEs in light of the current status of the Health Information Technology for Economic and Clinical Health (HITECH) Act with respect to deployment of the national plan for interoperability and HIEs.

3. Compare and contrast different models of HIEs in terms of technical and business models.

4. Assess the current state of HIEs, barriers to success, and factors associated with success.

5. Examine evaluation models for informing successful models of interoperability and exchange.

6. Examine important challenges that are pivotal to success using proper identification of patients with a master patient index as an example of a significant issue with trust and patient safety implications.

7. Evaluate case studies, thus amplifying the need for trust frameworks to protect security and privacy of information and reinforcing the value of HIE once trust and sharing are established.

KEY WORDS

health information exchange, interoperability

INTRODUCTION

In 2001, the Institute of Medicine (IOM) established a vision for 21st-century health care that could include safe, effective, patient-centered, timely, efficient, and equitable care (IOM, 2001). Blumenthal (2010), former director of the Office of the National Coordinator for Health Information Technology (ONC-HIT), described the goals of the Health Information Technology for Economic and Clinical Health Act as follows: "to create an electronic circulatory system for health information that nourishes the practice of medicine, research and public health, making health professionals better at what they do and the American people healthier" (Blumenthal, 2010, p. 385).

The infrastructure envisioned under the HITECH Act has also been described as the Nationwide Health Information Network (NHIN) or the NwHIN, and it has the purpose of connecting the nation through health information exchanges at both regional and state levels and finally at the federal level. The fundamental goal of the HIE, according to Williams, Mostashari, Mertz, Hogin, and Atwal (2012, p. 527), is that "health information follows the patient wherever and whenever they seek care, in a private and secure manner so that teams of doctors, nurses and care managers can provide coordinated, effective, and efficient care." The vision for the NwHIN is to create its own infrastructure that is capable of transforming the delivery of health care and wellness by providing efficient, secure, and accurate access to health information (Fridsma, n.d.).

Exchange of health information is a fundamental concept under the HITECH Act and is also vital for establishing meaningful use (MU) of electronic health records (EHRs). HIEs are generating significant value to patients, providers, and health care systems; however, there are also significant technical and financial issues that hamper success. In this chapter, we examine the history and current state of HIEs, the value being generated, and implications for MU; discuss business and technical models; and outline factors indicative of success, as well as common challenges, including financial and technical considerations such as proper patient identification. Finally, a case study evaluates patient safety, privacy, and the importance of establishing trust frameworks to ensure success across the nation.

HISTORY OF HIEs COMPARED WITH CURRENT HIEs

Exchange of health care information within a community is not a new concept, as significant initiatives started in the early 1990s in the form of community health management information systems (CHMIS), followed by community health information networks (CHINs) in the mid- to late 1990s and, more recently, under the HITECH Act's regional health information exchanges (HIEs). We compare and contrast these three efforts and compare these community-based initiatives with the purpose of the NwHIN outlined in the ONC's plans for future exchange of health information.

Community Health Management Information Systems

CHMISs date back to work established in the early 1990s under the Hartford Foundation. CHMISs were established primarily as a payer-driven model to assess eligibility and address rising health care costs. They were supported by centralized data repositories containing eligibility, administrative claims data, and some clinical information for a geographically defined area within a community supported by stakeholders, including local agencies, payers, employers, and researchers. Although the purpose of the CHIMSs was similar to the intent of the HIEs of this decade—to use health care data to drive down costs and address quality—the technology constraints were significantly different than those faced today. The Internet was not as robust in terms of speed and reliability; software and hardware were expensive, requiring costly network connections; and integration of data sources presented significant issues because of lack of interoperability standards (Vest & Gamm, 2010).

Community Health Information Networks

CHINs emerged in the mid- to late 1990s and were commercially driven endeavors with intents that were similar to those of our current HIEs. They focused on exchanging data across a community; however, these initiatives lacked payer and community stakeholders. CHINs were primarily transaction-based, provider-based data exchanges that did not store data within a centralized repository. A number of issues presented sustainability problems for the CHINs, including competitor organizations with limited commitment to share data, vendor transaction-based fees that were not cost justified, and questionable return on investment (ROI; Barach & Small, 2000; President's Council of Advisors on Science and Technology, 2010; Woolf, Kuzel, Dovey, & Phillips, 2004).

Regional Health Information Organizations

RHIOs were the next concept to arise and were related to exchange of regional data. RHIOs were defined as "neutral, third-party organizations that facilitate information exchange between providers within a geographical area to achieve more effective and efficient healthcare" (Vest & Gamm, 2010, p. 290). The RHIOs across the country vary in their approach to architecture and may use federated, centralized, or hybrid approaches for storage and exchange of health care information. Table 11.1 outlines these three types of community-based initiatives and compares and contrasts their purpose, stakeholders, architecture, and challenges.

TABLE 11.1 Comparing and Contrasting CHMIS, CHIN, RHIO, and HIE			
Type of Exchange	Stakeholders	Purpose	Technical Architecture
CHMIS	Payers, health care consumers	Eligibility, payer assessment, cost reduction	Central repository
CHIN	Providers	Cost reductions for providers through shared information	Transactions based, decentralized
RHIO	Providers	Quality improvement and cost reductions	Varies by community
HIE	Varies depending on initiative	Quality improvement and cost reductions, improvement in public health	Varies by community

CHIN, community health information network; CHMIS, community health management information systems; HIE, health information exchange; RHIO, regional health information exchange.

Source: Vest and Gamm (2010).

Health Information Exchange

HIEs could be defined as a combination of the previously mentioned initiatives that have the exchange of health care information as their core purpose; however, comparing and contrasting historical initiatives with what currently constitutes an HIE is the authors' purpose within this section. HIEs under the HITECH Act were largely funded by federal initiatives to lay the architecture for exchange, where communities lack the infrastructure, and to promote further infrastructure and exchange in communities that historically had some infrastructure established (Pre-HITECH Act).

Nationwide Health Information Network

The purpose of the NwHIN has several objectives that were noted in 2010 as follows: (a) develop capabilities for standard-based and secure data exchange; (b) enable data exchange for coordination of care information among hospitals, laboratories, physicians' offices, pharmacies, and other providers; (c) ensure appropriate information is available at the point of care; (d) enable secure and accurate information exchange; (e) provide consumers with a choice as to how their personal health information is handled; (f) reduce medical errors and support evidence-based care; and (g) reduce health care costs arising from inefficiencies, medical errors, and incomplete health information. This vision for the national network was presented by Doug Fridsma, MD, PhD, director, Office of Interoperability and Standards, ONC, and is reflected in Figure 11.1.

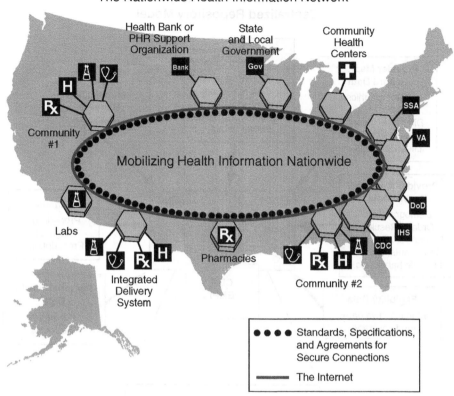

FIGURE 11.1. ONC vision for the NwHIN.

PHR, personal health record.

Source: Fridsma, n.d.

ARCHITECTURAL AND DATA-EXCHANGE MODELS FOR HIE

HIE can vary depending on whether data are managed in a centralized or decentralized manner or whether a combined approach with both methods of managing data is used, typically referred to as a "hybrid" approach. These models are noted in Figure 11.2. Decentralized data management is also called a "federated model." A decentralized or federated approach maintains control of the source data at the originating organization, and data are cached and transmitted to the provider as needed at the point of care. A record-locator service is needed within this model to identify and retrieve records accurately to support a point-to-point exchange of data between provider organizations. In this model, no data are stored in a centralized data repository. In the centralized data repository, HIE data sharing is protected through data-sharing agreements, and data are stored for use by organizations through the data repository. This approach typically fosters use of data within the community or region in a collaborative manner, supporting initiatives to improve quality, patient safety, population health, and care coordination. Later in this chapter, we discuss a case study on readmissions that is supported by this

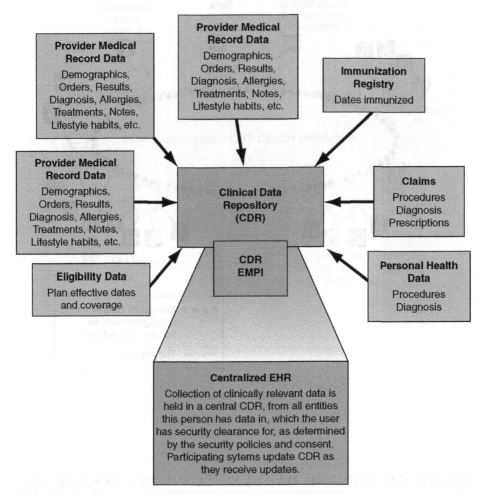

FIGURE 11.2. HIE models.

EHR, electronic health record; EMPI, enterprise master patient index; HIE, health information exchange.

Source: Gaebel (2011). Reproduced courtesy of HIMSS.

type of HIE model. This model requires a high degree of trust and collaboration within a community to allow a central data repository model to develop.

Technical Exchange

There are various models supporting technical exchange of data. Two common models used throughout the nation are the direct-messaging and the query-based transactions models. ONC-supported direct messaging is a basic function needed across the nation to allow secure messaging between and among providers; it is very similar to e-mail in that it is currently exchanged in the private sector, but with additional security requirements because of the required protected health information (PHI) and Health Insurance

Federated or Decentralized Model

FIGURE 11.2. (continued)

Portability and Accountability Act (HIPAA) protection. As HIEs reach higher levels of functionality, the interoperability of exchange of data increases in terms of ability to exchange structured data ubiquitously, both between and across care settings. Table 11.2 depicts examples of moving from the paper-based to a more advanced HIE model that fully exchanges machine-readable and -interpretable data using standards such as Health Level Seven (HL7; machine readable) and Logical Observation Identifiers Names and Codes (LOINC, machine interpretable). Figure 11.3 reflects how an exchange operates to manage machine-readable data using HL7 exchange standards to secure messages across the HIE both between and among providers.

Direct Messaging Project

The Direct Messaging Project is a project supported by ONC to provide a means for organizations to exchange secure data at the point of care at a reduced cost. The Direct Project itself neither runs nor provides services of an HIE, but it instead convenes stakeholders

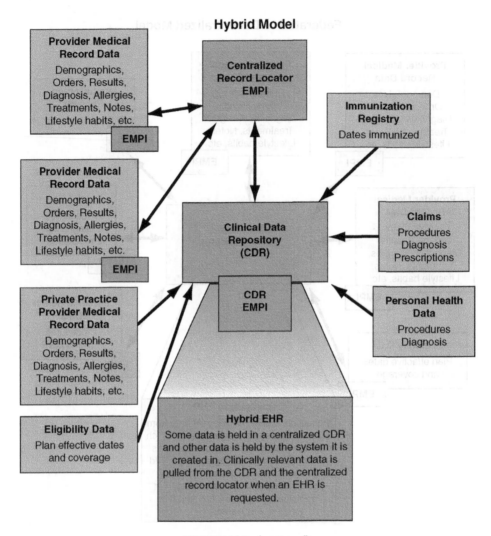

FIGURE 11.2. *(continued)*

to help establish the standards and service descriptions needed to address the key requirements for MU required to successfully attain financial incentives. According to the
National Learning Consortium posted on HealthIT.gov (HealthIT.gov, n.d.): "For Stage 2
MU, EHR vendors are required to either (a) certify their transitions-of-care modules or
complete EHR product offerings to include Direct to meet certification requirements,
or (b) work with a third party to provide Direct services." ONC cautions providers that
the tools an EHR vendor provides may or may not include the word "Direct," so it is
important to have a conversation with the EHR vendor to understand the tools available
within an EHR product (HealthIT.gov, 2014a). Within this approach, there are Direct
addresses that are required. Health information service providers (HISPs) can provide
support for services needed to undergird this type of exchange.

The Direct Project develops specifications using an "open government" approach
to enable collaboration for the development of a secure, scalable, and standard-based
approach for transporting health care data over the Internet to and from participants

TABLE 11.2 Descriptions of Interoperability Levels

Level	Description	Examples
1	Nonelectronic world	Mail, phone
2	Machine-transportable data	Manual fax, secure e-mail, and scanned documents
3	Machine-organizable data	Secure e-mail of free text, incompatible or proprietary file formats, and HL7 message
4	Machine-interpretable data	Automated entry of LOINC results from an external lab into a primary care provider's EHR

EHR, electronic health record; HL7, Health Level Seven; LOINC, Logical Observation Identifiers Names and Codes.

Source: Bennett, Tuttle, May, Harvell, and Coleman (2007).

Data Sources and HIE Approach

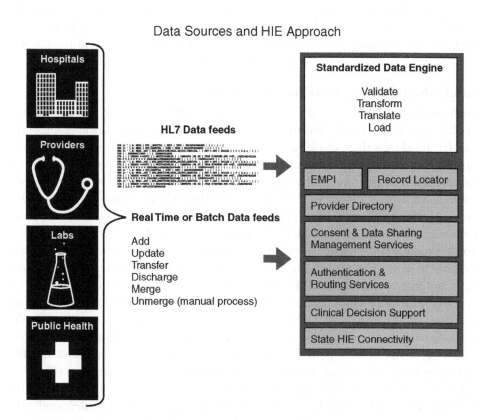

FIGURE 11.3. Sample of an approach for data exchange that is common in HIEs.

HIE, health information exchange; HL7, Health Level Seven.

(including providers, laboratories, hospitals, pharmacies, and patients). This process uses platforms similar to secure e-mail that encrypt data and support a cryptographic validation process. The Direct Project was initiated to help providers meet Stage 2 MU requirements and to foster the development of the NwHIN.

The Direct Project provides services to exchange data at lower costs than a fully functional HIE that supports the query-based technical approach to exchange. Many new HIE initiatives start their services with the Direct Project protocols and expand the development of services over time. This project helped many HIEs with an easy "on-ramp" for a wide set of providers and organizations looking at exchanging data. The vision for the Direct Project is to establish "one nationwide exchange, consisting of the organizations that have come together in a common policy framework to implement the standards and services" (directproject.org, 2015). The Direct Project is an exchange model providing a community with the ability to support health care providers who need to send and receive electronic information, such as lab results, patient referral, or discharge summaries, both easily and securely to support coordinated care (Williams et al., 2012).

Query-Based HIE

Query-based exchange provides the community and providers with the ability to find information when they are delivering potentially unplanned care. This is common in scenarios within the emergency department (ED), such as in the case of a patient with myocardial infarction (MI) where cardiac history is needed or an unresponsive patient for whom basic medical history is helpful. In a fully functional query-based exchange, a provider can electronically query external EHR systems for patient medical records and electronically respond to searchers from external EHR systems (HealthIT.gov, 2014b).

Standards and Interoperability Framework

Harmonization of efforts to enable exchange of data across the nation is likely the largest challenge related to effective and accurate data exchange to fulfill the vision of the NwHIN. To address these challenges, ONC has adopted an open access and communications platform to foster a community of sharing to address "real-world" problems encountered with interoperability and standards. The community includes standards development organizations (SDOs), vendors, and the HIT community, including HIEs across the country. These partners come together to share ideas and strategize to improve harmonization of standards. "The S&I Framework was established in order to enable health care stakeholders to drive higher interoperability and greater health information exchange to improve quality of care" (siframework.org, 2014). Initiatives under the Standards and Interoperability (S&I) Framework are focused projects that address specific areas where development is needed. Initiatives as of January 2015 include the following: (a) transitions of care, (b) laboratory results interface, (c) provider directories, (d) query health, (e) data segmentation, (f) electronic submission request for medical document (esMD), (g) certificate interoperability, (h) longitudinal coordination of care, and (i) public health reporting. All of these areas constitute challenges with the ability to effectively and seamlessly exchange data and information to support the goals outlined under the HITECH Act related to HIE. Harmonization of standards is focused on developing the seamless communication needed for data exchange. Table 11.3 provides an overview of these initiatives outlined in the S&I initiatives.

TABLE 11.3 S&I Framework Initiatives

Initiative	Description
Transitions of care	Initiative addresses the exchange of core clinical information among providers, patients, and other authorized entities electronically in support of MU and IOM-identified needs for improvement in the quality of care.
Laboratory results interface	This is focused on the challenge of lab reporting to ambulatory primary care providers; this not only is driven primarily by the needs of internal medicine, family practice, and pediatrics but may also be leveraged by other providers and settings.
Provider directories	This initiative has two purposes: 1. To determine the standards and specifications that should be used to enable discovery of a digital certificate when a recipient's direct address is known (read more about the Direct Project) 2. To determine the requirements, core data set, and data model needed to query provider directories for electronic service information (such as SOAP address, direct address, etc.) when some basic provider attributes are known
Query health	The initiative defines the standards and services for distributed population health queries from certified EHRs and other sources of patient records.
Data segmentation	This addresses the implementation and management of varying disclosure policies in an electronic HIE environment in an interoperable manner; the goal is to enable a pilot project that allows providers to share portions of an EMR while not sharing others, in line with applicable policy.
esMD	Initiative offers providers a new mechanism for submitting medical documentation to review contractors, such as the CMS Improper Payments auditors.
Certificate interoperability	This initiative aims at enabling providers to electronically exchange and protect electronic health information created or maintained by the certified EHR technology through the implementation of appropriate technical capabilities; the preliminary focus was on developing an analysis of the issues related to complying with digital certificate requirements for exchanging data with federal agencies.
Longitudinal coordination of care	The purpose of this initiative is to support and advance patient-centric interoperable HIE across the long-term and post-acute care spectrum.
Public health reporting	The purpose of this initiative is to harmonize HIT standards and implementation guides for bidirectional interoperable communication between clinical care and public health entities for selected use cases.

CMS, Centers for Medicare & Medicaid Services; EHR, electronic health record; EMR, electronic medical record; esMD, electronic submission request for medical document; HIE, health information exchange; HIT, health information technology; IOM, Institute of Medicine; MU, meaningful use; S&I, Standards and Interoperability Framework; SOAP, simple object access protocol.

Adapted from siframework.org (2014).

Business Models

The various business models for HIEs differ across the country. HIEs as conceptualized under the federal mandate push for an information highway or a circulatory system for exchange of health care data; HIEs vary largely across the nation in terms of both architecture and business model purposes. Some of the common-use cases for exchange tend to align with the value proposition and business drivers for the exchange. Common-use cases include public health initiatives, quality reporting, and shared information on high-risk populations such as indigent patients and those receiving emergency medical care. These HIEs, as conceptualized under the HITECH Act, are intended to shape the NwHIN by connecting the regional and state HIEs to the national network. An advantage of this model is that providers within a region can frequently align on needs of the community and develop RHIOs and HIEs within states to meet those specific needs. Often, services provided relate to requirements valued by providers and the community, and, depending on the demands of the community, may dictate the type of infrastructure needed for the HIE. Table 11.4 reflects some examples of value-based services that can be provided by HIEs and the description of the value proposition provided with the services.

TABLE 11.4 Valued Services Associated With HIEs and RHIOs	
Service	Value
Referral management	Allows users to efficiently manage referrals with electronic forms that are simpler and easier to fill out, as patient information can be pre-populated from the regional exchange
EMR publishing and transfer	Secure electronic document publishing with the ability to upload and transfer documents; allows a provider to securely share patients' medical records with any connected health care provider individually or publish them to the regional community
Provider of clinical messaging and notifications	Secure communication for connected health care providers
Demographic and clinical data exchange	Access to demographic and clinical data from connected health care providers; has the ability to view medical records from a secure HIPAA-compliant web portal, download and print patient information or in some cases, import directly into the EHR
Data feed and interfacing	System interface with HL7 compliance can provide ability to deliver discrete data elements and help connect to health care partners across a regional exchange

EHR, electronic health record; EMR, electronic medical record; HIE, health information exchange; HIPAA, Health Insurance Portability and Accountability Act; HL7, Health Level Seven; RHIO, regional health information exchange.

MASTER PATIENT INDEX AND RECORD LINKAGE

To provide accurate identification of patients across care settings within an HIE, a regional master patient index (MPI) and a record locator system are necessary. The purpose of an MPI is to identify unique patients within a delivery system maintaining disparate information systems or across institutions within regions. An MPI is an important element for effective management of patient care across institutions, particularly for HIE, and it has the ability to properly identify whether the records queried or retrieved belong to the correct individual.

Electronic and comprehensive linking of records has proved to be challenging. The routine matching of a unique identifier (e.g., Social Security number) is not enough to accurately identify multiple records associated with the same individual. Such linking assumes a high level of quality in the underlying data (Fernandes et al., 2007). Many health care organizations have an MPI application, which is provided as either passive or active functionality to identify individuals within the hospital or integrated delivery system. A passive system is seamless to the end user, whereas an active system requires active participation by the end user in the registration or scheduling system. Both methods are deployed to identify patients at the corporate or local level (Altendorf, 2007). These same types of systems can be used within a region and on a larger scale within an HIE.

Different Methods for Record Linkage in HIEs

Deterministic, rule-based, and probabilistic linkage methods are the three primary methods used for linking with systems deploying a combination of two or more methods. Probabilistic methods are considered the most sophisticated and use complex mathematical models to weight (assign a score) the match probability. Record linkage methods can be deterministic, probabilistic, or a combination of both. Probabilistic linkage takes into account the uncertainty that can exist in comparing the values being used for comparison (Grannis, Overhage, Hui, & McDonald, 2003). The uncertainty is related to the "rareness" of the characteristic used for comparison and how much confidence we have in the characteristic's ability to contribute toward uniqueness and hence a higher probability match (Krumholz et al., 2008). For example, a name, such as Jones or Smith, is likely to have a smaller match weight than more unusual names. Common or consistent names in a region can create challenges with record linkage and proper identification of individuals.

Record Linkage for Managing Clinical Quality

Regional HIE can support regional exchanges of information for managing quality of care within the region. One example of this is addressing transitions of care across institutions and care settings. This is an essential capability needed to perform well within new payer models requiring at-risk contracts, pay for performance, and efficient management of chronic illnesses. One example of a benefit that can be realized with the support of regional HIE relevant to record linkage in a central data repository model is tracking and trending outcome measures such as 30-day readmissions across care settings. Many institutions and health care systems can track readmissions within their own organizations, but they cannot track a readmission that occurs outside their institution (Altendorf, 2007).

In order to calculate readmission rates and effectively examine factors contributing to readmissions, multiple encounters by the same patient need to be linked together to provide a complete picture of care for patients. It is important to examine chains of readmissions to determine factors that might be targets for improvement within health care delivery systems (McBride, Pine, Goldfield, Hernandez, & Kennerly, 2008). Record linkage creates a single record from two or more records that belong to the same person. Historically, in a paper-based record system, the linking of personal records has been handled manually through record requests among providers. Many of the centralized data repository models have record locator features within the repository that allow identity matching to locate not only a record belonging to an individual patient but also the ability to link records across care settings.

The challenge to properly track patients within and across health care organizations to identify which patients are readmitting for conditions, such as heart failure, diabetes, mental health, and other chronic conditions, is becoming increasingly important to communities, particularly under new payment models. In addition, as organizations implement and utilize EHRs to support delivery of care, it is important that these systems be developed to capture the information and confounding factors to better understand the chains of readmissions such that interventions can be designed to effect change. Many of these systems are developed for point-of-care delivery and have not been developed to allow easy and accurate tracking of such information between providers. These systems typically require the combination of an additional component in the form of a clinical repository. These systems have enormous potential to expand and deliver additional information to clinicians, but they need further development and are costly to configure to meet the needs of supporting improvement processes, such as addressing readmissions. The modifications should be planned based on evidence, input from end users, and designed with clinical and technical input. Because many EHRs are missing the ability to robustly query quality data, one significant value proposition for HIEs is to provide support using a centralized data repository approach to track, trend, and report data on quality indicators such as readmissions.

VALUE OF HIE COUPLED WITH EHRs

The increasing use of EHRs and HIEs is beginning to demonstrate value to doctors, hospital systems, and patients. Studies have demonstrated that giving physicians access to patients' data from EHRs through HIEs results in fewer repeat procedures and reduces the number of medication errors. Data also indicate that diagnostic tests and follow-up visits decrease, whereas cost savings increase with greater use and exchange of EHRs. In addition to the cost savings of HIEs, their value in providing immediate access to vital patient health information can be a critical tool in delivering timely and appropriate care. Further, studies reflect the growing satisfaction of end users typically coupled with improved quality of care resulting from the use and exchange of data from EHRs. Some examples of these findings are included in the bulleted studies noted as follows:

► The University of Michigan found that patients visiting emergency rooms using EHRs and connected to an HIE were 59% less likely to have a redundant CT scan,

44% less likely to get a duplicate ultrasound, and 67% less likely to have a repeated chest x-ray (Lammers, Adler-Milstein, & Kocher, 2014).

► A St. Luke's Hospital (Cedar Rapids, IA) study found that use of HIE reduced hospital readmissions by 14% in their 500-bed hospital with more than 17,000 annual admissions (Bradke, 2009).

► A study published in *Applied Clinical Informatics* found that the odds of a hospital admission were 30% lower when HIE was accessed during the patient's ED visit (Vest, Kern, Campion, Silver, & Kaushal, 2014).

► In October 2013, researchers from the Medical University of South Carolina reported that HIE use resulted in a total savings of $1,035,654 for the state's patients, based on Medicare-allowable charges, or $1,947 per patient. They found that having access to an HIE for emergency patients produced savings that included $476,840 from reduced radiology testing (298 patients) and $551,282 as a result of patients avoiding admission to the hospital (56 patients). The study also found that nearly 90% of the 231 participating clinicians said using HIE improved the quality of patient care, with 82% saying valuable time was saved, reporting a mean time savings of 105 minutes per patient (Carr, 2013, October 14).

► Sharing of electronic health information across every major ED in the Memphis, TN, area, resulted in reduced hospital admissions, reduced radiology tests, and an annual cost savings of nearly $2 million, according to a Vanderbilt University study released by the *Journal of the American Medical Informatics Association* (Frisse et al., 2012).

► A 2011 study from Humana and the Wisconsin HIE found that with a $10 savings per impacted patient, the total decrease in ED expenditures under conservative estimates was still more than $4 million (Tzeel, Lawnicki, & Pemble, 2011).

► The Rochester (NY) RHIO found that when health care providers use the RHIO to query patient information as a part of care, the likelihood of duplicate image testing is reduced by 35%. The RHIO also found that when it is accessed by health care providers after hospital discharge, there is a 55% reduction in 30-day readmission rates. Furthermore, when the RHIO is accessed in the ED, study findings indicate that the odds of being admitted to the hospital from the ED are reduced by 30% (Vest et al., 2014).

► Research published by the National Center for Biotechnology Information shows that having complete patient information available at the point of care reduces adverse drug events and patient safety errors. According to a study by Smith et al. (2005), incomplete information at the point of care has been shown to adversely affect care in 44% of clinic visits and delay care in 59% of visits. A second report found that 18% of patient safety errors and 70% of adverse drug events could be eliminated if the right information were consistently available at the right time (Kaelber & Bates, 2007). The findings of a third study concluded that poor communication of medical information at transition points is responsible for as much as 50% of all medication errors and for up to 20% of adverse drug events (Bates et al., 1997).

▶ A 2013 study published in *BMC Medical Informatics and Decision Making* found that when external medical histories were consulted, the likelihood of 7-day readmissions decreased by 48% overall and by 27.2% when compared with viewing only information available in the local electronic medical record (EMR) system (Ben-Assuli, Shabtai, & Leshno, 2013).

▶ A 2012 survey from Accenture found that 53% of doctors surveyed also believed the introduction of EHRs improved the quality of care for their patients (Kern et al., 2008).

▶ Research published in the *Journal of General Internal Medicine* found in a study of small, group practices that electronic access to laboratory results across the exchange network was associated with higher performance in preventive care, chronic disease management, and patient satisfaction (Kern et al., 2008).

▶ A National Center for Health Statistics study found that 85% of the physicians who use EHR systems reported being satisfied with their system. Seventy-four percent believed that using their system enhanced overall patient care in certain areas, such as being alerted to critical lab values (52%), identifying potential medication errors (43%), and ordering fewer tests because lab results were available (30%). Ninety-two percent of patients were happy with E-Prescribing, and 63% reported fewer medication errors (Jamoom et al., 2012).

These studies demonstrate the increasing use of EHRs and HIEs within the health care industry and indicate their value as demonstrated by improved quality and reduced cost through reduced utilization of supplies and services.

MAINTAINING PRIVACY OF THE NwHIN

The privacy of personal health information and the accuracy of the information within the exchange is critical to the overall success of the nationwide exchange of health information. Health care consumers and providers must be able to trust that protected health information (PHI) is accurate and exchanged in a secure and private series of organized networks throughout the nation. Under statutory law, the ONC was required to not only develop the NwHIN but also to work with the chief privacy officer appointed by the Health and Human Services secretary to protect privacy and security of personal health information within the NwHIN (U.S. Congress, 2009, TitleXIII Section 3001b and 3001e). In 2012, administration of the eHealth Exchange transferred to the nonprofit now known as the Sequoia Project (previously Healtheway; http://sequoiaproject.org/ehealth-exchange/about/history).

Framework for Success of HIE

This section covers the trust frameworks needed to secure the privacy of personal health information and to maintain accuracy of the data within the exchanges. Various HIEs across the country have established mechanisms for developing trust within the regional and state exchanges through programs that certify HIEs and the provision of services through sufficient infrastructure, policy, and procedure to constitute a trusting organization. One example of this approach is established in Texas.

CASE STUDY OF TEXAS'S TRUST FRAMEWORK

The Texas Health Services Authority (THSA) was created in 2007 by the Texas legislature as a public–private entity to promote and coordinate electronic HIE in the state. In 2009, the federal HITECH Act created the State HIE Cooperative Agreement Program to fund state planning and implementation of HIE. The Texas Health and Human Services Commission (HHSC) contracted with THSA to coordinate implementation of the state HIE plan. Alongside HHSC, THSA worked on the State HIE Cooperative Agreement to support the planning, development, and implementation of local HIE networks with HITECH Act funding. THSA continues to provide support and coordination for local HIE development, including the creation of HIETexas—the state HIE hub that connects to the eHealth Exchange, administered by the Sequoia Project. The Sequoia Project is a nonprofit organization that was created to advance the implementation of HIE across states and was formerly Healtheway (The Sequoia Project, 2012).

As a part of the trust framework for Texas, THSA partnered with the Electronic Healthcare Network Accreditation Commission (EHNAC) in 2013 to develop an HIE accreditation program for all Texas HIEs. Public and private HIE organizations operating in the state are recognized for meeting and maintaining accepted and uniform standards in the handling of PHI. The program is designed to increase trust in HIE efforts and improve interoperability within the state, with the goal of increasing the number of physicians and patients participating in HIEs through emphasis on security, privacy, and accuracy of information exchanged within the state.

A model for the Texas program is shown in Figure 11.4. Many states, including Texas, have more stringent requirements to protect PHI than exists at the federal level under HIPAA requirements (see Chapter 14 for more information on federal HIPAA requirements). Texas defines a "covered entity" in a much broader sense than HIPAA does: "Any person who: (A) for commercial, financial, or professional gain, monetary fees, or dues, or on a cooperative, nonprofit, or pro bono basis, engages, in whole or in part, and with real or constructive knowledge, in the practice of assembling, collecting, analyzing, using, evaluating, storing, or transmitting PHI. The term includes a business associate, health care payer, governmental unit, information or computer management entity, school, health researcher, health care facility, clinic, health care provider, or person who maintains an internet site; (B) comes into possession of PHI; (C) obtains or stores PHI under this chapter [the Texas Medical Privacy Act]; or (D) is an employee, agent, or contractor of a person described in (A), (B), or (C) insofar as they create, receive, obtain, maintain, use or transmit PHI" (Texas Health Services Authority, 2012).

Texas, in partnership with the Health Information Trust Alliance (HITRUST), established a certification program called "SECURETexas: Health Information Privacy and Security Certification." Benefits of certification are as follows: (a) Certification builds consumer confidence in the entity's maintenance and exchange of PHI; (b) risk assessments are a component of the certification, thereby allowing

(continued)

CASE STUDY OF TEXAS'S TRUST FRAMEWORK (*continued*)

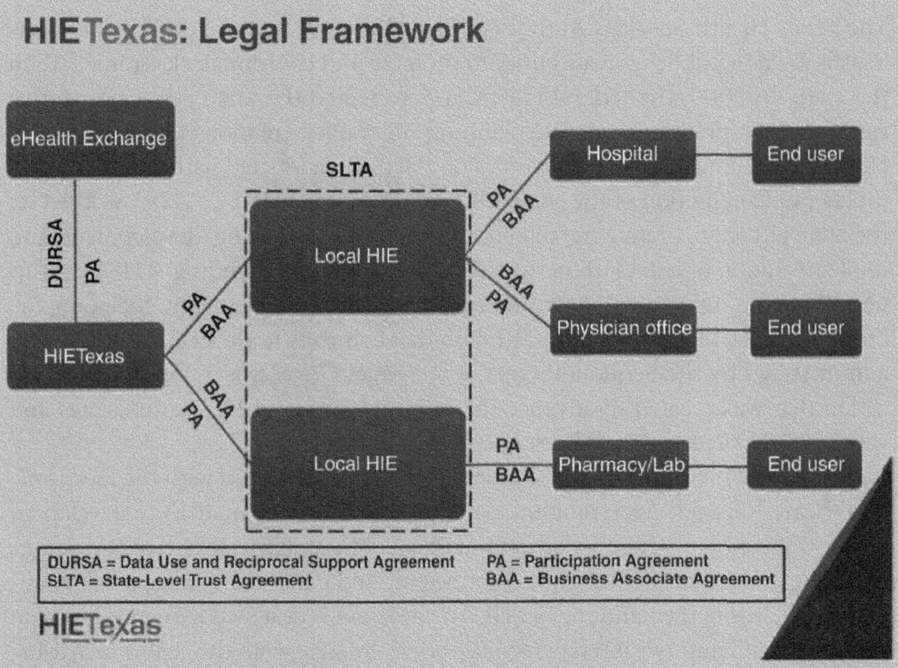

FIGURE 11.4. THSA trust framework.

entities to meet HIPAA/HITECH security requirements; and (c) certification can mitigate state penalties in the event of a breach of privacy or security, as the Texas statute indicates that fees associated with levying a civil or administrative penalty consider whether the covered entity maintained SECURETexas certification at the time of the violation. The certification report card provides objective, third-party evidence of compliance with two significant benefits for providers and health care organizations regarding mitigation under the Texas Medical Records Privacy Act, and another for mitigation under HIPAA at 45 CFR 164.408.

Figure 11.4 reflects the Texas Trust Framework and the legal documentation supporting private and secure exchange of health information in Texas. Within this framework, there are a number of legal documents required that are typical of exchange requirements throughout the nation. We describe these agreements in Table 11.5 with definitions of the legal documents outlined and included in the Federal Data Use and Reciprocal Support Agreement (DURSA), participation agreements (PAs), state-level trust agreement (SLTA), and business associate agreements (BAAs).

The purpose of this infrastructure is to instill confidence in the health care consumers within the state that their PHI is maintained properly and securely. Without that assurance, providers and health care consumers are unlikely to support HIEs within their states and communities.

(*continued*)

CASE STUDY OF TEXAS'S TRUST FRAMEWORK (*continued*)

Type of Agreement	Stakeholders	Purpose
Federal DURSA	Signed by all eHealth exchange participants, including HIETexas	Federal document; contains information on privacy, security, and technology standards
PAs	Agreements between THSA and HIETexas participants, and between HIETexas participants and their end users	Contains information on business issues such as timing, pricing, etc.
SLTA	Signed by HIETexas participants	State-level document maintained by THSA; contains information on privacy, security, and technology standards
BAAs	Agreements between THSA and HIETexas participants, and between HIETexas participants and their participant users	Contains details on the proper use, disclosure, and protection of PHI

TABLE 11.5 Legal Agreements Typical for Trust Frameworks and HIEs

BAAs, business associate agreements; DURSA, Data Use and Reciprocal Support Agreement; HIE, health information exchange; PAs, participation agreements; PHI, protected health information; SLTA, state-level trust agreement; THSA, Texas Health Services Authority.

SUMMARY

We have discussed the importance of HIE to the nation's strategic plan to fully maximize the nationwide health information infrastructure in improving patient safety and quality, creating efficiency with cost reductions, and improving the health of the nation. The history of the concept of HIE as well as barriers to success with prior initiatives have been discussed. The value of exchange has been noted through various studies that have produced results, indicating that HIE can produce results that achieve many of the goals for the NwHIN. HIEs are different in both form and business intent depending on the state's or region's needs. The business model that establishes success typically establishes how the HIE is constructed and what model it takes on, including a central data repository, a decentralized/federated model, and a hybrid approach. All three models have been defined with figures that give the reader a sense of how these different approaches work with respect to exchange of data. Finally, a case study has been described that presents the reader with an opportunity to place him- or herself in a community leadership role and to make decisions for the community as to how exchanges should materialize to meet the community's needs.

EXERCISES AND QUESTIONS FOR CONSIDERATION

You are in the chief nursing officer role and have been asked by your health care system to represent the hospital on a board of a new not-for-profit entity established by your community to build and manage the HIE within your region. Your region has been awarded a federal grant of $250,000 to build the HIE to serve the community. At the first board meeting of diverse stakeholders, including payers, providers, hospitals, public health, and health care consumers, the group must advise the chief executive on what type of exchange the group believes is needed. The chief executive indicates that a basic exchange using the Direct Project protocols for the size of the community is likely to exceed the federal grant dollars, and, as such, the group needs to align on a value proposition of what the community needs. This is hoped to result in the community being willing to pay for the additional costs.

The community has a population of more than 250,000 with a significant indigent population that tends to use the ED as an access to care for routine health care needs. Hospital staff also suspect that they have drug seekers going from one ED to the next seeking additional medications, yet do not have the information to confirm this suspicion or to track patients from one institution to another.

The community has two major health care systems that are heatedly competitive and unlikely to be willing to share data in a central data repository. Providers in the community comprise one large-practice consortium and multiple independent providers. The large group of providers is demanding that some sort of exchange be established to support their referral base. As a result, there is heated debate as to whether the community aligns on a business and infrastructure strategy. Based on information within the chapter, your group must consider the following questions:

1. Based on the needs of the community noted in the case study, what is your recommendation as to the best infrastructure and technical exchange model that the community should promote?

2. What are some of the barriers consistent with other communities' failures that might be issues for your community and how do you overcome those issues?

3. What type of exchange might support the needs of the providers in the community?

4. What does the region need to accurately track patients across care settings?

5. What is the most cost-effective model to be considered, and is it generating value for the community?

REFERENCES

Altendorf, R. (2007, October). *Establishment of a quality program for the master patient index*. Paper presented at the AHIMA's 79th National Convention and Exhibit Proceedings, Philadelphia, PA. Retrieved from http://library.ahima.org/xpedio/groups/public/documents/ahima/bok1_039331.hcsp? dDocName=bok1_039331

Barach, P., & Small, S. D. (2000). Reporting and preventing medical mishaps: Lessons from nonmedical near miss reporting systems. *British Medical Journal, 320,* 759–763. doi:http://dx.doi.org/10.1136/bmj.320.7237.759

Bates, D. W., Spell, N., Cullen, D. J., Burdick, E., Laird, N., Petersen, L. A., . . . Leape, L. L. (1997). The costs of adverse drug events in hospitalized patients. *Journal of the American Medical Association, 277*(4), 307–311. doi:10.1001/jama.1997.03540280045032

Ben-Assuli, O., Shabtai, I., & Leshno, M. (2013). The impact of EHR and HIE on reducing avoidable admissions: Controlling main differential diagnoses. *British Medical Council/Medical Informatics and Decision Making, 13*(49). doi:10.1186/1472-6947-13-49

Bennett, R., Tuttle, M., May, K., Harvell, J., & Coleman, E. (2007). *Health information exchange in post-acute and long-term care case study findings: Final report.* U.S. Department of Health and Human Services Report #HHS-100-03-0028. Retrieved from http://aspe.hhs.gov/daltcp/reports/2007/HIE case.htm

Blumenthal, D. (2010). Launching HITECH. *New England Journal of Medicine, 362*(5), 382–385. doi:10.1056/NEJMp0912825

Bradke, P. (2009). *Transition home program reduces readmissions for heart failure patients.* Retrieved from http://collab.fha.org/files/TransitionHomeProgram.pdf

Carr, C. (2013, October 14). *Health information exchange saves $1 million in emergency care costs for medicare.* Retrieved from http://newsroom.acep.org/2013-10-14-Health-Information-Exchange-Saves-1-Million-in-Emergency-Care-Costs-for-Medicare

directproject.org. (2015). *The Direct Project: Home.* Retrieved from http://wiki.directproject.org/

Fernandes, L., Brandt, M., Fetcher, D., Grant, K., Hatton, L., Postal, S., . . . American Health Information Management Association MPI Task Force. (2007). Building an enterprise master person index. *Journal of AHIMA, 75*(1), 56A–56D.

Fridsma, D. (n.d.). *NW-HIN: Past, present and future.* Unpublished manuscript.

Frisse, M. E., Johnson, K. B., Nian, H., Davison, C. L., Gadd, C. S., Unertl, K. M., . . . Chen, Q. (2012). The financial impact of health information exchange on emergency department care. *Journal of the American Medical Informatics Association, 19*(3), 328–333. doi:10.1136/amiajnl-2011-000394

Gaebel, H. (2011). *HIMSS common HIE technical infrastructure.* Retrieved from https://himsshie.pbworks.com/w/page/4777793/HIEModels

Grannis, S. J., Overhage, J. M., Hui, S., & McDonald, C. J. (2003). *Analysis of a probabilistic record linkage technique without human review.* Paper presented at the AMIA Annual Symposium Proceedings 2003: 259–263.

HealthIT.gov. (2014a). *Direct basics: Q&A for providers.* Retrieved from http://www.healthit.gov/sites/default/files/directbasicsforprovidersqa_05092014.pdf

HealthIT.gov. (2014b). *What is HIE?* Retrieved from http://www.healthit.gov/providers-professionals/health-information-exchange/what-hie#query-based_exchange

HealthIT.gov. (n.d.). *Eligible hospital tip sheet for meaningful use stage 2: Implementation tips for summary of care objective.* Retrieved from https://www.healthit.gov/sites/default/files/meaningful_use/EH_TOC_TipSheet.pdf

Institute of Medicine. (2001). *Crossing the quality chasm: A new health system for the 21st century* (No. IOM2001). Washington, DC: Author. Retrieved from http://www.iom.edu/~/media/Files/Report%20Files/2001/Crossing-the-Quality-Chasm/Quality%20Chasm%202001%20%20report%20brief.pdf

Jamoom, E., Beatty, P., Bercovitz, A., Woodwell, D., Palso, K., & Rechtsteiner, E. (2012). *Physician adoption of electronic health record systems: United States, 2011* (NCHS Data Brief No. 98). Hyattsville, MD: National Center for Health Statistics. Retrieved from http://www.cdc.gov/nchs/data/databriefs/db98.pdf

Kaelber, D. C., & Bates, D. W. (2007). Health information exchange and patient safety. *Journal of Biomedical Informatics, 40*(Suppl. 6), S40–S45. doi:http://dx.doi.org/10.1016/j.jbi.2007.08.011

Kern, L. M., Barrón, Y., Blair, A. J., Salkowe, J., Chambers, D., Callahan, M. A., & Kaushal, R. (2008). Electronic result viewing and quality of care in small group practices. *Journal of General Internal Medicine, 23*(4), 405–410. doi:10.1007/s11606-007-0448-1

Krumholz, H., Normand, S.-L., Keenan, P., Lin, Z., Drye, E., Bhat, K., . . . Schreiner, G. (2008). Hospital 30-day heart failure readmission measure methodology. Prepared by Yale New Haven Health Services Corporation/Center for Outcomes Research & Evaluation for the Centers for Medicare & Medicaid Services. Baltimore, MD: CMS.

Lammers, E., Adler-Milstein, J., & Kocher, E. (2014). Does health information exchange reduce redundant imaging? Evidence from emergency departments. *Medical Care, 52*(3), 227–234. doi:10.1097/MLR.0000000000000067

McBride, S., Pine, M., Goldfield, N., Hernandez, A., & Kennerly, D. (2008, October). *Clinically specific conditions and considerations for tracking readmissions.* NAHDO: Tracking Hospital Readmissions, Research and Reporting Conference, San Antonio, TX. doi:https://www.nahdo.org/node/314

President's Council of Advisors on Science and Technology. (2010). *Realizing the full potential of health information technology to improve healthcare for Americans: The path forward* (Report to the President). Washington, DC: Executive Office of the President, The White House. Retrieved from http://www.whitehouse.gov/sites/default/files/microsites/ostp/pcast-health-it-report.pdf

Public Health Service Act 3001, Sec. 3001. Retrieved from http://www.hipaasurvivalguide.com/public-health-service-act/section-3001.php

The Sequoia Project. (2012). *About the Sequoia Project.* Retrieved from http://sequoiaproject.org/about-us

siframework.org. (2014). *S&I framework: Home.* Retrieved from http://www.siframework.org/

Smith, P. C., Araya-Guerr, R., Bublitz, C., Parnes, B., Dickinson, L. M., Van Vorst, R., . . . Pace, W. D. (2005). Missing clinical information during primary care visits. *Journal of the American Medical Association, 293*(5), 565–571. doi:10.1001/jama.293.5.565

Texas Health Services Authority. (2012). *Who should get certified?* Retrieved from http://securetexas.org/about/who-should-get-certified

Tzeel, A., Lawnicki, V., & Pemble, K. R. (2011). The business case for payer support of a community-based health information exchange: A humana pilot evaluating its effectiveness in cost control for plan members seeking emergency department care. *American Health & Drug Benefits, 4*(4), 207–216. Retrieved from http://www.ahdbonline.com/issues/2011/july-august-2011-vol-4-no-4/732-feature-732

U.S. Congress. (2009). Health Information Technology for Economic and Clinical Health (HITECH) Act, Title XIII of Division A and Title IV of Division B of the American Recovery and Reinvestment Act of 2009 (ARRA), Pub. L. No. 111-5, 123 Stat. 226 (Feb. 17, 2009), codified at 42 U.S.C. §§300jj et seq.; §§17901 et seq

Vest, J. R., & Gamm, L. D. (2010). Health information exchange: Persistent challenges and new strategies. *Journal of the American Medical Informatics Association, 17*(3), 288–294. doi:10.1136/jamia.2010.003673

Vest, J. R., Kern, L. M., Campion, T. R., Silver, M. D., & Kaushal, R. (2014). Association between use of a health information exchange system and hospital admissions. *Applied Clinical Informatics*, 5(1), 219–231. doi:http://dx.doi.org/10.4338/ACI-2013-10-RA-0083

Williams, C., Mostashari, F., Mertz, K., Hogin, E., & Atwal, P. (2012). From the Office of the National Coordinator: The strategy for advancing the exchange of health information. *Health Affairs*, 31(3), 527–536. doi:10.1377/hlthaff.2011.1314

Woolf, S. H., Kuzel, A. J., Dovey, S. M., & Phillips, R. L. (2004). A string of mistakes: The importance of cascade analysis in describing, counting, and preventing medical errors. *Annals of Family Medecine*, 2(4), 317–326. doi:10.1370/afm.126

CHAPTER 12

National Standards for Health Information Technology

Susan H. Fenton and Susan McBride

OBJECTIVES

1. Discuss the history of health care data standards and the importance of the standards to the overall national health information technology (HIT) plan for the United States.

2. Discuss the historical development of the Nationwide Health Information Network (NwHIN) standards and their relationship to the Public Health Information Network (PHIN).

3. Understand the four different methods of standards creation.

4. Identify which electronic health record (EHR) standards are required for meaningful use (MU).

5. Perform a gap analysis to determine where standards might need to be created.

6. Determine potential positive and negative consequences of mapping between data standards.

7. Define the different nursing data standards and their potential use within EHRs.

KEY WORDS

data standards, Health Level 7, SNOMED, interoperability, data mapping, NIC, NOC, NANDA, ASTM, CPT, Digital Imaging and Communications in Medicine, HISB, IEEE, IOM Patient Safety Data Standards, ICD-9CM/ICD-10CM, LOINC, NCPDP, NDF-RT, RxNorm, UMLS, X12, messaging, code sets, ad hoc standards, de facto standards, government-mandated standards, common data standards, clinical document architecture, continuity-of-care record, continuity-of-care document, current procedural terminology, ICD-9-CM, ICD10-CM, Multipurpose Internet Mail Extensions

---

CONTENTS

INTRODUCTION

Health care data standards are a fundamental building block that the industry must address to fully realize the potential of the information technology (IT) infrastructure implemented under the Health Information Technology for Economic and Clinical Health (HITECH) Act and to capitalize on subsequent development, including global expansion of standards. This chapter covers the history of health care data standards under the NHIN and the PHIN, and the effort to "harmonize" or tie these efforts together under federal agencies, including the Centers for Medicare & Medicaid Services (CMS), the Office of the National Coordinator for Health Information Technology (ONC), and the Centers for Disease Control and Prevention (CDC). In addition, we review the various methods used to develop the national HIT data standards, identify important standards relevant to reaching Stage 3 of MU, and identify potential gaps that may represent barriers to fully realizing the entire potential of the national infrastructure for HIT. Finally, how the momentum to create a common language used to describe the contribution of nursing fits within the national and international agenda to create interoperability worldwide is explored.

HISTORICAL BACKGROUND

In a world that wants to, or even must exchange health information to improve the quality of health care delivery and reduce costs, standards are essential. Anyone who remembers the emergence of cell phones and e-mail can attest to this. In the beginning, cell phones only worked on the carrier network. Soon, standards were introduced and cell phones now roam the country. The same evolution happened with e-mail, when initially one was limited to exchanging e-mails with other people using the same e-mail service. Now, because of standards, e-mails are exchanged at will among different e-mail providers. This ability of a system to work with or use the parts of another system is known as "interoperability" (Interoperability, n.d.). This chapter explores the myriad standards needed for health care to become "interoperable" for the NwHIN, as well as for the PHIN. The development of standards by the different standards development organizations (SDOs), the role played by the ONC Standards Committee (U.S. Congress, 2010), MU, data mapping, and nursing data standards are also discussed. Standards are essential for the successful use of HIT.

NwHIN Standards

The U.S. NwHIN is intended to support the interoperable exchange of health information across the country. Codified in the HITECH Act that was a part of the American Recovery and Reinvestment Act of 2009 (U.S. Congress, 2010), it is important to note that health information exchange (HIE) efforts actually began in the 1990s. Community health management information systems (CHMISs) focused on the development of a centralized repository of clinical, demographic, and eligibility data. CHIMISs were first established in 1990 through grants from the Hartford Foundation (Vest & Gamm, 2010). Unfortunately, the technology was still rudimentary and CHMISs faced too many obstacles to become widespread (Vest & Gamm, 2010). Community health information networks (CHINs) emerged a few years later, and they were focused primarily on financial savings for providers (Vest & Gamm, 2010). This proved to be unsustainable; however, efforts did not stop there. In the late 1990s and early 2000s, regional health information organizations (RHIOs), facilitating HIE among providers in a geographical area, began to emerge. These HIE precursors experienced the same problems that are still encountered by HIEs. They encountered problems in identifying a sustainable business model, assuring privacy and security of the data, and overcoming the issue of competitor distrust.

However, standards for the exchange of health information have continued to evolve. The ONC Office of Standards and Interoperability (S&I) launched the S&I Framework project. More commonly called the S&I Framework, the ONC describes the project as follows:

> The S&I Framework empowers health care stakeholders to establish standards, specifications, and other implementation guidance that facilitate effective health care information exchange. The S&I Framework creates a forum—enabled by integrated functions, processes, and tools—where health care stakeholders can focus on solving real-world interoperability challenges. (Office of the National Coordinator for Health Information Technology, 2014)

The S&I Framework development effort is quite dynamic, and its different aspects are discussed. However, readers are encouraged to go to www.siframework.org to ensure they have the latest information. The S&I Framework functions are depicted in the abstract model reflected in Figure 12.1.

The specific NwHIN-related artifacts developed by the S&I Framework have been grouped into three areas: (a) content structure specifications, (b) transport and security specifications, and (c) vocabulary and code set specifications (So & Hebel, 2014). A substantial number of standards are required for effective HIE. The one explored here in depth is the Direct Project messaging standard. This initiative uses Multipurpose Internet Mail Extensions (MIME) for content packaging, with MIME for security and signatures, whereas X.509 digital signatures are used to establish sender and receiver authenticity (Directproject.org, 2014). Messages are routed using Simple Mail Transfer Protocol (SMTP). Additional details are available at www.directproject.org. Although the Direct Project solution does not provide all of the functionality ultimately desired and demanded for full interoperability, it is definitely a step in the right direction. Figure 12.2 reflects an abstract model demonstrating how the Direct Project sends messages securely from the sender to the receiver.

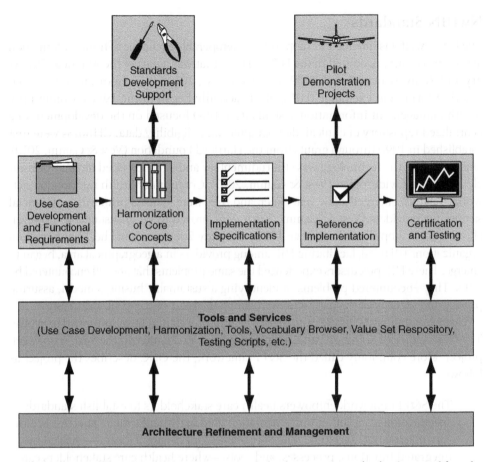

FIGURE 12.1. Set of functions for the S&I Framework development across the development life cycle.
Source: Office of the National Coordinator for Health Information Technology (2014).

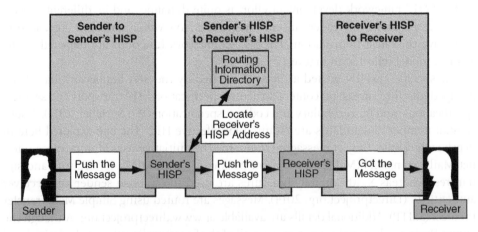

FIGURE 12.2. The Direct Project Abstract Model.
HISP, health information service provider.
Source: Directproject.org (2014).

To deal with the challenges already mentioned, HIE standards continue to evolve quickly and in previously unanticipated ways. Readers of this text should refer to the websites already mentioned to ensure they are utilizing the most up-to-date information given the rapid expansion of this capability and the dynamic nature of this development.

PHIN Standards

One of the most anticipated and useful applications of health information standards and HIE is in the public health arena. Syndromic surveillance and immunization registries are just two examples of the need for public health standards and HIE. Syndromic surveillance is a mechanism that is used to identify disease clusters early, before diagnoses, to confirm and report findings to public health agencies (Henning, 2004).

The PHIN began as a formal initiative in the early 2000s, with the original PHIN Preparedness Functional Requirement released in April 2005 (CDC, 2007). The initial specifications were targeted at early event detection, outbreak management, connecting laboratory systems, and partner communication and alerting, among other functionalities (CDC, 2007). As is often the case with initial specifications, these were found to need clarification and further refinement. Thus, the greater part of the year 2006 was spent in restructuring the PHIN requirements to reflect the public health workflow of identification, analysis, communication, and intervention. By February 2007, the specifications were revised and reissued as PHIN, Version 2. However, because nothing remains static in HIT, the standards continue to be updated.

In 2010, PHIN released their Cascading Alert Checklist, along with certification criteria for cascading alerts. Most recently, the S&I Framework has added the Public Health Reporting Initiative (PHRI). Initiated in 2013, this project seeks to:

▶ Select/harmonize the standards facilitating electronic reporting from clinical information systems to public health agencies

▶ Create/harmonize implementation specifications

▶ Create/harmonize reference implementations for standards testing, certification, criteria, and processes

▶ Create recommendations for public health reporting functions that are to be considered for Stage 3 of MU

Without a doubt, maintenance and improvement of public health, including syndromic surveillance of diseases, are among the main reasons for developing and utilizing effective standards for the transmission and exchange of health information.

STANDARDS DEVELOPMENT

It is helpful and important for people who work with health care data standards to understand the process by which the standards are developed. In addition, advanced practice clinicians, particularly clinical informaticists, are important contributors to the development of standards, policies, and practices related to standards implementation and use. The four basic methods of standards development are as follows:

1. *Ad hoc standards* are those that are established by a group of stakeholders without a formal adoption process.

2. *De facto standards* have evolved over time to become universally used without governmental or other mandates.

3. *Government-mandated standards* are specified or established by the government for certain purposes.

4. *Consensus standards* are those that are developed through a formal process of comment and feedback by interested stakeholders (Hammond & Cimino, 2001).

These four methods of standards development are not mutually exclusive. For example, many standards that are now either de facto or government-mandated standards were originally consensus standards.

Common Data Standards

This section reviews the common data standards and their purpose in health care. In addition, we cover how these standards relate to MU and the overall strategy used to achieve the full intent of MU of electronic health records. Many types of standards, as well as many different standards within each type, are needed to develop EHRs that are capable of interoperability. A goal of the industry is also to attain semantic interoperability. Semantic interoperability requires that the meaning of the information is understood as the data are exchanged. This may sound very simple; however, this is not always so. For example, if one simply receives the word "cold" in a transmission, the meaning cannot be known. The patient may have a cold. The patient may feel cold. The patient may be hypothermic from being left in the cold. This section describes some of the most common types of standards, as well as those most often used within each type.

Readers should look at the ONC Standards Hub website at www.healthit.gov/policy-researchers-implementers/meaningful-use-stage-2-0/standards-hub, as well as at the previously mentioned S&I Framework website for the most current information regarding standards and their relationship to EHR certification as well as the MU program. Within each standard, there are many values that can be used. The National Library of Medicine (NLM) has been designated as the national Value Set Authority Center (VSAC, pronounced V-sak). The VSAC maintains and provides access to all official versions of vocabulary value sets contained in the MU of clinical quality measures (CQMs).

Standards can generally be grouped into vocabulary and nonvocabulary standards. There are nonvocabulary EHR standards that include EHR functional specifications, messaging, clinical document standards, and medical imaging standards. We review a few of these in greater detail in the next section.

Functional Specifications of EHRs

The HL7 EHR-System Functional Model is "balloted by multiple standards organizations" and offers specific criteria for what constitutes a functional EHR (Health Level Seven [HL7] International, 2014a). The functional specifications have driven a large component of what constitutes a certified EHR in the United States under the MU technical requirements. The standards organizations involved in this process are expansive and include the following international entities:

► **International Organization for Standardization (ISO)**: A voluntary membership international standards group: www.iso.org/iso/home.html

► **European Committee for Standardization (CEN)**: A national standards body comprising 33 European countries

► **International Health Terminology Standards Development Organization (IHTSDO)**: An international not-for-profit standards group based in Denmark that owns the rights to Systematized Nomenclature of Medicine—Clinical Terms (SNOMED-CT). www.ihtsdo.org/

► **Clinical Data Interchange Standards Consortium (CDISC)**: A global, open, multidisciplinary, non-profit organization that has established standards to support the acquisition, exchange, submission, and archive of clinical research data and metadata. www.cdisc.org/

► **The Global Language of Business (GS1)**: An international standards group largely responsible for bar code standardization worldwide. www.gs1us.org/

► **Health Level 7 (HL7)**: A not-for-profit, American National Standards Institute (ANSI)-accredited standards development, as in standards development organization. www.hl7.org/

This model defines a standardized structure that must be present in the EHR systems to be constituted "an EHR" by these organizations. An important distinction is that this group does not define a functional model as "one system," but instead can consist of multiple components that constitute the system. MU certification of EHRs for the MU Incentive Program followed this definition in that "a certified EHR" under the CMS EHR Incentive Program can use either a modular approach or a complete system (HealthIT.gov, 2014).

Messaging

The most common health care messaging standard for text information is HL7. Two HL7 standards are focused on messaging: HL7 v2.x and HL7 V3. Version 2.x focuses on 12 different functions within health care, ranging from patient administration to order entry to medical records management to personnel management, among other functions. HL7 V3 utilizes similar domains as version 2; however, it uses extensible markup language (XML) and the HL7 Reference Information Model based on object-oriented principles.

Clinical Document Standards

The two leading clinical document standards are the HL7 Clinical Document Architecture (CDA) and the American Society for Testing Materials (ASTM) Continuity of Care Record (CCR). These two standards were merged, with the result being the Continuity of Care Document (CCD). The CDA provides the markup standardization that indicates the structure and semantics of the clinical document specifically for the purpose of standardizing clinical information to be exchanged both between and across care settings. The CDA can contain information such as admissions and discharge summaries, imaging, and pathology reports. The CCR is a data set that specifies important components, including administrative, demographic, and clinical information or facts about an individual patient's health care (Kibbe, 2005).

The CCD is a joint effort of HL7 International and ASTM to further promote exchange and interoperability through use of XML-based standards with the goal of sending clinical information from one provider to another without losing clinical meaning (HL7 International, 2014b). The Quality Reporting Document Architecture (QRDA) is an evolving standard created specifically for capturing and reporting quality measures. This standard will be covered in Chapter 28. QRDA and the Health Quality Measures Format (HQMF) are, essentially, the framework in which the measures reside within the EHR.

Medical Imaging and Communication

Digital Imaging and Communications in Medicine (DICOM) is also an international standards organization with the express purpose of establishing a global standard for the exchange of medical imaging and related information according to ISO standards. DICOM is a messaging standard that is used to communicate diagnostic and therapeutic information on digital images and associated data (DICOM, 2014).

Code Sets, Vocabularies, and Values

Content is included within each of the categories or types of standards. For example, patient records have demographics such as race and gender, as well as drugs, clinical laboratory results, diagnoses, and procedures. Common code sets, vocabularies, or values must be utilized for data to be exchanged using the HL7 standard and understood between different organizations and providers. Some of these important code sets include International Classification of Diseases (ICD-10-CM/PCS). Current Procedural Terminology (CPT) Code sets, Logical Observation Identifiers Names and Codes (LOINC), and Systematized Nomenclature of Medicine—Clinical Terms (SNOMED-CT). We cover these code sets in the next section.

ICD and CPT Code Sets

The most common code sets used are the diagnostic and procedural coding or classification systems. The oldest, most established system is the ICD, which is promulgated and maintained by the World Health Organization (WHO). The United States converted to ICD-10-CM on October 1, 2015. An international standard does not exist for procedures. In the United States, there are separate standards for inpatient procedures and ambulatory care procedures. ICD-9-CM, volume 3, was historically used for inpatient procedures, with a new system, ICD-10-PCS, adopted on October 1, 2015. Ambulatory care procedures are coded using the American Medical Association (AMA)'s CPT® (AMA, n.d.). The primary purpose of these classification systems in the United States is reimbursement or claims processing. These systems are classification systems, meaning they classify diseases or procedures into groups or categories. Categorization, though, is not often adequate to meet other needs requiring more detail.

LOINC and SNOMED-CT

The more detailed coding systems include vocabularies. Two of the most commonly used are the LOINC and the SNOMED-CT. The LOINC standard provides identifiers, names, and codes for representing clinical observations and laboratory test results in a way that allows them to be exchanged effectively and efficiently. SNOMED-CT provides a broad clinical vocabulary that includes clinical findings, procedures, and diseases.

EHRs, MU, AND THE IMPORTANCE OF DATA STANDARDS

To fully achieve the strategies envisioned by the U.S. national plan promulgated under the HITECH Act and to create the NwHIN throughout the nation with full interoperability, standards are crucial. Stage 1 of MU laid the foundation of EHRs implemented with a common set of metrics established through the certification criteria for vendors under the certification rules. Within these rules were specifications related to data standards that must be met to be fully certified. Stage 2 pressed harder on creating mechanisms within the EHRs to exchange data across care settings. This has proved to be challenging. The Agency for Healthcare Research and Quality (AHRQ) report, *A Robust Health Data Infrastructure*, prepared by JASON (AHRQ, 2013), calls on the industry to design an overarching data architecture for MU of Stage 3 that would provide logical organization of all functions to support full interoperability, while simultaneously protecting privacy and security of data exchanged. We cover exchange more fully in Chapter 11, and the requirements for privacy and security in Chapter 14. However, the identified barriers to realizing the full potential of interoperability are noted as follows by the JASON report:

> Although current efforts to define standards for EHRs and to certify HIT systems are useful, they lack a unifying software architecture to support broad interoperability. Interoperability is best achieved through the development of a comprehensive, open architecture. (AHRQ, 2013, p. 40)

The report calls on the ONC to create a committee structure that will oversee this effort to design the right infrastructure to meet these interoperability needs. The ONC has excellent resources available to fully understand the evolving standards and how these standards fit within the strategy to fully realize the NwHIN with a fully interoperable U.S. infrastructure. Important data standards are noted in Table 12.1. A more comprehensive list of data standards and their relationship to MU certification criteria is maintained by the ONC under the Standards and Certification Regulations website the "Standards Hub." On this site, www.healthit.gov/policy-researchers-implementers/meaningful-use-stage-2-0/standards-hub, one can access a table containing the publisher of the standards, the precise standard, and the exact notation within the certification criteria where the standard fits within the regulatory text. One can visit the ONC website and review a few of the standards. As one can see from this expansive list, there are many layers of standards with oversight from a number of national organizations, including the AMA, American Dental Association, CDC, CMS, HL7, and ASTM International, among others.

Stage 2 of Meaningful Use

Stages 1 and 2 of MU require certification of EHRs that are dependent on meeting the national standards with respect to content, transport, and security data. In Stage 2

TABLE 12.1 Standards Organizations and Important National Standards	
Technology Standards for Health Care	
Messaging Standards	**Used for**
HL7	Clinical data
X12N	Financial data, HIPAA-mandated transactions, transport of data
DICOM	Images
NCPDP	Standards for pharmacy business functions, HIPAA-mandated transactions
IEEE	Bedside instruments, medical information bus
Terminology Standards	
LOINC	Lab interoperability/data exchange
Drugs	NLM/FDA/VA collaboration on RxNorm, NDF-RT
Billing	CPT, ICD-9-CM
Clinical	UMLS, SNOMED, and others

CPT, Current Procedural Terminology; DICOM, Digital Imaging and Communication in Medicine; FDA, Food and Drug Administration; HIPAA, Health Insurance Portability and Accountability Act; HL7, Health Level Seven; ICD-9-CM, International Classification of Diseases, 9th edition, Clinical Modification; IEEE, Institute of Electrical and Electronics Engineers; LOINC, Logical Observation Identifiers Names and Codes; NCPDP, National Council for Prescription Drug Programs; NDF-RT, National Drug File-Reference Terminology; NLM, National Library of Medicine; SNOMED, Systematized Nomenclature of Medicine; UMLS, Unified Medical Language System; VA, Veterans Administration.

Source: National Health Information Infrastructure (n.d.).

of the MU Rule, the measureable objectives align with policy priorities for the National Health Plan. An important aspect of Stage 2 of MU that has proved to be the most difficult to reach for hospitals and providers is the requirement for care coordination. Not only is this difficult to attain from a clinical and practice workflow standpoint, but this requirement is also heavily reliant on data standards and, as such, provides an excellent example of how the data standards discussed in this chapter come together to produce a patient-centered, engaged health care consumer. Figure 12.3 reflects this requirement under the care coordination measure of Stage 2 of MU (ONC-HIT, 2013). One should note the dependency on multiple data standards reflected in this diagram. In addition, the requirements for documenting smoking status provide an excellent example of the complexity of utilizing the requirement for SNOMED-CT to assign a unique value to a clinical concept. Table 12.2 reflects these values.

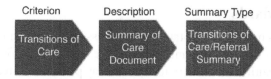

Criterion	Description	Summary Type
Transitions of Care	Summary of Care Document	Transitions of Care/Referral Summary

Common MU Data Set

- Patient name
- Sex
- Date of birth
- Race**
- Ethnicity**
- Preferred language**
- Care team member(s)
- Medications**
- Medication allergies**
- Care plan
- Problems**
- Laboratory test(s)**
- Laboratory value(s)/result(s)
- Procedures**
- Smoking status**
- Vital signs

Criterion-Specific Data Requirements

- Provider Name & Office Contact Information (Ambulatory Only)
- Reason for Referral (Ambulatory Only)
- Encounter Diagnoses**
- Cognitive Status
- Functional Status
- Discharge Instructions (Inpatient Only)
- Immunizations**

> Data requirements marked with a double asterick (**) also have defined vocabulary, which must be used

170.314(b) MU Certification Criterion Stage 2

FIGURE 12.3. Care coordination requirement for meeting Stage 2 of MU.
MU, meaningful use.

TABLE 12.2 SNOMED-CT Smoking Status Codes Required With Stage 2 of MU

Description	SNOMED-CT code
Current everyday smoker	449868002
Current some-day smoker	428041000124106
Former smoker	8517006
Never smoker	266919005
Smoker, current status unknown	77176002
Unknown whether ever smoked	266927001
Heavy tobacco smoker	428071000124103
Light tobacco smoker	428061000124105

MU, meaningful use; SNOMED-CT, Systematized Nomenclature of Medicine—Clinical Terms.

Source: Office of the National Coordinator for Health Information Technology (2013).

Potential Gaps in Standards

Although the use of standards in the United States has progressed and accelerated since the HITECH Act was passed in 2009, much remains to be done. This section covers some of the potential gaps in the health care industry today that may prohibit full realization of the national health care strategy to improve care through use of technology.

The first gap identified is the lack of data quality standards. One of the main concerns in this area is that of "copy and paste." There is a general consensus that copy and paste has led to a deterioration in the quality of clinical documentation. This is a very serious problem because it has the potential to decrease rather than increase the quality of clinical care. One problem that this would begin to address would be standards regarding which data fields should be static and which should be dynamic. Static fields would be those that are automatically copied forward from encounter to encounter, being updated only rarely, as needed. Dynamic fields would be those that need to continually be entered as new data. Examples of static fields include gender, race, and even something such as personal health history. Examples of dynamic fields include temperature, current conditions, and blood pressure. Recognizing and institutionalizing the copying of data that should rarely, if ever, change would ease the data-entry burden on clinicians and reduce the incentives to copy and paste other data.

Although there are many standards around required data elements and value sets for different data elements, many free-form data elements, such as height, weight, or other free-text fields, come with formatting requirements but with no other constraints or data quality standards. It would be beneficial to have standardized constraints on data elements whenever logical. For example, the weight field for adults should trigger alarms if a weight below 90 or above 500 is entered. That is not to say that the outlier weights could never be correct, but only that those entering the data should be alerted to the possibility of incorrect data. Without standardized constraints such as these, it is much easier for data that are clearly incorrect to not only be entered into EHRs but also be transmitted and shared across the health care industry.

Another desperately needed standard is in the area of advanced directives. This one is much more difficult, because state laws govern the legal implementation of advanced directives for health care. However, the current state of recording advanced directives, a simple "yes or no," makes it impossible to incorporate the desires of the patient into the EHR and any orders or clinical decision support. Until we can effectively incorporate patient and family preferences into health care, we cannot claim to fully deliver "patient-centered care."

As one can see from these two examples, the work to develop standards for EHRs in the United States is incomplete. We challenge our readers to think of other standards that both could and should be developed for EHRs.

DATA-MAPPING CONSIDERATIONS

There is a wide variation in the needs of providers and the health care industry at large with respect to data standards and architecture to support full exchange of data from the EHR. As a result, there are a variety of uses for the standards. For example, there are multiple code sets and data sets that necessitate data mapping between the code sets and data sets.

Data mapping is defined as the process of linking interoperable components from one system to another, involves mapping "one component to another," and is an essential component for interoperability (McBride, Gilder, Davis, & Fenton, 2006). The ISO defines *data mapping* as "the process of associating concepts or terms from one coding system to concepts or terms in another coding system and defining their equivalence in accordance with a documented rationale and a given purpose" (International Organization for Standardization [ISO], 2010). Data mapping is not only attempted between terminologies and classification systems but can also be done between the data elements or data fields in different applications or systems. There are both positive and negative consequences to mapping data. This section discusses the concept of data mapping, when and how it is currently utilized, and some of the challenges and undesirable consequences that occur along with it.

The development of any data map must begin with a clearly defined purpose. Maps can be created for data integration, clinical care, or other purposes. Each map with a variability in purpose will be different even if identical coding or data sets are used. Any map includes a source and a target. Each map originates from a data or code set known as the source. The code or data set in which one is attempting to find a code or data representation with an equivalent meaning is known as the target. When the map moves from an older source code (or data set) to a newer target code (or data set), it is a forward map. A map that goes from a newer source code or data set to an older target code or data set is a reverse map. For a map to be complete, its source, target, and direction should be specified.

The relationships in any map are often determined and defined by the purpose of the map. Examples of types of map relationships might include:

▶ *One to one*: The source entry has an exactly matching target entry

▶ *One to many*: The source entry has many potential target entry matches

▶ *No match*: The source entry has no matches in the target system

The level of equivalence can indicate the relationship between two code or data sets. Equivalence in a map is determined by the distribution of the map relationships for a given map. For example, a map containing 50% one-to-one maps would have a higher level of equivalence than one containing 20% one-to-one maps (AHIMA, 2011).

Additional considerations for mapping include the reasons for the project, or "the use case," as well as who is expected to benefit and use the map. As a result, data-map ownership and governance of the data maps are critical considerations, as someone has to maintain the map in the long term within the clinical information system. As code sets change and are updated, mapping maintenance considerations are important to data integrity. In addition, updates to code sets are not always on the same time schedule. For example, SNOMED-CT is updated every year in January and July (NLM, 2014), whereas ICD codes in the United States are updated annually on October 1 of every year. There are a number of considerations that a project team should work through when methodically developing a data map. The steps will help organizations develop and manage the reliability, validity, and long-term use of data maps within organizations. According to AHIMA, the data-mapping use case should be documented prior to implementation and include the reasons or purpose for the map, benefit or business case for the map, costs associated with the map, risks and benefits, end users, standards necessary and an indication of whether any are proprietary, and any document dependencies that might rely on the maps. Once this is done and the map is ready to be conceptualized, AHIMA advises that the heuristics or rules related to the map be developed. These rules include data sources to be mapped, inclusion and exclusion criteria, reliability procedures that need to be addressed, quality parameters to measure effectiveness, pilot testing procedures, implementation and iterative testing strategies for maintenance, and communication plans for stakeholders (AHIMA, 2011).

DESIRED CHARACTERISTICS FOR CONTROLLED MEDICAL VOCABULARIES

Cimino (1998) published "Desiderata" for controlled medical vocabularies while emphasizing the importance of a number of "desirable" characteristics. These characteristics include the following important areas: content, concept orientation, concept permanence, nonsemantic concept identifier, polyhierarchy, formal definitions, rejection of "not elsewhere classified (NEC)," recognized redundancy, multiple granularities, multiple consistent views, and graceful evolution. These terms are defined in Table 12.3. As the industry considers standards with respect to data, data maps, and the use of controlled medical vocabularies, it will be important to align development with the priorities noted by Cimino's classic work to specify what is needed in controlled medical vocabularies (Cimino, 1998).

NURSING DATA STANDARDS

Nursing data standards are important to the practice of nursing to document care provided and the contributions made by nursing to improve patient care quality, safety, efficiency, and population health. A number of national and international activities are promulgated to develop and expand useful standardized languages for direct patient care (bedside care), as well as home health and various interprofessional activities.

National Data Standards for Nursing

The American Nursing Association (ANA) recognized the importance of standardized nursing taxonomy and established a standing committee, the Committee for Nursing Practice Information Infrastructure (CNPII), to review and recognize standardized languages that support nursing practice. Many of these standards recognize the importance of capturing details and characteristics about the health care consumer that are not available in other terminologies; create an understanding of the context of care; and promote patient-centric care planning, care coordination, and outcomes evaluation across all settings. Throughout its history, CNPII identified two minimum data sets, seven interface terminologies, and two multidisciplinary terminologies, which are listed in Table 12.4. Initially, CNPII's recognition efforts focused solely on nursing-specific content developed by the profession. As the environment changed and other multidisciplinary terminologies evolved, codes for SNOMED-CT, LOINC, and alternate billing codes (ABC) became relevant to nursing practice and received ANA recognition.

TABLE 12.3 Desired Characteristics for Controlled Medical Vocabulary	
Characteristic	Description
Content	Content matches the purpose and is complete with expandability to add content as needed
Concept orientation	Terms must correspond to at least one meaning ("nonvagueness")
Concept permanence	Concept meaning must remain regardless of expansion or retirement of the concept
Nonsemantic identifier	Concept must have a unique identifier
Polyhierarchy	There are multiple ways of organizing the clinical vocabulary with hierarchy
Formal definitions	These definitions clarify concepts with a clear definition of characteristics
Reject NEC	"Not elsewhere classified," no specific code to classify the condition
Recognized redundancy	Synonomy or naming similarities
Multiple granularities	Multiple levels of detail
Multiple, consistent views	Same or similar views across use
Graceful evolution	Plan evolutionary paths for expansion and development

Adapted from Cimino (1998).

The CNPII identified existing relationships both between and among the various recognized terminologies as depicted in Table 12.5 (American Nurses Association [ANA], 2007b). Today's health care environment presents a very different picture as reflected in a later discussion of the collaborative and evolutionary efforts of the International Council of Nurses (ICN) and IHTSDO related to International Classification of Nursing Practice (ICNP®) and SNOMED-CT®.

International Nursing Standards

In a joint effort, the ICN and the IHTSDO, owner of SNOMED-CT, created a collaboration to ensure that nursing standards are not omitted from the international agenda to create a global international infrastructure for HIT, and that nurses worldwide have the

TABLE 12.4 ANA-Recognized Data Sets and Terminologies

Terminology	Description	Date Recognized by ANA	Oversight and Ownership	Website
Data Element Sets				
NMDS	Nursing Minimum Data Set; the minimum essential data elements necessary to describe clinical nursing practice	1999	ICN-Accredited Research and Development Center University of Minnesota	www.nursing.umn.edu/icmp/minimum-data-sets/
NMMDS	Nursing Management Minimum Data Set	1998	NMMDS School of Nursing	http://ana.nursingworld.org/npii/nmmds.htm
Interface Terminologies				
CCC	Clinical Care Classification System, formerly Home Health Care Classification System (HHCC)	1992	Virginia K. Saba, EdD, RN, FAAN, FACMI, LL	www.clinicalcareclassification.com
ICNP®	International Classification for Nursing Practice; provides an international standard to facilitate the description and comparison of nursing practice locally, regionally, nationally, and internationally	2000	International Classification for Nursing Practice	www.icn.ch/icnp.htm
NANDA	Nursing Diagnoses, Definitions, and Classifications	1992	NANDA International	www.nanda.org/
NIC	Nursing Interventions Classification System	1992	The Center for Nursing Classification and Clinical Effectiveness, University of Iowa	www.nursing.uiowa.edu/excellence/nursing_knowledge/clinical_effectiveness/index.htm

NOC	Nursing Outcomes Classification	1997	Center Director, Center for Nursing Classification and Clinical Effectiveness, University of Iowa	www.nursing.uiowa.edu/excellence/nursing_knowledge/clinical_effectiveness/index.htm
Omaha system	Classification, Intervention, and Problem Outcomes Rating Schemas for home health	1992	Board of Directors, the Omaha System	www.omahasystem.org
PNDS	Perioperative Nursing Data Set	1999	Association of Perioperative Registered Nurses	www.aorn.org/Clinical_Practice/EHR_Periop_Framework/EHR_Perioperative_Framework.aspx/
Multidisciplinary Terminologies				
ABC codes	Intervention codes used for clinical care, including integrative practices	2000	ABC Coding Solutions	www.abccodes.com
LOINC®	Logical Observation Identifiers Names and Codes; used for clinical care, outcomes management, and research	2002	Regenstrief Institute	http://loinc.org
SNOMED-CT	Systematized Nomenclature of Medicine—Clinical Terminology	1999	SNOMED Terminology Solutions—A Division of the College of American Pathologists	www.ihtsdo.org/snomed-ct/

Courtesy: (American Nurses Association, 2007a) ANA disclaimer on these standards: This information is historical in nature and does not reflect the continuing evolution of standardized nursing terminologies http://ana.nursingworld.org/npii/terminologies.htm

TABLE 12.5 Relationships Among ANA-Recognized Terminologies

	1	2	3	4	5	6	7	8	9	10	11	12	13
	NMDS	NMMDS	CCC	ICNP®	NANDA	NIC	NOC	OMAHA	PCDS	PNDS	ABC	LOINC®	SNOMED CT
									retired				
Data Element Sets													
1. NMDS (Nursing Minimum Data Set)			•	•	•	•	•	•		•	•		
2. NMMDS (Nursing Management Minimum Data Set)													
Interface Terminologies													
3. CCC (Clinical Care Classification)	•			•							•		•
4. ICNP® (International Classification of Nursing Practice)	•		•										
5. NANDA (NANDA International)	•					•	•			•			•
6. NIC (Nursing Intervention Classification)	•				•		•				•		•

Terminology										
7. NOC (Nursing Outcome Classification)	•	•		•					•	•
8. OMAHA (Omaha Home Health Care System)	•	•							•	
9. PCDS (Retired; Patient Care Data Set)										
10. PNDS (Perioperative Nursing Data Set)	•	•		•					•	
Multidisciplinary Terminologies										
11. ABC (Alternative Billing Codes)	•	•		•				•		
12. LOINC® (Logical Observation Identifiers Names and Codes)						•	•			
13. SNOMED-CT (Systematic Nomenclature of Medicine–Clinical Terms)		•		•	•	•	•			•

Courtesy: (American Nurses Association, 2007b) ANA disclaimer on these standards: This information is historical in nature and does not reflect the continuing evolution of standardized nursing terminologies http://ana.nursingworld.org/npii/relationship.htm

data, information, and tools needed to provide care to patients and communities. Under this effort, IHITSDO and the ICN have agreed to expand the work to align the data within SNOMED-CT and the ICNP through a joint publication of mappings (tables) between SNOMED-CT and ICNP diagnosis and nursing interventions. This joint effort will improve the interoperability internationally with respect to nursing data standards and the harmonization of nursing data standards with the international HIT infrastructure (NLM, 2012).

SUMMARY

Data and information standards are essential for the U.S. health care industry to meet clinical quality and public health goals for the nation. Standards are required to achieve semantic interoperability, as well as to achieve the important public health aim of effective biosurveillance with international implications. It is important to understand the different types of standards, as well as how different standards were developed so as to understand fully how they can and cannot be utilized. Although there are many health information standards in use and development continues, there are gaps that remain. Because health care and the IT supporting it continue to evolve, the standards need to continue to be developed. In this chapter we have covered some of the important standards, oversight organizations, and the national and international strategies used to establish standards to fully realize the interoperability for the NwHIN with global considerations. This chapter not only reflects how far we have come with respect to data standards over a fairly short period of time but also points to the work that is yet to be done to fully harmonize and create complete interoperability of standards within an architecture that is fully functional and can eventually expand to include global considerations.

EXERCISES AND QUESTIONS FOR CONSIDERATION

Identify one of the data standards discussed in the chapter or within the tables or website resources provided. Examples could include SNOMED-CT®, LOINC, HL7, CCD, DICOM, Continuity of Care Record Standard (CCR), Quality Reporting Document Architecture (QRDA), Digital Imaging and Communications in Medicine (DICOM), and standardized nursing terminologies (NIC, NOC, NANDA).

Identify the following important considerations related to the standard selected:

1. Introduction of the standard

2. Information as to where the standard fits in the national HIT infrastructure

3. Status of the standard with respect to current or future use

4. Implications for MU and interoperability

5. Implications for patient safety, quality, and population health

6. Challenges and/or barriers for implementation

7. Source of the standard, oversight of the development and use of the standard, history of the standard, references of where to electronically locate the standard, and

if the standard is not available, electronically identify where the standard can be located

8. Examine the standard in light of Cimino's desired characteristics for controlled medical vocabularies, and determine which of these concepts align with the standard reviewed.

REFERENCES

Agency for Healthcare Research and Quality. (2013). *A robust health data infrastructure.* (No. AHRQ Publication No. 14-0041-EF). Rockville, MD: Author.

American Health Information Management Association. (2011). Data mapping best practices. *Journal of American Health Information Management Association, 82*(4), 46–52.

American Medical Association. (n.d.). *CPT—Current procedural terminology.* Retrieved from http://www.ama-assn.org/ama/pub/physician-resources/solutions-managing-your-practice/coding-billing-insurance/cpt.page

American Nurses Association. (2007a). *Recognized data sets and terminologies.* Retrieved from http://ana.nursingworld.org/npii/terminologies.htm

American Nurses Association. (2007b). *Relationships among ANA recognized data element sets and terminologies.* Retrieved from http://ana.nursingworld.org/npii/relationship.htm

Centers for Disease Control and Prevention. (2007). *PHIN requirements: Version 2.* Retrieved from http://www.cdc.gov/phin/library/archive_2007/111759_requirements.pdf

Cimino, J. J. (1998). Desiderata for controlled medical vocabularies in the twenty-first century. *Methods of Information in Medecine, 37*(4–5), 394–403.

Digital Imaging and Communication in Medicine. (2014). *Strategic document.* Retrieved from http://dicom.nema.org

Directproject.org. (2014). *The direct project: Overview.* Retrieved from http://directproject.org/content.php?key=overview

Hammond, E. W., & Cimino, J. J. (2001). Standards in medical informatics. In E. H. Shortliffe & L. E. Perreault (Eds.), *Medical informatics computer applications in health care and biomedicine* (2nd ed., pp. 212–256). New York, NY: Springer-Verlag.

Health Information Technology for Economic and Clinical Health Act; *code of federal regulations § 3004(b)(1).* (2010).

Health Level Seven International. (2014a). *Section 4: EHR profiles—HL7 EHR-system functional model, R2.* Retrieved from http://www.hl7.org/implement/standards/product_brief.cfm?product_id=269

Health Level Seven International. (2014b). *Section 5: Implementation guide: HL7/ASTM implementation guide for CDA R2, continuity of care document (CCD) release 1.* Retrieved from http://www.hl7.org/implement/standards/product_brief.cfm?product_id=6

HealthIT.gov. (2014). *EHR incentives & certification: Certification process for EHR technologies.* Retrieved from http://www.healthit.gov/providers-professionals/certification-process-ehr-technologies

Henning, K. J. (2004). Overview of syndromic surveillance: What is syndromic surveillance? *Morbidity and Mortality Weekly Report, 53*(Supplement), 2014-5-11.

International Organization for Standardization. (2010). Mapping of Terminologies to Classifications. 05-31-2010 ISO TC 215/SC N, ISO 2010.

Interoperability. (n.d). In *Merriam-Webster's online dictionary*. Retrieved from http://www.merriam-webster.com/dictionary/interoperability

Kibbe, D. C. (2005). *Unofficial FAQ of the ASTM Continuity of Care Record (CCR) Standard*. Washington, DC: American Academy of Family Physicians. Retrieved from http://continuityofcarerecord.org/x6454.xml

McBride, S., Gilder, R., Davis, R., & Fenton, S. (2006). Data mapping. *Journal of American Health Information Management Association, 77*(2), 44–48.

National Health Information Infrastructure. (n.d). *Standards and standards organization*. Retrieved from http://www.aspe.hhs.gov/sp/nhii/standards.html

National Library of Medicine. (2012). *Nursing problem list subset of SNOMED-CT*. Retrieved from http://www.nlm.nih.gov/research/umls/Snomed/nursing_problemlist_subset.html

National Library of Medicine. (2014). *SNOMED-CT® release files*. Retrieved from http://www.nlm.nih.gov/research/umls/licensedcontent/snomedctfiles.html

Office of the National Coordinator for Health Information Technology. (2013). *Implementing consolidated-clinical document architecture (C-CDA) for meaningful use stage 2*. Retrieved from http://www.healthit.gov/sites/default/files/c-cda_and_meaningfulusecertification.pdf

Office of the National Coordinator for Health Information Technology. (2014). *S & I Framework update: HIT standards committee*. USA: HealthIT.gov.

So, E., & Hebel, L. (2014). *NwHIN portfolio*. Retrieved from http://confluence.siframework.org/display/SR/NwHIN+Portfolio

Vest, J. R., & Gamm, L. D. (2010). Health information exchange: Persistent challenges and new strategies. *Journal of the American Medical Informatics Association, 17*(3), 288–294. doi:10.1136/jamia.2010.003673

CHAPTER 13

Public Health Data to Support Healthy Communities in Health Assessment Planning

Lisa A. Campbell, Susan McBride, and Sue Pickens

OBJECTIVES

1. Discuss factors that influence the need for communities to provide community health needs assessments, including regulatory requirements and voluntary programs within the United States.

2. Outline the community needs assessment process and how data can be converted into information to knowledgably notify the planning process by providing models and tools that can be used in communities to structure the process.

3. Describe community health assessment data analysis methods, including both primary and secondary data analysis, metrics, and triangulation of the information to notify assessment, planning, intervention, and evaluation of health within communities.

4. Discuss a case study of a community and tools used to assess the health community needs and to develop a community health improvement plan.

5. Outline a road map for clinicians to utilize in approaching community health assessment and improvement by utilizing available health information technology within the industry.

6. Review steps to assessment, planning, intervention design, and evaluation.

7. Identify gaps in available resources and how those gaps will be addressed within the National Health Information Network and the harmonization of Public Health Information Network standards.

KEY WORDS

---

public health, community health needs assessment,* community health improvement plan, public health performance standards, outcomes, evaluation, and assessment, primary data, secondary data, community health report cards

---

CONTENTS

INTRODUCTION

Historically, it has been challenging to access information available to communities when performing community health assessments, interventions, and evaluations. However, as a result of rapidly expanding data sources under the emerging national health information technology (HIT) infrastructure, this challenge has become more manageable and population health has subsequently improved. Thus, to effectively utilize this new national infrastructure, one must comprehend not only HIT but also Public Health Infrastructure (PHI) and Community Health Assessment (CHA) strategies. This chapter examines how the expanded HIT infrastructure can be used in tandem with electronic health records (EHRs) and health information exchanges (HIEs) to bolster public health in communities across the United States. This information is placed within the context of how these essential tools can inform new payer reform models of care under the Patient Protection and Accountable Care Act (ACA) and the approach of various states to expand Medicaid. It is essential that under these risk contract models of payment we manage the health of at-risk individuals. To accomplish that goal, community assessment and intervention that impact health are critical. This chapter provides foundational information to accomplish the goal. In addition, a community assessment case study is examined to demonstrate how new sources of information can support this public health improvement goal.

PHI, HIT, and community assessment strategies are the focus of this chapter. These three fundamental building blocks are critical in effectively utilizing HIT and the rapidly expanding data sources under the emerging national HIT infrastructure to improve population health. Considering this infrastructure, we examine how new sources of information can be accessed to effectively support communities and public health in using new sources of information through the EHR and HIEs within the communities across the

---

*Community Health Assessment (used by local and state health departments) and Community Health Needs Assessment (as outlined in the ACA) are used with slightly different intent; however, for the sake of consistency we will use Community Health Needs Assessment (CHNA).

United States. We also examine a case study of a community assessment and witness how new sources of information can support effectiveness of these kinds of assessments.

COMMUNITY HEALTH NEEDS ASSESSMENT BACKGROUND

A community health needs assessment (CHNA) is the process of collecting and analyzing data to mobilize communities, empower citizens, engage stakeholders, set priorities, and identify resources to improve population health (Public Health Accreditation Board [PHAB], 2013) or "the outcomes of a group of individuals, including the distribution of such outcomes within the group" (Kindig & Stoddart, 2003, p. 380). Findings from the CHNA form a core of information that is an inextricable part of any community health improvement plan (CHIP). The CHIP is a process of realistic priority setting and long-range planning that includes action plans to achieve the goals and objectives of a plan. Action plans identify target areas to be addressed, the organization responsible, timelines, and actionable next steps. Each step in the action plan is critical to ensure its goals and objectives are accomplished. CHNAs and CHIPs are the foundation for improving a population's health.

Purpose of a CHNA

How well is your community doing? What are its strengths and assets? How do you know what is needed to improve the health of your community? CHNAs are tools that help us answer these questions. In recent years, community needs assessments have become essential documents for public health departments, as well as nonprofit and public hospitals to help address and improve the health of the populations they serve. A CHNA can be defined as an evidence-based analysis of the health-related strengths, weaknesses, opportunities, and threats for a specified community. "Community" can be defined not only geographically but also demographically by alternate groupings such as linguistic (Spanish-speaking children), work status (chemical plant workers), legal status (immigrant, visiting worker, incarcerated individual), or other characteristics such as veterans, refugees, HIV status, or sexual orientation.

Historical and Current Policy-Driven Requirements for CHNAs

CHNAs became essential under the proliferation of community benefit laws that began being passed by states in the late 1980s and 1990s (Hilltop Institute, n.d). Many states require nonprofit hospitals to conduct a community needs assessment; however, 37 states do not require nonprofit hospitals to conduct this assessment. In 2010, the ACA was passed and it established new standards that nonprofit hospitals must meet for federal tax exemption (Internal Revenue Service [IRS], 2014). These include conducting a CHNA and developing an implementation strategy every 3 years (Somerville, Nelson, & Mueller, 2013). These assessments and strategies create an important opportunity to improve the health of communities. They ensure that hospitals have the information they need to provide community benefits that meet the needs of their communities. They also provide an opportunity to improve the coordination of hospital community benefits along with other efforts to improve community health. By statute, the CHNAs must take into account input from "persons who represent the broad interests of the community served by the hospital facility, including those with special knowledge of or expertise in public health" (Association of State and Territorial Health Officials [ASTHO], 2015).

The ACA outlines the processes, methods, and contents required to conduct a CHNA, which broadly include the following elements:

▶ A description of the community service by the hospital

▶ An assessment of the health needs of the defined community

▶ Input of people representing the broad interests of the community

▶ Input from regional, state, or local health departments

▶ Input from medically underserved, low-income, and minority populations

▶ Written comments received from the public (IRS, 990)

Centers for Disease Control and Prevention Voluntary Accreditation Program

The Centers for Disease Control and Prevention (CDC) and the Robert Wood Johnson Foundation (RWJF) support the implementation of the national voluntary accreditation program for local, state, territorial, and tribal health departments. These standards are meant to strengthen the PHI of our communities (CDC, 2014). The public health model reflected in Figure 13.1 includes three core functions with 10 essential health services (CDC, 2010a). The core functions are assessment, policy development, and assurance. Under each core function are subcomponents to the process that outline the 10 essential health services. These functions and the essential health services are noted as follows:

1. Assessment

   a. Monitor health

   b. Diagnose and investigate

2. Policy development

   a. Inform, educate, and empower

   b. Mobilize community partnerships

   c. Develop policies

3. Assurance

   a. Enforce laws

   b. Link to/provide care

   c. Assure a competent workforce

   d. Evaluate

A CHNA conducted every 5 years is a part of the voluntary standards. It contributes to the core function of the local health department through identifying the assessment, policy development, and evaluation (CDC, 2010a; 2010b).

A third type of CHNA is required in communities that have a 1115 Medicaid Waiver. The Medicaid Waivers are methods that states are deploying to test ways to expand

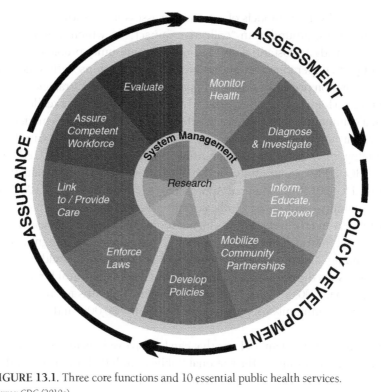

FIGURE 13.1. Three core functions and 10 essential public health services.
Source: CDC (2010a).

Medicaid to meet the needs of their specific state (Medicaid.Gov, 2014). Under the Waiver, states are required to develop a community needs assessment for each of their Waiver regions. Waiver projects that are developed should address the gaps and needs found in this assessment.

The confluence of these standards requiring CHNAs favors collaboration and coordination to meet all the requirements by different governing bodies and to improve the health of the community. The fundamental tenet of a community assessment is that local data and local criteria are essential to the solution of local problems that affect the health of a community. A CHNA helps establish community health goals and public health interventions, provides a starting place for regional health care planning, establishes goals and objectives for grant funding, and creates implementation strategies for local institutions to measure and evaluate health improvement.

COMMUNITY NEEDS ASSESSMENT PROCESS

A literature review is the necessary first step in the development of a community assessment. This review encompasses various assessment methods from the public health sector, hospital/health care systems, and other areas such as civic indices. The review is conducted on an ongoing basis to provide the most up-to-date methods for assessing community needs and assets. The review encompasses assessments from the public health sector, hospital and health care systems, and other areas such as municipalities and community-based organizations.

A review of various models of community assessments shows that the most effective assessments are grounded in "collective impact," in which a highly structured collaboration yields a substantial impact on large community problems. Collective impact focusing on cooperation, collaboration, and partnerships with stakeholders to help achieve common priorities and inform partners' investment strategies is foundational to the process (Kania & Kramer, 2011). In addition, there are excellent tools based on which a community can structure its efforts. Table 13.1 contains models of community assessment, including the National Association of County and City Health Officials Mobilizing for Action through Planning and Partnerships (NACCHO-MAPP) model (NACCHO, 2009), Community Health Assessment aNd Group Evaluation (CHANGE) model (CDC, 2013), the Planned Approach to Community Health (PATCH) model, and the Community Health Status Indicators model (see Table 13.1 for more information on these models and the website links for additional information). These resources provide foundational information based on which a community can design its overall strategy for community assessment. However, careful consideration should be taken as to what model best suits the community. For example, CHANGE is ideal for a community population less than 100,000 and takes approximately 3 months to complete. MAPP is best suited for a community population greater than 100,000 and has a timeline of 18 months.

There are also excellent tool sets that can be deployed, including the tools highlighted in Table 13.2. For example, the National Public Health Performance Standards (NPHPS) instrument version 2.0 and the CHANGE tool from the CDC (CDC, 2013) can be combined to fully assess a community using a combination of a structured model approach with tools readily available. These tools reflect the development of federal agencies, hospitals, health care systems, universities, and associations across the country working with stakeholders to develop tools and strategies available as examples of best practices. Tools such as these can be considered a framework when examining data and information available within communities working with stakeholders in the community to design community health assessment strategies. Figure 13.2 reflects the University of Wisconsin's County Health Rankings model. The County Health Rankings model provides a systematic approach for communities to identify opportunities to improve their health, engage and activate local leaders, and connect and empower community leaders. It is a road map for understanding data and developing strategies for community change.

Since enactment of the ACA, nonprofit hospitals are now required to conduct CHNAs. Pursuant to these requirements, hospitals have begun partnering with local public health departments (LPHDs) and stakeholders from local public health systems (LPHSs) to form intersectoral partnerships. Figure 13.3 reflects this public health system model. The partnerships that encourage collaboration among organizations (Adeleye & Ofili, 2010) and leverage resources are ideal to accomplish the CHNA and develop the CHIP. The success of these partnerships is the future of public health practice and it serves as a reminder that effective stakeholder engagement has become increasingly important, because many communities face a shortage of public health professionals (ASTHO, 2014; Beck, Boulton, Lemmings, & Clayton, 2012; University of Michigan, 2013). The tools and resources reflected in Tables 13.1 and 13.2 are a result of this type of sharing and development within communities.

TABLE 13.1 Models of Community Assessment		
Model	**Description**	**Additional Information**
MAPP	MAPP is focused on helping communities improve health and quality of life through community-wide strategic planning. MAPP uses four methods for creating the assessment and community plan, including (a) themes, (b) measures, (c) analytics, and (d) forces.	www.naccho.org/topics/infrastructure/mapp/framework/mappbasics.cfm
CHANGE	CHANGE was developed by the CDC to guide assessment and planning. The CHANGE tool helps a community in determining the overall health of the community and in identifying existing gaps for improvement. CHANGE is an Excel-based data collection tool developed by the Division of Healthy Communities Program at the National Center for Chronic Disease Prevention and Health Promotion of the CDC.	www.cdc.gov/nccdphp/dch/programs/healthycommunitiesprogram/tools/change.htm
PATCH	PATCH is a capacity-building model that uses a board-based advisory group, such as the State Bureau of Health, as well as community participation to design and model assessment plans.	www.lgreen.net/patch.pdf
CHSI	CHSI is a model that fosters development of key health indicators for local communities and encourages stakeholder groups' dialogues and actions that can be taken to improve a community's health. The CHSI report has more than 200 measures for each of the 3,141 U.S. counties.	http://wwwn.cdc.gov/communityhealth

CHANGE, Community Health Assessment aNd Group Evaluation; CHSI, Community Health Status Indicators; MAPP, Mobilizing for Action through Planning and Partnerships; PATCH, Planned Approach to Community Health.

The challenge in developing a plan is the uniqueness of every community with respect to things such as the prevalence of disease, a community's layout, city ordinances, county laws, human capital, existing prevention efforts, and leadership support. All of these factors must be taken into account as a community considers a plan for health improvement, along with the HIT, HIE, penetration of EHRs in the community, and availability of clinical data to inform the plan. Although the plurality of variables that need to be accounted for is challenging, development and execution of CHNAs and CHIPs can be done with a very systematic approach to examining information within the community.

TABLE 13.2 Resources and Tools for Assessment From Hospitals, Health Systems, Universities, and Associations

Tool	Description	Additional Information
NPHPS instrument version 2.0	The NPHPS instrument was used to obtain a high-level systems evaluation of how well the LPHS was meeting the 10 essential public health services.	www.cdc.gov/nphpsp/theinstruments.html
HCI platform	The HCI developed an easy-to-use platform, including tools and information for organizations and community groups. It is a customizable web-based information system that enables a constantly updated "living" needs assessment and helps hospitals meet health care reform and IRS 990 requirements for conducting community health needs assessments. The platform is designed to give stakeholders access to high-quality CHNA data and health indicators.	www.healthycommunitiesinstitute.com/spotlight-making-community-benefit-programs-vital-and-strategic/?gclid=COj2pYWQxsACFehj7AodggcA1Q
Association for Community Health Improvement Toolkit	This toolkit is a guide for planning, leading, and using CHNAs to better understand and improve the health of communities. It presents a suggested assessment framework with a six-step process, including a practical guide with a structured systematic approach.	www.assesstoolkit.org/
University of Wisconsin/RWJ County Health Rankings	The County Health Rankings include vital health factors, such as high school graduation rates, obesity, smoking, unemployment, access to healthy foods, the quality of air and water, income, and teen births in nearly every county in the United States. The annual rankings provide a revealing snapshot of how health is influenced by where we live, learn, work, and play. They provide a starting point for change in communities. The County Health Rankings model provides a road map that offers guidance and tools to understand the data, and strategies that communities can use to move from education to action.	www.countyhealthrankings.org

UCLA (University of California, Los Angeles)–HIA toolkit	*HIA* is most often defined as "a combination of procedures, methods and tools by which a policy, program or project may be judged as to its potential effects on the health of a population, and the distribution of those effects within the population" (World Health Organization [WHO], 2015). This broad definition from the WHO-ECHP, presented in the Gothenburg Consensus paper on HIA, reflects the many variants of HIA. A more precise definition is that HIA is a multidisciplinary process within which a range of evidence about the health effects of a proposal is considered in a structured framework.	www.hiaguide.org/methods-resources
Kaiser Permanente Community Health Assessment Toolkit	This toolkit was developed to ensure compliance with the new federal requirements of the ACA. It provides a detailed federal requirements checklist that encompasses pre-assessment planning to implementation planning.	www.communitycommons.org/groups/community-health-needs-assessment-chna/
CHA	CHA brought together stakeholders, including hospitals, local health departments, and federally qualified health centers, to align goals and develop a process that fosters improvements in health outcomes. The basis of the toolkit utilizes the Association for Community Health Improvements framework, which includes six steps for completing a CHNA.	http://documents.cthosp.org/documents/community-health/cha-chna-master-document_final.pdf
Cook Children's Hospital Community Assessment	This Children's Hospital Approach begins with community surveys, focus groups, key informant surveys, and community meetings. The basis for their community participatory survey toolset is for each community to take on responsibilities for the issues and solutions within their county.	www.cookchildrens.org/AboutUs/Pages/Community-Health-Needs-Assessment-Report.aspx
Dignity Health's CNI	Dignity Health's CNI provides a numerical indicator that accounts for the underlying socioeconomic and access barriers that affect a population's health status. In developing the CNI, Dignity Health identified five prominent barriers related to income, culture/language, education, insurance, and housing. It has been developed at a ZIP (Zone Improvement Plan) code level. A score of 1.0 indicates a ZIP code with the least socioeconomic barriers, whereas a score of 5.0 represents a ZIP code with the most socioeconomic barriers.	www.dignityhealth.org/Who_We_Are/Community_Health/STGSS044508

ACA, Accountable Care Act; CHA, Connecticut Hospital Associations; CHNA, Community Health Needs Assessment; CNI, Community Need Index; ECHP, European Center for Health Policy; HCI, Healthy Communities Institute; HIA, health impact assessment; IRS, Internal Revenue Service; LPHSs, local public health systems; NPHPS, National Public Health Performance Standards; WHO-ECHP, World Health Organization European Center for Health Policy.

317

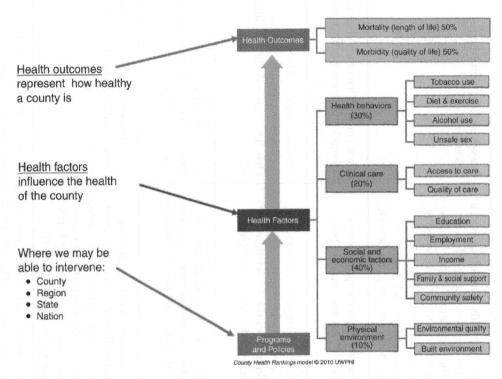

FIGURE 13.2. University of Wisconsin's County health rankings model.

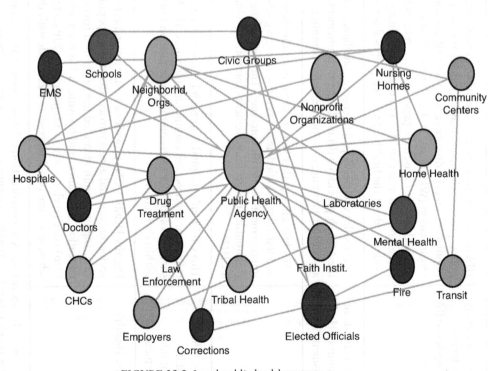

FIGURE 13.3. Local public health systems.

CHCs, community health centers; EMS, emergency medical services.

Source: CDC (2010b).

Community Asset Mapping and Geomapping Methods for Assessment

Community assessments should function as a tool that helps rebuild communities. In *Building Communities from the Inside Out* (Kretzmann & McKnight, 1993), John McKnight and John P. Kretzmann propose that communities are not developed based on their deficiencies but on their strengths. The combination of community strengths and assets is a critical component of a community assessment, with identification of strengths and assets used to build on within each community. This helps identify community competencies and organizations that can help improve community health. It also brings community ownership to the issues. Assets to be mapped are resources such as libraries, parks, recreation centers, businesses, churches, block clubs, cultural groups, associations, and schools.

Looking even deeper into community competencies, one finds the individual and household capacities that exist in each neighborhood. It may be very difficult to identify these assets. However, these are the assets that change communities (ABCD Institute, 2009). An example is the Neighborhood Health Status Improvement project by Deborah Puntenney (ABCD Institute, 2010). The approach is a place-based strategy and is designed by the residents of the community with a grassroots orientation. It includes mapping local health assets, mobilizing local residents and associations, and leveraging the resources within the community to implement the plan. Figure 13.4 reflects a community assessment map completed in Texas (Edwards, Suchltz, Erickson, & Pickens, 2013). This is an example of community assets by mapping location of hospitals and charitable care clinics, as well as other community resources that impact health. These types of data visualizations are powerful representations of data that can focus communities on the available resources demonstrating strengths, as well as areas that reflect lack of available resources within the community demonstrating weaknesses.

Geomapping methods that reflect disease prevalence and comorbidities in the population are also a powerful illustration of where at-risk populations may reside. Figure 13.5 reflects the analysis of trends related to methycillin-resistant *Staphylococcus aureus* (MRSA). This illustration indicates MRSA rates by county in Texas for the year 2004, indicating where primary and secondary clusters of MRSA rates of infection reside (McBride, 2005, 2006).

Data-Analytic and Statistical Approaches

A community health assessment uniquely blends different types of data that relate to the health status of individuals, communities, and populations. The community assessment methodology is an epidemiological-based process that is used for identifying populations with a predisposition to poor health. The goal of a community assessment is to locate communities that have common characteristics. It must be statistically valid, nonjudgmental, and specific to geographic locations and health criteria. The assessment process described here blends four different data-analytic strategies to identify community needs.

The first data-analysis method begins with the compilation of secondary data. These data are demographic variables, birth statistics, the leading causes of death, access to primary care, social factors such as food insecurities, policies and programs, physical

Dallas County

Community Health Needs Assessment Service/Provider Locations

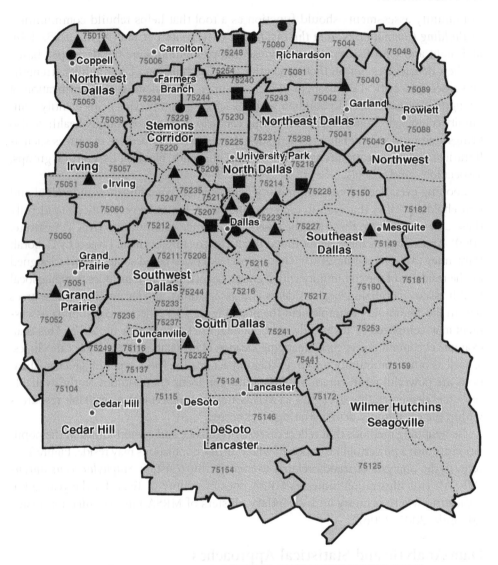

Total in Dallas County	Service/Provider Type
10	● Farmers' Market
29	▲ Recreation
9	■ Walking/Bike Trails

Locations are approximate and based on street address.

FIGURE 13.4. A map of community assets.

Source: Edwards et al. (2013).

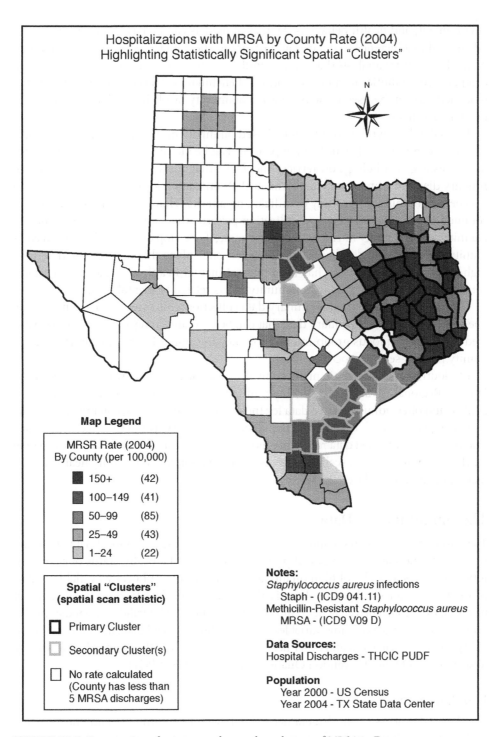

FIGURE 13.5. Geomapping of primary and secondary clusters of MRSA in Texas.

MRSA, methicillin-resistant *Staphylococcus aureus*; THCIC, Texas Health Care Information Collection; PUDF, Public Use Data File.

Source: McBride (2005).

environment, and health behaviors. Statistical models can be based on ranking methods related to adherence to policies and programs, health factors and health outcomes, hierarchical cluster analysis that groups similar communities together, or a method that compares communities to state and national benchmarks. All these statistical and analytic methods can be used to help identify community needs in an objective, nonjudgmental data-driven process.

The second analytic method can be based on inpatient utilization patterns of each identified community. The utilization patterns can be viewed in terms of different product lines (e.g., cardiology, obstetrics, oncology), diagnosis-related groups (DRGs), or primary diagnosis. Emergency department (ED) utilization for nonemergency care can also be part of this second study of utilization patterns. This type of analysis generates common disease factors based on utilization patterns that can inform assessment and planning for community intervention. For example, if one's top diagnoses for a given community are cardiovascular disease and diabetes, one's plans should be directed at those high-risk populations. If one has high rates of mental health-associated admissions, consideration should be paid to community needs related to mental health.

The third analytic method is primary data collection; this can come from more than one source. Examples of primary data that can be used are survey data, preferably gathered by telephone; focus group information; key informant interviews; and/or a community priority-setting process.

The fourth type of analytic method involves capitalizing on new data sources from HIEs or Regional Data Initiatives. These initiatives involve the collection of electronic clinical and often administrative data for the purpose of improving collaboration in the region on patient safety, quality, and population health initiatives. HIEs that deploy data warehouse or centralized data repository models generate data and analytics in the region for that purpose and are excellent sources of information for community health assessment and planning (Glaser, 2006).

The Importance of Data

The basis for a successful community assessment is contingent on local data and criteria to aid in the solution of regional problems that affect the health status of a community. The data should be of high quality and sourced from publically available and/or privately held data (in the case of the HIE or regional collaborative), or the data might be purchased from a privately held third party. Data needed for valid assessment involve population statistics, economic variables, birth and birth-related data, mortality and morbidity data, access to care, and other health indicators such as the Agency for Healthcare Research and Quality Prevention Quality Indicators (AHRQ-PQIs).

Population Variables

Population density is a core element needed to reflect the community and may be noted as the total number of individuals living in a specific area per square mile. Many conditions that produce impacts on community health are related to density. An example of this type of health impact is the contagion of communicable diseases occurring at higher population densities. With lower population densities, the availability of medical care tends to decrease. Other factors that should be noted within the community assessment include age, race, and ethnicity. Age groups are important, because children are more susceptible to communicable disease and injury, the elderly to chronic and degenerative disease, and young adults to injuries. An example of the importance of race and ethnicity can be seen by the higher prevalence rates of diabetes generally found in the Hispanic population. With respect to racial groups, American Indians and Alaska Natives are more than twice as likely to develop diabetes as are White Americans (Johns Hopkins Medicine, 2014).

Economics—Income

It is also important to consider economic data on the community. The effect of income can determine housing conditions, nutritional status, social standing, social ties, education, access to health services, and other social and health problems or social determinants of health. According to research from the California Endowment, "your ZIP code shouldn't predict how long you live" (California Endowment, 2014; Davis, Cohen, & Rodriguez, 2010).

Birth and Birth-Related Information

Birth rates and neonatal mortality are specific indicators that reflect growth in the community, as well as potential health risks. For example, neonatal mortality is correlated with low birth weight with a direct impact on an infant's ability to survive and develop. Maternal factors, such as a mother's age and educational levels (available in birth certificate data), have been shown to affect health status of both mother and baby (Office of Adolescent Health, 2014).

Mortality and Morbidity—Death-Rate Variables

Age-adjusted death rates for leading causes of death are standard metrics in a health assessment, and these can be comparable over time and among geographic areas. Mortality and morbidity (disease prevalence) are important factors to be considered when assessing a community's health status. What is the burden of disease? How could mortality rates for various comorbid conditions be compared with state and national rates? It is important to examine these questions in data analysis and reports within a CHNA. The AHRQ Inpatient Quality Indicators for mortality and utilization can be used to examine morbidity and mortality for a region. These indicators are noted in Table 13.3. These indicators are sensitive not only to morbidity within the community but also to the quality of health care services provided in the community, and they are frequently used by states to report quality measures to the public (AHRQ, 2014a). Figure 13.6 presents an example of this type of quality analysis using the congestive heart failure (CHF) risk-adjusted mortality rate showing a trend over time. This indicator reflects a downward trend on mortality rates for this community (McBride, 2007).

Access to Primary Care

In conjunction with preventive services, access to primary care has been shown to reduce early onset of disease and death (Bauer, Briss, Goodman, & Bowman, 2014; Haughton & Stang, 2012; Nicholas & Hall, 2011; Starfiled, So, & Macinko, 2005; Stevens et al., 2014). The AHRQ has developed an algorithm for determining preventable hospitalizations. Applying these data to local geography can help in identifying communities where access

TABLE 13.3 AHRQ Quality Indicators

Mortality rates for conditions
AMI
AMI without transfer
Congestive heart failure
Gastrointestinal hemorrhage
Hip fracture
Pneumonia
Acute stroke

Mortality rates for procedures
Abdominal aortic aneurysm repair
Coronary artery bypass graft
Craniotomy
Esophageal resection
Hip replacement
Pancreatic resection
Percutaneous transluminal coronary angioplasty
Carotid endarterectomy

Hospital-level procedure utilization rates
Cesarean section delivery
Primary cesarean delivery
Uncomplicated vaginal birth after cesarean delivery (VBAC)
Total rate for vaginal birth after cesarean delivery (VBAC)
Incidental appendectomy in the elderly
Bilateral cardiac catheterization
Laparoscopic cholecystecomy

Area-level utilization rates (e.g., county, state)
Coronary artery bypass graft
Hysterectomy
Laminectomy or spinal fusion
Percutaneous transluminal coronary angioplasty

Volume of procedures
Abdominal aortic aneurysm repair
Carotid endarterectomy
Coronary artery bypass graft
Esophageal resection
Pancreatic resection
Percutaneous transluminal coronary angioplasty

AHRQ, Agency for Healthcare Research and Quality; AMI, acute myocardial infarction.
Source: AHRQ (2014a).

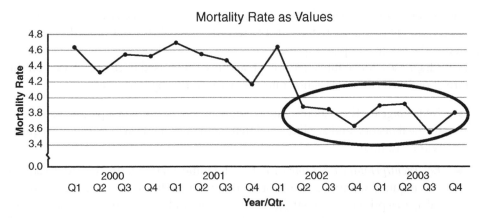

FIGURE 13.6. Congestive heart failure mortality rates—an example of AHRQ quality indicators used in community assessments reflecting a trend line with reduced overall rates of mortality.
AHRQ, Agency for Healthcare Research and Quality.

TABLE 13.4 AHRQ-PQIs
Bacterial pneumonia
Dehydration
Urinary tract infections
Perforated appendix
Low birth weight
Angina without procedure
Congestive heart failure
Hypertension
Adult asthma
Chronic obstructive pulmonary disease
Uncontrolled diabetes
Diabetes, short-term complications
Diabetes, long-term complications
Lower-extremity amputations among patients with diabetes

AHRQ-PQIs, Agency for Healthcare Research and Quality Prevention Quality Indicators.

Source: AHRQ (2014b).

to care may be influencing the utilization patterns measured within the indicators. The Prevention Quality Indicators (PQIs) are a set of measures that can be used with hospital inpatient discharge data to identify quality of care for "ambulatory care sensitive conditions." These are conditions for which good outpatient care can potentially prevent the need for hospitalization or for which early intervention can prevent complications or more severe disease. The PQIs are population based and are adjusted for covariates such as age, sex, and risk. Table 13.4 reflects the AHRQ-PQI measures (AHRQ, 2014b).

The New York University (NYU) Center for Health and Public Service Research has developed an algorithm to help classify ED utilization. The algorithm was developed with the advice of a panel of ED and primary care physicians, and it is based on an examination of a sample of almost 6,000 full ED records. Data abstracted from these records included the initial complaint, presenting symptoms, vital signs, medical history, age, gender, diagnoses, procedures performed, and resources used in the ED. Based on this information, each case is classified into one of the following categories:

▶ *Nonemergent*: The patient's initial complaint, presenting symptoms, vital signs, medical history, and age indicated that immediate medical care was not required within 12 hours.

▶ *Emergent/primary treatable care*: Based on information in the record, treatment was required within 12 hours, but care could have been provided effectively and safely in a primary care setting. The complaint did not require continuous observation, and no procedures were performed or resources used that are not available in a primary care setting (e.g., CT scan or certain lab tests).

▶ *Emergent*: ED care needed—preventable/avoidable—ED care was required based on the complaint or procedures performed/resources used, but the emergent nature of the condition was potentially preventable/avoidable if timely and effective ambulatory care had been received during the episode of illness (e.g., the flare-ups of asthma, diabetes, congestive heart failure).

▶ *Emergent*: ED care needed—not preventable/avoidable—ED care was required and ambulatory care treatment could not have prevented the condition (e.g., trauma, appendicitis, myocardial infarction; NYU, 2014).

Pulling It All Together

The final summary of data analysis that informs the community assessment is a complete view of the community from the standpoint of the data and information available. Pulling it all together in a complete picture involves the use of multiple data sources related to both primary data (collected by the community for a specific purpose) and secondary data (data collected for a different purpose, but used secondarily to inform assessment). It is helpful to have a point of reference in a checklist to ensure all sources of information are covered. Table 13.5 provides a tool that can be used for this purpose in the form of a needs assessment checklist for variables to be considered in a community needs assessment.

Triangulation of Data

With the use of these types of public domain data and indicators highlighted earlier, these data can be used in combination with primary data collected in the community to triangulate the information using a method that results in effectively informing a community health intervention program. An example of this type of triangulation might be a community needs index, preventable hospitalizations, and avoidable ED visits. Figure 13.7 reflects such an analysis done by Parkland Health and Hospital System (Parkland Hospital System, 2008).

One of the strengths of a needs assessment is that the data can provide objectivity when statistically valid and can also provide a complete analysis of the community. Such

TABLE 13.5 Needs Assessment Checklist for Variables to Be Considered in a Community Needs Assessment	
Health risk variables	*Inpatient discharges per 1,000 population*
Population variables	☐ Discharges per 1,000 population for each service area or the county as a whole (excluding newborns)
☐ Population	☐ Discharges per 1,000 population for each service area or the county as a whole for the top five dischargers
☐ Total population density	
☐ Population by age groups (0–4 years of age, 5–17 years of age, 18–64 years of age, 65 years and older)	☐ Potentially avoidable hospitalizations
	☐ ED use by type of visits— nonemergent, emergent/ treatable primary care, emergent/ED care needed/preventable avoidable, emergent/ED care needed
Ethnicity	
☐ Percentage of Whites	
☐ Percentage of African Americans	
☐ Percentage of Hispanics	
☐ Percentage of Asians, etc.	*Public health data*
Socioeconomic data	☐ Rates of communicable diseases
☐ Percentage of people below federal poverty guidelines	☐ Rates of sexually transmitted diseases
☐ Total number of households	**Survey Data**
☐ Estimated per capita income	*Health risk data*
☐ Estimated average household income	☐ Behavioral Health Risk Factor Surveillance Survey (includes risk behaviors such as smoking, obesity, exercise, fruits and vegetables, bicycle helmets, poor health days, poor mental health days, etc.)
☐ Percentage of households with incomes <$15,000	
☐ Unemployment rate	
☐ Occupational status	
☐ Value of housing	
☐ Educational level	
☐ Percentage of households in food deserts	☐ National Health Interview Survey, National Health and Nutrition Examination Survey
☐ Density of liquor stores	

ED, emergency department.

methods can include using national benchmarks such as Healthy People 2020 goals, American health rankings or state health rankings, comparisons to similar communities as is provided in the community health status indicators, comparing trends over time, or a hierarchical cluster analysis that clusters similar communities together (U.S. Department of Health and Human Services, n.d.). Mapping is a useful process that is used to help find like communities or combine contiguous counties (side by side), creating an expanded community approach. This approach can be used to compare and contrast counties and cities within the larger community. Figure 13.8 reflects a comparison of a community to other services areas in the region and to past performance on health risk behaviors. This visual also depicts the power of analytic tools for community assessment.

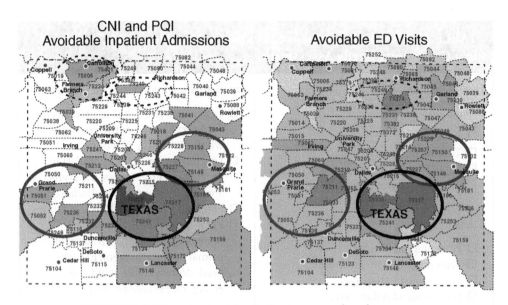

FIGURE 13.7. Triangulation of data indicating areas of need.

CNI, community need index; ED, emergency department; PQI, Prevention Quality Indicator.

Source: McBride (2005).

Priority Setting Based on the Data Analysis

It is not possible to be effective in improving the health of the community by imposing solutions from outside. Stakeholders must be involved and committed to the strategies. Public health professionals and other content experts have unique knowledge that assists communities in assessment, planning, intervention, and evaluation of community health initiatives, but they do not always have firsthand knowledge of the community. There is greater success in improving community health when the community establishes the priorities and claims ownership of its strengths and weaknesses (Brown, Feinberg, & Greenberg, 2012; Foster-Fishman, Berkowitz, Lounsbury, Jacobson, & Allen, 2001; Roussos & Fawcett, 2000; Zakocs & Edwards, 2006). The community priority setting process focuses on areas of the most concern to the residents of targeted communities. Although data analysis and analytic reporting can inform these decisions, the community must decide what it believes are the top priorities to be addressed. For the Dallas County CHNA, data were triangulated from the regional primary and secondary data analyses. In addition, focus group data, primary informant surveys, and the consensus of the planning committees from each community helped create the final plan. Figure 13.9 reflects a dashboard of the Dallas County assessment. Using these types of data to inform the community, all stakeholders involved in the process organized and approved priorities.

Special Considerations for Rural and Small Communities

When assessing rural and small communities, there is often a lack of reliable and valid data at the ZIP code level. Public domain data that are available often mask data with small cell sizes in rural and small communities to protect the confidentiality of individuals

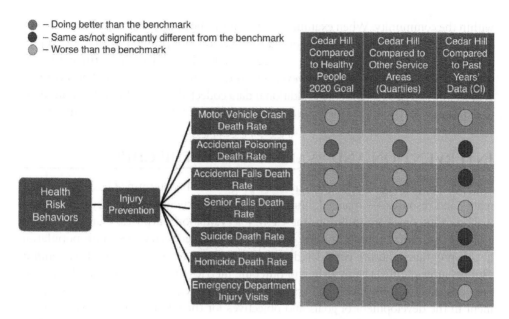

FIGURE 13.8. Community comparative analysis and analytic score card.

Source: Parkland Hospital System (2013).

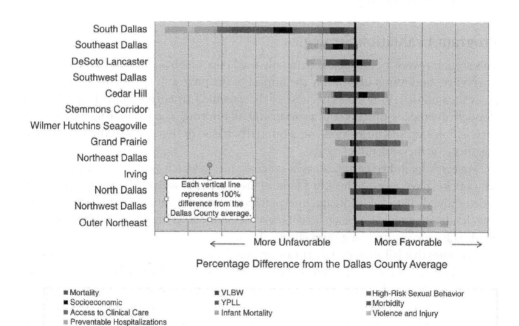

FIGURE 13.9. Dashboard for Dallas County assessment on triangulated primary and secondary data within the community assessment.

Note: All data are from the years 2009–2012; years available vary by topic.

within the community. When examining data within these types of communities, assessment and planning frequently rely on data collected from primary sources within the community or compare data at higher aggregate levels, such as the entire county, to examine patterns and trends. However, when data are used in regional and country aggregation, it is important to use additional data collected directly from the community to determine whether identified patterns and trends are relevant to the community.

INTERVENTION AND EVALUATION OF THE CHIP

The goals and objectives of a CHIP must be pragmatically determined based on current reality and resources—financial, human capital, and structure—and they must also be realistic. Outcomes are built into the CHIP for evaluation purposes. Outcome metrics address environmental and policy changes that are necessary to sustain population health programs and are considered priorities that are manageable based on community resources. Thus, the inclusion of outcome metrics provides a measure for overall program effectiveness during the evaluation phase (CDC, 1999). A stakeholder's alignment in the development of goals and objectives for the CHIP should be based on the results from the data analysis and tools used to assess the community. Objectives include action steps or evidence-based population strategies aligned with current best practices in public health to address environmental and behavioral conditions contributing to disease in the community.

Program Evaluation Strategies

This section covers the strategies commonly used once one has assessed the community, intervened, and wants to examine the impact of the program. In the case of the CHIP, an evaluation determines effectiveness of the executed strategies and is best achieved through an ongoing process of evaluation and monitoring. The monitoring progress for each action step should be done on a quarterly basis. Action steps in the CHIP work together to achieve identified goals.

Strategies are linked to indicators or outcome metrics such as the percentage of those who smoke, have access to healthy foods, or are physically active. Effectiveness of CHIP is determined after evaluation and interpretation of the outcomes of data analysis by all stakeholders, because it is stakeholders who cement ownership in a CHIP and ensure its ultimate success and long-term effectiveness.

Outcomes that fall short of the plan are analyzed and included in recommendations for future iterations of the CHIP. Outcome data should be contextualized in light of several contributing factors: barriers such as limited resources (stakeholders, funding, etc.), lack of program support (organizational, political will, or community), and population change (inward or outward migration). Evaluation should provide necessary community feedback on progress of the CHIP. Evaluation is a vital part of planning, improving existing programs, adding to the evidence that supports prevention strategies, and demonstrating a return on investment (CDC, 1999). However, caution should be exercised by not generalizing results beyond the community being evaluated.

The following case study reflects the use of the models, tools, and techniques for a community health assessment, planning, intervention, and evaluation.

CASE STUDY

In 2012, a public health nurse was approached by a local county judge to develop a proposal for improving the health of a county in a southern state. The proposal included background information, rationale for conducting a CHNA, steps for developing a CHIP, identification of evidence-based practices in population health, a timeline for each phase of the process, and actionable information to justify the project. Data analysis within the small communities identified the following high-priority areas:

▶ 90 per 1,000 preventable hospitalizations based on ambulatory care sensitive conditions for Medicare patients
▶ 11% prevalence of diabetes in those older than 20 years
▶ 31% prevalence of adult obesity
▶ 6.1% prevalence of heart disease

Building a business case, linking the prevalence of disease, and reporting the cost of hospitalizations to commissioners who oversee a local county hospital were fundamental strategies used by public health professionals in selling recommended community health improvement activities. The final proposal was presented during the commissioners' court and unanimously approved by the county commissioners.

Phase one of the public health professional's approach involved completion of the NPHPS instrument. In keeping with this purpose, the NPHPS instrument was used to obtain a high-level system evaluation of how well the local public health service was meeting the 10 essential public health services and a baseline for assessment (CDC, 2010a; 2010b). The baseline measurements from the NPHPS were evaluated concurrently with the results yielded from the CHANGE (CDC, 2013) tool in phase two. The CHANGE tool helps a community in determining the overall health of the community and in identifying existing gaps for improvement. The NPHPS assisted the stakeholders and the LPHS in identifying areas for improvement and in strengthening stakeholder partnerships. The NPHPS instrument helped community stakeholders in answering the following two questions:

1. What capacity does the LPHS have?
2. How well is the LPHS meeting the 10 essential public health services?

Stakeholders from all sectors of the county, including work sites, schools, community organizations, community institutions, and health care systems, were invited to attend a daylong retreat to complete the NPHPS instrument. The public health professional invited organizations to participate though direct telephone calls and e-mail invitations.

Before administration of the NPHPS instrument, an information session was conducted to provide contextually relevant information about the LPHS and a community health report. Demographics from census data were presented by ZIP

(continued)

CASE STUDY (*continued*)

code as well as by rates of top comorbidities, including diabetes, heart disease, and obesity (Robert Wood Johnson [RWJ], 2014; U.S. Census Bureau, 2013).

Careful evaluation with respect to time and resources was important for the public health professional and appropriate for the community. The CHANGE instrument was identified as an ideal fit for the community of 86,000 people in this case study. Successful completion of the CHANGE tool requires stakeholder collaboration to conduct sector assessments. In keeping with this necessity, stakeholder groups were formed and eventually reached a consensus on how decisions would be made, the number of sites to be assessed for each sector, and who would be responsible for sector assessments. The sectors and corresponding number of sites were as follows: community at large (1), community organizations (3), the health care sector (5), school sectors (2), and work-site sectors (3). Responses to environmental and policy questions were entered into the CHANGE sector Excel files. Responses for each of the sector questions range from 1 (issue has not been identified or no elements in place in the environment) to 5 (evaluation of policy enforcement or all elements are in place in the environment) or 99 (policy or environmental change not appropriate for community; CDC, 2013). As an example for the physical activity portion of the evaluation, sites are asked whether they promote stairwell use. Some organization or sites do not have stairs, so they should be instructed to use 99 for missing data. Monthly stakeholder meetings are conducted to help monitor progress and provide technical support during the assessment period.

Once the NPHPS instrument was completed, responses were entered into the NPHPS county profile of the CDC. The overall scores provided a systems view of how well the community is meeting the 10 essential public health services (EPHS). Each score is a composite assigned to the activities for each of the 10 EPHS standards. The scores range from 0% (no activity) to a maximum of 100% (all activities associated with the standard are being performed at a maximum level). Performance scores for each of the EPHS and range bars with minimum and maximum values assist in identifying gaps (Figure 13.6). Essential public health services with wide range bars indicate gaps in services and warrant a closer look when conducting the CHNA and consideration for integration into the CHIP. While rounding out the evaluation using the NPHPS instrument, stakeholders can review and discuss results and set priorities using the optional Priority Setting Instrument. Values for priority-setting questions are entered into the NPHPS priority-setting link of the CDC on the website to generate the report. It should be noted that high-priority and low-performing EPHSs can be evaluated and integrated into the CHNA and CHIP planning process.

CHANGE results were entered into a sector data grid to evaluate assets and needs. These scores are not benchmarked against national or state data but provide a community benchmark that is used to measure progress of CHIP goals and objectives over time. This information was used to identify gaps and needs for the community. For example, in the scores, we obtained and determined that areas

(*continued*)

CASE STUDY (*continued*)

receiving scores of 60% or less would be gaps and would be considered for inclusion in the CHIP. In contrast, areas receiving scores of 61% to 100% would be classified as assets and would, therefore, not be a priority to be addressed in the CHIP.

Additional county data were gathered to support findings from the CHANGE tool and to assist stakeholders with the development of the CHIP. One of the principal challenges to the collection of these data was finding data at the county level because of data protection constraints in public domain data, as many health indicators, such as social determinants of health and rates of chronic disease, either were difficult to locate or were simply not available. One issue relates to sample size of the state Behavioral Risk Factor Surveillance Survey. The absence of county benchmark data makes it difficult to accurately reflect success of the CHIP. To supplement for these data insufficiencies at the county level, data from the County Health Rankings and the state as well as regional data for cardiovascular disease and for social determinants of health. The report card for the community assessment in the case study is reflected in Figure 13.10, and the goals established for the community based on the assessment are noted in Figure 13.11.

After a review of the case study, one should reflect on the following questions:

1. What tools were deployed in this case study?
2. How effective was the assessment and goal planning? Defend your position using elements of the chapter to reinforce your position.
3. Why do you think the public health professional selected the tools and the model for assessment used?
4. What data challenges were evident in this case?
5. How might an HIE in the region have helped this community?

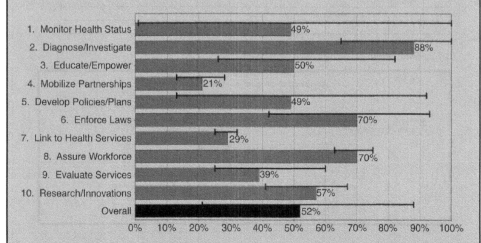

FIGURE 13.10. Community report card with data triangulation demonstrated. Essential service summary of performance scores by essential public health service.

(*continued*)

CASE STUDY (*continued*)

Essential Service	Priority Rating	Performance Score (level of activity)
Quadrant I (High Priority/Low Performance) - These important activities may need increased attention.		
1. Monitor health status to identify community health problems	9	49 (Moderate)
4. Mobilize community partnerships to identify and solve health problems	10	21 (Minimal)
5. Develop policies and plans that support individual and community health efforts	7	49 (Moderate)
7. Link people to needed personal health services and assure the provision of health care when otherwise unavailable	9	29 (Moderate)
9. Evaluate effectiveness, accessibility, and quality of personal and popuation-based health services	10	39 (Moderate)
Quadrant II (High Priority/High Performance) - These activities are being done well, and it is important to maintain efforts.		
6. Enforce laws and regulations that protect health and ensure safety	7	70 (Significant)
Quadrant III (Low Priority/High Performance) - These activities are being done well, but the system can shift or reduce some resources or attention to focus on higher-priority activities.		
2. Diagnose and investigate health problems and health hazards	5	88 (Optimal)
8. Assure a competent public and personal health care workforce	4	70 (Significant)
10. Research for new insights and innovative solutions to health problems	4	57 (Significant)
Quadrant IV (Low Priority/Low Performance) - These activities could be improved, but are of low priority. They may need little or no attention at this time.		
3. Inform, educate, and empower people about health issues	2	50 (Significant)

Summary of the EPHS performance scores and overall scores

EPHS		Score
1	Monitor health status to identify community health problems	49
2	Diagnose and investigate health problems and health hazards	88
3	Inform, educate, and empower people about health issues	50
4	Mobilze community partnerships to identify and solve health problems	21
5	Develop policies and plans that support individual and community health efforts	49
6	Enforce laws and regulations that protect health and ensure safety	70
7	Link people to needed personal health services and assure the provision of health care when otherwise unavailable	29
8	Assure a competent public and personal health care workforce	70
9	Evaluate effectiveness, accessibility, and quality of personal and population-based health services	39
10	Research for new insights and innovative solutions to health problems	57
Overall performance score		52

Group Evaluation

Community Health Assessment and Group Evaluation

COMMUNITY-AT-LARGE

Additional infromation about the community can be included in the comment box denoted by the red tab.

COMMUNITY'S NAME: Southern County

Module Score Summaries		
Policy (%)	Environment (%)	Module
69.70	52.31	Physical Activity
56.45	61.19	Nutrition
52.73	54.55	Tobacco Use
64.44	75.56	Chronic Disease Management
52.73	43.64	Leadership

FIGURE 13.10. (*continued*)

(continued)

CASE STUDY (*continued*)

Needs and Assets

	Low		NEEDS	ASSETS	High
	0–20%	21–40%	41–60%	61–80%	81–100%
Community at Large (CAL)					
Physical Activity			CALE	CALP	
Nutrition			CALP	CALE	
Tobacco			CALP, CALE		
Chronic Disease Mgt.				CALP, CALE	
Leadership			CALP, CALE		

Assessment Data on Health Outcomes and Behavioral Risk Factors

Health Outcome	County	State	Measure
Diabetes	11.0%	9%	Prevalence for those > 20 yrs.
Cardiovascular Disease	7.8%	6.6%	Percentage of heart disease > 18yrs 2005–2008
Adult Obesity	30%	29%	Percentage of adults reporting BMI ≥ 30
Preventable Hospital Stays	90	68	Hospitalization rate per ambulatory care-sensitive condition per 1,000 Medicare enrollees
Environmental Conditions			
Limited Access to Healthy Foods	14.0%	9%	Percentage of low-income individuals who do not live close to a grocery store
Access to Parks	14%	33%	Percentage of those living within .5 miles of a park
Access to Exercise Opportunities	68%	74%	Percentage of population with adequate access to locations for physical activities
Behavioral Conditions			
Tobacco Use	25%	17%	Percentage of adults reporting smoking ≥100 cigarettes & currently smoking
Physical Inactivity	24%	24%	Percentage of adults > 20 yrs. reporting no leisure time or physical activity

FIGURE 13.10. (*continued*)

(*continued*)

CASE STUDY (*continued*)

Goal 1.0	Decrease the number of residents without access to healthy food from 14% to 9% by December 31, 2017.
Objective 1.1	Expand & develop existing farmers' market program to include locations accessible to all community members by December 31, 2017.
Objective 1.2	Establish and promote a county-wide community garden program, increasing number of sites accessible to outlying areas from 0 to 4 by December 31, 2017.
Objective 1.3	Initiate the Expanded Food and Nutrition Education Program by December 31, 2017.
Goal 2.0	Reduce tobacco use in the county from 25% to 17.5% by December 31, 2017.
Objective 2.1	Develop a county-wide tobacco-cessation program by May 31, 2015.
Objective 2.2	Develop a county Smoke-Free Order, with community stakeholders, for adoption by December 31, 2017.
Objective 2.3	Implement a tobacco use awareness campaign with community partners to reach all sectors of the county by December 31, 2016.

FIGURE 13.11. Goals and objectives for the community.

SUMMARY

In today's environment of cost containment, accountable care organizations (ACOs), and health care reform, financial viability of health care providers depends on creating and maintaining healthy communities. The community assessment methodology described within this chapter is provided to outline a systematic approach to use data and information available within the community to pinpoint community service locations and public health outreach activities, as well as to measure the health status outcomes of the residents of those communities. Community assessments are valuable methods used by health care institutions nowadays for strategic planning to support healthy communities and outreach programs; however, to well inform the process, methods such as those described within the chapter are required. This chapter has provided models, tools, metrics, and data-analysis approaches to inform community health assessment and planning. Finally, the chapter has provided a case study to demonstrate how to effectively apply these methods within a community.

EXERCISES AND QUESTIONS FOR CONSIDERATION

You are approached by your local community to provide leadership in a community assessment and planning process. Consider the content covered with respect to community
assessment and planning, models and tools presented, and primary and secondary data
sources and reflect on the following questions:

1. What is the first step in this process in aligning stakeholders for planning? Why
   is it important to consider this as the first step in the process?

2. What model(s) will you use to structure the process and why are models such as
   these important to the process?

3. What data will you need to collect as primary data? What data are available in
   the public domain that you may be able to use to inform the assessment and
   planning?

4. Why are data important to the community health assessment?

5. If you are assessing a rural community, what might be the constraints with respect
   to data availability that you need to factor into the analysis? How will you address
   these constraints?

REFERENCES

ABCD Institute. (2009). *About us*. Retrieved from http://www.abcdinstitute.org

ABCD Institute. (2010). *Research*. Retrieved from http://www.abcdinstitute.org/research

Adeleye, O. A., & Ofili, A. N. (2010). Strengthening intersectoral collaboration for primary health care
in developing countries: Can the health sector play a broader role? *Journal of Environmental and
Public Health* (Article ID 272896), 6. doi:10.1155/2010/272896

Agency for Healthcare Research and Quality. (2014a). *Inpatient quality indicators overview*. Retrieved
from http://www.qualityindicators.ahrq.gov/modules/iqi_resources.aspx

Agency for Healthcare Research and Quality. (2014b). *Prevention quality indicators overview*. Retrieved
from http://www.qualityindicators.ahrq.gov/modules/pqi_resources.aspx

Association of State and Territorial Health Officials. (2014). *ASTHO profile of state public health*
(Vol. 3). Arlington, VA: Author. Retrieved from http://www.astho.org/Profile/Volume-Three

Association of State and Territorial Health Officials. (2015). *Community health needs assessments*.
Retrieved from http://www.astho.org/Programs/Access/Community-Health-Needs-Assessments

Bauer, U. E., Briss, P. A., Goodman, R. A., & Bowman, B. A. (2014). Prevention of chronic disease in
the 21st century: Elimination of the leading preventable causes of premature death and disability in the
USA. *The Lancet*, 384(9937), 45–52. doi:http://dx.doi.org/10.1016/S0140-6736(14)60648-6

Beck, A. J., Boulton, M. L., Lemmings, J., & Clayton, J. L. (2012). Challenges to recruitment and retention of the state health department epidemiology workforce. *American Journal of Preventive Medicine*,
42(1), 76–80. doi:http://dx.doi.org/10.1016/j.amepre.2011.08.021

Brown, L. D., Feinberg, M. E., & Greenberg, M. T. (2012). Measuring coalition functioning: Refining
constructs through factor analysis. *Health Education & Behavior*, 39(4), 486–497. doi:10.1177/1090198
111419655

California Endowment. (2014). *Life expectancy health happens here*. Retrieved from http://www
.calendow.org/zipcode-or-genetic-code-which-is-a-better-predictor-of-health/

Centers for Disease Control and Prevention. (1999). *Framework for program evaluation in public health:
Morbidity and Mortality Weekly Report*, 48(RR-11), 1–40. Retrieved from http://www.cdc.gov/
mmwr/PDF/RR/RR4811.pdf

Centers for Disease Control and Prevention. (2010a). *The public health system and the 10 essential
public health services: Overview*. Retrieved from http://www.cdc.gov/nphpsp/essentialservices.html

Centers for Disease Control and Prevention. (2010b). *National public health performance standards*.
Retrieved from http://www.cdc.gov/nphpsp/theinstruments.html

Centers for Disease Control and Prevention. (2013). *Community health assessment and group evaluation (CHANGE): Building a foundation of knowledge to prioritize community needs*. Retrieved from
http://www.cdc.gov/nccdphp/dch/programs/healthycommunitiesprogram/tools/change.htm

Centers for Disease Control and Prevention. (2014, December). *STLT public health professionals gate-
way: National voluntary accreditation for public health departments*. Retrieved from http://www.cdc
.gov/stltpublichealth/accreditation

Centers for Medicare & Medicaid Services. (2014). *Waivers*. Retrieved from http://www.medicaid.gov/
medicaid-chip-program-information/by-topics/waivers/waivers.html

Davis, R. A., Cohen, L., & Rodriguez, S. (2010). Toward health equity: A prevention framework for
reducing health and safety disparities. In B. J. Healey & R. S. Zimmerman (Eds.), *The new world of health
promotion: New program development, implementation, and evaluation*. Sudbery, MA: Jones & Bartlett.

Edwards, J., Suchltz, L., Erickson, N., & Pickens, S. (2013, August). *Horizons: The Dallas County
community health needs assessment*. Retrieved from http://www.parklandhospital.com/Uploads/
Public/Documents/PDFs/Community/Community-Health-Needs-Assessment.pdf

Foster-Fishman, P. G., Berkowitz, S. L., Lounsbury, D. W., Jacobson, S., & Allen, N. A. (2001). Building
collaborative capacity in community coalitions: A review and integrative framework. *American Journal
of Community Psychology*, 29(2), 241–261. doi:10.1023/A:1010378613583

Glaser, J. (2006). *Health information exchange (HIE) business models: The path to sustainable financial
success*. Deloitte Center for Health Solutions. Retrieved from http://www.providersedge.com/ehdocs/
ehr_articles/Health_Info_Exchange_Business_Models.pdf

Haughton, B., & Stang, J. (2012). Population risk factors and trends in health care and public policy.
Journal of the Academy of Nutrition and Dietetics, 112(Suppl. 3), S35–S46. doi:http://dx.doi.org/
10.1016/j.jand.2011.12.011

Health.gov. (1994). *U.S. public health functions steering committee: Public health in America*. Retrieved
from http://www.health.gov/phfunctions/public.htm

Hilltop Institute. (n.d). *Community benefit state law profiles: A 50-state survey of state community benefit
laws through the lens of the ACA*. Retrieved from http://www.hilltopinstitute.org/hcbp_cbl.cfm

Internal Revenue Service. (2014). *New requirements for 501(c)(3) hospitals under the Affordable Care
Act*. Retrieved from http://www.irs.gov/Charities-%26-Non-Profits/Charitable-Organizations/New-
Requirements-for-501(c)(3)-Hospitals-Under-the-Affordable-Care-Act

Johns Hopkins Medicine. (2014). *Health library: Diabetes*. Retrieved from http://www.hopkinsmedicine
.org/healthlibrary/conditions/diabetes/diabetes_statistics/diabetes/diabetes_home_85,P00343

Kania, J., & Kramer, M. (2011). *Standford social innovation review: Collective impact* (Review No.
LSU-2011). Washington, DC: LeLand Standford Jr. University. Retrieved from http://c.ymcdn.com/
sites/www.lano.org/resource/dynamic/blogs/20131007_093137_25993.pdf

Kindig, D., & Stoddart, G. (2003). What is population health? *American Journal of Public Health,* 93(3), 380–383.

Kretzmann, J. P., & McKnight, J. L. (1993). *Building communities from the inside out: A path toward finding and mobilizing a community's assets.* Evanston, IL: ACTA Publications.

McBride, S. (2005). Geo-map trending of the MRSA infections in hospital discharge data. In *Combining the AHRQ indicator sets to assess the health of communities: Powerful information for planning purposes* (1st ed., pp. 20–28). Dallas, TX: Dallas-Fort Worth Hospital Council Data Initiative. Retrieved from http://www.qualityindicators.ahrq.gov/Downloads/Resources/Presentations/2005/2005AHRQQI_McBride_Combining_Sets_to_Assess_Health_of_Communities.ppt

McBride, S. (2006). *Epidemiologic evaluation of rising MRSA in Texas.* Paper presented at the Poster Session of the CDC Assessment Conference, Atlanta, GA.

McBride, S. (2007, November 13). *AHRQ conference: A regional commitment to improve the healthcare workforce, patient safety, quality & the health of populations served, presented.* Washington, DC: Agency for Healthcare Research and Quality.

National Association of County and City Health Officials. (2009). *Integrating performance improvement processes: MAPP, National Public Health Performance Standards, and Accreditation.* Retrieved January, 5, 2013, from http://www.naccho.org/topics/infrastructure/mapp/framework/mapppubs.cfm

New York University. (2014). *Algorithm to help classify ED utilization.* Retrieved from http://wagner.nyu.edu/faculty/billings/nyued-background

Nicholas, J. A., & Hall, W. J. (2011). Screening and preventive services for older adults. *Mount Sinai Journal of Medicine,* 78(4), 498–508. doi:10.1002/msj.20275

Office of Adolescent Health. (2014). *Trends in teen pregnancy and childbearing.* Retrieved from http://www.hhs.gov/ash/oah/adolescent-health-topics/reproductive-health/teen-pregnancy/trends.html

Parkland Hospital System. (2008). *Community health checkup 2008: Trends, highlights and new features.* Dallas, TX: Parkland Hospital System.

Parkland Hospital System. (2013). *Community health assessment: Cedar hill service area.* Dallas, TX: Parkland Hospital System. Retrieved from http://www.parklandhospital.com/Uploads/Public/Documents/PDFs/Health-Dashboard/Cedar-Hill-Dashboard-2013.pdf

Public Health Accreditation Board. (2013). *Public Health Accreditation Board: Standards & Measures Version 1.0.* Retrieved from http://www.phaboard.org/accreditation-overview/getting-started

Robert Wood Johnson. (2014, January). *County health rankings.* Retrieved from http://www.countyhealthrankings.org

Roussos, S. T., & Fawcett, S. B. (2000). A review of collaborative partnerships as a strategy for improving community health. *Annual Review of Public Health,* 21(1), 369–402. doi:10.1146/annurev.publhealth.21.1.369

Somerville, M. H., Nelson, G. D., & Mueller, C. H. (2013). *Hospital community benefits after the ACA: The state law landscape.* (Issue Brief No. 6). Baltimore, MD: The Hilltop Institute at UMBC. Retrieved from http://www.hilltopinstitute.org/publications/HospitalCommunityBenefitsAfterTheACA-StateLawLandscapeIssueBrief6-March2013.pdf

Starfiled, B., So, L., & Macinko, J. (2005). Contribution of primary care to health systems and health. *MilBank Quarterly,* 93(3), 1–76. Retrieved from http://www.commonwealthfund.org/usr_doc/Starfield_Milbank.pdf

Stevens, C. D., Schriger, D. L., Raffetto, B., Davis, A. C., Zingmond, D., & Roby, D. H. (2014). Geographic clustering of diabetic lower-extremity amputations in low-income regions of California. *Health Affairs,* 33(8), 1383–1390. doi:10.1377/hlthaff.2014.0148

University of Michigan. (2013). *Enumeration and characterization of the public health nursing workforce: Findings of the 2012 public health nursing surveys* (No. RWJ-062013). Ann Arbor, MI: University of Michigan Center for Excellence in Public Health Workforce Studies. Retrieved from http://www.sph.umich.edu/cephw/docs/Nurse%20Workforce-RWJ%20Report.pdf

U.S. Census Bureau. (2013). *State and county quickfacts*. Retrieved from http://quickfacts.census.gov/qfd/states/48000.html

U.S. Department of Health and Human Services. (n.d.). Healthy People 2020. Retrieved from http://healthypeople.gov

World Health Organization. (2015). *Health impact assessment*. Retrieved from http://www.who.int/water_sanitation_health/resources/hia/en

Zakocs, R. C., & Edwards, E. M. (2006). What explains community coalition effectiveness? A review of the literature. *American Journal of Preventive Medicine, 30*(4), 351–361. doi:10.1016/j.amepre.2005.12.004

CHAPTER 14

Privacy and Security in a Ubiquitous Health Information Technology World

Susan McBride, Annette Sobel, and Helen Caton-Peters

OBJECTIVES

1. Discuss the need, history, and principles of the Health Insurance Portability and Accountability Act (HIPAA), including transactions, privacy, and security components.

2. Discuss the increased requirements of the HIPAA outlined in the Health Information Technology for Economic and Clinical Health (HITECH) Act and the purpose of increased protections.

3. Discuss the importance of clinicians fully understanding and being the trusted agents who protect patients' health care information.

4. Describe common issues seen in the clinical setting that constitute privacy and security violations and how to mitigate these issues.

5. Describe cybersecurity threats and the need to enhance security in the health informatics (HI) environment as a result of these threats.

6. Evaluate a case study magnifying the importance of protected health information (PHI) protections and violations to the trust of consumers.

7. Develop a strategy and plan to address privacy and security with an exercise outlined for the reader.

KEY WORDS

Health Insurance Portability and Accountability Act, transactions, privacy, security, PHI, 837 institutional, covered entity, texting, social media, trust, health informatics environment, cloud, ubiquitous computing, cybersecurity, vulnerabilities, telehealth, robotics, decision assisting

CONTENTS

INTRODUCTION

In recent years, the significance of safeguarding the privacy and security of health information has become a primary and critical issue for health care providers and informatics professionals. Though not a new issue, the relevance to practice is more pressing than ever as new ways in which health data are collected, used, and shared not only promise innovation but also increase the potential for misuse and breach. Adoption of electronic health records (EHRs) and other forms of health technology has grown at such a rapid rate that existing privacy policy protections are not sufficient and gaps in safeguards are evident as data flow across and through this ever-changing health care ecosystem. Studies have shown that patients generally have a large amount of trust in providers but that trust can very quickly erode if a breach of any magnitude occurs with their health information (Hall et al., 2002). Consequences stemming from system disruption and data theft and loss can lead to significant patient harm and result in organizational, reputational, and financial damage. Patients and providers must be able to trust the technology they use to make the most gains in health care. It is up to all nursing professionals and particularly nurse informaticists (NI) to establish and maintain this trust so that the benefits of a fully interoperable and learning health system can be realized (Eden, Wheatley, McNeil, & Sox, 2008). The IOM defines a *learning health care system* as one "that links personal and population data to researchers and practitioners, dramatically enhancing the knowledge base on effectiveness of interventions and providing real-time guidance for superior care in treating and preventing illness" (IOM, 2013, p. ix).

Regulatory Environment

To begin to understand how to appropriately safeguard health information, one must understand the regulatory environment as it applies to the type of data and its intended use. Perhaps the most recognizable health privacy regulation is the Health Insurance Portability and Accountability Act (HIPAA). Enacted in 1996, this regulation is considered a seminal event in health privacy regulation and sets a floor for privacy and security practices for defined "covered entities" (CEs).[1] In addition, providers and organizations participating in the government meaningful use (MU) program are required to attest that they meet certain privacy and security measures. However, there are numerous other policy-related considerations that a health care professional must take into account when ensuring that patient rights to confidentiality are respected and upheld, including understanding the entire regulatory picture and maintaining awareness of the capabilities and weaknesses of the technological environment in which he or she practices.

Federal protections for the privacy and security of health data beyond the HIPAA apply depending on circumstances, and nurse informaticists need to be aware of the implications for practice.

Federal Trade Commission

Nurses practice in many different health care settings and in ever-expanding roles. The traditional approaches to privacy and security may require a broader understanding of how health data may be regulated. The Federal Trade Commission (FTC) enforces privacy and security practices and describes its mission as follows:

> The Federal Trade Commission (FTC) is an independent U.S. law enforcement agency charged with protecting consumers and enhancing competition across broad sectors of the economy. The FTC's primary legal authority comes from Section 5 of the Federal Trade Commission Act, which prohibits unfair or deceptive practices in the marketplace. The FTC also has authority to enforce a variety of sector-specific laws, including the Truth in Lending Act, the CAN-SPAM Act, the Children's Online Privacy Protection Act, the Equal Credit Opportunity Act, the Fair Credit Reporting Act, the Fair Debt Collection Practices Act, and the Telemarketing and Consumer Fraud and Abuse Prevention Act. This broad authority allows the Commission to address a wide array of practices affecting consumers, including those that emerge with the development of new technologies and business models. (FTC, 2014)

The recent 2014 case of LabMD versus FTC demonstrates how the FTC uses its enforcement authority to hold companies accountable for the protection of personal medical information. In this case, the FTC alleges that LabMD failed to reasonably protect the security of consumers' personal data, including medical information. The complaint alleges that in two separate incidents, LabMD collectively exposed the personal information of approximately 10,000 consumers. The complaint alleges that LabMD billing information for more than 9,000 consumers was found on a peer-to-peer file-sharing network and then, in 2012, LabMD documents containing sensitive personal information of at least 500 consumers were found in the hands of identity thieves. This case is ongoing, but it highlights an important lesson for health care professionals to heed. Health data deserve special attention and protection regardless of location or form, and we are challenged to continually address these concerns in light of all possible regulatory requirements.

---

[1]Covered entities (CE) are defined as "health care providers who conduct covered health care transactions electronically, health plans, and health care clearinghouses" (Federal Register/Vol. 78, No. 17/Friday, January 25, 2013/ Rules and Regulations, p. 5567).

Food and Drug Administration

Another federal regulatory agency with a role in the privacy and security of health care data is the Food and Drug Administration (FDA). The FDA oversees the safety of medical devices, which includes addressing the management of cybersecurity risks and hospital network security. Recent guidelines issued (FDA, 2013) recommend that medical device manufacturers and health care facilities take steps to ensure that appropriate safeguards are in place to reduce the risk of failure caused by cyberattack. This could be initiated by the introduction of malware into the medical equipment or unauthorized access to configuration settings in medical devices and hospital networks. The consequences of not adequately addressing these risks could be dire. As medical devices are increasingly integrated within health care environments, there will be a need for vigilance toward cybersecurity practices to ensure all systems are adequately protected and patients remain safe from harm. Nurse informaticists are frequently called on to evaluate safety and effectiveness of new devices and software. Considerations of cybersecurity must be included in any evaluation process.

Substance Abuse and Mental Health Services Administration

Certain types of health data considered especially sensitive enjoy special protection under the law. In the case of substance abuse treatment data, there are heightened confidentiality protections afforded by 42 CFR Part 2 enforced by the Substance Abuse and Mental Health Services Administration (SAMHSA, 2014). These regulations exist to protect patients receiving substance abuse treatment in federally funded facilities against possible discrimination. Patients must give their consent to share data collected from these facilities with other health care providers, and those protections persist in that a patient must give express consent for any future disclosures as well.

State Regulatory Requirements

A discussion of privacy regulations would not be complete without mentioning that health care professionals need to also be aware of specific state and international laws that impact data use. State privacy laws differ widely, sometimes conflicting with and preempting federal privacy regulations by establishing greater protections (Health Information Law [HIL], 2012). This situation adds a layer of complexity that must be navigated carefully to ensure adherence with federal requirements while at the same time respecting the timely and secure sharing of patient data across state lines. In many cases, special protection exists for data such as HIV and sexually transmitted disease diagnoses, mental health records, and information related to minors. Informatics professionals must be familiar with what state law requires and understand potential consequences of sharing data in new models of care such as accountable care organizations (ACOs) and health information exchanges (HIEs).

International Law

International law will play an increasing role in privacy protections for patients as data are shared across U.S. borders (Healthcare Information and Management Systems Society [HIMSS], n.d). Data can be stored offshore and fall under international law, which may affect rights and use. Health technology developers are based across the globe and are challenged with incorporating privacy and security practices that must meet a complex web of regulatory requirements. Frequently, those developers are innovative nurses and providers who are addressing patient care and building mechanisms for clinical decision support (CDS) by designing creative and simple-to-use applications and tools. Building privacy and security best practices, such as strong authentication procedures and encryption, into these tools as a part of the software development cycle will prevent many potential vulnerabilities. Using the regulatory framework in place will guide developers toward key practices and robust risk assessment procedures that will circumvent a vast array of possible negative consequences.

Health Insurance Portability and Accountability Act

The fundamentals of HIPAA, including its history, requirements of the Act, additions to the regulatory requirements under the Act, implications for clinicians, and how EHRs, MU, and emerging innovative technologies are likely to push the constraints of the regulations are described in this section. HIPAA was passed into law in 1996 and was subsequently amended and expanded to address increasing privacy of personal health information (PHI).

We review the HIPAA regulations passed in 1996 and discuss updates to the regulation examining why additions to requirements under the Health Information Technology for Economic and Clinical Health (HITECH) Act with updated protection of privacy, security, and enforcement penalties are described as having "put teeth in HIPAA" (Clearwater Compliance, 2012). A number of resources are available that support organizations in adhering to HIPAA regulations, including guidance developed by the Office for Civil Rights (OCR) and the Office of the National Coordinator (ONC). We provide information on how to access and utilize these expansive resources to help understand and adhere to HIPAA regulations. Finally, we discuss the significance of added security related to cyber threats and the importance of all health care professionals in maintaining a heightened awareness related to this relatively new threat.

HEALTH INSURANCE PORTABILITY AND ACCOUNTABILITY ACT BACKGROUND

The HIPAA of 1996 is also known as the Kennedy–Kassenbaum Act after former senators Nancy Kassebaum (R-Kansas) and Edward M. Kennedy (D-Massachusetts). Before the passage of the Affordable Care Act (ACA), HIPAA was considered the most significant federal health care reform since the enactment of Medicare and Medicaid in 1965 (Atchinson & Fox, 1997). This expansive Act covered health insurance reform in five titles. Titles I and II of the Act focus on health insurance reform around the portability of health insurance between jobs and limitations to preexisting conditions and, through administrative simplification, to contain fraud, waste, and abuse within health care. For the purpose of this chapter, title II is the emphasis of discussion because it deals primarily with protection of clinical data.

Title II of HIPAA required the Department of Health and Human Services (HHS) to establish national standards for electronic health care transactions and national identifiers for providers, health plans, and employers (CMS, 2013). With the increased use of electronic claims and billing transactions data came the understanding of the need to protect the privacy and security of the health data captured within those transactions and, more broadly, by the entities responsible for the collection and use of those data. Therefore,

HHS was also required to develop rules for privacy and security that would apply when the electronic transactions and codes sets were used. Finally, it was important to establish enforcement procedures that HHS would follow to investigate reports of noncompliance and fines that organizations would be subject to. These rules are outlined in 45 CFR Part 160, 45 CFR Part 162, and 45 CFR Part 164. The transaction and code set, employer identifier, and National Provider Identifier (NPI) rules are administered and enforced by the Centers for Medicare & Medicaid Services (CMS), whereas the privacy and security rules are administered and enforced by the Office for Civil Rights (OCR; HHS.gov, 2014).

The HIPAA regulations apply to organizations defined as covered entities (CEs). Under the regulations, CEs include health plans, health care clearinghouses, and certain health care providers. To be considered a CE and therefore subject to the HIPAA regulations, a health care provider must be conducting certain transactions in electronic form. Key dates for HIPAA enactment are noted in Table 14.1. The initial stages of HIPAA involved a complicated regulatory requirement with extensive comment periods in the rule-making process, modifications to the final rules, delays, and final effective dates that were often accompanied with considerable efforts at compliance by CEs within the industry. Figure 14.1 provides an overview of HIPAA, which notes that the Administrative Simplification sections of the Act are more applicable to health care providers, whereas the Insurance Reform sections are the most relevant to payers. We focus more here on covering the sections relevant to health care providers and focus minimally on the insurance reform components.

TABLE 14.1 Key HIPAA Dates and Deadlines

Date	Deadline for Noted Action
August 21, 1996	HIPAA Public Law 104–191 signed
November 3, 1999	HIPAA Privacy Rule proposed
December 28, 2000	HIPAA Final Privacy Rule initially posted but underwent revisions
October 16, 2002	Electronic health care transactions and code sets—all CEs except those that filed for an extension and small health plans
April 14, 2003	Privacy Rule in effect for all CEs except small health plans
April 16, 2003	Electronic health care transactions and code sets—all CEs must have started software and system testing
April 14, 2004	Privacy Rule in effect for small health plans
April 20, 2005	Security Rule comes into effect
March 16, 2006	Enforcement Compliance in effect

CEs, covered entities; HIPAA, Health Insurance Portability and Accountability Act.

Source: CMS (2013).

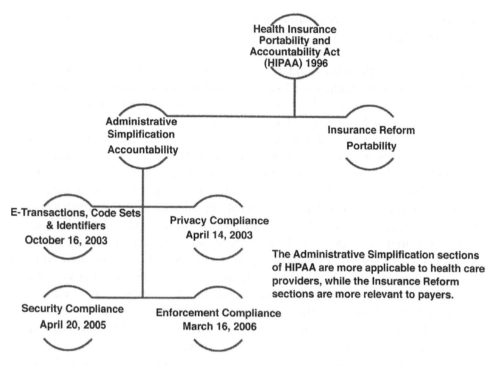

FIGURE 14.1. HIPAA sections and important dates.

Electronic Transactions and Code Sets Requirements

According to the CMS, transactions "are electronic exchanges involving the transfer of information between two parties for specific purposes" (CMS, 2003). The transactions component of HIPAA requires that the Department of Health and Human Services adopt national standards for electronic health care transactions, which constitute a large part of the administrative simplification component. The transactions formats and standards are specified in the regulation, and they are aimed at creating administrative simplification so that payers, providers, and claims adjudication third parties are aligned on standard formats for processing claims and payments as well as for the maintenance and transmission of electronic health care information and data. These standards include the following specifications:

- ▶ Eligibility for Health Plan Inquiry and Response (270/271)
- ▶ Healthcare Claim (837)
- ▶ Healthcare Claim Status Request and Notification (276/277)
- ▶ Referral Certification and Authorization (278)
- ▶ Healthcare Claims Payment and Remittance Advice (835; McCormick & Gugerty, 2013, p. 108)

The HIPAA transaction standards require that any provider or payer transmitting information as noted earlier must do so in the format specified by the most current regulations dictating the code sets within the format for the type of electronic transaction.

For example, the standardized billing format for a hospital is the 837 intuitional (837i) format. The American National Standards Institute (ANSI) ASC X12 837 is the claim or encounter format. Specified code sets fall within that standard, and the data within the form must conform to the standards, including rigorous edits that ensure the data within the form meet compliance. CEs are required to use the format if they submit the transaction electronically, and the claims payer is required to receive the format. Claims that are not considered complete or that contain errors must be corrected before they can be processed, or receive denial, rejection, or remittance advice, all of which have their own electronic ANSI transactions formats to automate the process. In the event the claim submitted by the hospital or provider does not meet the definition of a "clean claim" or lacks complete or correct information, the claim will be rejected and sent back to the hospital through this process. The International Classification of Diseases, 9th Revision, Clinical Modification (ICD-9-CM) codes are an example of a code set that the hospital must use within the 837i electronic format. These codes will be updated to ICD-10-CM on October 1, 2015, with hospitals and providers expected to use the new code set starting in October (CMS, 2015). The X12 formats are messaging standards developed for the purpose of transmitting data between two entities referred to as "trading partners" in the HIPAA legislation. These file formats are periodically updated, for example, the ASC X12 837 has revisions that include a 5010 version providing a mechanism for allowing the use of ICD-10-CM, as well as other improvements. In the example given, trading partners are the hospital, the clearinghouse transmitting the claim to the payer, and the payer entity. All CEs must be able to utilize up-to-date HIPAA standards under the electronic transactions and code sets requirements. In addition to the institutional formats for hospitals, there is a professional format for provider billing (837 Professional or 837P), as well as dental (837 Dental or 837D) and retail pharmaceutical transactions (National Council for Prescription Drug Programs; CMS, 2003). Figure 14.2 depicts the

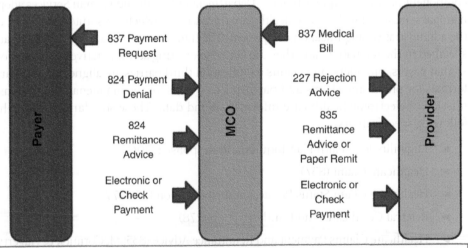

FIGURE 14.2. Provider electronic transaction process.

Source: Ohio Bureau of Workers' Compensation (n.d.).

typical claims processing and electronic billing provider flow. The claims payer can be Medicare, Medicaid, or private payers; this process follows federal billing transaction requirements regardless of the payer. The electronic data transmission (EDT) services for a managed care organization (MCO) are often managed by clearinghouse intermediary service providers.

Privacy Rule

Although Congress passed HIPAA in 1996, the Privacy Rule was not promulgated until 2003. The Privacy Rule is intended to protect the rights of individuals with respect to the confidentiality of PHI while simultaneously allowing legitimate use of these data by governing disclosure of PHI. According to the U.S. Department of Health and Human Services, the purpose of the Privacy Rule was as follows:

> The HIPAA Privacy Rule establishes national standards to protect individuals'
> medical records and other personal health information and applies to health
> plans, health care clearinghouses, and those health care providers that conduct
> certain health care transactions electronically. The Rule requires appropriate
> safeguards to protect the privacy of personal health information, and sets limits
> and conditions on the uses and disclosures that may be made of such informa-
> tion without patient authorization. The Rule also gives patients rights over their
> health information, including rights to examine and obtain a copy of their health
> records, and to request corrections. (HHS.gov, n.d.-b)

An important distinction to be made between the Privacy Rule and the Security Rule is that the provisions within the Privacy Rule apply to all PHI regardless of form, whereas the Security Rule governs electronic PHI. The Privacy Rules have undergone modifications after the final rules posted in 2003, the most recent of which are a part of omnibus legislation in the HITECH Act provisions (discussed next). However, the goals of the Privacy Rule remain true to initial intent by mandating federal protections for personally identifiable health information, establishing rights to access and control over health information, and preservation of important uses of PHI, such as through research, to improve quality of care. The key elements of the Privacy Rule include comprehensive specifications about CEs and Business Associates (BAs), permitted uses and disclosures, research, individual rights, administrative requirements, and compliance and enforcement.

Guidance Regarding Methods for De-identification of PHI

There are two different methods recommended for de-identifying protected health information (PHI) in compliance with HIPAA. *PHI* is defined as individually identifiable health information that is transmitted or maintained by a covered entity or its business associates in any form or medium (45 CFR 160.103). The definition exempts a small number of categories of individually identifiable health information, such as individually identifiable health information found in employment records held by a covered entity in its role as an employer.

The two methods recommended are (a) expert determination through applying statistical or scientific principles (algorithms) to de-identify the PHI, and (b) Safe harbor methods, including the removal of 18 types of identifiers with no ability for residual information to identify the person (HHS.gov, 2015). The 18 elements that must be protected are as follows:

1. Names
2. All geographical subdivisions smaller than a state, including street address, city, county, precinct, zip code, and their equivalent geocodes, except for the initial three digits of a zip code, if according to the current publicly available data from the Bureau of the Census: (a) the geographic unit formed by combining all zip codes with the same three initial digits contains more than 20,000 people; (b) the initial three digits of a zip code for all such geographic units containing 20,000 or fewer people are changed to 000.
3. All elements of dates (except year) for dates directly related to an individual, including birth date, admission date, discharge date, and death date; all ages older than 89 and all elements of dates (including year) indicative of such age, except that such ages and elements may be aggregated into a single category of age 90 or older.
4. Phone numbers
5. Fax numbers
6. Electronic mail addresses
7. Social Security numbers
8. Medical record numbers
9. Health plan beneficiary numbers
10. Account numbers
11. Certificate/license numbers
12. Vehicle identifiers and serial numbers, including license plate numbers
13. Device identifiers and serial numbers
14. Web Universal Resource Locators (URLs)
15. Internet Protocol (IP) address numbers
16. Biometric identifiers, including finger and voice prints
17. Full face photographic images and any comparable images
18. Any other unique identifying number, characteristic, or code (note this does not mean the unique code assigned by the investigator to code the data). (HHS.gov, 2015)

Security

The Security Rules were issued by the Department of Health and Human Services (DHHS) in 2003 with a compliance date of 2005. The Security Rules are applicable to electronic health information created, received, used, and maintained by CEs and contain scalable and flexible measures that CEs must address as a part of their electronic PHI security-related activities. Security safeguards fall into three areas of compliance: (a) administrative, (b) physical, and (c) technical. The administrative component requires policies and procedures to be in place within protected entities to demonstrate how the entity complies with the Act. The physical requirements relate to controlling physical access or inappropriate access to protected information. Finally, the technical component requires that CEs protect PHI when the data are transmitted or exchanged.

Enforcement

In 2006, HHS issued the rules that specify enforcement of HIPAA by setting civil penalties for violating HIPAA rules. In addition, procedures for investigations and hearings for violations were defined. Until this point, the rules and regulations were in place, but no clear enforcement requirements were spelled out. There are a number of recent examples of enforcement cases with issues related to unpatched and unsupported software resulting in a $150,000 fine, a medical records dumping case resulting in a $800,000 fine, and larger fines ranging from $1.7 million to $3.3 million for settlements on potential violations (HHS.gov, n.d.-a).

Business Associate Agreements

The HIPAA privacy law applies to CEs that are health plans, health care clearinghouses, or health care providers; however, many health care providers require the services of organizations under contract for certain functions that may require the handling of PHI. The Privacy Rule allows for these contractual relationships with a BA (HHS.gov, 2003). Under HIPAA, a BA is considered an extension of a covered identity, meaning that the requirements to protect PHI are considered to extend to the BA. A BA conducts activities on behalf of the CE. Activities that are considered BA activities are things such as claims processing or administration, data analysis, processing or administration, utilization review, quality assurance, billing, benefit management, practice management, and repricing. Examples of some Business Associate Agreements (BAAs) that are becoming more prevalent are cloud or service providers for EHR or data repository hosting and developers outside of organizations. Organizations, such as the Health Information Exchanges, ePrescribing Gateways, or any other organization that manages transmission of PHI or requires access to PHI on a routine basis, are considered a BA under the definitions noted in 45 Code of Federal Regulations (CFR) 160, Subpart A in Section 160.103 (eCFR.gov, 2014).

The use of a contract is required to ensure the relationship between and CE and BA is clearly defined. For HIPAA, this contract is also known as a BAA. This contract between the CE and BA must comply with certain privacy rule and security rule requirements and the BA is directly liable for violations (HHS.gov, 2003).

A discussion of the HIPAA rules would be incomplete without remarking on the identifier standards and their significance to the transactions conducted in health care. As mentioned earlier, HHS has developed an Employer Identifier number (EIN) and an National Patent Identifier (NPI) for use in health care transactions. Use of such identifiers provides a means for standardized identification of employers, providers, and others, both within and across health information technology (HIT) systems. This simplifies the process of electronic data sharing, leading to greater efficiencies and improved care delivery. An early plan for identifier standards under HIPAA was the development of a patient identifier that was also intended for use with electronic transactions. This rule has never been developed, and organizations are challenged with finding alternative solutions for dealing with the very important task of correct patient identification, not only within an electronic transaction used under HIPAA, but also across all electronic health technology and care delivery systems where patients seek care. The consequences of mismatched and misrouted health information represent a real threat to patient safety that cannot be ignored in the absence of federal regulation. A Master Patient Index (MPI) is one strategy that care delivery organizations employ to connect patient identities across their systems and maintain the integrity of data they collect, use, and share.

Advanced practice nurses should engage in developing and adopting safe and secure practices for patient identity matching to improve coordination of care while upholding patients' rights. Consumer privacy advocates have voiced serious concerns over the implications of an NPI. As uses of electronic health information expand, so do the potential abuses. All efforts aimed at solving this complex problem should seek to engender patient and provider trust and balance this with safety and security risks associated with increased HIE.

HITECH ACT INCREASED PROTECTIONS

With the passage of the HITECH Act of 2009 as a part of the American Recovery and Reinvestment Act (see Chapters 1 and 4), the movement from paper-based records to EHRs and the expansion of HIE anticipated under the HITECH Act constituted unprecedented amounts of PHI data being exchanged in electronic format and, as such, new vulnerabilities of exposure were anticipated. As a result, along with the HITECH Act came additional provisions for HIPAA that went above and beyond the original protections established in 1996. Also known as the Omnibus HIPAA rule, these changes significantly expand individual rights and provide increased protection and control over health information. The HITECH Act requires HHS to perform audits, increases penalties for noncompliance based on level of negligence, and outlines breach notification requirements. These substantial modifications have been described as HHS "putting teeth in HIPAA," meaning that these provisions or violations of them are likely to be much more painful economically and with penalty subject to jail time for organizations or individuals who violate these protections intentionally.

2013 Modifications

Modifications to the HIPAA Privacy, Security, Enforcement, and Breach Notification Rules Under the HITECH Act and the Genetic Information Nondiscrimination Act (GINA) along with other modifications to the HIPAA regulations were filed in the *Federal Register* in a final ruling on January 25, 2013, with entities required to comply with the final rules by September 23, 2013 (HHS, 2013).

So what changed with this new regulation, and why did additional protections need to be put into place? In 2013, HHS Secretary Kathleen Sebelius stated the following regarding these final rule changes: "Much has changed in health care since HIPAA was enacted over fifteen years ago. The new rule will help protect patient privacy and safeguard patients' health information in an ever expanding digital age" (HHS.gov, 2013). The final rules filed in 2013 further reinforced the HITECH Act changes, including the following modifications to:

► Privacy, Security, and Enforcement Rules to strengthen privacy and security protections for health information and to improve enforcement originally provided for by the HITECH Act in 2009

► Breach Notification Rule, which replaces the interim final rule originally published with the HITECH Act in 2009

► Increase privacy protections under the Privacy Rules for genetic information as required by the GINA of 2008

► Changes to the rules that are intended to increase workability and flexibility by decreasing the burden and better harmonizing the requirements with those under other HHS Departmental regulations (HHS, 2013)

One of the most important things to note with the latest 2013 changes is that they indicate that regulations continue to evolve and change within the landscape of health information and are responsive to needs of the health care consumer in the digital age. The changes related to genomic data are reflective of this ever-expanding landscape. The final rule is based on statutory changes under the HITECH Act, enacted as part of the American Recovery and Reinvestment Act of 2009, and the GINA of 2008, which clarifies that genetic information is protected under the HIPAA Privacy Rule. The most important aspect of these changes is that this rule prohibits most health plans from using or disclosing genetic information for underwriting purposes. Additional requirements that may be particularly relevant to advanced practice nurses and others providing health care services and billing for those services include the following:

► Restrictions on disclosures of PHI

► Information about services paid for out of pocket must be withheld from the payer on the patient's request.

► Treatment, payment, and health care operations disclosures must be tracked and records should be maintained for 3 years.

► CEs with EHRs must provide or transmit PHI in electronic format as directed by the patient.

► Limits for uses and disclosures related to marketing and fund-raising

► Extension of accountability to BAs and subcontractors (HHS.gov, 2013)

The privacy and security changes in the final rulemaking provide the public with increased protections and control of PHI, and individual rights are expanded in important ways. Patients can ask for a copy of their record in electronic form. When individuals pay in cash, they can instruct the provider not to share information about their treatment with their health plan. The final omnibus rule sets new limits on how information is used and disclosed for marketing and fund-raising purposes and prohibits the sale of an individual's health information without his or her permission. BAs and subcontractors must now comply of the requirements and are directly liable for violations.

An additional emphasis of the HITECH Act is patient engagement. The patient-engagement movement will continue to drive for new and innovative ways to involve patients in care. Patients wishing to incorporate applications and technological tools for health and fitness into their health-care regimen should be able to feel secure in the knowledge that these tools have built-in safeguards and that providers have evaluated the safe and secure use of such tools. This will require involvement of nurses in all stages of development, including representation at the federal policy level. These new advances will also require enhanced cybersecurities, because the majority of these applications are Internet based.

ENHANCING CYBERSECURITY IN THE HEALTH INFORMATICS ENVIRONMENT

New and emerging computing environments in health informatics (HI) referred to as "the HI Environment" create additional threats with respect to security of the nation and present a significant risk to organizations that manage health care data. We are responsible to individuals represented within the data for managing and protection. We live in a world of ubiquitous or pervasive computing, made more dramatic and powerful by its direct connection to critical life decision making under frequently stressful and time-critical conditions. What this means is a world redefined by access to information "anytime and anywhere," bereft of the physical devices or formatting constraints. The human–system interface is continuously adaptive, self-organizing, complex, and intended to conform to the user's needs. "User" is continuously redefined in this environment, and it is sometimes elusive as when representing a hospital or insurance company entity or function, such as accounting.

The Landscape

The health care informatics landscape is enormous. We now understand that intellectual property theft is rampant, and theft in the health care and public health sectors comprised 43% of all data breach-associated identify thefts, as noted by a 2014 report by the Identify Theft Resource Center. We also recognize that medical devices and other consumer electronics comprise approximately 30 billion of the 50 billion Internet-connected devices worldwide (Cisco, 2013). We place a strong emphasis on security of medical informatics when considering the expanding online footprint when combined with the rapidly growing malicious activity of "botnets" and other autonomous attackers, with the United States in the lead in terms of protections against such acts worldwide (Tim, 2014).

Review of Basic Terms

Introduction to some basic concepts is in order at this time. Ubiquitous computing requires an evolving sophisticated technical base, defined by a matrix-based taxonomy of functional properties as opposed to specific physical device-centered requirements. Elements may include sensing, data analytics, decision assisting, communication protocols, and so forth. By definition, a myriad of sorts of data will be accessible to multiple users performing multiple tasks, ranging from personal genetic information analysis to manipulation and overlays of radiologic images to travel and geospatial data for determination of forensic epidemiologic risk of disease. Patterns will continuously emerge and reemerge in individual and aggregate patient records, and this trend analysis will help define who and what we are, and most important, when, how, where, and what risk or vulnerability we have to established or predicted medical conditions and/or diseases. Probabilities of exposure will be calculable and accessible to the patient, and potential medical and therapeutic interventions may or may not be recommended as possible or likely to be successful. Regardless, the data will be accessible to multiple users, and those who care for us, observe us, either directly or tangentially, all of the time. Like it or not, ubiquitous or pervasive computing implies data access and knowledge at some level.

A rapidly evolving research and development base nurtures this technocentric world of medical and health-related informatics and expanding cybersecurity concerns. This base consists of many components, which include operating systems (the management of hardware), mobile code, input/output devices, networks, communication protocols, and materials. Operating systems must support multiuser and multitasking environments and include users, applications, and hardware. Operating systems evoke a continuum of security concerns across processes, which include memory protection, user access, networks, World Wide Web, and information integrity, just to name a few at-risk vulnerabilities. The more the multiuser, multitasking environment expands, so does the threat environment.

In an effort to systematically understand the threats and vulnerabilities of the HI environment, the environment may be broadly characterized as one dictated by the parameters of risk = vulnerability × access × motivation. The overall intent of security is to mitigate risk. For all intents and purposes, risk can never equal zero, and risk increases as the complexity of the HI environment increases. We attempt to boost information security through controlling the attributes of confidentiality, integrity, and availability by means of layered security. Layered security is augmented through awareness and education and includes personal, physical, and organizational security. Although standards of security are established organizationally, ultimately, the weakest link in any system is the human–system interface. Vulnerabilities are exploited by many, including actions such as eavesdropping, exploitation through Trojans, worms/viruses, denial-of-service attacks, malware, payloads, rootkits, and key-loggers, which are among the more commonly referred to categories. Table 14.2 defines these vulnerability terms for the reader. This list is not meant to be exhaustive, but it provides the reader with a foundation to understand some of these basic terms. We encourage the reader to examine these and other similar terms, as this is an ever-evolving area with new threats developing almost daily in the worldwide communications network of the Internet.

Although our primary concerns include protection of patient-specific data and identity of individuals, the HI environment characterized by "data, information (and knowledge) on demand" has other tolls to exact that are beyond individual security and scale to financial sabotage and potential intellectual property theft. Property theft in terms of

TABLE 14.2 Security Vulnerability Terms	
Term	Description
Trojans	A program that is similar to a virus but does not replicate; it appears to be legitimate when presented to the user but performs illicit activity when it runs and stays on the computer until properly removed, allowing unauthorized users to take control of the computer
Worms	Destructive program that replicates itself on a computer or network that is either wired or wireless, doing damage by reproduction and consuming memory and internal disk space
Viruses	General term indicating software that infects a computer, the code of which is typically buried in an existing program that the end user unintentionally loads, thereby infecting the computer with the virus; infected programs can propagate throughout a network
Denial-of-service attacks	An intentional attack on a system, preventing legitimate users from using the service by flooding the network, causing disruptions, and targeting a specific individual or system from using the service
Malware	Malicious software loaded to a computer and intended to destroy data, steal information, or aggravate the user
Payloads	A term used to describe malicious software, viruses, Trojans, and worms that produce harmful results; examples of payloads include data destruction, or spurious e-mails or texts sent to a large number of people
Rootkits	A type of Trojan that hides from detection, allows the attacker to have access to "the root" of the computer, and commonly intercepts application program interface calls
Key-loggers	Also called "Keystroke logger," a program or hardware device installed to capture key strokes of the end user

DMR, digital rights management.

Source: McDowell (2013).

new and emerging PHI, such as pharmacotherapeutics, represents a new type of PHI and identity theft for individuals (Identity Theft Resource Center, 2015).

We begin by posing questions to establish a framework for security implementation and operations. First and foremost in establishing a framework for critical information and information protection, we must consider the following questions:

1. Who (or what functional group) in the HI environment needs to know and should have access?

2. What entity grants access and monitors adherence and compliance with security policies?

3. What entity enforces security policy and standards?

4. Who really "owns" our data and controls access as data evolves in complexity and integration?

Even though data trace back to "me," they may be generated by a hospital, secondary provider of services, a pharmaceutical company, or others and may actually be "proprietary" and have implications regarding intellectual property. Each of these issues poses another security concern and challenge, presents another layer for consideration, and, ultimately, requires standardization and watchfulness. No matter how complex security is, security is the responsibility of the user and the manipulator of the data. Organizationally, policies are put in place in an effort to preempt security breaches and collateral damage to networks and other data sources and to ensure confidentiality.

Necessity for Enhanced Security in the Health Information Environment

For the purposes of this discussion, the authors will simplify the cybersecurity discussion to a high-level description of the computing landscape and the major at-risk issues/system components that the reader should be aware of and that he or she may take proactive actions to protect. The authors assume that the future will consist of increasingly complex HI environments that store, retain, manipulate, and share health data and information with the end result of "knowledge" that is useful to individual entities and society as a whole. The assumption is also made that the clients/users of the data and information sets comprising the HI environments are both public and private and thus classified as "hybrid."

Complex systems are dynamic security sieves. When we consider the shear amount of health care information today, we are astounded by an estimated 5 exabytes (5×10^{18}) bytes of data currently stored and readily accessible on the Internet and described as health information (Eric Schmidt, Executive Chairman of Google, personal communication, August 2010). Functionally, this information is manipulated, analyzed, and used in multiple functions, sometimes in parallel. These functions include personal identification, archiving, financial application, health diagnostics, and analysis, just to name a few. When we consider the world of HI, we are describing a world of intertwined specialization and generalization and a continuum of data leading to information to knowledge to ultimately wisdom, with and without human intervention. When considering this paradigm, we consider security as an absence of technological surprise or compromise of information and/or function. Functionally, security is a toolkit (not a lock) that enables mitigation of the effects of surprise or compromise when it occurs. Security is truly a ubiquitous function of the HI environment.

Defining the Environment and Its Uniqueness

When discussing security, we need to understand the future of communications infrastructure beginning with today's ubiquitous computing systems. "Ubiquitous computing" refers to everywhere and anywhere/anytime computing that is enabled by a significant underlying infrastructure. This computing scheme enables the use of open source data coupled with big data and cloud computing. In an ideal world, this concept seems wonderful. In reality, this scheme is fraught with security nightmares. To begin with, especially when considering the sensitivity of some medical data, the lines between a "need to know" and "need to share" becomes increasingly challenging. When compounded with the need for time-critical access to data and decision making, the security challenges may become untenable.

Cloud Computing Vulnerabilities

Cloud computing creates a set of vulnerabilities for a number of reasons. Of course, we know that all sorts of data reside in the cloud. For the intents and purposes of this discussion, all data in the cloud have a certain amount of exposure from a security standpoint. For example, data that are networked and distributed may be considered easily targeted. So, one alternative to improved security is tighter control of data access and hence more difficult use to legitimate users. Although tighter control sounds good on the surface, the end result may be contrary to what we are trying to achieve: improved accessibility for patient management and improved outcomes.

Other significant entities that we care about reside in the cloud as well. These include "pay as you go" functions such as servers, apps, databases, health care data, and mobile servers. In addition, typically someone else manages and owns the cloud and controls and decides its protection strategies for us.

One approach to security in the cloud is called unified data protection (UDP). This approach treats all data as the same; all data in the cloud may be accessed and manipulated by multiple applications and users, and this may be occurring simultaneously. So instead of limiting access to data to specific trusted users, which is a traditional approach, we may consider limiting access to trusted functions. This approach enables access anywhere and supports the evolving paradigm of personalized medicine in a ubiquitous computing environment.

The key to security centers includes verification of the data sender, source, and the consumer of the data. A proactive approach to security requires continuous trolling for anomalies in patterns and established security parameters. In a sea of complex data analytics and use and sometimes novel data manipulation by multiple users, assumption of trustworthiness seems a more rational approach to security than an initial assumption that every entity must prove trustworthiness. Reverting to the new paradigm of subsequent limitation of access will enable the open environment of cloud computing and access to social media and open source information in personalized medicine and patient education. Previously stove-piped functions will be more readily integrated in a seamless manner.

The Next-Generation Health Information Environment and Its Challenges

As health care continues to evolve in terms of its technological sophistication and personalization, so does the complexity of associated security challenges. For example, health care continues to push the limits of information readily available to patients on their health, susceptibility to disease, and, most recently, genetic composition. Some of these sources of information are through commercially available genomics and proteomics services. In theory, every patient can assess his or her own genetic susceptibility to disease, and probability of response and recovery within certain error parameters to select therapeutic options. Through the use of social media and other tools, group assessments, validation, social norms, and discussion result in an understanding of optimized diagnostics and therapeutics. However, user beware! The looming concern of misinformation, misrepresentation, and misinterpretation of data and clinical implications are omnipresent. Hence, an important component of the world of total access and open HIE is patient education and expectation management.

Security Implications for the HI Professional

The rapidly evolving world of telehealth, telepresence, and robotics is upon us. Serious security implications arise in a world of decision-assisted technology applications. Although the complexity of information that is necessary for effective and optimized decision making in health care benefits to a great extent from layered security, security measures should be balanced with information access issues. Having an exceedingly complex health information security environment that ensures security creates a dysfunctional operational environment. It is best to determine the level of acceptable risk for an integrated system of hardware, software, automation, and users, and to proceed to develop the optimal security system requirements and criteria that also meet end user needs to an acceptable level. It behooves each and every health care provider and researcher, especially those responsible for data and information analytics, to be actively involved in this process. In addition, the authors believe that each HI researcher-practitioner should be keenly encouraged to understand the intricacies of health information security and its challenges.

Challenges for the Future

The challenge for health care providers and informatics nurses will be to understand data flow and exchange in a constantly changing and dynamic ecosystem where the traditional privacy boundaries provided by HIPAA and other regulations either overlap or do not provide sufficient protection thereby creating gaps. New demands for privacy and security will arise given the rapid evolution of technology, and standards to address them may not be clear. Policy making will not keep pace with technological change, so it will be especially important to understand how to keep abreast of security vulnerabilities and weaknesses within systems where data are exchanged across traditional and nontraditional settings. More health data are captured and used outside of the realm of HIPAA in today's environment, which challenges us to be more familiar with appropriate security and privacy practices.

ROLE OF THE CLINICIAN IN PROTECTION OF PHI

Surveys indicate that the majority of privacy and security breaches often result from human error or negligence. In fact, the fourth annual benchmark study on privacy and data security released by the Ponemon Institute in March 2014 indicates that 75% of organizations surveyed say that employee negligence is their biggest concern (Ponemon Institute, 2014). Organizations recognize that there are gaps in policy, technology, and education that can lead to negligence. This is an area that nurses must be cognizant of and look for ways to mitigate.

Clinicians' Responsibilities

What can clinicians do to help protect the health care consumers' PHI? Steps that all clinicians should take to comply with HIPAA include awareness of the different components of HIPAA, professional commitments to advocacy for health care consumers and patients, and heightened awareness of where PHI might be exposed. Text messages that constitute unsecure messaging (routine mobile phone texts), photos taken with mobile devices in the workplace with the potential for exposing computer screens with subsequent posting to Facebook and other social media pages, and student nurses taking photos of the first injection given with patient labels on syringes may constitute HIPAA violations. These actions, though seemingly innocent, violate patients' rights under HIPAA. The profession of nursing is responsible to patients for those protections. In 2014, the American Association of Nurses issued a privacy and confidentiality statement for members:

> Ongoing advances in technology, including computerized medical databases, telehealth, social media and other Internet-based technologies, have increased the likelihood of potential and unintentional breaches of private/confidential health information. The purpose of this position statement is to speak on the role of nurses in protecting privacy and confidentiality and in providing recommendations to avoid a breach (ANA, 2015, p. 1 of ANA Revised Position Statement on Privacy and Security).

In addition, one should stay up to date with all changes to HIPAA, including new provisions under the HITECH Act with an understanding of how MU measures relate to privacy and security regulations under HIPAA and the increased protections under the HITECH Act. CMS defines the EHR incentive program, and ONC defines the EHR certification criteria. Use of certified EHR technology ensures that the technology can support the requirements of MU.

Privacy, Security, MU, and the HITECH Act

MU requires that electronic health information created or maintained in a certified EHR be protected with appropriate technical capabilities. Stage 2 of MU sets requirements for privacy, security, and patient access through secure electronic messaging that supports the idea that patient–provider communication is protected and technology should be used to communicate regardless of whether health-related information is maintained. Building on the concept of a more engaged patient, the view, download, and transmit capabilities required by MU provide patients with the ability to view online information, download and transmit their health information within 4 business days of the information being available. To meet MU requirements, all CEs must conduct a risk assessment in accordance with the requirements under 45 CFR 164.308(a)(1). If any deficits are noted in the risk assessment, the CE must address the deficiencies and put a plan in place to address all areas that may be in violation of the HIPAA. This requirement is a core objective for meeting stage 1 of MU (CMS, 2014a). In stage 2, requirements increase with the expectation that encryption/security of data stored in certified EHR technology be addressed in accordance with requirements under the HIPAA security rule. It is important to note that the requirements on encryption must now be considered regardless of whether the data are being transmitted (sent) or stored (at rest; CMS, 2014b). Once a risk assessment is conducted, identified deficiencies must be corrected and security updates must be implemented as necessary. Thus, the privacy and security criteria for certified EHR technology to meet stage 2 of MU are more detailed and include authentication, access control, authorization, auditable events and tamper resistance, audit reports, auto log off, emergency access, end-user device encryption, integrity, and optional accounting of disclosures.

Nurses play a role in each of these MU scenarios; they should ensure that they understand and support the patient access requirements and educate themselves on appropriate ways to secure data in their work environments. Nurses may be involved in data collection for risk-analysis procedures, should be aware of the environment, and should suggest changes to improve protections where needed.

The Basics of a Security Risk Assessment

A security risk assessment (SRA) is an important step a hospital or clinic can take to identify risks and vulnerabilities to PHI (e.g., breaches of HIPAA requirements). Such incidents might include roles within the organization that are not properly assigned, allowing individuals to see PHI inappropriately and in misuse of portable devices that store PHI. The basic steps for an assessment recommended by the ONC include:

1. Review existing security of PHI

2. Identify threats and vulnerabilities

3. Assess risks for likelihood and impact

4. Mitigate security risk

5. Monitor results (HealthIT.gov, 2015a)

Risk Assessments—an Important Role for the Nursing Informaticist

The role of the nursing informaticist and other clinical informatics professionals involves several important responsibilities such as knowing and implementing the requirements of MU and HIPAA. One of those requirements is a security risk assessment. The Office of the National Coordinator for Heath Information Technology (ONC-HIT) and the OCR, recognizing the challenging task of security risk assessments, have provided an online tool that can be downloaded in Windows or mobile device applications. The tool walks the end user through the process of assessing the organization. It is a self-contained tool that is question-based, guiding the organization through a series of 156 questions. In addition to the software application, the ONC has provided a comprehensive user's guide

(HealthIT.gov, 2015a). This tool was designed for small providers to use and helps in complying with requirements of HIPAA and MU. The authors recommend that readers review the SRA tool along with this chapter (www.healthit.gov/providers-professionals/security-risk-assessment-tool).

The clinical informaticist requires additional expertise as to how a security audit might take place and awareness of what constitutes a full audit. Generally, in larger institutions, security professionals are responsible for conducting and analyzing audits and the NI may be involved with gathering data for the actual audit. However, in small clinics, Critical Assess Hospitals (CAHs), and small rural community hospitals, nurses may be responsible for conducting the audit. With this type of assessment tool, scrutiny of how the organization adheres to policy is critical, with an important step in assessment being observation of practices in place, not simply a policy stating that the staff are adhering to policy and procedures.

The staff must be aware of all policy and procedures to protect PHI, maintain security of PHI, and follow the policies and procedures. As noted earlier, the human factor is often the largest challenge in organizations' violations of HIPAA law. Training and education of all staff may also be the responsibility of nursing leadership, particularly in smaller facilities with limited resources.

THE NURSE'S ROLE IS IMPORTANT IN ESTABLISHING PUBLIC TRUST

Beyond state and federal implications, nursing boards are also taking actions regarding issues related to disclosures and on events related to social media breaches, and they are ensuring nurses are accountable for their actions related to patient health information (American Nurses Association, 2014). Nurses should familiarize themselves with the changes underway and demonstrate behaviors that exemplify these standards.

Nurses play an important role in establishing and maintaining patient trust. To preserve that special relationship, we must take steps to understand the rules that exist, implement ways to protect and secure information, and educate staff and patients. To maintain and protect the confidentiality of patient information, it is critical that nurses understand the intersection of HIT and how it contributes to the clinician–patient trust relationship.

Nurses should educate themselves on federal and state regulations and policies that impact their patient populations and, where possible, become involved in policy-making activities to ensure the voice of nursing is represented. Formulating institutional and organizational policies that represent the rights of patients guaranteed by the law and implementing them accurately can be highly effective for mitigating the damaging effects that result without rules being articulated clearly for health care providers and patients to understand.

One should take time to understand the security potential and limitations related to technology that are a part of one's work environment. One should think through the workflows and how they impact the security of patient information and work with vendors to build solutions that work and that providers and patients can trust. Other roles that nursing leaders may play include national standards work on security and transport of data, maintaining institutional policies, particularly in areas that relate to things such as encryption and use of e-mail, texting, and mobile devices. Nursing leadership is also responsible for the education of the nursing staff at all levels, acting as a role model and mentor by demonstrating effective actions and steps to protect the PHI of the public. These responsibilities are significant in terms of maintaining the public trust.

POPULATION HEALTH AND RESEARCH DATA

Although provisions for research are clearly stated in the Privacy Rule, access to data has, in some respects, become more restrictive as public and private entities, including research repositories, have tightened access to data in the name of maintaining secure and protected PHI. Other avenues have opened up public domain data in remarkable ways under federal initiatives for open access to data; this can improve the health, safety, and strength of the nation. Under the Open Government Initiative established by the Obama Administration, the president states:

> My administration is committed to creating an unprecedented level of openness in Government. We will work together to ensure the public trust and establish a system of transparency, public participation, and collaboration. Openness will strengthen our democracy and promote efficiency and effectiveness in Government. (The White House, 2015)

We encourage the reader to access www.data.gov and explore sources available in the health care domain. The website is home to the U.S. Government's open data with data, tools, and other resources for researchers and developers. However, penalties increasing under the HITECH Act and audits occurring result in organizations being less likely to take any risks associated with managing access to data that may identify individuals within the research repository or data set in the private sector. Although advances in technology have vastly improved the amount and quality of data collected and could facilitate probing analyses not done three decades ago, researchers are rarely given access even when detailed protocols are provided (Wartenberg & Thompson, 2010).

Examples of public domain data are the National Center of Health Statistics (NCHS) compilation of de-identified birth, death, and fetal death data for the entire country. Many attest to significant value in these types of de-identified sources as recently reflected in public testimony provided in December 2014 to the ONC Health Information Technology Policy Committee, Privacy and Security Work Group (HealthIT.gov, 2015b). Others express concern that the de-identification provides limited use for epidemiologic studies, particularly with respect to people with chronic illness (McGraw, 2009; Wartenberg & Thompson, 2010). An example of expressed concern is reflected in Wartenberg and Thompson's claim (2010) that the Department of Veterans Affairs had instructed its hospitals to protect patient privacy, and as a result of these protections no longer provide cancer surveillance data at federal and state levels. These researchers indicate that the lack in submission creates a gap in the overall interpretation of data and is a disservice to our veterans in the prevention and treatment of cancer (Wartenberg & Thompson, 2010).

Researchers have voiced their concerns regarding the negative impact that the HIPAA Privacy Rule has on access to data that are necessary to perform credible and viable results, however, measurable proof in the protection of data is still lacking (Nass, Levit, Gostin, & Institute of Medicine, 2009). As patient advocates, health care providers, and researchers, we must strike a balance between patient privacy protection and the research process (Bova, Drexler, & Sullivan-Bolyai, 2012), and we should gain the trust of patients by possessing a thorough understanding of the protection of personal information (Rho, Jang, Chung, & Choi, 2013). There is work underway to define the permitted uses under HIPAA for research in a big data world with initiatives such as Patient Centered Outcomes Research. The goal is to build a trust framework to support such data uses (PCORI, 2015).

SUMMARY

We have reviewed background information on the protection of health care data under the HIPAA regulatory requirements established in 1996 and updates to that regulation enacted with the HITECH Act to increase protection of data. Each component of HIPAA was discussed, including transactions, privacy, and security rules. We have discussed the enforcement component and how enforcement and audits have increased with sizable penalties for disclosures by organizations across the United States. In addition, we have examined other regulatory requirements, including state laws that can override federal law when considered more stringent with respect to protections.

We have also discussed the importance of public trust and nursing roles that are important for establishing strong policies and procedures in protecting the PHI and identity of individuals whom we care for on a daily basis. Most issues with security breaches are related to vulnerabilities created by human errors; therefore, we also related common incidences of HIPAA violations and reviewed why they occurred and how to mitigate these types of incidents while emphasizing the importance of security risk assessments in that process.

Population health data and the "push and pull" between protecting privacy and disclosing adequate information to address epidemiologic and other research questions were noted, comparing and contrasting the various positions on whether we, as a nation, have the right balance between open government and public disclosure of health care data for common good versus potential risks of disclosing public domain data that might be used to identify individuals.

New threats in terms of cybersecurity were reviewed with special attention as to why these new threats are occurring, what they are, and what we can do as an industry to guard against these exposures. Technical terms related to cybersecurity were noted and used within the context of threats that all health care professionals should be aware of to help guard against disclosures. Finally, an exercise is presented to consider the SRA tool established by the ONC and the Office of Civil Rights to assess organizations for adequate protections.

EXERCISES AND QUESTIONS FOR CONSIDERATION

Considering information related in this chapter, identify a clinical environment in which PHI or personal identifiers might be vulnerable to exposure. Download the SRA tool available on the Health IT.gov website: www.healthit.gov/providers-professionals/security-risk-assessment-tool.

The SRA takes you through each HIPAA requirement by presenting questions about your organization's activities. Your "yes" or "no" answer will show you whether you need to take corrective action for that particular item. There are a total of 156 questions. Use the SRA to assess the health care organization you have chosen and write a report for the organization as to areas it needs to consider.

Consider the following questions:

1. Which areas do you consider as high risk and what actions should be taken with these vulnerabilities?

2. Whose responsibility is it to address vulnerabilities and risks to PHI?

3. In the event an audit occurs at this point in time, what do you believe the organization would do regarding adherence to HIPAA? What recommendations would you make to the organization to prepare for such an audit?

4. How important are policies and procedures to adherence to the HIPAA protections of PHI? Is having a policy in place adequate evidence of meeting requirements under HIPAA of protecting PHI?

REFERENCES

American Nurses Association. (2014). *6 tips for nurses using social media*. Retrieved from www.nursing world.org/FunctionalMenuCategories/AboutANA/Social-Media/Social-Networking-Principles-Tool kit/6-Tips-for-Nurses-Using-Social-Media-Poster.pdf

American Nurses Association. (2015). *Revised privacy and confidentiality position statement*. Retrieved from http://www.nursingworld.org/MainMenuCategories/EthicsStandards/Ethics-Position-Statements/ PrivacyandConfidentiality.html, p. 1.

Atchinson, B. K., & Fox, D. M. (1997). The politics of the health insurance portability and accountability act. *Health Affairs, 16*(3), 146–150. Retrieved from www.library.armstrong.edu/eres/docs/eres/ MHSA8635-1_CROSBY/8635_week2_HIPAA_politics.pdf

Bova, C., Drexler, D., & Sullivan-Bolyai, S. (2012). Reframing the influence of the Health Insurance Portability and Accountability Act on research. *Chest, 141*(3), 782–786. doi:10.4103/0255-0857.90155

Centers for Medicare & Medicaid Services. (2003). Overview of electronic transactions & code sets. *HIPAA Information Series 1*(4), 1–8. Retrieved from www.cms.gov/Regulations-and-Guidance/HIPAA-Administrative-Simplification/EventsandLatestNews/Downloads/Whateelectronictransactionsand codesets-4.pdf

Centers for Medicare & Medicaid Services. (2013). *HIPAA: General information*. Retrieved from https://www.cms.gov/Regulations-and-Guidance/HIPAA-Administrative-Simplification/HIPAA GenInfo/index.html

Centers for Medicare & Medicaid Services. (2014a). *2014 definition: Stage 1 of meaningful use*. Retrieved from cms.gov/Regulations-and-Guidance/Legislation/EHRIncentivePrograms/Meaningful_ Use.html

Centers for Medicare & Medicaid Services. (2014b). *Stage 2: Meaningful use*. Retrieved from www.cms .gov/Regulations-and-Guidance/Legislation/EHRIncentivePrograms/Stage_2.html

Centers for Medicare & Medicaid Services. (2015). *ICD-10*. Retrieved from www.cms.gov/Medicare/Coding/ICD10/index.html?redirect=/icd10

Cisco. (2013). *Cisco CIO summit 2013: Summary*. Retrieved from www.cisco.com/web/offer/ciosummit 2013-london/CIOSummit2013_Summary.pdf

Clearwater Compliance. (2012). *Preparing for the HIPAA security rule again; now, with teeth from the HITECH Act!* (White Paper for Health Care Professionals). Retrieved from clearwatercompliance.com/wp-content/uploads/HIPAA-HITECH-Security-Rule-FAQ_WhitePaper_v6.pdf. (HIPAA)

eCFR.gov. (2014, December). *Electronic code of federal regulations*. Retrieved from www.ecfr.gov/cgi-bin/text-idx?SID=6476a9ffd68705614e3599e553a393fe&node=se45.1.160_1103&rgn=div8

Eden, J., Wheatley, B., McNeil, B., & Sox, H. (2008). *Knowing what works in health care: A roadmap for the nation* (Brief). Washington, DC: National Academies Press. Retrieved from books.nap.edu/openbook .php?record_id=12038

Federal Trade Commission. (2014). *2014 privacy and data security update*. Retrieved from https://www.ftc.gov/system/files/documents/reports/privacy-data-security-update-2014/privacydatasecurity update_2014.pdf

Food and Drug Administration. (2013). *Cybersecurity for medical devices and hospital networks: FDA safety communication*. Retrieved from http://www.fda.gov/medicaldevices/safety/alertsandnotices/ucm356423.htm

Hall, M., Dugan, E., Camacho, F., Kidd, K., Aneil, M., & Balkrishnan, R. (2002). Measuring patients' trust in their primary care providers. *Medical Care Research and Review, 59*, 293–318.

Healthcare Information and Management Systems Society. (n.d). *Security and privacy of electronic medical records* (White Paper). Chicago, IL: Author. Retrieved from http://www.himss.org/files/himssorg/content/files/securityandprivacyofelectronicmedicalrecords.pdf

HealthIT.gov. (2015a). *Security risk assessment tool*. Retrieved from https://www.healthit.gov/providers-professionals/security-risk-assessment-tool

HealthIT.gov. (2015b). *HITPC Health Big Data Report*. Retrieved from https://www.healthit.gov/sites/faca/files/HITPC_Health_Big_Data_Report_FINAL.pdf

Health Information Law. (2012). *Health information and the law: States*. Retrieved from http://www .healthinfolaw.org/

HHS.gov. (2003). *OCR HIPAA privacy: Business associates*. Retrieved from http://www.hhs.gov/ocr/privacy/hipaa/understanding/coveredentities/businessassociates.pdf

HHS.gov. (2013). *New rule protects patient privacy, secures health information*. Retrieved from http://www.hhs.gov/news/press/2013pres/01/20130117b.html

HHS.gov. (2014). *Office for civil rights*. Retrieved from http://www.hhs.gov/ocr/office/index.html

HHS.gov. (2015). *Guidance regarding methods for De-identification of protected health information in accordance with the health insurance portability and accountability act (HIPAA) privacy rule*. Retrieved from http://www.hhs.gov/ocr/privacy/hipaa/understanding/coveredentities/De-identification/guidance .html#_edn2

HHS.gov. (n.d.-a). *Health information privacy: Stolen laptops lead to important HIPAA settlements*. Retrieved from http://www.hhs.gov/ocr/privacy/hipaa/enforcement/examples/stolenlaptops-agreements .html

HHS.gov. (n.d.-b). *Health information privacy: The privacy rule*. Retrieved from http://www.hhs.gov/ocr/privacy/hipaa/administrative/privacyrule/index.html

Identity Theft Resource Center. (2015). *Identity theft resource center breach report hits record high in 2014.* Retrieved from http://www.idtheftcenter.org/Press-Releases/2014breachstatistics.htm

Institute of Medicine. (2013). *Best care at lower cost: The path to continuously learning health care in America.* Washington, DC: The National Academies Press.

McCormick, K. M., & Gugerty, B. (2013). Human factors in healthcare IT. *Healthcare information technology exam guide.* New York, NY: McGraw-Hill.

McDowell, M. (2013). *Security tip (ST04-015): Understanding denial-of-service attacks.* Retrieved from http://www.us-cert.gov/ncas/tips/ST04-015

McGraw, D. (2009). Privacy and health information technology. *Journal of Law Medicine & Ethics, 37*(3), 121–149. doi:10.1111/j.1748-720X.2009.00424.x

Nass, S. J., Levit, L. A., Gostin, L. O., & IOM. (2009). *Beyond the HIPAA privacy rule: Enhancing privacy, improving health through research.* Washington, DC: National Academies Press. Retrieved from http://www.ncbi.nlm.nih.gov/books/NBK9576/

Ohio Bureau of Workers' Compensation. (n.d.). EDI implementation guide. Provider billing flow. Retrieved from https://www.bwc.ohio.gov/provider/services/techlevel.asp

Patient Centered Outcomes Research Institute. (2015). *About us.* Retrieved from http://www.pcori.org/about-us

Ponemon Institute. (2014). *Learn to manage your privacy & security risks.* Retrieved from http://www2.idexpertscorp.com/ponemon-report-on-patient-privacy-data-security-incidents

Rho, M. J., Jang, K. S., Chung, K. Y., & Choi, I. Y. (2013). Comparison of knowledge, attitudes, and trust for the use of personal health information in clinical research. *Multimedia Tools and Applications, 67*(3), 1–4. doi:10.1007/s11042-013-1772-6

Substance Abuse and Mental Health Services Administration. (2014). *Laws and regulations.* Retrieved from http://www.samhsa.gov/about-us/who-we-are/laws-regulations

Tim, G. (2014). *Renting a zombie farm: Botnets and the hacker economy.* Retrieved from http://www.symantec.com/connect/tr/blogs/renting-zombie-farm-botnets-and-hacker-economy

U.S. Department of Health and Human Services. (2013). *Modifications to the HIPAA privacy, security, enforcement, and breach notification rules under the Health Information Technology for Economic and Clinical Health Act and the Genetic Information Nondiscrimination Act; other modifications to the HIPAA rules: Final rule.* Retrieved from www.gpo.gov/fdsys/pkg/FR-2013-01-25/pdf/2013-01073.pdf

Wartenberg, D., & Thompson, D. W. (2010). Privacy versus public health: The impact of current confidentiality rules. *American Journal of Public Health, 100*(3), 407–412. doi:10.2105/AJPH.2009.166249

The White House. (2015). *State of the union.* Retrieved from http://www.whitehouse.gov/Open/

CHAPTER 15

Personal Health Records and Patient Portals

Mari Tietze, Cristina Winters, and Stephanie H. Hoelscher

OBJECTIVES

1. Appraise the relationship among the personal health record (PHR)/portal, patient engagement/activation, and patient safety and quality.

2. Identify factors associated with increased patient PHR/portal use.

3. Examine advantages and disadvantages of patient-generated health information.

4. Identify components of the ideal patient portal.

5. Predict achievable levels of patient engagement/activation in one's practice.

6. Model the PHR/portal implementation using the interprofessional approach to increase patient use.

KEY WORDS

patient safety, quality, population health, meaningful use, patient engagement, patient activation

---

CONTENTS

INTRODUCTION

The *Federal Strategic HIT Plan 2015–2020* report had a clear message for patients and providers, "collect data, share data and use data" (Office of the National Coordinator for Health Information Technology [ONC-HIT], 2014, p. 5). Not only is this so at the individual level but, more important, at the community level. This approach firmly supports the effort of personal health record (PHR) data use and aligns all the people involved (ONC-HIT, 2014). This strategy appears to be an evolution from the 2010 efforts to implement electronic health record (EHR) systems in provider facilities to a broader infrastructure of EHRs and PHRs to include the community at large.

The use of EHRs has risen dramatically in recent years. EHR use has increased in private practice from 17% in 2008 to 34% in 2011 (Goldzweig, 2012). Important to this growth is the PHR, a component associated with the EHR that provides specific access via an electronic portal, for the patient's view of his or her own information. A PHR is defined by the Social Security Act (42 U.S.C. 1320d(6)) as "individually identifiable health information, and includes, with respect to an individual, information (A) that is provided by or on behalf of the individual; and (B) that identifies the individual, or with respect to which there is a reasonable basis to believe that the information can be used to identify the individual" (see Congressional Record—House, February 12, 2009, p.H1348, which is available online at www.ssa.gov/OP_Home/ssact/title11/1171.htm).

The National Learning Consortium indicated that a patient portal, on which a PHR exists, is a "secure online website that gives patients convenient 24-hour access to personal health information from anywhere with an Internet connection" (National Learning Consortium, 2014, p. 1). Using a secure username and password, patients can view health information, such as the following:

- Recent doctor visits
- Discharge summaries
- Medications
- Immunizations
- Allergies
- Lab results

Some patient portals also allow patients to do the following:

- Exchange secure e-mails with their health care teams
- Request prescription refills
- Schedule nonurgent appointments
- Check benefits and coverage
- Update contact information
- Make payments

► Download and complete forms

► View educational materials

With patient portal implementation, an organization can enhance patient–provider communication, empower patients, support care between visits, and, most important, improve patient outcomes (National Learning Consortium, 2014, p. 1). As illustrated in Figure 15.1, the components of the PHR/patient portal typically include (a) patient record/history (from the provider's main EHR); (b) educational/training documents; (c) collaboration methods such as e-mail 24 hours a day, to communicate with health care professionals; and (d) quality metrics, such as outcome measures, that demonstrate progress over time (Cognator.com, 2014).

In terms of efficiencies, the portal provides a means for the provider to send messages to the patient and to ease workflow by reducing phone messages and unscheduled visits by the patient (Clarke et al., 2013). Patients benefit from portal use, as they are allowed to use the services provided rather than having to wait for long periods for phone calls to be returned by the clinic. Portal use may also be cost-effective, in that it may decrease the need for repeated tests and procedures by specialists or emergency care providers, as the patient has the ability to access diagnostic procedures and interventions from a laptop, computer, tablet, or smartphone (Di Maio, 2010).

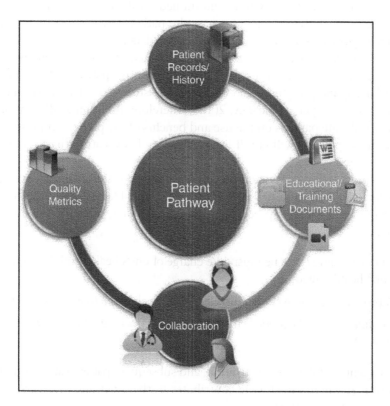

FIGURE 15.1. Patient pathway (portal) and associated sources of health improvement information and professionals.

Source: Cognator.com (2014).

MEANINGFUL USE REQUIREMENTS FOR
THE PATIENT PORTAL

According to the U.S. Department of Health and Human Services (2013, p. 1), meaningful use (MU) refers to the "set of standards defined by the Centers for Medicare & Medicaid Services (CMS) Incentive Programs that governs the use of EHRs and enables eligible providers and hospitals to earn incentive payments by meeting specific criteria." During Stage 2 of MU, health care providers had to implement a patient portal as a part of the EHR in 2014. The requirements are that the eligible provider must provide patients with the ability to view online, download, and transmit their health information. An eligible provider is any physician or midlevel provider who participates in the Medicare or Medicaid EHR incentive program (McGraw, 2012). The eligible provider must provide "50% of all unique patients seen within a reporting period access within four business days of when the information is available to them" (Netti, 2013, p. 1). The requirements for Stage 2 of MU are that 5% of patients must download and/or transmit information via the portal (Netti, 2013).

Not every patient will enroll in and use the portal. As the portal is a relatively new concept, many patients are unfamiliar with it and the benefits that it can provide. Providers, on the other hand, are often reluctant to engage in the use of the portal for various reasons, with many fearing that patient portal access will increase their workload or worry that their notes will be questioned (Walker et al., 2011). Nevertheless, as the Stage 2 of MU requirements exists, the patient portal must be implemented and utilized by patients and providers for the providers to continue to receive financial reimbursements for services. These services are based on submitted allowable Medicare charges or a set payment for the Medicaid incentive pathway. A penalty will be imposed for eligible providers who do not successfully report EHR-MU criteria by 2015 (Harrison, Koppel, & Bar-Lev, 2007). Therefore, it is financially important for providers to educate patients on the use and benefits of the patient portal so providers hope that these patients will enroll in and use this EHR feature that has been made available to them.

From a clinical perspective, and the approach used for this chapter, the underlying rationale for PHRs and associated patient portals is to facilitate the patient's engagement/activation in the care delivery process. Specifically, as noted, patient activation is defined as follows:

▶ Understanding that one must take charge of one's health and that actions determine health outcomes

▶ A process of gaining skills, knowledge, and behaviors to manage health

▶ Confidence to make needed changes (Hibbard, Stockard, Mahoney, & Tusler, 2004, p. 1010)

As such, patient portal, patient activation, and subsequent patient safety and quality of care delivery are intertwined. One contributes to the other and vice versa (National Learning Consortium, 2013).

DIGITAL DIVIDE AND HEALTH LITERACY

As noted, patient portals are online applications that allow the patient access to his or her medical information and enable communication with his or her health care provider (National Learning Consortium, 2014). According to Emont (2011), the use of health information technologies (HITs) and online resources has great potential to boost care quality by improving care access, efficiency, chronic disease management, and patient and family involvement. Barriers to the use of the portal exist, despite advantages of the service. Many patients do not know about the service, as implementation of a patient portal is a relatively new concept.

One aspect of patient portal use that has been debated is the notion of access to the Internet. In one study (Kruse et al., 2012), 638 family practice clinic patients completed questionnaires about their use of the Internet. Of these, 499 (78%) were Internet users and 139 (22%) were nonusers. Lack of computer access and not knowing how to use e-mail or the Internet were the most common barriers to Internet use. Younger age, higher education and income, better health, and absence of a chronic illness were associated with Internet use. The major factor associated with Internet use among patients with chronic conditions was age. As such, authors suggested that if older adults with chronic illness are to reap the benefits of HIT, their Internet access will need to be improved and institutions that are planning to offer consumer HIT should be aware of groups with lower Internet access (Kruse et al., 2012).

Despite access, the patient portal and associated PHR must be presented at a low reading level and understandability should be matched to the target population. A 2010 report by the U.S. Office of Disease Prevention and Health Promotion defined *health literacy* as "The degree to which individuals have the capacity to obtain, process, and understand basic health information and services needed to make appropriate health decisions" (Office of Disease Prevention and Health Promotion, 2010, p. 6). The report claims that limited health literacy affects people of all ages, races, incomes, and education levels, but the impact of limited health literacy disproportionately affects lower socio-economic and minority groups. It affects people's ability to search for and use health information, adopt healthy behaviors, and act on important public health alerts. Limited health literacy is also associated with worse health outcomes and higher costs (Berkman et al., 2004).

The national action plan to improve health literacy contains seven goals aimed at improving health literacy and suggests strategies for achieving them. They are as follows:

1. Develop and disseminate health and safety information that is accurate, accessible, and actionable

2. Promote changes in the health care system that improve health information, communication, informed decision making, and access to health services

3. Incorporate accurate, standards-based, and developmentally appropriate health and science information and curricula in child care and education at the university level

4. Support and expand local efforts to provide adult education, English language instruction, and culturally and linguistically appropriate health information services in the community

5. Build partnerships, develop guidance, and change policies

6. Increase basic research and the development, implementation, and evaluation of practices and interventions to improve health literacy

7. Increase the dissemination and use of evidence-based health literacy practices and interventions (Office of Disease Prevention and Health Promotion, 2010, p. 7)

An accompanying report by the Agency for Healthcare Research and Quality (AHRQ) published extensive guidelines for developers of materials and websites for the low-literacy population (AHRQ, 2007). In the Appendix, the report provide a comprehensive "yes/no" checklist for developers that can guide them in written materials, PHRs, and patient portal creations. A few representative items for consideration are as follows:

▶ Words are short, simple, and familiar (1–2 syllables, no jargon, acronyms, abbreviations)

▶ Unavoidable technical terms are explained

▶ Sentences are short

▶ Written in "active" voice rather than "passive" voice (use "Mary visited the clinic" rather than "The clinic was visited by Mary")

▶ Consistent use of words throughout

▶ Reading level is not above sixth grade (AHRQ, 2007, A-1)

The National Learning Consortium has supported providers with guidance and materials to optimize patient engagement in their care. One fact sheet specifies how to optimize patient portals for patient engagement and to meet MU requirements (National Learning Consortium: Advancing America's Health Care, 2013). The materials list the following actions:

1. Make sure the portal engages patients

2. Have providers learn the benefits of patient portals

3. Understand the relationship between the patient portal and MU

4. Implement portal features that support engagement

5. Implement the portal systematically via provider control, team focus, and efficiency

6. Promote and facilitate patient use (National Learning Consortium: Advancing America's Health Care, 2013, p. 1)

Others have emphasized the relationship between health care literacy and patient safety and quality (Berkman et al., 2004; Sarkar et al., 2010; Tomsik & Briggs, 2013). Common findings are that patients with low-level literacy are at high risk for unintended health care events and unsuccessful care delivery. For example, compared with those who did not report any health literacy limitation, even among those with Internet access, patients with diabetes reporting limited health literacy were less likely to both access and navigate an Internet-based patient portal than those with adequate health literacy (Sarkar et al., 2010). Thus, although the Internet has potential to greatly expand the capacity and reach of health care systems, current use patterns suggest that, in the absence of participatory design efforts involving those with limited health literacy, those most at risk for poor diabetes health outcomes will fall further behind if health systems increasingly rely on Internet-based services alone.

Compounding this issue, a review of literature has suggested that although effective interventions integrate strategies that motivate, empower, and encourage patients to make informed decisions and assume responsibility for self-care, gaps in current evidence lack information on how to improve adherence and self-care for patients who are at an increased risk of poor adherence, including those with cognitive and functional impairments and low health literacy (Evangelista & Shinnick, 2008).

PHR/PORTAL IMPACT ON PATIENT SAFETY, UNINTENDED CONSEQUENCES

As noted in a previous chapter, the book by James details events in which a failure of integrated care ended in the death of his 19-year-old son. Among many other observations, James claimed that in a truly patient-centered medical system "laws must be written to require providers to offer medical records to their patients after every office visit and hospital stay" (James, 2007, p. 122). The PHR and associated patient portal are platforms where patient-generated data, management of the portal, and bidirectional interaction are exemplars of such patient-centered medical systems. However, in addition to putting the patient in the center of the medical record system, the PHR/patient portal tool, when actively used, improves the safety and quality (effectiveness and efficacy, if you will) of care delivery (James, 2013).

Other studies have indicated that the level of communication between patient/family members and providers is inversely related to unintended consequences of health care delivery (Sittig & Ash, 2007). Historically, in 1999, with the first Institute of Medicine (IOM) report on errors in health care delivery, the need for increased communication of patients to health care providers and health care providers to health care providers was a key recommendation (Institute of Medicine [IOM], 2000) reiterated in further IOM (IOM, 2001, 2012) reports.

CONTRIBUTION OF PERSONAL DATA— TELLING THE PATIENT'S STORY

A Patient's Questions Are the Answer

The AHRQ campaign to encourage communication between patients and providers puts the focus on patient-generated questions and associated follow-ups (AHRQ, 2014). Figure 15.2 represents the campaign's home web page where the campaign slogan displays, "Questions Are the Answers." The web page highlights the main features, such as "The 10 Questions You Should Know" before attending your next appointment with your provider. Patients are offered an option to customize those questions according to their specific needs through the "Build Your Own Question List" feature. The website

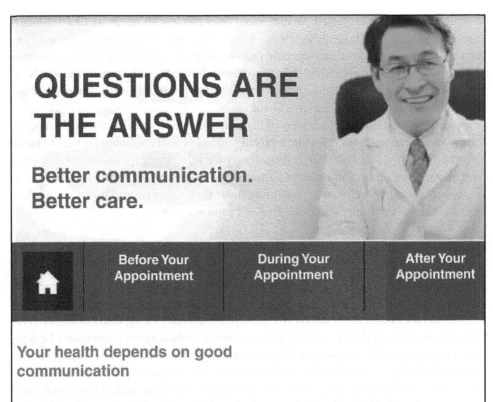

FIGURE 15.2. AHRQ campaign, "Questions Are the Answer."
Source: Agency for Healthcare Research and Quality (2014).

also guides patients with details about what to do both during and after the appointment with their providers.

Give the federal government's emphasis on importance of communication (see Federal HIT Strategic Plan 2015–2020, Figure 15.3), it is suggested that, at minimum, this web page should be prominently displayed on any PHR/patient portal for patient support in communicating optimally with providers. For those without Internet access, written materials, such as pamphlets, should be provided.

Patient-Generated Health Information

The question of whether or not patients should be able to control the information in their EHR is an ongoing debate (Blumenthal & Squires, 2014). Some say that information belongs to patients, and they alone have the right to decide who can access their data.

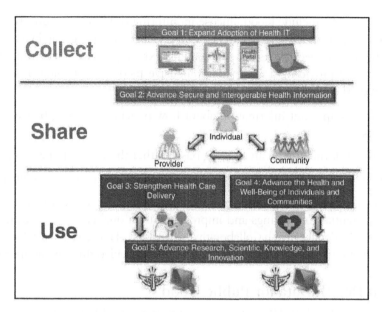

FIGURE 15.3. Five goals of the federal HIT strategic plan 2015 to 2020.
Source: ONC (2014).

Others, mainly clinicians, counter that the clinician needs unfettered access to patient information to provide the bests care possible. Regardless of this, health professionals should realize that if patients do not trust that their EHR data are well protected and used to their advantage, the relationship with clinicians will suffer and patients will withhold information (Blumenthal & Squires, 2014).

The shift toward a more patient-centered medical record and associated patient engagement/activation in care delivery has opened the discussion of "patient-generated health information." Patient-generated health data (PGHD) are health-related data created, recorded, or gathered by or from patients (or family members or other caregivers) to help address a health concern (HealthIT.gov, 2014c; National eHealth Collaborative, 2013). PGHD (HealthIT.gov, 2014c) include but are not limited to:

► Health history

► Treatment history

► Biometric data

► Symptoms

► Lifestyle choices

PGHD are distinct from data generated in clinical settings and through encounters with providers in two important ways:

1. Patients, not providers, are primarily responsible for capturing or recording these data.

2. Patients decide how to share or distribute these data to health care providers and others (HealthIT.gov, 2014c).

Examples of PGHD include blood glucose monitoring or blood pressure (BP) readings using home health equipment, or exercise and diet tracking using a mobile application. PGHD is important, because its use supplements existing clinical data, filling in gaps in information and providing a more comprehensive picture of ongoing patient health. PGHD can do the following:

► Provide important information about how patients are doing between medical visits

► Gather information on an ongoing basis, rather than only at one point in time

► Provide information that is relevant to preventive and chronic care management

The use of PGHD offers an opportunity to capture needed information for use during care, with potential cost savings and improvements in quality, care coordination, and patient safety (National eHealth Collaborative, 2013; ONC-HIT, 2014). PGHD significantly reflects the patient's story by reflecting information provided directly by the patient.

Personal Health Data for Public Good

Closely associated with PGHD is the notion of personal health data (PHD) that are used by others beyond the role of actual health care delivery. As its primary value, PGHD contributes such data to health care decision making for the patient, whereas PHD has the broader purpose of knowledge acquisition to optimize health care decision making, most generally through research studies (California Institute for Telecommunication and Information Technology, 2014). At issue is the fact that health-related data are being tracked more often as the number of mobile-wearable devices and smartphone applications increase. Subsequently, an understanding of the nature of such data and its use would seem fundamental.

An example of the value for such PHD is a study that examined attitudes toward PHD from the individuals who track PHD, the companies involved in self-tracking devices, apps, or services, and the researchers who might use the data (California Institute for Telecommunication and Information Technology, 2014). In 2013, online surveys and interviews of three relevant stakeholder groups were conducted: individuals, researchers, and companies and key informants. Online surveys of 465 self-selected individuals and 134 self-selected researchers who participated and a sampling of interviews were also conducted.

Key findings indicated that:

► Individuals were very willing to share their self-tracking data for research. However, the dominant condition (57%) for making their PHD available for research was an assurance of privacy for their data. More than 90% of respondents said that it was important that the data be anonymous.

► The current methods of informed consent are challenged by the ways in which PHD is being used and reused in research.

► Researchers are enthusiastic about using PHD in research but are the most concerned about the validity of PHD and lack of standardization of devices (California Institute for Telecommunication and Information Technology, 2014).

Despite sampling bias, the report concludes that to enhance the potential to generate knowledge out of PHD, creative solutions enabling individual rights to be respected, while providing access to high-quality and relevant PHD for research, must be developed (California Institute for Telecommunication and Information Technology, 2014). Thus, PHD contributes to overall efforts at telling the patient's story and, as such, although validity and confidentiality characteristics of the data are of concern, PHD should be highly valued as a data source.

Industry Trends and Community Involvement

Studies have suggested that the health of individuals is directly impacted by the health of the individual's community (Rein, 2012). In fact, the community has a central role in the 2014 HIT federal strategic plan, as indicated in the diagram reflecting the overall plan (ONC-HIT, 2014). Goal 2 of the plan is to "Share Advance Secure and Interoperable Health Information," which is depicted as the interrelationship among individual, provider, and community (see Figure 15.3; ONC-HIT, 2014).

As the importance of patients/people and their associated communities become more evident in practice improvement efforts, HIT professionals must embrace the role of organizational systems design that guides the HIT professional in designing systems that are conducive to patient safety and quality practice, including telling the patient's story. Nelson, Batalden, Godfrey, and Lazar (2011) outline steps to take to partner with patients to design and improve care, viewing patients as informants and advisors.

Considering the desire to tell the patient's story in systems such as the EHR and the PHR, an imperative exists to capture not only physical and physiological data but also social and behavioral data. The capture of such valuable data is addressed by an IOM report (IOM, 2014). The report depicts a comprehensive set of factors to be considered in the social and behavioral domain, including sexual orientation, housing insecurities, health literacy, patient activation status, self-efficacy, and neighborhoods/communities. All of the factors, collected in an organized framework, would support telling the patient's and the community's story.

INTERPROFESSIONAL INFORMATICS TO INCREASE PHR/PORTAL USE

The observation that PHRs are not working as expected is fairly common knowledge; however, trends are improving. More than four in five patients with online access to their health records (86%) used their online records at least once, according to the National Partnership for Women and Families study; more than half (55%) used them three or more times a year (Milliard, 2014; National Partnership for Women and Families, 2014).

In spite of this low level of PHR/portal use, providers who use EHRs in their practice are interested in meeting the CMS-MU reimbursement incentives, of which patient use of PHR/patient portals is one. As noted, Stage 2 of MU is intended to "provide patients the ability to view online, download and transmit their health information within four business days of the information being available to the EP (eligible provider)" (McCarty, 2013, p. 4). Specifically, health information must be made available to 50% of patients within 4 business days of receiving the information, and "5% of unique patients, or their authorized representative, must view, download, or transmit their health information to a third party" (McCarty, 2013).

One ambulatory clinic attempted to increase their rate of patient access to the patient portal and PHR. The clinic's doctor of nursing practice (DNP) practitioner and colleagues conducted a study that compared two methods of teaching patients about the portal (Winters, 2014). The study research question was: Does one-on-one education on the benefits and use of the patient portal increase the proportion of participants who obtain portal access compared with those who receive a handout only within a 2-week period after being offered access to the patient portal at check-in/registration? Using a convenience sample, a total of 176 participants were divided into two groups using random assignment. Results of a chi-square analysis conducted on the two groups found no significant difference between patient portal use. Findings suggested that one-on-one education on the use and benefits of the patient portal was not associated with an increase in patient portal use (Winters, 2014).

Methods of Portal Adoption

As evidenced by the results of the research study mentioned earlier, introduction of a new technology for patient use can present unique challenges. For example, sources on PHR/portal use have indicated that marketing and brochures in waiting rooms and exam rooms are an important first step (Wald, 2010). Numerous other approaches for increasing patient PHR/portal use exist and, based on the non-significance of the research study mentioned earlier, approaches involving multi-method interventions may work better than single-method interventions.

One of the key interventions for successful PHR/portal use is staff involvement. In a study by Ketterer et al. (2013), it was suggested that the positive attitudes of providers and staff about the patient portal made a difference in the number of patients who obtained portal access. Similarly, Wald (2010) found that portal adoption was low without key marketing approaches and thorough staff involvement. Wald also found that higher levels of enthusiasm among staff and health care providers proved to be successful in increasing portal use among patients. At the study site mentioned earlier, with only one provider discussing the benefits and use of the portal, patients may not have felt that the portal was that important and this may have been a limitation to the study, contributing to the low numbers of patients who obtained portal access in the study (Winters, 2014).

Similar to staff involvement, interprofessional collaboration can be associated with increased PHR/portal use by patients. Interprofessional collaboration means that all health care professionals on the team are working toward the same goals and contribute to each other's components of the team goals for the patient (Interprofessional Collaborative Expert Panel, 2011). Thus, encouragement and enthusiasm about the PHR/portal can be exhibited by the interprofessional collaborative team in an effort to increase patient portal use rates.

Characteristics for Success

Efforts to increase rates of patient PHR/portal use have been extensively studied (Ancker et al., 2011; Britto, Hesse, Kamdar, & Munafo, 2013; Goel et al., 2013; Zsolt,

Aspy, Chou, & Mold, 2012). In addition, studies have suggested that increased patient PHR/portal use was associated with positive patient outcomes for management of diabetes (HealthIT.gov, 2014a), smoking cessation (HealthIT.gov, 2013), and medication adherence (HealthIT.gov, 2014b), to name a few. Subsequently, attention to characteristics for success provided through other efforts at PHR/portal implementation should be considered as follows.

Computer-Literacy Level

Depending on the patient's level of computer literacy, some people may require more time to be educated than others. Kruse et al. (2012) found that lack of both computer access and computer literacy were barriers to portal enrollment, which can be mitigated by one-on-one computer training and support.

Education Level of Patients

Individuals with higher education and higher income were associated with a higher rate of Internet use (Kruse et al., 2012). An inability to understand participant education level could be a barrier in the effort to increase portal adoption.

Patient Satisfaction With Portal Use

One of the main goals of the patient portal is to improve patient satisfaction and access to care, patient–provider communication, and patient outcomes (Di Maio, 2010), which lead to patient satisfaction. Providers should measure patient satisfaction with their portal as a part of the preplanning process.

Enrollment Process

Pertinent factors, including barriers to enrollment, methods of portal adoption, and information on the objectives of MU, were found to hinder successful implementation (Hurtado, Swift, & Corrigan, 2001; Page, 2004).

Assessment of Internet Access

One study did not first determine whether the patient had Internet access before attempting to recruit participants for portal use, which would most likely skew the results of the study (Yen & Bakken, 2012). If the patient does not have Internet access, other access sources, such as family members, should be considered.

Time Frame for Adoption

There were no studies related to the portal that studied a 2-week time frame as a limit for patients to sign up for the patient portal. One study reported that a 2-day to 2-week time frame was believed to be a reasonable compromise between recollection bias and unwanted clinical change (Dahm, 2008). Identifying a realistic time frame between patient education/recruitment and measurement of patient portal adoption is warranted.

Reading-Level Assessment for Patient and Materials

Most adults read between an eighth- and ninth-grade level (Safeer & Keenan, 2005). For patients whose primary language is not English, the problem is even greater

(Safeer & Keenan, 2005). Thus, Safeer and Keenan believe that having educational material at the sixth-grade or lower level enhances understanding, as even those with adequate health literacy prefer to read patient education materials at this level.

Severity of Patient Illness

Severity of patient illnesses should be a consideration in planning for patient PHR/portal use. Patient education is essential in achieving effective outcomes and, if the patient is not receptive to learning for reasons such as illness, the educational experience will most likely be ineffective (Roberts, 2004).

Knowledge of Portal Use Trends

Studies have indicated that patient characteristics, such as age and gender, affect the type of PHR/portal features that a given patient might access. This means that knowing which patients are accessing which portal features can guide portal development. Therefore, offering features that patients are most likely to be interested in may increase portal adoption in the clinic (Sanders et al., 2013). As such, reports from the PHR/portal that provide details of patient use trends are imperative to successful design and implementation of the PHR/portal.

SUMMARY

According to the literature, few studies on measuring the effectiveness of teaching patient portal use have been reported. The most significant was the study by Wald (2010), in which marketing strategies along with enthusiasm from all staff, including the providers, was an effective means of increasing portal use.

EXERCISES AND QUESTIONS FOR CONSIDERATION

Organizations have focused on increasing patient engagement using electronic tools. For example, Steven Rush, director of the Health Literacy Innovations Program at United-Health Group, cautioned that in the rush to ask patients to use websites, portals, smartphones, and other forms of electronic communication, it is important to teach them how to use these valuable tools. He mentioned research showing that unless there is a personal touch that accompanies these electronic tools, many people will stop using them in about 2 weeks (Alper & Hernandez, 2014).

1. Describe a scenario in your practice in which lack of personal touch has impacted the patient's engagement in care.

2. Explain what technology can be used to enhance rather than hurt a patient's engagement in care.

3. Identify two other professionals on the typical health care team to collaborate with in adding a personal touch to technology-enhanced patient engagement efforts.

4. Summarize the problem and associated solutions in a protocol for optimal implementation of a technology-enhanced patient engagement project.

CASE STUDY

MyChartCare

Consider this case study on patient portals and consumer engagement. Complete the suggested case study activity.

In a city with a population of just less than 300,000, there are two major health care systems in place. Of these two, University Medical Center (UMC) is recognized as the county hospital and it works directly with two of the largest ambulatory systems in the area. The hospital has more than 400 beds and houses the area's only level-one trauma and burn centers, as well as other major specialties.

Secure and effective communication and engagement with their patients was a collective goal. Keeping up with MU was another expectation. Thus, the development of a patient portal system with its EHR was vital to achieving these goals. MyChartCare was successfully launched in 2013. This case study reflects the development of this patient portal and how it relates to patient safety and engagement; it describes the functions and benefits of a patient portal as well as the role of MU.

Description of Patient Portal

So what exactly is a patient portal? HealthIT.gov defines it as "a secure online website that gives patients convenient 24-hour access to personal health information from anywhere with an Internet connection" (HealthIT.gov, 2014d, p. 1).

When establishing a patient portal, there are two routes to be considered: basic access and advanced functionality. Basic access is the minimum of what MU expects when developing a patient portal. The more advanced functionality is more of the "bells and whistles" that can be implemented within the patient portal.

While maintaining strict site security, most portals can provide the patient access to the following information on

- Recent doctor visits
- Discharge and clinical summaries
- Medications and prescription renewals
- Immunizations records
- Allergies (drug, environmental, or food)
- Lab results—quick access (radiology and labs)

More advanced portal construction can also provide access to the following information:

- Exchange secure e-mails with their health care teams via a secure portal.
- Request prescription refills.
- Schedule nonurgent appointments.
- Check benefits and coverage.
- Update contact information.
- Make payments.

(continued)

CASE STUDY (*continued*)

> ► Download and complete forms.
> ► View educational materials (patient specific).

Relationship to MU

One view of MU is that it was developed in direct response to the Affordable Care Act (ACA) of 2010. MU consists of objectives and measures laid out by the CMS. The CMS defines *MU* as "using certified EHR technology to: Improve quality, safety, efficiency, and reduce health disparities. Engage patients and family. Improve care coordination, and population and public health" (CMS, 2014). The word "engage" is frequently used when working with MU standards. This is because the goal is to engage the patient and his or her family in the patient's safety and health care.

All of this allows providers or facilities to apply or "attest" for MU incentive monies. To qualify, the organizations must meet certain core and menu Stage I and II objectives and measures. For example, in relation to the patient portal, the most simplified list could be narrowed down to lab results, problems lists, medication lists, and medication allergies lists.

Put simply, the main requirements of meeting CMS-MU standards for patient engagement using a portal are:

1. Patient portal is required to provide access to PHRs.
2. Patient portal is required to have secure messaging between the patients and their providers/facilities for questions, medication refills, appointment requests, and so forth.

Case Study Activity

In terms of history, patient portals have advanced from simple web pages, used for patient registration or for patients to e-mail their providers, into the complex multifaceted tools they are today. Given the importance of patient engagement through the patient portal, describe three technology vendors you can find on the Internet who are marketed as being integrated with a "patient portal" and/or the "PHR," and who have a focus on patient engagement. List the components of their systems that are showcased to "engaged patients" that should be considered for the MyChartCare patient portal.

REFERENCES

Agency for Healthcare Research and Quality. (2007). *Accessible health information technology (IT) for populations with limited health literacy: A guide for developers and purchasers of health IT*. Washington, DC: U.S. Department of Health and Human Services. Retrieved from http://www.healthit.ahrq.gov/health-it-tools-and-resources/health-it-literacy-guide

Agency for Healthcare Research and Quality. (2014). *Questions are the answer: Better communication, better care*. Retrieved from http://www.ahrq.gov/patients-consumers/patient-involvement/ask-your-doctor/index.html

Alper, J., & Hernandez, L. J. (2014). *Facilitating patient understanding of discharge instructions: Workshop summary* (No. ISBN978-0-309-30738-3). Washington, DC: National Academies Press. Retrieved from http://www.nap.edu/catalog/18834/facilitating-patient-understanding-of-discharge-instructions-workshop-summary

Ancker, J., Barrón, Y., Rockoff, M., Hauser, D., Pichardo, M., Szerencsy, A., & Calman, N. (2011). Use of an electronic patient portal among disadvantaged populations. *Journal of General Internal Medicine, 26*(10), 1117–1123. doi:10.1007/s11606-011-1749-y

Berkman, N. D., DeWalt, D. A., Pignone, M. P., Sheridan, S. L., Lohr, K. N., & Lux, L. (2004). *Literacy and health outcomes* (No. AHRQ Publication No. 04-E007-2). Rockville, MD: Agency for Research and Quality.

Blumenthal, D., & Squires, D. (2014). Giving patients control of their EHR data. *Society of General Internal Medicine, 30*(Suppl. 1), S42–S43. doi:10.1007/s11606-014-3071-y

Britto, M., Hesse, E., Kamdar, O., & Munafo, J. (2013). Parents' perceptions of a patient portal for managing their child's chronic illness. *Journal of Pediatrics, 163*, 280–281.

California Institute for Telecommunication and Information Technology. (2014). *Personal data for the public good: New opportunities to enrich understanding of individual and population health, final report of the health data exploration project* (No. PHDrwjf2014). Princeton, NJ: Robert Wood Johnson Foundation. Retrieved from www.rwjf.org/en/research-publications/find-rwjf-research/2014/03/personal-data-for-the-public-good.html

Centers for Medicare & Medicaid Services. (2014). *Meaningful use definition & objectives.* Retrieved from http://www.healthit.gov/providers-professionals/meaningful-use-definition-objectives

Clarke, M. A., Belden, J. L., Koopman, R. J., Steege, L. M., Moore, J. L., Canfield, S. M., & Kim, M. S. (2013). Information needs and information-seeking behaviour analysis of primary care physicians and nurses: A literature review. *Health Information and Library Journal, 30*(3), 178–190. doi:10.1111/hir.12036

Cognator.com. (2014). *Empowering the patient, transforming healthcare.* Retrieved from http://www.cognitor.com/patient-pathway

Dahm, R. (2008). The first discovery of DNA. *American Scientist, 96*(4), 320. doi:10.1511/2008.73.3846

Di Maio, A. (2010). *Gartner launches open government maturity model* (No. GI2010). Gartner Inc. Stanford, CT. Retrieved from http://www.blogs.gartner.com/andrea_dimaio/2010/06/28/gartner-launches-open-government-maturity-model

Emont, S. (2011). *Measuring the impact of patient portals: What the literature tells us* (No. CHF2011). Oakland, CA: California Healthcare Foundation.

Evangelista, L. S., & Shinnick, M. A. (2008). What do we know about adherence and self-care? *Journal of Cardiovascular Nursing, 23*(3), 250–257.

Goel, M., Brown, T., Williams, A., Cooper, A., Hasnain-Wynia, R., & Baker, D. (2013). Patient reported barriers to enrolling in a patient portal. *Journal of the American Medical Informatics Association, 18*, i8–i12. doi:10.1136/amiajnl-2011-000473

Goldzweig, C. L. (2012). Pushing the envelope of electronic patient portals to engage patients in their care. *Annals of Internal Medicine, 157*(7), 525–526.

Harrison, M. I., Koppel, R., & Bar-Lev, S. (2007). Unintended consequences of information technologies in health care: An interactive sociotechnical analysis. *Journal of the American Medical Informatics Association, 14*(5), 542–549. doi:10.1197/jamia.M2384

HealthIT.gov. (2013). *Improving tobacco use screening and smoking cessation in a primary care practice* (No. CaseStudy2013). Washington, DC: Author. Retrieved from http://www.healthit.gov/providers-professionals/improving-tobacco-use-screening-and-smoking-cessation-primary-care-practice

HealthIT.gov. (2014a). *Improving blood pressure control for patients with diabetes in 4 community health centers.* Retrieved from http://www.healthit.gov/providers-professionals/improving-blood-pressure-control-patients-diabetes-4-community-health

HealthIT.gov. (2014b). *Issues brief: Medication adherence and health IT* (No. CaseStudy2014). Washington, DC: Author. Retrieved from http://www.healthit.gov/sites/default/files/medicationadherence_and_hit_issue_brief.pdf

HealthIT.gov. (2014c). *Patient generated health data.* Retrieved from http://www.healthit.gov/policy-researchers-implementers/patient-generated-health-data

HealthIT.gov. (2014d). *What is a patient portal?* Retrieved from https://www.healthit.gov/providers-professionals/faqs/what-patient-portal

Hibbard, J. H., Stockard, J., Mahoney, E. R., & Tusler, M. (2004). Development of the patient activation measure (PAM): Conceptualizing and measuring activation in patients and consumers. *Health Services Research, 39*(4), 1005–1026.

Hurtado, M. P., Swift, E. K., & Corrigan, J. M. (2001). *Crossing the quality chasm: A new health system for the 21st century* (No. IOM 2001). Washington, DC: Institute of Medicine.

Institute of Medicine. (2000). *To err is human: Building a safer health system* (No. ERR-1999). Washington, DC: Author. Retrieved from http://www.iom.edu/~/media/Files/Report%20Files/1999/To-Err-is-Human/To%20Err%20is%20Human%201999%20%20report%20brief.pdf

Institute of Medicine. (2001). *Crossing the quality chasm: A new health system for the 21st century* (2001). Washington, DC: National Academies Press. Retrieved from http://www.nap.edu/openbook.php?isbn=0309072808

Institute of Medicine. (2012). *Health IT and patient safety: Building safer systems for better care.* Washington, DC: Author.

Institute of Medicine. (2014). *Capturing social and behavioral domains in electronic health records: Phase 1.* Washington, DC: National Academies Press.

Interprofessional Collaborative Expert Panel. (2011). *Core competencies for interprofessional collaborative practice: Report of an expert panel* (No. ICEP-2011). Interprofessional Education Collaborative. Retrieved from www.ipecollaborative.org/uploads/IPEC-Core-Competencies.pdf

James, J. T. (2007). *A sea of broken hearts: Patient rights in a dangerous, profit-driven health care system.* Bloomington, IN: AuthorHouse.

James, J. T. (2013). A new, evidence-based estimate of patient harms associated with hospital care. *Journal of Patient Safety, 9*(3), 122–128. doi:10.1097/PTS.0b013e3182948a69

Ketterer, T., West, D., Sanders, V., Jossain, J., Kondo, M., & Sharif, I. (2013). Correlates of patient portal enrollment and activation in primary care pediatrics. *Academic Pediatrics, 13*(3), 264–271. doi:10.1016/j.acap.2013.02.002

Kruse, R., Koopman, R., Wakefield, B., Wakefield, D., Keplinger, L., Canfield, S., & Mehr, D. (2012). Internet use by primary care patients: Where is the digital divide? *Family Medicine, 44*(5), 342–347.

McCarty, Z. S. (2013). Stage 2 meaningful use: Are you ready? *Optometry Times, 5*(6), 22–23.

McGraw, M. (2012). EHR: Embracing the next phase of meaningful use. *Review of Optometry, 149*(11), 36–39.

Milliard, M. (2014). *Patients want more from their EHRs.* (No. HcITnews2014). Retrieved from http://www.HelathcareITnew.com

National eHealth Collaborative. (2013). *Patient generated health information: Technical expert panel final report December 2013* (No. Grant#7U24AE000006-02). Washington, DC: Author. Retrieved from http://www.himss.files.cms-plus.com/FileDownloads/pghi_tep_finalreport121713_1394215078393_9.pdf

National Learning Consortium. (2013). *Patient portal implementation leads to better messaging, greater efficiency, and improved patient engagement at desert ridge family physicians.* Washington, DC: HealthIT.gov. Retrieved from http://www.healthit.gov/providers-professionals/desert-ridge-family-physicians

National Learning Consortium. (2014). *What is a patient portal?* Retrieved from http://www.healthit.gov/providers-professionals/faqs/what-patient-portal

National Learning Consortium: Advancing America's Health Care. (2013). *Fact sheet: How to optimize patient portals for patient engagement and meet meaningful use requirements* (No. NLC2013). Washington, DC: HealthIT.gov. Retrieved from http://www.healthit.gov/sites/default/files/nlc_how_to_optimizepatientportals_for_patientengagement.pdf

National Partnership for Women and Families. (2014). *Engaging patients and families: How consumers value and use health IT* (No. NPWF2014). Washington, DC: National Partnership.org. Retrieved from http://www.nationalpartnership.org/research-library/health-care/HIT/engaging-patients-and-families.pdf

Nelson, E. C., Batalden, P. B., Godfrey, M. M., & Lazar, J. S. (2011). In Authors (Ed.), *Value by design: Developing clinical microsystems to achieve organizational excellence* (1st ed.). San Francisco, CA: Jossey-Bass.

Netti, J. (2013). *Engaging patients via portals: Major focus of meaningful use in 2014.* Retrieved from http://www.netticonsulting.com/articles/Engaging-Patients-via-Portals-Major-Focus-of-Meaningful-Use-in-2014.pdf

Office of Disease Prevention and Health Promotion. (2010). *National action plan to improve health literacy* (No. USDHHS2010). Washington, DC: U.S. Department of Health and Human Services. Retrieved from http://www.health.gov/communication/hlactionplan

Office of the National Coordinator for Health Information Technology. (2014). *Federal health IT strategic plan 2015–2020: Collect, share, use* (No. ONCplan2014). Washington, DC: U.S. Department of Health and Human Services. Retrieved from http://www.healthit.gov/sites/default/files/federal-healthIT-strategic-plan-2014.pdf

Page, A. (2004). *Keeping patients safe: Transforming the work environment of nurses.* Washington, DC: National Academies Press.

Rein, A. (2012). *Beacon policy brief 1.0: The beacon community program: Three pillars of pursuit* (Report Brief No. BPB-2012). Retrieved from https://www.healthit.gov/sites/default/files/pdf/beacon-brief-061912.pdf

Roberts, D. (2004). Advocacy through patient teaching. *MEDSURG Nursing, 13*(6), 363–382.

Safeer, R. S., & Keenan, J. (2005). Health literacy: The gap between physicians and patients. *American Family Physician, 72*(3), 463–468.

Sanders, M., Winters, P., Fortuna, R., Mendoza, M., Berliant, M., Clark, L., & Fiscella, K. (2013). Internet access and patient portal readiness among patients in a group of inner-city safety-net practices. *Journal of Ambulatory Care Management, 36*(3), 251–259. doi:10.1097/JAC.0b013e3182970219

Sarkar, U., Karter, A. J., Liu, J. Y., Adler, N. E., Nguyen, R., Lopez, A., & Schillinger, D. (2010). The literacy divide: Health literacy and the use of an internet-based patient portal in an integrated health system—results from the diabetes study of Northern California (DISTANCE). *Journal of Health Communication, 15,* 183–196. doi:10.1080/10810730.2010.499988

Sittig, D. F., & Ash, J. S. (2007). *Clinical information systems: Overcoming adverse consequences.* Boston, MA: Jones & Barlett.

Tomsik, E., & Briggs, B. (2013). *Empowering patients through advanced EMR use: The role of patient education and health literacy in patient portals.* Retrieved from http://www.healthmgttech.com/empowering-patients-through-advanced-emr-use.php

Wald, J. (2010). Variations in patient portal adoption in four primary care practices. *American Medical Informatics Association, 13,* 837–841.

Walker, J., Leveille, S. G., Ngo, L., Vodicka, E., Darer, J. D., Dhanireddy, S., . . . Delbanco, T. (2011). Inviting patients to read their doctors' notes: Patients and doctors look ahead. *Annals of Internal Medicine, 155*(12), 811–819.

Winters, C. (2014). *Increasing the use of patient portals in a primary care setting.* (Unpublished doctoral dissertation). Dallas, TX: Texas Woman's University.

Yen, P., & Bakken, S. (2012). Review of health information technology usability study methodologies. *Journal of the American Medical Informatics Association, 19*(3), 413–422. doi:10.1136/amiajnl-2010-000020

Zsolt, N., Aspy, C., Chou, A., & Mold, J. (2012). Impact of a wellness portal on the delivery of patient-centered preventive care. *Journal of the American Board of Family Medicine, 25*(2), 158–167. doi:10.3122/jabfm.2012.02.110130

CHAPTER 16

Telehealth and Mobile Health

Mari Tietze and Georgia Brown

OBJECTIVES

1. Apply the telemedicine approach to patient care assessment in a description of one's own clinical environment.

2. Demonstrate an understanding of the professional licensure requirements applicable to telehealth-based care delivery.

3. Predict the trend in remote patient monitoring/management for patients with heart failure who are at a risk for readmission.

4. Describe the growth of mobile health (mHealth) and list the top two categories for health care providers.

5. Identify a strategy involving mHealth that is applied to existing patient services to enhance care delivery for both supplier and patient.

6. Compare the privacy and security needs in telehealth with traditional health care delivery services.

KEY WORDS

telehealth, telemedicine, telemetry, mobile health, remote patient monitoring, remote patient management, telehome care, teledermatology, telegenomics

---

CONTENTS

INTRODUCTION

Telecommunication technologies are changing ways of thinking, acting, and communicating throughout the world. This involves new, multidisciplinary ways of working and can bring health care directly to patients. It is bringing a new generation of information scientists in touch with the hardware and software technologies they generate. In terms of the financial future of telemedicine, one industry expert predicts that the U.S. telehealth market will grow from $240 million today to $1.9 billion in 2018, an annual compounded growth rate of 56% (Wood, 2013).

Telecommunication reaches out to the previously unreachable rural areas of our country (Darkins & Cary, 2000). Remote care, as pointed out in *The Future of Nursing*, a report by the Institute of Medicine/Robert Wood Johnson Foundation (IOM/RWJF, 2010), predicted that shifts in time and place of care have significant implications for nursing, suggesting that nursing may be delivered remotely similar to electronic health records (EHRs), computer provider order entry (CPOE) systems, lab results, imaging systems, and pharmacies that are linked in the exchange networks (IOM/RWJF, 2010). This chapter focuses on care delivery that is "away" from the patient. This is in contrast to care delivery in the direct vicinity of the patient. It is about the use of telemetry technology that transmits digital components regarding the patient's physical, physiological, and psychological status.

For the purpose of this book, the term "telehealth" is intended to encompass three broad methods of digital care delivery that are "away" from the patient:

1. Telemedicine (stationary scheduled remote diagnostics of health status)
2. Remote management/monitoring/coaching (stationary home or facility based with scheduled and as-needed remote transmission of health status)
3. Mobile health (mHealth) "community" groups/social media (wearable mobile patient-generated health data with scheduled and as-needed remote transmission of health status)

Characteristics that may be typical of these digital methods of care delivery relate to the mode of technology transmission, the type of reporting and the report's recipient, approach to patient engagement, and outcome measures. Some examples, illustrated in Table 16.1, are videoconferencing, sensor-based data collection, manual input-based data collection, health coaching, other significant involvement, cost–benefit analysis, data-collection database, data-collection portal, security, reporting to patient, reporting to provider, reporting to insurer/payer, reporting to community/groups/social media, direct patient engagement/activation, inherent interprofessional collaboration, and inherent reportable outcome measures. Note that mHealth is not marked for HIPAA regulation because some of these apps have been generally available and may be used by consumers to collect their own health data. As such, they would simply be considered consumer-based health data, even if the data are associated with a specific cell phone number (and are not, technically speaking, personally identifiable information; Practice Fusion Blog, 2012).

TABLE 16.1 Characteristic by Telehealth Method			
Characteristic	Telemedicine	Remote Management	mHealth
Video conference	X	X	X
Provider-to-provider consultation	X		
Sensor-based data collection		X	X
Data-collection database		X	X
Data-collection portal/sharing/social media		X	X
Social media applications		X	X
HIPAA privacy and security focused	X	X	
Reporting directly to patient		X	X
Reporting directly to provider	X	X	
Reporting directly to insurer	X	X	
Direct patient engagement/activation		X	X
Inherent interprofessional collaboration		X	
Inherent reportable outcome measures		X	
Commonly reimbursable by insurance	X	X	

HIPAA, Health Insurance Portability and Accountability Act; mHealth, mobile health.

TELEMEDICINE

History, Current Use, and the Future

"Telemedicine," a term coined in the 1970s, which literally means "healing at a distance" (Strehle & Shabde, 2006, p. 956), signifies the use of information and communication technology (ICT) to improve patient outcomes by increasing access to care and medical information. Recognizing that there is no one specific definition of telemedicine—a 2007 study found 104 peer-reviewed definitions of the word (Sood, 2007)—the World Health Organization (WHO, 2010, p. 9) has adopted the following broad description:

> The delivery of health care services, where distance is a critical factor, by all health care professionals using information and communication technologies for the exchange of valid information for diagnosis, treatment and prevention of

disease and injuries, research and evaluation, and for the continuing education of health care providers, all in the interests of advancing the health of individuals and their communities.

The many definitions highlighted in the WHO report indicated that telemedicine is an open and constantly evolving science, as it incorporates new advancements in technology and responds and adapts to the changing health needs and contexts of societies. For the purpose of the WHO report (WHO, 2010), telemedicine and telehealth are synonymous and are interchangeably used. Four elements noted to be germane to telemedicine were the following:

1. Its purpose is to provide clinical support.
2. It is intended to overcome geographical barriers and connects users who are not in the same physical location.
3. It involves the use of various types of ICT.
4. Its goal is to improve health outcomes (WHO, 2010, p. 9).

Exemplars of Use for Health Promotion

Basic Types and Trends

Telemedicine applications can be classified into two basic types, according to the timing of the information transmitted and the interaction between the individuals involved—be it health professional to health professional or health professional to patient (Patterson, 2005). Store-and-forward, or asynchronous telemedicine involves the exchange of prerecorded data between two or more individuals at different times. For example, the patient or referring health professional sends an e-mail description of a medical case to an expert who later sends back an opinion regarding diagnosis and optimal management (Lombardi, 2009). In contrast, real time, or synchronous telemedicine requires the involved individuals to be simultaneously present for immediate exchange of information, as in the case of videoconferencing (Lombardi, 2009). In both synchronous and asynchronous telemedicine, relevant information may be transmitted in a variety of media, such as text, audio, video, or still images. These two basic approaches to telemedicine are applied to a wide array of services in diverse settings, including teledermatology, telepathology, and teleradiology (Currell, 2008; Wootton, Menzies, & Ferguson, 2009).

Telemedicine and Nursing

At times, technologic advances in health care have often outpaced the ability to integrate the technology efficiently, establish best practices for its use, and develop policies to regulate and evaluate its effectiveness. These may be insufficient reasons to put the brakes on innovation, particularly those "disruptive innovations" (Grady, 2014, p. 38). In terms of nursing practice, for example, telemedicine is growing rapidly (Grady, 2014; Trossman, 2014). One common area for telemedicine in nursing is in the tele-ICU (intensive care unit), where nurses can monitor ICU patients in a remotely located hospital (Trossman, 2014). Another is for nurses to reach rural residents to accomplish health assessments in an effort to keep elderly patients in their homes rather than coming to the hospital (Trossman, 2014).

Implementation, Financing, and Sustainability

WHO Report

Health system transformation requires the involvement of all stakeholders. Partnerships usually facilitate change, and the telemedicine sector is no different. Community leaders, health professionals, academic institutions and educators, health administrators, and policy makers represent the best alliance to make necessary changes to reflect and react to societal needs. Figure 16.1 represents this principle (WHO, 2010, p. 23).

Figure 16.1 shows five sectors, namely, health policy, administration, academic institutions, health providers, and community. Via these sectors, development, implementation, evaluation, and sustainability of telemedicine in developing countries were reviewed during a thematic search of the literature. Five key lessons were drawn from this review, and they are in line with the U.S. national health care strategies reflected in the annual reports of the National Prevention Council (2014) and the U.S. Department of Health and Human Services (2014). As such, the five key lessons of the WHO report, which inform social accountability in health practice across the sectors, are provided for consideration in this chapter (WHO, 2010).

> Lesson 1: Collaboration, participation, and capacity building are fundamental to the success and sustainability of telemedicine initiatives. (p. 24)
>
> Lesson 2: Organizations and individuals engaging in telemedicine initiatives in developing countries [and rural areas] need to be aware of the local context in which they work, i.e. available resources, needs, strengths, and weaknesses. (p. 24)

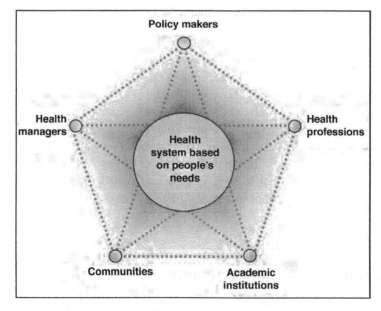

FIGURE 16.1. Social accountability partnership program.
Source: World Health Organization (2010).

Lesson 3: Use simple solutions that appropriately meet the needs of a clinical context or community to optimize cost-effectiveness and minimize complexity in change management. (p. 25)

Lesson 4: Evaluation is vital for scalability, transferability, and continuing quality improvement of telemedicine; it should include documentation, analysis, and dissemination. (p. 24)

Lesson 5: The social benefits of telemedicine contribute to the health of communities and human development, and are important goals unto themselves. (p. 26)

American Medical Association Policy on Telemedicine

Members of the American Medical Association (AMA) believe that the appropriate use of telemedicine to deliver care to patients could greatly improve access and quality of care while maintaining patient safety. During its annual 2014 meeting, the AMA voted to approve a list of guiding principles for ensuring the appropriate coverage of and payment for telemedicine services. The principles aim to help foster innovation in the use of telemedicine, protecting the patient–physician relationship and promoting improved care coordination and communication with medical homes (AMA, 2014, June 11).

The guiding principles stem from a policy developed by the AMA's Council on Medical Service that addresses coverage and payment for telemedicine, which provided a robust background on the delivery of telemedicine. Eight specific statements outline care delivery, collaboration, and payment guidelines (AMA, 2014, June 11).

Regional Telehealth Resource Centers

Telehealth resource centers (TRCs), funded primarily by the federal government and Office of Rural Health Policy, have been established to provide assistance, education, and information to organizations and individuals who are actively providing or interested in providing medical care at a distance. The simple charter from the Office for Advancement of Telehealth is used to assist in expanding the availability of health care to underserved populations, and the assistance we provide is generally free of charge.

Nationally, there are 14 TRCs: 12 regional centers, all with different strengths and regional expertise, and two national centers, which focus on areas of technology assessment and telehealth policy. Twelve of the TRCs have a regional focus, whereas all TRCs participate as a consortium to provide information and assistance to all requests. Contact information related to each TRC is available at the TRCs website at the Office of the National Coordinator (ONC; Office of the National Coordinator for Health Information Technology [ONC-HIT], 2014b). In reviewing the established TRCs, it appears that most geographic areas of the United States are adequately covered.

REMOTE MANAGEMENT

History, Current Use, and the Future

Remote monitoring and management of patients in their homes is another popular telehealth methodology. Remote patient monitoring (RPM) refers to a wide variety of technologies designed to manage and monitor a range of health conditions. Point-of-care monitoring devices, such as weight scales, glucometers, and blood pressure monitors, whether stand-alone or fully integrated within a health data reporting system, provide alerts when health conditions decline. These technologies are particularly useful for the elderly, chronically ill, and people in rural areas who have trouble accessing traditional sites of care (Center for Technology and Aging, 2012c). In addition to improved management of the health conditions, remote management programs have been found to reduce overall cost of care delivery and improve patient safety and quality (Centers for Disease Control and Prevention [CDC], 2014).

Remote monitoring/management methodology is also commonly associated with telephone interaction between health care professionals, such as nurses, and patients and/or family members who are in their homes. For example, a book on telehealth nursing practice indicated that telehealth is:

> Delivery, management, and coordination of care and services that integrate electronic information and telecommunication technologies to increase access, improve outcomes, and contain or reduce costs of health care, an umbrella term used to describe the wide range of services delivered across distances by all health-related disciplines. (Espensen, 2012, p. 5)

Telephone triage is sometimes considered a subcomponent of telehealth (Rutenberg & Greenberg, 2012). Telephone triage is a "process between the nurse and the client that occurs over the telephone and involves identifying the nature and urgency of client health care needs and determining the appropriate disposition" (Rutenberg & Greenberg, 2012, p. 5).

Regardless of the care delivery term used, that is, telehealth or telephone triage, RPM/management involves some kind of telephone interaction. In terms of oversight for professional practice of this mode of health care delivery, professional standards and credentialing have been developed in disciplines such as nursing. Professional organizations, such as the American Academy of Ambulatory Care Nursing (AAACN), for example, developed standards, continuous education programs, and a special interest group (SIG) specific to the practice of telehealth nursing (Rutenberg & Greenberg, 2012). In fact, in 2007, the AAACN adopted the position that telehealth nursing, instead of being a practice that is separate and apart, is an integral element of ambulatory care nursing. Because the AAACN recognized that to be effective in practice, nurses must have a broad base of knowledge in ambulatory care, the AAACN worked with the American Nurses Association (ANA) to represent telehealth/telephone triage content in the Ambulatory Care Nurses Certification Exam (AAACN Board of Directors, 2007). Subsequently, the ANA's Ambulatory Care Nurses Certification Exam is considered the professional certification for telehealth nursing (AAACN Board of Directors, 2007).

Exemplars of Use for Health Promotion

As noted, care of the patient outside of the acute care setting has historically been represented by the home health care industry. With the spread of telemetry technology, home health care has evolved to a new industry of RPM and management. The organizations comprising this new industry are quite varied in their capabilities, services offered, size, and outcomes. The care standards that regulate and oversee the remote monitoring industry have been borrowed from the home health care industry.

Beginning in January 2010, home health agencies have been required to collect a revised version of the OASIS (Outcome and Assessment Information Set) data set (OASIS-C). OASIS-C includes data items supporting measurement of rates for use of specific evidence-based care processes. From a national policy perspective, the Centers for Medicare & Medicaid Services (CMS) anticipate that these process measures will promote the use of best practices across the home health industry (CMS, 2014).

According to the AAACN in their 2007 guidelines document, the components of decision support tools should define the ongoing care management of a broad problem or issue in six areas:

1. Assessment/data collection/caller interview process
2. Classification/determination of acuity
3. Nature/type/degree of advice/intervention/direction to the caller
4. Information/education of caller
5. Validation of patient understanding/verbal contracting
6. Evaluation/follow-up/effectiveness of advice or intervention (Espensen, 2012, p. 99)

These six areas encompass the nursing process that is essential to telehealth nursing practice. If any of these components are missing from the decision support tools, the nursing process is incomplete, thereby possibly allowing a potential gap in the quality of care. Many decision support tools do not include the steps to validate the patient's understanding or to evaluate the follow-up/effectiveness of advice or intervention given. Validation is an important part of the nursing process and should be part of the telehealth encounter. No matter how decision support tools are defined, they serve as an essential tool in telehealth nursing practice. Well-written guidelines provide standardization, decision support, legal protection, and documentation ease to the nurse (Espensen, 2012).

Commonly, the use of technology for database creation and support has been limited except for the reporting of the OASIS-C data requirements. One exception to this pattern is CareCycle Management (CCM; see www.carecycle.com). CCM uses a full EHR system, a clinical decision support system (CDSS), a clinical predictive analytics tool, and its own warehouse of patient, operational, and financial data. As such, CCM has an optimal understanding of patients in their care and associated trends. The organization boasts of a 6.7% all-cause readmission rate (64% lower than national averages) and reflects a readmission rate that continues to decrease over time.

How does CCM maintain a lower-than-industry standard for all-cause postacute readmission rate? Their model of care delivery is likely a factor. It involves evidence-based protocols, high telecommunication skills of practitioners, high family engagement levels, consistent attention to medications, and targeted home health visits that are specific to actual or predicted negative outcomes. Minimum data collection from the patient's home involves weight, blood pressure, pulse, temperature, blood glucose (if appropriate), and oxygen saturation percentage. CareCycle Navigator® is the decision support engine that gathers hundreds of more patient parameters to guide the case manager toward

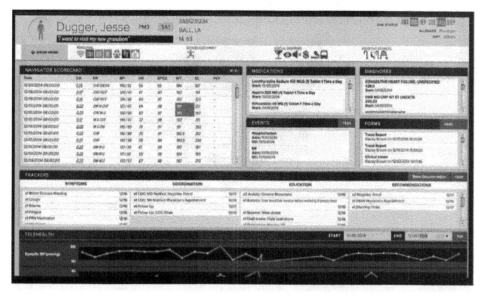

FIGURE 16.2. CareCycle management's Navigator® tool.
Source: CareCycle.com (2015).

the ideal evidence-based practice, real-time decision making. The CareCycle Navigator®, illustrated in Figure 16.2, provides user-friendly, color-coded clinical and psychosocial information in a logical workflow pattern with readily available drill downs to detail desired by the case manager. This level of data sophistication yields clinical actions at the prevention stage rather than the intervention stage of care delivery, an ideal approach for readmission reduction and health care improvement.

Implementation, Financing, and Sustainability

Professional Licensure

In examining the practice of telephone triage from a regulatory perspective, a key consideration is licensure and regulation of interstate practice. Because the practice of telephone triage transcends the geographic boundaries associated with face-to-face nursing care, jurisdictional questions have surfaced about the locus of responsibility in telephone triage and other forms of telehealth nursing. In other words, if a nurse, or other health care professional, is providing care over the telephone to a patient in another state, where is that care delivery taking place? Is the professional practicing in the state in which the patient is located at the time of the interaction or in the state in which the professional is located when the encounter takes place (Rutenberg & Greenberg, 2012, p. 82)?

Most states have taken the position that the locus of responsibility rests with the state in which the patient is physically located during his or her interaction with the nurse, rather than the site at which the nurse is located while providing care to the patient. This issue and the need for consistency, and application of the law, led to the development in 1998 of the Nurse Licensure Compact (NLC; National State Boards of Nursing, 2014). Figure 16.3 indicates states that are a part of the NLC.

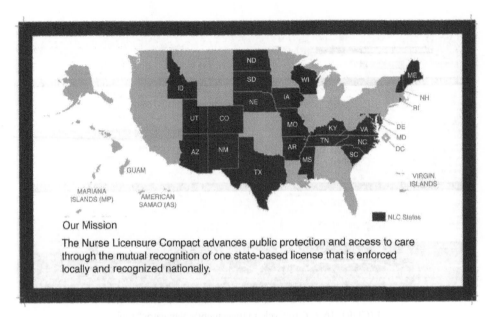

FIGURE 16.3. NLC states.

Source: National State Boards of Nursing (2014).

Financing and Sustainability

Revenues for RPM solutions reached $5.8 billion in 2013, including revenues from medical monitoring devices, mHealth connectivity solutions, care delivery software platforms, and monitoring services, according to a report from information technology (IT) research firm Berg Insight (Eddy, 2014). In terms of the scope of RPM, the report found that around 3 million patients worldwide were using connected home medical monitoring in 2013. Much of the funding rationale for such programs is the associated decrease in acute, ambulatory, urgent, and emergency care needed for these patients.

Patients with heart failure are of particular interest for management by remote monitoring not only because of the high rate of readmission to acute care hospitals but also because of the CMS adjustment in reimbursement for hospitalizations that results within 30 days of a previous hospitalization (Berwick & Hackbarth, 2012; Davis, Schoen, & Guterman, 2013; Schoen et al., 2007). Numerous studies have indicated that these readmissions can be avoided with added postacute care remote management (CDC, 2014. Center for Technology and Aging, 2012b); Subsequently, financing and sustainability of such programs has been associated with a sound return on investment (ROI) approach.

Understanding the basics of ROI is fundamental to success for most technology projects. As such, Appendix 16.1 includes content from an ROI primer focused on the RPM market (Center for Technology and Aging, 2012a). As illustrated, details, such as benefits, costs, labor, technology, volume of patients, and regional economic characteristics, must be considered. In the final equation, benefits divided by costs provide per patient/per year (PPPY) net savings and the associated proportion of the ROI.

One of the many ROI approaches used for remote monitoring of patients with heart failure is provided by the Center for Technology and Aging. The study compared outcomes for two groups of patients: one receiving remote monitoring services (intervention group) and one that was not receiving such services (control group). Statistically significant study results indicated the following:

▶ A decline in all-cause hospitalizations among intervention group patients was observed after the use of home telehealth technology (a mean of 1.5 hospitalizations per patient was observed in the 12-month period before the intervention versus a mean of 0.9 hospitalizations per patient during the intervention period).

▶ The number of ED visits declined for both groups during the study period, but the decline in ED visits was greater in the intervention group.

▶ Among intervention group patients, declines in the number of urgent care visits, cardiology visits, and home health visits were also observed in the pre- and post-intervention periods (Center for Technology and Aging, 2012b).

Final results of this study indicated that the total cost to plan and implement this project (more than 2 years) was approximately $575,000 and that ROI for patient experience and cost savings was warranted. Given the importance of ROI approaches, the Center for Technology and Aging has provided a publicly available toolkit for setting up, implementing, and calculating ROI for technology-focused improvement studies (Center for Technology and Aging, 2015). Figure 16.4 lists the eight critical "workstreams" provided by the toolkit, including the ROI calculator via the financial management workstream.

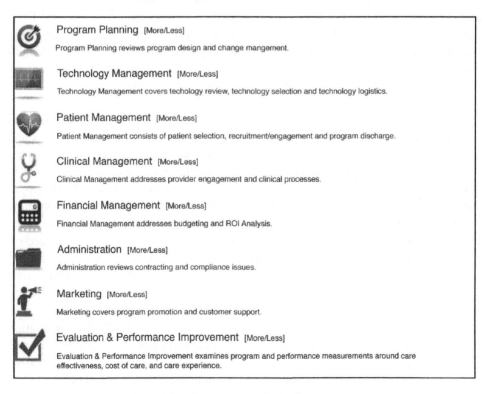

FIGURE 16.4. RPM toolkit workstreams.
Source: Center for Technology and Aging (2015).

MOBILE HEALTH

History, Current Use, and the Future

In addition to being the most common way to communicate health data, mHealth technology is also the most promising way to engage patients in their health care. mHealth is defined as generation, aggregation, and dissemination of health information via mobile and wireless devices (Healthcare Information and Management Systems Society, 2014, p. 1).

In 2012, a Mobile Devices Roundtable of industry experts and consumers was convened by the Department of Health and Human Services (Pritts, 2012). The meeting confirmed that mobile technology is a great equalizer in the delivery of health care, although there are still privacy and security concerns regarding its use. Privacy and security challenges associated with accessing, storing, and/or transmitting health information were also discussed. Specific topics in the roundtable discussion included the following:

▶ Bringing your own device (BYOD)

▶ Texting patient-specific information

▶ Sending images

▶ Security training of personnel

▶ Using mobile applications

During the Mobile Devices Roundtable, government officials across various federal agencies, including the Federal Communications Commission, the Food and Drug Administration, the Federal Trade Commission, the National Institute of Standards and Technology, and the Office of Civil Rights (OCR) explored their agency's role in mHealth and how that role intersects with protecting and safeguarding health information in the context of mobile devices and health care delivery (Pritts, 2012). The potential roles are illustrated in Figure 16.5.

Top mHealth publishers manage to generate more than 3 million free and 300,000 paid downloads in the United States on the iOS platform. The reach on other platforms and in other countries not only differs a great deal but also shows the increase of business potential for mHealth apps. Not only are consumers taking advantage of smartphones to manage and improve their own health, but a significant number (15%) of mHealth applications are also primarily designed for health care professionals. These include continuing medical education (CME), remote monitoring, and health care management applications. Figure 16.6 illustrates the distribution of mHealth app categories with fitness, medical references, and wellness being the largest three categories (research2guidance, 2014).

As for the future of mHealth, the mHealth market is expected to reach $26 billion by 2017 (Informa Exhibitions, 2013). Currently, there are 97,000 mHealth applications in major app stores: Only 9% of the total market revenue in the next 5 years will come from application download revenue, whereas 84% of the total mHealth application market revenue will come from related services and products such as sensors (Informa Exhibitions, 2013).

The Internet of Things (IoT) is one of the most important technological developments of this generation and a natural step in the evolution of mobile-connected solutions. Today, there are roughly two Internet-connected devices for every man, woman, and

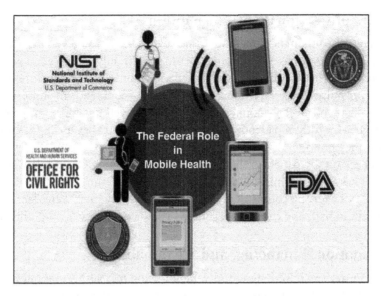

FIGURE 16.5. Federal role in mHealth.
Source: Pritts (2012).

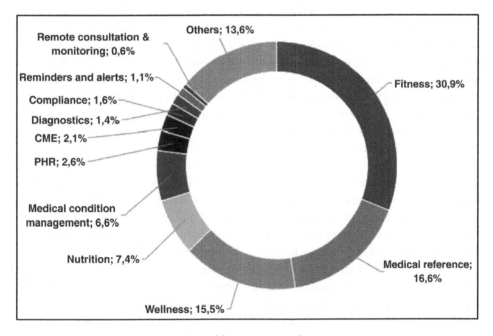

FIGURE 16.6. mHealth app category share percentages.
CME, continuing medical education; PHR, personal health record.
Source: research2guidance (2014).

child on the planet. By 2025, analysts are forecasting that this ratio will rise past six. This means we can expect to grow nearly 50 billion Internet-connected devices in the next decade (Savitz & Humphreys, 2012). This will also be the trend in health care, so management for patients is key to success.

Exemplars of Use for Health Promotion

In health care, mHealth in the form of wearable devices has been known to reduce mortality rates by 35% in some cases (Sullivan, 2014). Most currently, patients can wear a monitor on their wrists that continually tracks their vital signs—blood pressure, respiratory rate, pulse rate, pulse oximetry, and body temperature—and sends the information to an EHR. The stats then travel to monitors that calculate a wellness index measured from a 0 to 5 scale. In one study, if patients' vitals rank from 0 to 2.9, they are in the clear "green" zone, but if they jump to 3.0 or above, a dangerous "red" zone, nurses on the unit are alerted to check on the patients. The tool helps combine information into a single value and makes it easy for the clinician to react accordingly (Sullivan, 2014, p. 1). While using this type of tool over the course of several years, mortality rates were decreased, code blues were cut in half, and the average length of stay was cut by 5.3% (Sullivan, 2014).

Implementation, Financing, and Sustainability

Health care providers have long found value in using mHealth to monitor patients at home 90 days after a hospital visit. But what happens after the reimbursements are gone and the hospital takes back its technology? Examples of creative strategies and new partnerships seek to keep that mHealth link going, and these are using the mobile personal emergency response services (mPERS) market as an entry point (Wicklund, 2015).

Specifically, Honeywell Life Care Solutions is joining forces with medical alert technology vendor MobileHelp to offer a consumer-facing platform that would allow patients to monitor their vital signs and share them with providers. Honeywell Life Care sees the mPERS field as an ideal entry point for providers who want to maintain a connection to patients beyond the reimbursable 30- to 90-day time period. Likewise, officials said many patients are reluctant to give up their home monitoring devices when the hospital asks for them back (Wicklund, 2015).

The partnership hits on an important strategy: For mHealth to succeed in the consumer market, it needs to attach itself to something that is already in place and a part of the consumer's lifestyle. Honeywell executives note that they are entering the home through mPERS solutions that are already established and are giving added value to the systems in place. This type of strategy benefits both supplier and consumer/patient. This plan shifts the cost to the consumer, and it may prove to be a key test in the willingness of the consumer market to pay for health monitoring services (Wicklund, 2015).

Given the fast paced growth of mHealth, knowledge and business focus are needed to manage the associated financial reimbursement. For the purposes of sustainability, one significant aspect of reimbursement is from the CMS. In fact, CMS touts that the trend to use accountable care organizations (ACOs) as the financial care delivery approach has actually slowed the growth in Medicare spending (Cavanaugh, 2014).

Federal health officials in December 2014 said that 89 new ACOs have joined the Medicare Shared Savings Program, bringing the total to 424 provider groups that now serve more than 7.8 million seniors. So far, ACOs have generated more than $417 million in savings, improving care in 30 out of 33 quality measures (Cavanaugh, 2014). Overall, Medicare spending per beneficiary has remained flat since 2010, growing at about 2% points lower than the gross domestic product (GDP) each year. "ACOs have driven progress in the way care is provided by improving the coordination and integration of healthcare, and improving the health of patients with a priority on prevention and wellness" (Cavanaugh, 2014, p. 1).

POLICIES, REGULATIONS, AND SECURITY

Medical Liability Coverage

A part of medical liability for telehealth is the equipment contractual agreement. One checklist to be considered for such an agreement includes three basic categories: equipment hardware, equipment–user–transmission interface, and backup systems (Darkins & Cary, 2000). The outline of such an agreement, at minimum, might include the following minimum criteria in contracting for telehealth:

1. Exact clinical and technical specifications
2. Financial viability linked to clear payment mechanisms
3. Clarification on competitive pricing arrangements and contract duration
4. Explicit outline and how to deliver the clinical service efficiently and effectively
5. Capacity to deliver remote consultations to specifications
6. Adequate premises and clinic space
7. Prearranged interface with other health care providers and billing arrangements
8. Regulatory requirements outlined and met
9. Clinical and financial risk management systems described
10. Quality standards agreed on and arrangements to monitor them outlined
11. Clear legal associations and indemnity arrangements
12. Contract monitoring and information requirements formalized
13. Emergency arrangements in place for the unexpected or disaster situations
14. Payment and conciliation processes in case of disagreements (Darkins & Cary, 2000, p. 195)

Health Information Portability and Accountability Act Compliance

The Health Information Portability and Accountability Act (HIPAA) includes provisions that address the security of health care information and protection of patient privacy. Patient confidentiality and HIPAA requirements apply to telehealth nursing. Privacy policies and informed patient consent remain the same for telehealth encounters as for in-person care (Rutenberg & Greenberg, 2012).

At one time, almost all of the data collected by the medical system was collected inside hospitals and clinics. This began to change with the introduction of devices, such as defibrillators and continuous positive airway pressure machines, that contain computers that collect telemetry about patients outside the provider facility. This telemetry is increasingly communicated by digital wireless links. Simultaneously, there has been an explosion of interest in wireless fitness devices that collect information, such as the number of calories used or the locations visited (by runners, for instance), on monitored subjects. Currently, the fitness systems commonly use communications with cell phones. The boundary between medical devices, such as defibrillators, and fitness devices, such as pedometers, has begun to blur with, for example, the introduction of devices that measure vitals such as blood pressure and pulse. Many of these trends raise concerns about security and privacy with respect to these devices (ONC-HIT, 2014a).

At the time that Strategic Health IT Advanced Research Projects (SHARPS) began, some members of the SHARPS team had shown security vulnerabilities of wireless communications with defibrillators. The SHARPS enabled a wide range of progress beyond the demonstration of these threats in terms of both the depth of analysis, such as the development of effective countermeasures and new platforms, and the breadth of analysis, such as studies for fitness devices, insulin pumps, and biosensors. The SHARPS are forging new areas in which the privacy and security of patient mobile data is safe (ONC-HIT, 2014a).

SUMMARY

Telehealth and mHealth represent fast growing areas of health care delivery that hold promise for basic care delivery, especially for those with limited access to care such as the underserved and those in rural areas. In the Nursing Education for Healthcare Informatics (NEHI) model, initially described in Chapter 1, telehealth and mHealth are aligned with the point-of-care technology concept. In addition, as per the NEHI model, the understanding of data analytics is imperative to success. This important understanding was reflected in the ROI for telehealth projects described in this chapter. Finally, patient safety and quality improvement with telehealth use has been demonstrated by the additional contact and monitoring of patients, yielding less untoward consequences (McBride, Tietze, & Fenton, 2013).

EXERCISES AND QUESTIONS FOR CONSIDERATION

Consider content covered with respect to ROI for telehealth projects in Appendix 16.1. Respond to the following questions:

1. What is the per patient per year (PPPY) benefit of the system?
2. What is the PPPY cost of the system?
3. What is the ROI percentage?
4. Create a telehealth project of your own and determine the associated ROI.

CASE STUDY

Consider the following case study.

Aims and Objectives: To evaluate the outcome of a grant opportunity for telehealth projects

Background: More than 30 telehealth projects in locations from West Virginia to Guam are receiving funding through the U.S. Department of Agriculture's Distance

(continued)

CASE STUDY (*continued*)

Learning and Telemedicine (DLT) program. Of the 65 grants awarded across 34 states, totaling more than $20 million, 31 grants valued at $8.6 million were telehealth related, with the rest going to educational services. An example of a typical grant is an almost $500,000 award that will enable the university to equip telemedicine carts with videoconferencing and cloud-based image sharing in more than 70 rural health care facilities in 46 counties (Wicklund, 2014).

Please respond to the following questions:

1. How would you use the $500,000 to enhance access to rural areas using telehealth?
2. What specific steps would you take to ensure success of the project?

REFERENCES

AAACN Board of Directors. (2007). *American Academy of Ambulatory Care Nursing (AAACN) holds telehealth visioning meeting: August 4, 2007* (No. AAACN2007). Pitman, NJ: American Academy of Ambulatory Care Nursing. Retrieved from http://www.aaacn.org/sites/default/files/documents/telehealth-mtg-summary.pdf

American Medical Association. (2014). *AMA adopts telemedicine policy to improve access to care for patients.* Retrieved from http://www.ama-assn.org/ama/pub/news/news/2014/2014-06-11-policy-coverage-reimbursement-for-telemedicine.page

Berwick, D. M., & Hackbarth, A. D. (2012). Eliminating waste in US health care. *Journal of the American Medical Association, 307*(14), 1513–1516. doi:10.1001/jama.2012.362

CareCycle.com. (2015). *Navigator®*. Dallas, TX: CareCycle Management. Retrieved from http://carecycle.com/navigator-video-form-page/

Cavanaugh, S. (2014). *ACOs moving ahead.* (No. CMSaco2014). Washington, DC: Centers for Medicare & Medicaid Services. Retrieved from http://www.blog.cms.gov/2014/12/22/acos-moving-ahead

Center for Technology and Aging. (2012a). *Determining the ROI from remote patient monitoring: A primer.* (No. CTArpmROI2012). Oakland, CA: Author. Retrieved from http://www.techandaging.org/ROI_Brief.pdf

Center for Technology and Aging. (2012b). *Management of heart failure patients using home telehealth: New England Healthcare Institute and Atrius Health.* (No. CTAhf2012). Oakland, CA: Author. Retrieved from http://www.techandaging.org/grants_NEHI.html

Center for Technology and Aging. (2012c). *Remote patient monitoring program.* Retrieved from http://www.techandaging.org/rpm_program_page.html

Center for Technology and Aging. (2015). *Remote patient monitoring toolkit.* Retrieved from www.toolkit.techandaging.org/toolkit/rpmtest

Centers for Disease Control and Prevention. (2014). *Chronic disease prevention and health promotion: Statistics and tracking.* Retrieved from http://www.cdc.gov/chronicdisease/stats/index.htm

Centers for Medicare & Medicaid Services. (2014). *Home health quality initiative.* Retrieved from https://www.cms.gov/Medicare/Quality-Initiatives-Patient-Assessment-Instruments/HomeHealthQualityInits/index.html?redirect=/homehealthqualityinits/

Currell, R. (2008). Telemedicine versus face-to-face patient care: Effects on professional practice and health care outcomes (No. CD002008, Issue 2). *Cochrane Database of Systematic Reviews*.

Darkins, A. W., & Cary, M. A. (2000). *Telemedicine and telehealth: Principles, policies, performance, and pitfalls*. New York, NY: Springer Publishing Company.

Davis, K., Schoen, C., & Guterman, S. (2013). Medicare essential: An option to promote better care and curb spending growth. *Health Affairs (Project Hope)* 32(5), 900–909. doi:10.1377/hlthaff.2012.1203

Eddy, N. (2014, July 1). Remote patient monitoring market to top $26 billion by 2018. *eWeek*, p. 1-1. Retrieved from http://www.eweek.com/it-management/remote-patient-monitoring-market-to-top-26-billion-by-2018.html#sthash.IRVHgAhE.dpuf

Espensen, M. (2012). *Telehealth nursing practice essentials*. Pitman, NJ: American Academy of Ambulatory Care Nursing.

Grady, J. (2014). Telehealth: A case study in disruptive innovation. *American Journal of Nursing, 114*(4), 38–45.

Healthcare Information and Management Systems Society. (2014). *mHealth*. Retrieved from http://www.himss.org/library/mhealth

Informa Exhibitions, L. (2013, March 8). The market for mHealth app services will reach $26 billion by 2017. *Mobile Health Today*, 1-1. Retrieved from www.mobilehealthcaretoday.com

Institute of Medicine/Robert Wood Johnson Foundation. (2010). *The future of nursing: Leading change, advancing health* (No. TFON2010). Washington, DC: National Academies Press. Retrieved from http://www.iom.edu/Reports/2010/The-Future-of-Nursing-Leading-Change-Advancing-Health.aspx

Lombardi, R. B. (2009). Telemedicine: Current status in developed and developing countries. *Journal of Drugs in Dermatology, 8*(4), 371–375.

McBride, S. G., Tietze, M., & Fenton, M. V. (2013). Developing an applied informatics course for a doctor of nursing practice program. *Nurse Educator, 38*(1), 37–42. doi:10.1097/NNE.0b013e318276df5d

National Prevention Council. (2014). *National Prevention Council: Annual report*. (No. NPC2014). Washington, DC: U.S. Department of Health and Human Services, Office of the Surgeon General. Retrieved from http://www.surgeongeneral.gov/initiatives/prevention/about/annual_status_reports.html

National State Boards of Nursing. (2014). *Nursing licensure compact information*. Retrieved from http://www.bon.state.tx.us/licensure_nurse_licensure_compact.asp

Office of the National Coordinator for Health Information Technology. (2014a). *Strategic health IT advanced research projects on security (SHARPS): Telemedicine cluster projects*. Retrieved from http://www.sharps.org/clusters/telemedicine-cluster

Office of the National Coordinator for Health Information Technology. (2014b). *Welcome to consortium of telehealth resource centers websites*. Retrieved from http://www.telehealthresourcecenter.org/overview/welcome-consortium-of-telehealth-resource-centers-website

Patterson, C. J. (2005). Introduction to the practice of telemedicine. *Journal of Telemedicine and Telecare, 11*(1), 3–9.

Practice Fusion Blog. (2012, February 7). *mHealth challenges around privacy and HIPAA*. Retrieved from http://www.practicefusion.com/blog/mhealth-challenges-around-privacy-and-hipaa/

Pritts, J. (2012). *HHS Mobile Devices Roundtable: Health care delivery experts discuss clinicians' use of and privacy & security good practices for mHealth* (No. mHrtbl2012). Washington, DC: U.S. Department of Health and Human Services. Retrieved from www.healthit.gov/buzz-blog/privacy-and-security-of-ehrs/mobile-devices-roundtable research2guidance. (2014). *mHealth app developer economics 2014: The state of the art of mobile health app publishing* (No. mH2014). Berlin, Germany: Author. Retrieved from http://www.research 2guidance.com/r2g/mHealth-App-Developer-Economics-2014.pdf

Rutenberg, C., & Greenberg, E. (2012). *The art and science of telephone triage: How to practice nursing over the phone*. Pitman, NJ: Anthony J. Jannetti.

Savitz, E., & Humphreys, J. (2012). How the Internet of things will change almost everything. *Forbes*. Retrieved from http://www.forbes.com/sites/ciocentral/2012/12/17/how-the-internet-of-things-will-change-almost-everything

Schoen, C., Guterman, S., Shih, A., Lau, J., Kasimow, S., Gauthier, A., & Davis, K. (2007). *Bending the curve: Options for achieving savings and improving value in U.S. health spending* (No. CWF2007). Washington, DC: Commonwealth Fund. Retrieved from http://www.commonwealthfund.org/publi cations/fund-reports/2007/dec/bending-the-curve-options-for-achieving-savings-and-improving-value-in-u-s-health-spending

Sood, S. P. (2007). Differences in public and private sector adoption of telemedicine: Indian case study for sectoral adoption. *Studies in Health Technology and Informatics, 130*, 257–268.

Strehle, E. M., & Shabde, N. (2006). One hundred years of telemedicine: Does this new technology have a place in paediatrics? *Archives of Disease in Childhood, 91*(12), 956–959.

Sullivan, K. (2014, October 21). Patient early warning detection system reduces mortality rates by 35 percent. *FierceHealthcare* p. 1-1. Retrieved from http://www.fiercehealthcare.com/story/patient-early-warning-detection-system-reduces-mortality-rates-35-percent/2014-10-21

Trossman, S. (2014). Back to the future? Telehealth services, tele-nursing are on the rise. *American Nurse, 46*(5), 1–6.

U.S. Department of Health and Human Services. (2014). *2014 Annual report to Congress: National strategy for quality improvement in health care* (No. AHRQ-2014). Washington, DC: Agency for Healthcare Research and Quality.

Wicklund, E. (2014, November 24). USDA awards $8 million in telehealth grants. *mhealthNews*. Retrieved from http://www.mhealthnews.com/news/usda-awards-8-million-telehealth-grants

Wicklund, E. (2015, January 12). Can mPERS bridge the gap between docs and home-based telehealth? *mhealthNews*. Retrieved from http://www.mhealthnews.com/news/can-mpers-bridge-gap-between-docs-and-home-based-telehealth?page=1

Wood, L. (2013, December 16). Research and markets: Global telemedicine market, which stood at US$ 14.2 billion in 2012, is expected to grow at a CAGR of 18.5% during 2012–2018. *Business Wire*.

Wootton, R., Menzies, J., & Ferguson, P. (2009). Follow-up data for patients managed by store and forward telemedicine in developing countries. *Journal of Telemedicine and Telecare, 15*(2), 83–88.

World Health Organization. (2010). *Telemedicine: Opportunities and developments in member states: Report on the second global survey on eHealth 2009: Global observatory for eHealth series, 2* (No. ISSN2220-5462). Geneva, Switzerland: WHO Press. Retrieved from http://www.who.int/goe/publica tions/goe_telemedicine_2010.pdf

APPENDIX 16.1 SAMPLE ROI FOR RPM

Center for Technology and Aging

What is the ROI?

For the purposes of this example, the gross benefit of the intervention is $4,000 per patient per year. The gross cost is $1,440. This would imply an ROI of 278%, meaning $2.78 would be returned for every dollar invested in the program. Seeing that the program would still produce a positive ROI even if the gross cost reduction were only half that of the 20% used in the analysis—or an ROI of 139%—the organization decides to implement a telehealth-based care-management program.

ROI Model Example	
Benefits of RPM program	
Average PPPY health care costs	$20,000
Estimated gross savings percentage	20%
Estimated PPPY gross savings	$4,000
Costs of RPM program	
Average labor cost PPPY	$600
Average technology cost PPPY	$600
Amortized implementation costs and other operating costs	$240
Total cost PPPY	$1,440
PPPY net savings	$2,560
ROI	278%

PPPY, per patient per year; ROI, return on investment; RPM, remote patient monitoring.
Source: www.techandaging.org/ROI_Brief.pdf

SECTION III

Data Management and
Analytics to Lay the Foundation
for Quality Improvement
(NEHI Model Component #2)

CHAPTER 17

Strategic Thinking in Design and Deployment of Enterprise Data, Reporting, and Analytics

Trish Smith and Susan McBride

OBJECTIVES

1. Discuss the importance of aligning data management, reporting, and analytics strategies with the enterprise strategic goals and objectives within a health care delivery organization (HDO).

2. Discuss a proposed framework for building an Enterprise Data Management, Reporting, and Analytics Program (E-DRAP) for creating a "single source of truth"—rather than disparate, siloed systems—for enhanced data, reporting, and analytic solutions regardless of the HDO's size, complexity, or budget constraints.

3. Define essential technology infrastructure required—including enterprise data warehouse and business intelligence tools—for integrating clinical, financial, operational, as well as research, and third-party databases.

4. Describe key people and organizational structures required for a successful program, including senior leadership sponsorship, information governance, business-led user requirements program, and data-driven culture.

5. Learn about processes that are essential for effectively building and deploying such a program within an HDO.

KEY WORDS

enterprise data warehouse, business intelligence, strategic plan, data models, program management, information governance, BI Competency Center, Agile, voice of customer, use-based data quality, business requirements, wireframes, prototyping, key performance indicators, standard reporting, ad-hoc reporting, scorecards, dashboards, data definitions, data dictionary, Master Data Management

CONTENTS

INTRODUCTION

The purpose of this chapter is to provide the advanced practice nurse and interprofessional teams with a practical, modular framework to engage their organization in developing trusted and meaningful data, reporting, and analytics to support their organization's enterprise strategic plan. The proposed framework is known as the Enterprise Data Management, Reporting, and Analytics Program and it is designed to integrate clinical, financial, operational, and one or more third-party data sources for robust reporting, analytics, and research. The framework is modular, scalable, and adaptable to meet the needs of the HDO regardless of its size, budget, organizational complexity, and/or level of maturity in developing stand-alone data marts, as well as more complex enterprise data warehouse (EDW) and business intelligence (BI) technology platforms.

Throughout this chapter, the phrase "reporting and analytics" is used to represent any type of report or analytics solution, including standard reports, ad-hoc reports, dashboards, scorecards, stand-alone analytic applications, or any other form of BI vendor tool, except where otherwise referenced by the authors.

BUSINESS NEED

Health care is not the only industry that is focused on use of data and analytics. In fact, a recent business report by the Massachusetts Institute of Technology (MIT) Center for Digital Business indicates that companies at large are making data and analytics a source of "competitive differentiation." It further indicates that those companies leading the "analytics revolution" are outperforming their competitors with respect to profitability by 26% and overall industry performance by as much as 9% compared with their industry peers (Kiron, Ferguson, & Prentice, 2013).

Capgemini and MIT Center for Digital Business categorize segmented surveyed organizations into three groups with respect to data and analytic use, including analytic innovators, analytic practitioners, and analytic challenged. Among the survey participants, only 11% were categorized as analytical innovators, defined by data and analytics and considered a core asset that permeates the organizational culture. Analytic practitioners predominately utilize data and analytics to address tactical and operational issues, whereas those organizations that are analytically challenged struggle to use data beyond their basic reporting applications (Kiron et al., 2013).

Many HDOs are likely to fall into the analytically challenged or analytic practitioner categories given the long, fragmented evolution of health care information technology (HIT) systems, starting with introduction of financial billing systems in the 1960s. Since mid-2000, a regulatory stimulus from the Health Information Technology for Economic and Clinical Health (HITECH) Act in 2009 and the Affordable Care Act (ACA) in 2010 has accelerated the national proliferation of electronic health record (EHR) data (as previously discussed in Chapter 4 of this book). Today, HDOs are flush with data from disparate transactional data sources (financial, EHR, operational). However, they are struggling to extract and use their data effectively for clinical operations improvement, cost-efficient care, and clinical research. Major challenges include system interoperability, disparate source with no data standards, inconsistent data definitions and terminology nomenclature, as well as rudimentary and multiple stand-alone analytic reporting and analytic capabilities that are incapable of meeting the ultimate, three broad aims of the National Quality Strategy (NQS)—better care, healthy people and communities, and affordable care.

To meet these national NQS goals and to competitively survive in the new health care payer market, HDOs must now make integrated data and analytics a core asset to meet the challenges of accelerating payment reform. HDOs compete based on how well they manage and use analytics within their organizations to achieve their strategic plan goals, including quality and efficient care, population health improvement, and often their research and education efforts.

The remainder of this chapter presents the proposed E-DRAP framework for creating technical, organizational, and process structures to achieve the HDO's strategic planning goals and position them as analytical innovators. Of utmost importance when embarking on this imperative journey, HDOs must always align with their strategic plan goals and address key questions in designing their reporting and analytics program, such as the following:

1. What is the intent or objective of the reporting and analytics program?
2. Why do you need it?
3. What is it you intend to do with the data and analytics?
4. Who will access the data and analytics?
5. What are the prioritized needs of both the organization and the key individuals?

FRAMEWORK: E-DRAP

This section describes the E-DRAP framework (Figure 17.1) developed by the authors working with other national organizations. This framework provides the foundation for organizations to become analytical innovators and to strengthen their analytic competitive position within their respective marketplace(s). As previously mentioned, the framework is modular, scalable, and adaptable to meet the needs of HDOs, regardless of their size, budget, organizational complexity, and/or level of maturity with regard to reporting and analytics.

The E-DRAP is designed to assist organizations in successfully operationalizing their reporting and analytics program by more tightly integrating the people, processes, and technologies associated with the effort. The remainder of this section describes the key considerations within the people, processes, and technology categories of the framework.

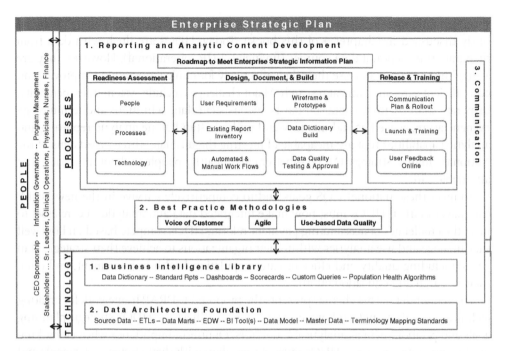

FIGURE 17.1. Framework: Enterprise Data Management, Reporting, and Analytics Program (E-DRAP).

Note: This figure identifies key components to consider in designing and building effective reporting and analytics to meet the organization's enterprise strategic goals and objectives. The framework is modular, scalable, and adaptable to meet the needs of health care delivery organizations, regardless of their size, budget, organizational complexity, and/or level of maturity with reporting and analytics.

Technology

The purpose of this section is to (a) identify key data architecture foundational components that are essential to launch and/or accelerate an HDO's reporting and analytics journey, (b) discuss importance of and options for sharing developed BI content within online BI libraries with end users, and (c) review alternatives for evaluating and selecting the optimum technology(s) among the myriad vendor options presented to HDOs.

Data Architecture Foundation

Depending on where the organization begins, HDOs should identify and understand the key technology components to be considered when developing their reporting and analytics program. The data architecture foundation must be designed and implemented to ensure effective integration of disparate data sources (clinical, financial, operational, research, third-party databases) using common data standards, definitions, and terminology, supported by enterprise master data management to align data definitions and data mapping. Ultimately, the goal in building an architecture foundation is to provide the end-user stakeholders with trusted, reliable, and accessible data to meet their respective needs in achieving the strategic plan goals. The key components to be considered are summarized in Table 17.1.

		TABLE 17.1 Key Technology Infrastructure Components for Enterprise Data Management, Reporting, and Analytics Program
Components	**Abbreviation**	**Description of Component**
Reporting and analytics		
Business intelligence	BI	Business intelligence is a set of methodologies, processes, architecture, and (software tools and) technologies that transform raw data into meaningful and useful information used to enable more effective strategic, tactical, and operational insights and decision-making (Evelson, 2010; Forrester Research, 2014).
BI library	Library	Business intelligence library is a centralized collection available electronically of all content developed by the organization to be used in reporting and analytics. Library includes KPI data definitions, standard reports, user-defined reports, and custom analyses and/or algorithms for analytics such as population health management.
Key performance indicator	KPI	Key performance indicators (aka measures and metrics) are quantifiable measurements reflecting the organization's goals. KPIs are organized typically into subject matter categories such as financial, operational, clinical, and satisfaction. Each KPI will have a documented data definition to ensure reliable reporting of that metric throughout the organization (see next).
KPI data definition	Dictionary	Data definitions are created for each KPI used in reporting and analytics by the organization. Data definitions will include both a business user and a technical definition.
Data stores		
Enterprise data warehouse	EDW	This is often referred to as an "analytic data management" system and is designed as a rational way to integrate and standardize disparate data sources (for multiple subject matters) while leveraging common data management and technologies to provide a trusted single source of truth for enterprise reporting and analytics (Beyer & Shaffer, 2014). It includes both hardware and software.

(continued)

TABLE 17.1 Key Technology Infrastructure Components for Enterprise Data Management, Reporting, and Analytics Program *(continued)*

Components	Abbreviation	Description of Component
Data marts	Mart	These may be either a subset of EDW or a separately developed mart for target end users and may contain a single subject matter of data. Examples of data marts include ambulatory visits or OR surgery marts.
Data management		
Data model	DM	Data modeling defines data elements and their structures and relationships among elements within the EDW. Data models are continually evolving with organizational needs, new data types, and technological innovations. Various data models discussed in the literature include star schema, early binding, late binding, and no binding (Sanders, Burton, & Protti, 2013).
Master data management	MDM	This includes the organization, management, and distribution of corporately adjudicated data with widespread use in the organization. It also includes processes that ensure that reference data are kept up to date and coordinated across an enterprise. Reference data are any data used to categorize other data or for relating data to information beyond the boundaries of the enterprise. These include data about patients, products, employees, vendors, and controlled domains (code values). Examples include master patient and master provider data (Data administration management association of NYC, 2009).
Terminology standards supporting interoperability	STDS	US national library of medicine is the central coordinating body for clinical terminology standards supporting the development, enhancement, and distribution of clinically specific vocabularies (i.e. SNOMED-CT, RxNorm, LOINC) to facilitate the exchange of clinical data and improve retrieval of health information (National Institutes of Health, U.S. National Library of Medicine, 2013).
Extract, translate, and load	ETL	This process is used for preparing and cleansing source system data for integration, transformation, and standardization into the EDW in coordination with the business requirements (Kimball & Caserta, 2004).

(continued)

Components	Abbreviation	Description of Component
TABLE 17.1 Key Technology Infrastructure Components for Enterprise Data Management, Reporting, and Analytics Program *(continued)*		
Source system data	Source data	Source systems include separately installed data systems, which may be integrated into either an EDW or a standalone data mart. Source examples include clinical transaction systems (patient accounting, EHR), standalone clinical applications (surgery, infection control, patient satisfaction), HRMS, FMS, SCM, CRM, and EPM software.

Note: This table provides an overview of key terms critical to implementing a successful technology infrastructure to support a healthcare delivery organization's enterprise data, reporting, and analytics program. The reader should refer to the IT literature for a more exhaustive discussion and for examples of each term.

CRM, customer relationship management; EHR, electronic health record; EPM, enterprise performance management; FMS, financial management solutions; HRMS, human resource management systems; LOINC, logical observation identifiers names and codes; OR, operating room; SCM, supply chain management; SNOMED-CT, systematized nomenclature of medicine—clinical terms.

BI Library

The BI library is a continually evolving, online collection of subject matter, reporting, and analytics (aka "content") that is readily available to and shareable with end users in a central location that is convenient within their reporting and analytics workflow. The library should be well organized by subject matter for quick access to a variety of content, including (a) standard reports (i.e., dashboards, scorecards, etc.) for easy drilling and filtering, (b) user-defined BI reports for personal and/or shared purposes, (c) data dictionary of key performance indicators (KPIs), and (d) custom queries and/or algorithms for analytics such as population health. The BI library represents the ultimate work product deliverables of the program management team (described in the People section—Business-Led Program Management), in conjunction with the team's IT (information technology) partners, data stewards, other domain subject matter experts, and the cross-functional work groups designing and documenting the user requirements (for more details, refer to the Processes section).

An example of BI library content is the data dictionary, which should contain all KPIs used in the enterprise reporting and analytics effort required to ensure data are being reported consistently, accurately, and reliably throughout the organization. In Table 17.2, the authors have provided an example of KPIs identified in March 2003 by Baylor Health Care System (now known as Baylor Scott & White Health System) to measure process of care measures for acute myocardial infarction (AMI) against specific target goals. Within the Data Definition Section of the BI library, each KPI has both business and technical data definitions, as well as other related information to be resolved, such as existing data source quality issues, point-of-care workflow documentation issues, and manual workflow processes on the back end before reporting.

TABLE 17.2 Example of KPIs to Be Defined in BI Library		
AMI—Clinical Preventive Services Measures (per Health Texas Provider Network)	**Health System's Current Performance**	**Goal**
Early aspirin use	98%	90%
Aspirin at discharge	96%	90%
Early beta-blocker use	85%	90%
Beta-blocker at discharge	90%	90%
Thrombolytics within 30 minutes of arrival	35	80%
Median time for thrombolytic administration	39.5 minutes	TBD
PTCA within 90 minutes of arrival	42%	
Median time for angioplasty administration	101 minutes	TBD
ACEI use for LVEF	84%	
Smoking-cessation counseling	94%	
Inpatient mortality	5.5%	TBD

Notes: Goals set by the VHA Inc. Chief Executive Officer Workgroup on Clinical Excellence.

This table is reproduced from an article published in March 2003 by Baylor Health Care System (now known as Baylor Scott & White Health System). The table includes KPIs that are used to measure the process of care measures for AMI with targets that are specific to their organization at time of publication.

This table can be viewed in color as supplementary data at *IJQHC* (*International Journal for Quality in Health Care*) Online.

ACEI, angiotensin-converting enzyme inhibitor; AMI, acute myocardial infarction; BI, business intelligence; KPI, key performance indicators; LVEF, left ventricular ejection fraction; PTCA, percutaneous transluminal coronary angioplasty.

Source: Ballard (2013).

Tools used to share the BI library content with end users include simple Excel files with embedded URL links to shared sites, Microsoft Sharepoint, and custom-designed interfaces. The optimum tool depends on the organization's size, budget, complexity, maturity, and IT resources available to support its library.

Evaluation and Selection of Technology Options

An enterprise strategic information plan should be developed and used to guide how the HDO implements its E-DRAP journey, EDW, BI, and analytics, including next-generation population health analytics. The plan should include clearly stated goals and objectives with a road map identifying workstreams of project work for people, processes, and technology. The road map should be based on the HDO's current state analysis and should identify the prioritized deliverables and target dates for each major workstream noted earlier. Information governance, program management, organization structures, and data stewards should be defined with timing specified for funding, roles and responsibilities, and policies and procedures. During the plan development, HDOs are encouraged to engage the vendor market as a learning process in either a formal or informal request for information (RFI) approach to understand the many market options available to HDOs (Beyer & Shaffer, 2014).

The authors have identified five general categories of analytic vendor options available in today's market for implementing data management, EDW, BI, and analytic products and solutions (Table 17.3). Ultimately, the final solution(s) implemented must include a flexible, open, and customizable EDW; data model; and extract, translate, and loads (ETLs) for continual data integration; as well as flexible BI reporting and analytic application(s) and/or tool(s), with the ultimate goal of migrating reporting and analytics to "self-service" over time where possible.

TABLE 17.3 Vendor Options: EDW/BI Products and Solutions for HDOs

EDW/BI Vendor Options	Option Description
1. Traditional EDW tech vendors	EDW technology vendors providing technical architecture, data modeling, ETL, master data management, and sometimes data dictionary and terminology mapping
2. Traditional BI tech vendors	BI tools vendors providing data presentation, querying and mining, and discovery and advanced visualization analytics solutions that are then customized to the organization's needs
3. Turnkey health care analytic vendors	Health care-focused technology vendors providing turnkey EDW, data model, ETLs and BI analytic reporting, dashboards, rules, and/or applications
4. EHR vendors	EMR transaction system vendors now migrating into the analytics field to protect market share; EDW, BI, and analytics are not core competencies for these vendors
5. Boutique analytic application vendors	Stand-alone HIT vendors providing "bolt on" specialty analytics applications; typically, these vendors may not provide a fully functional EDW and BI enterprise solution

Note: This table summarizes five high-level categories of vendor options providing EDW and BI commercial products and solutions to HDOs.

BI, business intelligence; EDW, enterprise data warehouse; EHR, electronic health record; EMR, electronic medical record; ETL, extract, translate, and load; HDO, health care delivery organization.

For those HDOs with adequate IT skills, resources, capital, time, and fortitude, building an infrastructure internally may be a feasible option. HDOs selecting this path may need to contract (at a minimum) with EDW and/or BI vendors (options 1 and 2 of Table 17.3) to deploy their EDW/BI technology foundation. These two stand-alone options are complex, expensive, and time-consuming and are not meant for the inexperienced or faint of heart. Data modeling constitutes a very significant percentage of work for these options, representing approximately 45% of the effort and requiring significant expertise in data modeling (Beyer & Shaffer, 2014).

Alternatively, HDOs may implement one or more combinations of commercial vendor packaged applications (options 3, 4, and/or 5), which may also entail implementing options 1 and 2 described earlier:

1. Turnkey HIT analytic vendor solutions provide packaged EDW, ETLs, data model, and BI analytic reporting, dashboards, rules, and/or applications to accelerate the HDO's analytic journey.

2. EHR vendor solutions provide new bolt-on, EDW/BI solutions to their existing EHR application(s) platform.

3. Boutique analytic application vendors providing specialty stand-alone analytics applications to meet needs, such as population health and predictive analytics, may not necessarily serve as a fully functional EDW/BI enterprise solution.

Often, organizations believe that these package solutions will more rapidly meet their needs through "vendor acceleration." A key appeal is the vendor's commercial data model, which many organizations believe will simplify their implementation efforts. However, organizations fail to take into account that these models must then be customized to the HDO's local environment, which may or may not be an easy process depending on the openness of the vendor's data model (Beyer & Shaffer, 2014).

Determining the optimum technology approach(es) for one's HDO may require support from experienced internal or external consultants in the evaluation, selection, contract negotiation, and implementation of the vendor(s), thereby providing the best solution to meet the specific needs and goals of the HDO environment.

People

The E-DRAP journey must be founded on a strong corporate culture of making data and analytics a core asset and source of competitive differentiation. Strong senior executive sponsor(s) must continually lead with clear communication of their message, while always aligning the use of data and analytics to the HDO's corporate strategy and goals (as diagrammed in Figure 17.2). Furthermore, a culture of data transparency must be key to the organization for all stakeholders, including administration and clinical providers, to collectively meet their clinical, quality, operational, and financial goals.

Information Governance Council

The need for information governance (Beyer & Shaffer, 2014) has accelerated as health care data have grown exponentially within HDOs, and as competitive pressures mount from the market, payers, and regulatory mandating agencies. To guide the E-DRAP effort, the Information Governance Council must be a business-led structure, including senior

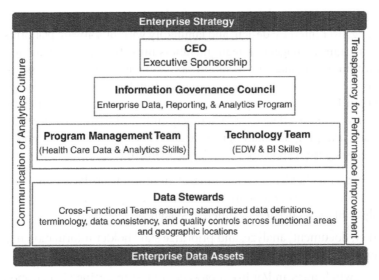

FIGURE 17.2. Key organizational components for an Enterprise Data Management, Reporting, and Analytics Program.

Note: This figure outlines organizational structures required to ensure data and analytics are core enterprise assets and sources of competitive differentiation.

leaders with expertise in health care data, analytics, as well as data-quality requirements. As described in Gartner's (2014) report to HDOs, it is recommended that the following elements of information governance be present:

1. CEO endorsement of effort with defined enterprise accountability and adequate funding

2. Governance named leaders accountable to business and clinical leaders for data standards, data quality, system integration, and to serve as advocates for the information needs of the business

3. Organizational structure designed with appropriate subcommittees, responsibilities, and accountability clearly documented and understood

4. Defined and documented processes for setting the enterprise vision, priorities, and road map decisions about information to drive important enterprise change

5. Established principles, policies, and procedures for data governance to guide the organization

Business-Led Program Management

A centralized and skilled business-led program management unit (often known as product management [Cagan, 2010]), or BI competency center (Di Maio, 2010) should be organized to lead and manage deployment of BI reporting and analytic content development. This centralized team is responsible for representing, gathering, and defining voice of customer (VOC) business user needs, as well as managing the E-DRAP road map (for more discussion, refer to the Processes section, which follows). This cross-functional team should include strong health care domain subject matter expertise (SME) and analytical skills, while including clinicians, clinical informaticists, quality-improvement specialists, statisticians, planning, finance, data exploration, statistical analysis techniques, data modeling, user interface design, and familiarity with BI software platforms. Furthermore, the program management team members must be organizational leaders, well respected within the organization, demonstrate excellent communication skills among all levels of the HDO, and be consummate consensus builders who are able to align business users and their IT development partners in delivering quality, optimum reporting and analytic solutions to the HDO users in a timely and meaningful manner (Cagan, 2010).

Specifically, the program management team represents the HDO's end-user stakeholders' interests with responsibility to do the following:

1. Organize stakeholders into meaningful groups of users based on their respective information needs and analytic skill sets (i.e., types of interactive reports and analytic BI views needed by different stakeholder segments).

2. Gather, document, analyze, and prioritize stakeholder information requirements to meet their respective operational and clinical needs.

3. Create wireframes and/or live prototypes to test reporting visualization before BI building and deployment.

4. Create a comprehensive online data dictionary with data definitions for each KPI used in wireframes and subsequent reports.

5. Own and manage the road map in partnership with its IT partners under the direction of the information governance council.

Processes

The development of effective reporting and analytics is a continual and iterative approach. This section describes the three main process components, including:

1. Road map, which documents the prioritized work streams of program management and IT sub projects

2. Key continuous and iterative process cycles designed to (a) assess readiness; (b) design, document, and build BI reporting and analytics; and (c) release and train end users

3. Supporting best practice methodologies to be employed throughout the continuous and iterative process cycles

Road Map

At the core of E-DRAP framework is the road map, which is a fluid planning document governed by the information governance council and managed by the business-led program management team, in partnership with its IT development partners. The road map reflects approved and prioritized business user requirements and guides the launch of enterprise reporting and analytic solutions to meet stakeholder needs. Furthermore, the road map is a living document, continually being refined, reprioritized, reviewed, and approved by the information governance council to meet the endless, emerging end-user feedback and business requirements for incremental functionality and new reporting and analytic solutions along the analytic continuum. An example of a road map is provided in Figure 17.3.

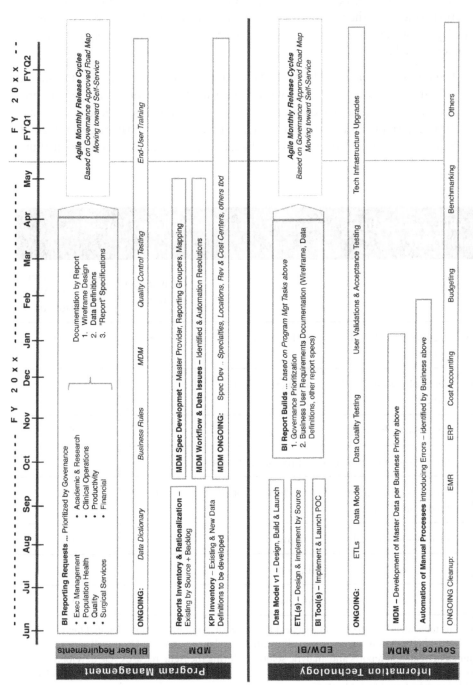

FIGURE 17.3. A roadmap example for an Enterprise Data Management, Reporting, and Analytics Program.

Note: This figure outlines potential "swim lanes" of program activity required to enhance an HDO's reporting use of the internally developed existing EDW and BI effort.

Key Continuous and Iterative Process Cycles

As previously noted, enterprise reporting and analytics needs to continually evolve as an organization matures with data use, as regulatory pressures change, and as technology innovations emerge in the market. The authors have identified three core and constant process cycles, which are constant in meeting business stakeholders' emerging reporting and analytic needs.

1. *Readiness assessment cycle*: As the HDO engages in the E-DRAP effort, it should continually assess where it is with respect to the maturity of its people, processes, and technology requirements. Several industry thought leaders (Di Maio, 2010; International Institute for Analytics [IIA], 2013; Kimball & Caserta, 2004; Sanders, Burton, & Protti, 2013; Stodder, 2013; The Data Warehousing Institute,

	TABLE 17.4 Readiness Assessment Checklist—Summary Categories for E-DRAP	# Checklist Items	Score (1 = Not Ready, 5 = Well Positioned)
1.0	Technology—Source system data accuracy & reliability	14	TBD
2.0	Technology—EDW/BI infrastructure & data model	4	TBD
3.0	People—Culture, governance, organization	11	TBD
4.0	Process—Communication of program & releases	4	TBD
5.0	Process—Existing reports & KPIs inventoried & reconciled for accuracy	6	TBD
6.0	Process—VOC & business requirements	5	TBD
7.0	Process—Agile design/build/deploy	4	TBD
8.0	Process—Use-based data quality	7	TBD

Note: This table identifies the summary checklist categories containing more detailed items to be considered when assessing an organization's readiness to launch an E-DRAP, as well as readiness to launch incremental reports and analytic solutions during the Agile release cycle development process. The user may customize this checklist to meet his or her respective needs. The detailed checklist may be found in Table 17.5.

BI, business intelligence; E-DRAP, enterprise data management and analytics program; EDW, enterprise data warehouse; KPIs, key performance indicators; VOC, voice of customer.

2009) have published their respective maturity models outlining the high-level components that organizations should evaluate. To help HDOs operationalize their ongoing maturity assessments, the authors have developed a more detailed readiness assessment checklist designed for HDOs to drill deeper into evaluating their people, processes, and technology components (summary readiness categories in Table 17.4). HDOs must continually "stress test" their existing structure to ensure there are no significant gaps that might hinder their ability to deliver valuable, usable, and feasible product solutions to end users. We recommend the reader stops and does a quick self-assessment of his or her organization's readiness using the Detail Readiness Assessment Checklist (Table 17.5).

TABLE 17.5 Readiness Assessment Checklist—Detail Items for E-DRAP		
		Score (1 = Not Ready, 5 = Well Positioned)
1.0	Technology—Source system data accuracy & reliability	
1	EDW single source of truth culture embraced—not silo sources	
2	Source system standards, terminology, & nomenclature	
3	Consistent data naming conventions for data model & reporting	
4	Source systems terminology—consistent & accurate	
5	Standardized data definitions within source systems or functional areas	
6	Master provider table developed	
7	Master person table developed	
8	Master data groupers or aggregators for reporting	
9	Cost accounting system integrated within EDW	
10	Benchmarking systems integrated within EDW	
11	Third-party analytics vendor systems integrated within EDW	

(continued)

	TABLE 17.5 Readiness Assessment Checklist—Detail Items for E-DRAP *(continued)*	Score (1 = Not Ready, 5 = Well Positioned)
12	Manual front- & back-end workflow processes identified	
13	Data quality controls from source systems → ETL → testing → production	
14	Source system IT accurate implementation	
2.0	Technology—EDW/BI infrastructure & data model	
1	EDW source of truth	
2	BI tool(s) evaluated	
3	Robust data model architecture	
4	Data quality control standards	
3.0	People—Culture, governance, organization	
1	Executive sponsorship of structured program	
2	Physician leadership & engagement	
3	Aligned incentives to promote accountability to program & enterprise goals	
4	Strategic plan identifies clear goals & objectives to align to reporting	
5	Lines of business defined with data structured and mapped for reporting/analytics	
6	Information governance council—leader & members named & organized	
7	Information governance council—charter, policies, & procedures drafted/approved	

(continued)

	TABLE 17.5 Readiness Assessment Checklist—Detail Items for E-DRAP (continued)	
		Score (1 = Not Ready, 5 = Well Positioned)
8	Information governance council—reporting prioritization & process approved	
9	Program management team formed & staffed as business-led organization structure	
10	Program management team partnered with staffed EDW/BI technology team	
11	Cross-functional team-based approach employed	
4.0	Process—Communication of program & releases	
1	Culture of data & analytics as a core asset	
2	Culture of transparency of physician information	
3	Single source of truth/enterprise data dictionary deployed; not silos of data	
4	Information governance council guiding oversight of E-DRAP effort	
5.0	Process—Existing reports & KPIs inventoried & reconciled for accuracy	
1	Board reports	
2	Leadership & management reports (monthly/weekly/etc.)	
3	Operational reports from disparate source systems	
4	Extracts provided from disparate source systems	
5	User-defined XLS used as custom reports	
6	Duplicate & inconsistent reporting eliminated	

(continued)

TABLE 17.5 Readiness Assessment Checklist—Detail Items for E-DRAP (continued)		Score (1 = Not Ready, 5 = Well Positioned)
6.0	Process—VOC & business requirements	
1	Cross-functional business requirements gathering & analysis	
2	Wireframing used to test stakeholder design & use requirements	
3	Data dictionary of KPI data definitions transparently created & available online	
4	Transparent report request process & prioritization employed	
5	Transparent online user feedback available	
7.0	Process—Agile design/build/deploy	
1	Agile methodology embraced & deployed for rapid cycle development	
2	Use of daily Scrums for team communications	
3	2- to 4-week release cycle development agreed to	
4	Iterative report build/revise cycles implemented with delivery dates adhered to	
8.0	Process—Use-based data quality	
1	Master data management of common data sets defined by business	
2	Terminology standards (SNOMED-CT, LOINC, RxNorm, etc.)	
3	Master data organized & cleaned for trusted reporting & analytics	
4	Business owner data stewards named & accountable for data definitions & quality	

(continued)

TABLE 17.5 Readiness Assessment Checklist—Detail Items for E-DRAP (continued)		Score (1 = Not Ready, 5 = Well Positioned)
5	Data stewards own KPI data definitions & user acceptance testing	
6	Workflow problems on front & back end identified & resolved	
7	Manual work-arounds to reporting identified and eliminated	

Note: This table identifies the detailed checklist categories of items to be considered when assessing an organization's readiness to launch an E-DRAP, as well as readiness to launch incremental reports and analytic solutions during the Agile release cycle development process. The user may customize this checklist to meet his or her respective needs.

BI, business intelligence; EDW, enterprise data warehouse; E-DRAP, enterprise data management, reporting, and analytics program; ETL, extract, translate, and load; KPI, key performance indicator; LOINC, Logical Observation Identifiers Names and Codes; SNOMED-CT, Systematized Nomenclature of Medicine—Clinical Terms; VOC, voice of customer.

2. *Design, document, and build cycle*: This cycle involves (a) gathering, documenting, and refining the business reporting and analytic needs; (b) developing wireframes and/or live prototypes for user feedback (refer to Supporting Best Practice Methodologies—VOC section for explanation about wireframing); (c) documenting the business rules (data definitions) for KPIs; (d) identifying issues impacting accurate reporting such as source data quality, front- and back-end workflow processes, and manual work-arounds; and (e) completing data testing and quality control with business user involvement and approval before release.

3. *Release and Training Cycle*: The release and end-user training of new BI reports must begin with a clear communication launch plan, including the organization's strategic commitment to data as a core asset and to the transparent use of data to becoming competitive analytics innovators. The information governance council and senior leadership are responsible for this communication messaging to physicians and all administrative business users to ensure alignment, commitment, and accountability throughout the organization. Depending on the size of the program management team, it may own the development communication plan, user training material development, end-user training, and feedback processes.

Supporting Best Practice Methodologies

Industry best practices should be integrated within and support the key continuous and iterative process cycles described earlier. Three best practices, in particular, are highlighted next, including Agile (AgileManifesto, 2001), Lean Six Sigma VOC (George & Vincent, 2002), and a Use-Based Data Quality Model (Orr, 1998).

1. *Agile*: This is a commonly used industry agnostic IT practice that promotes continual, iterative, and rapid-cycle releases to realize a quicker return on information investment to quickly meet end-user needs. Agile was formally defined in 2001 in the "Agile Manifesto" (AgileManifesto, 2001) and subsequently embraced and modified within the technology industry (Ambler & Lines, 2012).

   Adoption of pure Agile methodology in health care may be challenged at the onset because of (a) stakeholders' lack of knowledge about their data, especially with the deluge of new EHR implementations; (b) inconsistent terminology (i.e., departments, locations, specialties, service lines, etc.) among source systems; (c) lack of data stewards from the business to document and approve enterprise data definitions; (d) source system data quality and integrity issue resolution delaying short development cycles; and/or (e) front- and back-end workflow issues as well as existing manual workflow work-arounds.

2. *VOC*: End-user business requirements must lead the wireframe/prototype design and building of reporting and analytics solutions. VOC (George & Vincent, 2002) is a Lean Six Sigma process that is used to capture the customers' requirements to inform the reporting and analytics solutions development. This process is all about being proactive and constantly innovating to capture the changing requirements of the customers over time. The key is for the end user's input to be at the forefront throughout BI design and the build process to ensure that valuable, usable, and feasible reporting and analytic solutions are continually released throughout the HDO.

   Although several structured VOC qualitative and quantitative methodologies may be used, several techniques should be consistently employed to test out user requirements. Wireframes (see e.g., in Figure 17.4) and/or live prototypes are often used to help prioritize features and functionality and test ideas, as well as to help prioritize the release cycles for the HDO's reporting and analytic solutions. Program management may mock up (or prototype) their releases of interactive standard reports and dashboards using Excel, PowerPoint, and industry vendor wireframing tools. This technique offers an easy way to quickly engage stakeholders in dialogue and to refine the proposed visualization so that it will in actuality meet their respective clinical, operational, and/or financial data requirements before deploying IT resources to build it out.

3. *Data Quality and Integrity*: To continually enhance confidence and trust in the BI reporting and analytics solutions released, rigid data quality control techniques must be applied before releasing them into production for stakeholder use. The Data Quality Control process must involve both the business users and the IT teams to ensure data accuracy and reasonableness. In Orr's (1998) time-tested publication, he aptly explains that data quality can only be obtained if the stakeholders "use it or lose it!" In his data integrity model, Orr outlines his Data Quality Rules (Table 17.6), which are equally critical and essential to today's successful health care E-DRAP rollout.

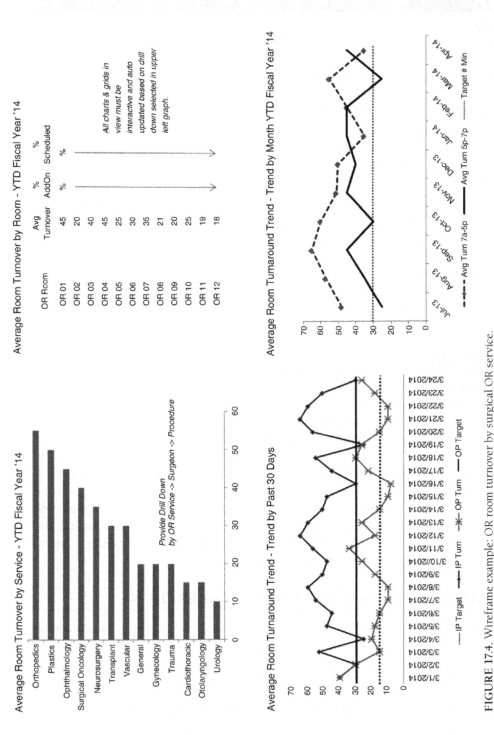

FIGURE 17.4. Wireframe example: OR room turnover by surgical OR service.

Note: This wireframe represents a draft layout of a BI dashboard layout based on numerous meetings with business stakeholders. Once the business has approved the final layout, the IT team will build this dashboard within the BI tool with the user-defined on the fly drill downs, filters, sorts, and other specified functionalities.

BI, business intelligence; IT, information technology; OR, operating room.

TABLE 17.6 Orr's Data Quality Rules	
Rule No.	Data Quality Rule
DQ1	Unused data cannot remain correct for very long.
DQ2	Data quality in an information system is a function of its use, not its collection.
DQ3	Data quality will, ultimately, be no better than its most stringent use.
DQ3	Data quality problems tend to become worse as the system ages.
DQ3	The less likely some data attribute (element) is to change, the more traumatic it will be when it finally does change.
DQ3	Laws of data quality apply equally to data and metadata (the data about the data).

Note: This table summarizes Kenneth Orr's Data Quality Rules established in his theoretical framework on data integrity described in Orr (1998, p. 68).

SUMMARY

In summary, this chapter has provided a practical framework for HDOs as they launch and/or enhance their EDW and BI strategy to become analytic innovators and competitive market leaders. The framework is modular, scalable, and adaptable to meet the needs of HDOs, regardless of their size, budget, organizational complexity, and/or level of maturity in developing stand-alone data marts, and more complex EDW and BI technology platforms. Health care leaders should consider how best to leverage components of this framework and techniques to succeed under new payment reform and pay-for-performance mandates to meet their respective enterprise strategic plan goals. The advanced practice nurse and interprofessional teams should identify, understand, and engage those responsible for reporting and analytics within their HDO order to ensure their end-user needs are being successfully met.

EXERCISES AND QUESTIONS FOR CONSIDERATION

Consider content covered with respect to data management, reporting, and analytics development, and respond to the following questions:

1. Why should people and processes be clearly structured and operationalized to meet your reporting and analytic business requirements?

2. Consider the assessment tool and use the tool to assess your clinical organization. Perform the assessment, consider the challenges identified in the chapter, and reconsider your assessment, as you interview key individuals in your organization, including the chief executive officer, chief financial officer, chief nursing

informatics officer, chief information officer, and chief medical informatics officer. Do their answers differ from yours? If so, why do you believe that is the case? What does that tell you about the readiness of your organization for an EDW/BI program?

3. Reflect on VOC described in this chapter for EDW/BI development and deployment. Determine which, if any, of these techniques are employed to meet your respective reporting and analytics requests. Evaluate the effectiveness of using these techniques within your organization.

4. Consider the options for selecting vendors to assist with your E-DRAP project and evaluate which options may be best for your organization and why.

REFERENCES

AgileManifesto. (2001). *The Agile manifesto.* Retrieved from www.agilemanifesto.org

Ambler, S., & Lines, M. (2012). *Disciplined Agile delivery: A practitioner's guide to Agile software delivery in the enterprise.* New York, NY: IBM Press.

Ballard, D. J. (2003). Indicators to improve clinical quality across an integrated health care system. *International Journal for Quality in Health Care, 15*(Suppl. 1), i13–i23. Retrieved from http://intqhc .oxfordjournals.org

Beyer, M. A., & Shaffer, V. (2014). *Top actions for healthcare delivery organization CIOs, 2014: Avoid 25 years of mistakes in enterprise data warehousing.* Retrieved from www.gartner.com/technology/ reprints.do?id=1-1R0QJVG&ct=140221&st=sb&mkt_tok=3RkMMJWWfF9wsRols67LZKXonjHpfs X56%2BUsW6G3lMI%2F0ER3fOvrPUfGjI4FScBhI%2BSLDwEYGJlv6SgFQrDDMaNy37gIUhE%3D

Cagan, M. (2010). *Inspired: How to create products customers love.* Sunnyvale, CA: Silicon Valley Product Group.

Data Administration Management Association of NYC. (2009). *Creating the golden record: Better data through chemistry.* Retrieved from http://damany.com/images/meeting/101509/damanyc_mdm print.pdf

Di Maio, A. (2010). *Gartner launches open government maturity model* (No. G12010). Retrieved from http://www.blogs.gartner.com/andrea_dimaio/2010/06/28/gartner-launches-open-government-maturity-model

Evelson, B. (2010). *Want to know what Forrester's lead data analysts are thinking about BI and data domain?* Retrieved from http://blogs.forrester.com/boris_evelson/10-04-29-want_know_what_ forresters_lead_data_analysts_are_thinking_about_bi_and_data_domain

Forrester Research. (2014). *Business intelligence.* Retrieved from https://www.forrester.com/Business-Intelligence

George, M. L., & Vincent, P. (2002). *Lean Six Sigma: Combining Six Sigma with Lean speed* (1st ed.). Madison, WI: McGraw-Hill.

International Institute for Analytics. (2013). *DELTA powered analytics maturity* (No. IIA2013). Retrieved from http://www.himssanalytics.org/docs/DELTA%20Suite%20Sell%20Sheet_October%202013.pdf

Kimball, R., & Caserta, J. (2004). *The data warehouse ETL toolkit: Practical techniques for extracting, cleaning, conforming, and delivering data.* Hoboken, NJ: John Wiley & Sons. Retrieved from http:// www.kimballgroup.com/data-warehouse-business-intelligence-resources/books/data-warehouse-dwetl-toolkit

Kiron, D., Ferguson, R. B., & Prentice, P. K. (2013). *From value to vision: Reimaging the possible with data analytics: What makes companies that are great at analytics different from everyone else*. (Research Report). Cambridge, MA: MIT Sloan Management Review. Retrieved from http://www.sas.com/content/dam/SAS/en_us/doc/whitepaper2/reimagining-possible-data-analytics-106272.pdf

National Institutes of Health, U.S. National Library of Medicine. (2013). *Supporting interoperability—Terminology, subsets and other resources from the NLM*. Retrieved from https://www.nlm.nih.gov/hit_interoperability.html

Orr, K. (1998). Data quality and systems theory. *Communications of the ACM, 41*(2), 66–71. Retrieved from http://www.ir.iit.edu/~dagr/DataMiningCourse/Research_Papers/p66-orr.pdf

Sanders, D., Burton, D. A., & Protti, D. (2013). *The healthcare analytics adoption model: A framework and roadmap* (White Paper). Salt Lake City, UT: HealthCatalyst. Retrieved from http://www.health catalyst.com/wp-content/uploads/2013/11/analytics-adoption-model-Nov-2013.pdf

Stodder, D. (2013). *Achieving greater agility with business intelligence: Improving speed and flexibility for BI, analytics, and data warehousing*. Retrieved from https://tdwi.org/articles/2013/01/04/achieving-greater-agility-with-business-intelligence-executive-summary.aspx

TDWI Research, Best Practices Report, 'Achieving Greater Agility with Business Intelligence: Improving Speed and Flexibility for BI, Analytics, and Data Warehousing', First Quarter 2013, David Stodder, Retrieved from http://www.tdwi.org

The Data Warehousing Institute. (2009). *TDWI's Business Intelligence Maturity Model poster*. Retrieved from https://knowledgeworks.wordpress.com/2009/02/17/the-tdwi-bi-maturity-model

CHAPTER 18

Data Management and Analytics: The Foundations for Improvement

Susan McBride and Mari Tietze

OBJECTIVES

1. Discuss the basics of database management and related items that health care organizations need to consider.

2. Discuss metrics development and the complexity of designing and well documenting measures for patient safety, quality, and population health improvement.

3. Examine levels of measurement and the importance of correctly analyzing health care data.

4. Describe the challenges of utilizing data from the clinical setting and outline specific steps to address those challenges.

5. Describe analytic software in the health care setting, including business intelligence (BI) tools and suites of products available to layer onto databases and data warehouses.

6. Discuss statistical analysis and common tests that are run for examining quality and patient safety issues.

7. Define and discuss *data mining*, what it is, and how it is utilized in health care.

KEY WORDS

databases, metrics, measures, analytics, analysis, levels of measurement, statistics, variables, independent variables, dependent variables, levels of measurement, string variables, cross tabulation, sampling methods, confidence intervals, normal distribution, power analysis, statistical control, common-cause variation, business intelligence tools, data warehouse, operational data repository, clinical data repository, data mining

CONTENTS

INTRODUCTION

Data management, measures, and analytics are the foundations of improvement. In health care, there are tremendous volumes of data available; however, very little of that data are matured into information and knowledge that generates the wisdom and critical thinking needed in the industry to fully capitalize on the electronic data being amassed. Value-based purchasing models are driving the industry to use data in significant new and innovative ways to compete in the health care industry. As with other industries, the health care industry is going to compete on analytics.

Davenport (2005) indicates that many companies have built their businesses on "the ability to collect, analyze and act on data" (p. 2). Health care will be no different, and this is particularly relevant with value-based purchasing models that will require that we compete on quality and efficiency. So, how does the health care industry establish a strong base within organizations to prepare organizations to be strategic in managing data effectively and analyzing it for success? Chapter 17 discussed data management and establishing a strategy on designing and deploying an enterprise data, reporting, and analytics-driven organization. This chapter covers the basics of data management needed to mature a data set and to analyze it for improvement purposes. We discuss how to approach a data analysis project, how to evaluate a data set for data integrity, and provide examples of common issues with data integrity. Levels of measurement and how those levels of measures are relevant to analytic approaches are discussed. Various analytic software applications are available for purchase for use with large data sets. Some of these common tools are examined, including spreadsheet applications, statistical packages, and business intelligence tool sets. We compare and contrast these tools and suggest applications for their use in common situations that are often encountered in the health care industry. Finally, we examine a case study using common statistical analysis and Microsoft Excel in an exercise to emphasize lessons learned.

DATA MANAGEMENT: FOUNDATIONS FOR ANALYSIS

Master data management is a coordination of people, practices, and automation, which was largely covered in Chapter 17. We cover data management within this chapter as an approach to fully understanding the data in preparation for analysis. The first step is to consider the data source and the integrity of the information. Areas to understand include the data structure, integration, metadata, and data modeling. We define these terms for the reader and discuss the importance of the terms related to analysis. This section covers the data warehouse operational data stores versus the historical data warehouse for analytics, the differences between them, and why one utilizes one versus the other.

Retrospective Data Warehouse, Operational, and Clinical Data Repository Defined

A data warehouse is a retrospective store of data set up to report trends, offer comparisons, and provide strategic analysis. It can include clinical, operational, and financial data (Englebardt & Nelson, 2002). It is typically considered a nonvolatile store of data that does not change with time. In contrast, a clinical or operational data repository accumulates clinical and operational data from many systems to assist clinicians in managing patient care at the point of care (Englebardt & Nelson, 2002). These types of data stores are expected to shift and change with time given the ever-changing nature of the patient. The clinical data repositories supporting the infrastructure of the electronic health records (EHRs) are examples of operational and clinical data stores. There are differentiating characteristics between a data warehouse and an operational data store that are important considerations for data management and analytic methods. To summarize the differences, a data warehouse refers typically to retrospective data, maintains both aggregate and detail-level data, centralizes data collection for the intended purpose, provides a common view of data reflecting the enterprise, supports analytic tools, is expandable to terabytes of data (20–100 terabytes of data are not uncommon), and provides data marts within the infrastructure (Imhoff, Galemmo, & Geiger, 2003). A data mart is a subsection of the data warehouse that stores data for a very specific intended purpose. For example, a data mart might be a subset of data for financial purposes that is isolated from clinical data that the end user does not need to have access to within the data warehouse. In contrast, a clinical or operational data store is subject oriented; in the case of the clinical data store, the subject would be the patient. In a financial data store, it might be an account number associated with "the subject." Data are fully integrated across time and events. Data are current and also volatile, meaning they change based on events occurring with the patient at that point in time, and are typically detailed data and not aggregate information (Imhoff et al., 2003). Differentiating detailed versus aggregate data, we can consider whether or not a patient who had died would be indicated in the clinical data store at the patient record level. Aggregate data for quality reporting purposes may contain a mortality rate, risk-adjusted mortality rate, and perhaps a risk of mortality by patient types.

There are a number of important considerations to remember when designing a data warehouse, and we cover some very basic design components that are important for data analysis and discovery. *Databases* are defined as a large collection of data organized for rapid search and retrieval (Database, n.d.). The design strategies are relevant to "the rapid search and retrieval" requirements for analysis. It is not an ideal use of workforce resources to have an analyst wait for hours or even minutes to return a query or report. When amassing large volumes of data, the way the structure of the database or data warehouse is constructed is very relevant. Analysts can be involved in design strategies if they are knowledgeable about what they want from the data and how they intend to use it. The authors advise a build that strategizes a "left to right" build strategy. In other words, the analyst needs to fully understand and operationalize (ability to measure) the outcomes and processes that he or she wants to retrieve from the data store before laying out the design. Frequently, organizations will design a data warehouse by depositing multiple data sources, including admissions, discharge and transactions data, financial data, clinical data, and supply chain data, without thinking in terms of what and how these data will be used. The informed analyst can help with the design strategy by being clear on what he or she needs from the data warehouse. In Chapter 17, we discussed strategies for convening the right people to design the enterprise data. This chapter addresses how an analyst determines what she or he wants from the data and how to think in terms of appropriate data-analysis methods.

BASICS OF DATA ANALYSIS

In designing a data-analysis strategy, the analyst wants to determine what it is that is needed for analysis. This might sound like a very basic notion, but designing accurate metrics and a data strategy that will populate the measure is often much more difficult than we initially think.

Measurement Theory

Measurement theory is a fundamental science used to understand data. Krebs (1987), in a classic article on measurement theory, notes: *"Measurement theory is the conceptual foundation of all scientific decisions. If the measurements are erroneous, no amount of statistical or verbal sophistry can right them"* (Krebs, 1987, p. 1834). In addition, Waltz, Strickland, and Lenz (2010) indicate that conceptual frameworks are critical to systematically guiding the measurement process by increasing the likelihood that concepts and variables universally salient to nursing and health care practice will be identified and explicated (Waltz et al., 2010).

Measurement theory can be considered the basis for evidence-based clinical practice and is an important consideration before any analysis of health care data. It is important to think from left to right—meaning we need to think about what it is we are intending to measure or the effect we want to examine and build systems and data-collection methods based on that outcome of interest. We identify what those elements or variables are by using conceptual and theoretical frameworks that many of us as clinicians know intuitively, but we are relying on theory we have learned over time and from the scientific literature to reinforce how we approach designing data-collection and analysis methods. *Measurement* can be defined as "the assignment of numbers to objects or events according to rules" (Stevens, 1959, p. 25). The goal of measurement is to accurately evaluate a phenomenon of interest and reduce concepts to operational definitions with numeric values. These numeric values can take on different levels of measurement.

Levels of Measurement

The levels of measurement can be classified into scale, nominal, ordinal, interval, and ratio data. Once classified, the level of measurement specifies which statistical operations can be properly used. These statistical analysis decision points are reflected in Figure 18.1.

These levels are defined as follows:

> ▶ *Nominal*: Numbers assigned represent an object's membership in one of a set of mutually exclusive, exhaustive, and unorderable categories.

▶ *Ordinal*: Numbers assigned represent an object's membership in one of a set of mutually exclusive and exhaustive categories that can be ordered according to the amount of the attribute possessed.

▶ *Interval*: Numbers assigned represent an object's membership in one of a set of mutually exclusive and exhaustive categories that can be ordered and are equally spaced in terms of the magnitude of the attribute under consideration.

▶ *Ratio*: Same as the interval but in addition the distance from an absolute zero point is known.

Nominal and ordinal data can be considered categorical data, whereas interval and ratio data can be considered a continuous variable or scale. Figure 18.1 reflects this more simplistic approach toward data analysis. The figure reflects the level of measurement and properties that can help an analyst determine how to approach analyzing variables.

Operationalizing a Measure

An operational definition clearly outlines precisely how a measure will be constructed. To clearly specify dependent measures or outcome measures and independent variables that might impact the outcome of interest is an important component to improving science, as well as to the fundamentals of research. To fully understand operational definitions, we need to define several terms, including (a) variable, (b) dependent variable, (c) independent variable, (d) confounder factors, (e) outcome measure, and (f) process measure. We start with defining the term "variable." A *variable* is defined as a quantity that may assume any of a set of values, such as the gender variable, which is either male or female; we can assign a value of 1 = male and 2 = female (variable, n.d.). A dependent variable in an analysis or study is the outcome of interest, such as mortality, total costs of a procedure, or 30-day readmissions. In many health care organizations today, "yes" or "no" are examples of variables of interest that can be considered dependent variables. Think in terms of these variables as dependent on independent variables. An independent variable is a variable that is related to the dependent variable of interest, or it may

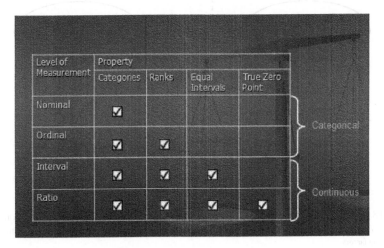

FIGURE 18.1. Four levels of measurement.

be an intervention that is manipulated in a research study or improvement process. The intervention would be considered a process measure that impacts the outcome measure. Figure 18.2 depicts a model frequently used in health outcome research and improvement science that was originally developed by Donabedian (1966). This model proposes relationships among components that are two dimensional, with interventions acting through characteristics of the system and of the client, and vice versa. The effect of an intervention in this study (e.g., induction of labor) is either mediated or modified by client and system characteristics. An example of these relationships in terms of primary cesarean delivery is that the effect of labor induction varies across parity and gestational age (McBride, 2005). The Donabedian (1966) health outcomes model is excellent for framing improvements and health care outcomes studies and for thinking through relationships and processes that may influence some outcomes of interest, such as examining the effect of inductions on primary cesarean delivery and what factors we believe will influence the relationship of the intervention (induction) with the outcome of interest (primary cesarean delivery). Independent variables, such as parity, gestation, race/ethnicity, maternal age, medical indication for induction, dystocia, fetal distress, and baby weight, were identified as significant factors related to induction of labor's influence on whether or not a successful primary cesarean or a successful vaginal delivery occurs. Confounding factors are situations or factors that influence the outcome of interest that a researcher or analyst must control for when examining the impact of an intervention on some outcome of interest (Hosmer & Lemeshow, 2000). For example, in the case of examining the impact on primary cesarean rates in a hospital, we would want to control for the inde-

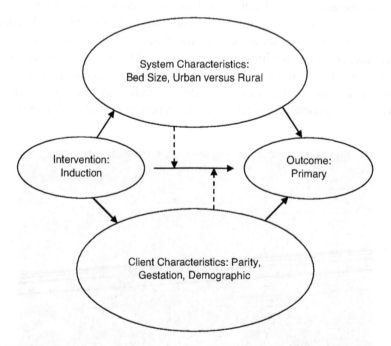

FIGURE 18.2. Examining odds of primary cesarean delivery using a quality health outcomes model.
Note: The dashed arrows represent interaction or effect modifiers, whereas the solid arrows depict the confounding effects or effect mediating factors.
Source: McBride (2005).

pendent variables noted as independent variables. But how will we define and measure the odds of a primary cesarean and the influence of induction of labor as "yes" or as "no"? By clearly defining what data will be used to measure these three factors, we are "operationalizing" the definitions. This was not intended to be a full discussion on research and improvement science, therefore, we refer the reader to a research text for full guidelines on research design and strategy. However, we are emphasizing that clearly defining measures and operationalizing precisely how you will measure variables in any analysis is a fundamental competency.

Conceptual models are visual diagrams, such as the health outcomes model noted in Figure 18.2, that are particularly helpful in clarifying how and what one will be analyzing. It is important to involve all stakeholders from interprofessional teams who fully understand the clinical domain one is examining. When approaching and operationalizing a measure, a relatively new technique is to convene the interprofessional team and map out the thought processes related to how the measure will be constructed using a mind map. Figure 18.3 presents an example of a mind map. A mind map is a visual depiction of some phenomenon of interest. In this case, it is a map of factors influencing an outcome of interest. Figure 18.3 reflects a map conceptualizing a measure for a catheter-associated urinary tract infection. In addition to conceptually mapping the process, more detail is needed to actually extract the data from the electronic environment for analyzing this outcome of interest. Figure 18.4 reflects the more detailed workflow map of the interprofessional departments that influence the outcomes of interest and have some impact on the actual data as they flow through the electronic environment.

Microsoft programs Excel and Word, along with several off-the-shelf applications, do a nice job of providing point-and-click tools with SmartArt features that support the construction of a mind map. Figure 18.3 presents an example of a measure mapped using a nice feature-functionality that helps create a mind map. Microsoft Excel, Word, and PowerPoint can be used to create conceptual models or "mind maps" of data elements and relationships to measures using SmartArt or other graphic features. Figure 18.4 uses Microsoft Visio to note workflow and roles related to the measure. The "traffic jam" notation in the figure presents the convergence of data into information to operationally define the numerator and denominator for the measure.

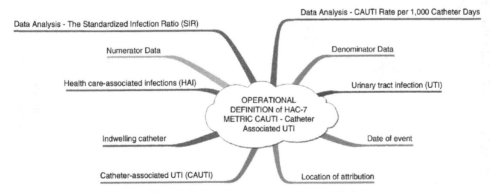

FIGURE 18.3. Mind map for operational definition of a measure for catheter-associated urinary tract infection.

Source: R. Gilder from McBride, Fenton, Valdes, and Gilder (2013).

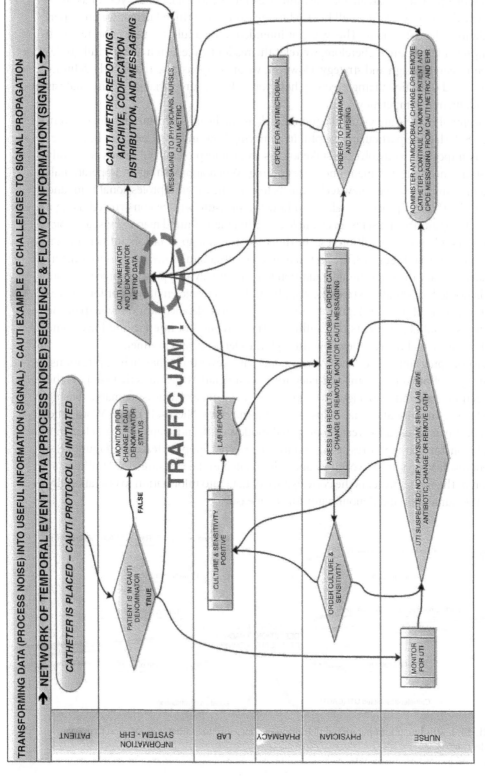

FIGURE 18.4. Transforming data into useful information and knowledge.

Note: Traffic jam notation presents the convergence of information into the operational definition of the numerator and denominator.

CAUTI, catheter-associated urinary tract infection; CPOE, computer provider order entry; EHR, electronic health records; UTI, urinary tract infection.

Source: R. Gilder from McBride et al. (2013).

Quality of the Data

Before using data, it is important to determine the quality of the data being used. Quality metrics for data are often a consideration for organizations and these metrics might include factors such as consistency of the information across the institution; completeness of the data; conformity to standard, accuracy, duplication, and overall integrity of the information. Let us take one of these types of data-integrity issues and walk through a process for identifying the issue. A duplicate records issue can create challenges involved in delivering patient care and in examining the data for outcomes analysis. For example, a cardiac patient presents to the emergency department (ED) with a myocardial infarction, and when the admitting clerk pulls up from the clinical data store within the EHR using a common look-up feature to search for patient records, the clerk notes two records that appear to be virtually the same individual but with different birth dates. This is a common problem within the EHR and is often an expensive issue to rectify within the clinical data store. The duplicate record must be merged into one master record.

When performing data analysis, duplicate records are a common problem; particularly when different sources or multiple extracts from the same data source are used, duplication of the cases can be introduced into an analysis file. Let us take the same example and consider that data have been extracted, translated, and loaded into a retrospective data warehouse for analysis of cardiac outcomes. A clinical analyst is analyzing retrospective outcomes data for patients with myocardial infarction, tracking and trending outcomes for the facility. If there are a number of duplicated medical records on the same individuals within the clinical data, the extracted data will inflate the overall denominator of total cardiac patients within the analytic files. Therefore, one of the first things an analyst should do before analyzing data is to inspect the data for data integrity on all factors noted earlier.

Exploring a Data Set

In addition to examining data for integrity of the information, an analyst should examine the data and explore the information before analysis.

Open the data file and visually inspect it.

▶ What rows and columns does the data set reflect?

▶ How are the data structured? Are the visibly missing data apparent in the file?

▶ Do they appear to be sorted in some order?

▶ What variables in the data set represent dependent, independent, and grouping variables?

If the software you are using has a feature to generate a data dictionary of file information, start with running the report that will provide you variable information, including position in the file, data labels on variables, measurement level (nominal, ordinal, scale, or string), column width, and variable labels, also referred to as "value sets." Examine all of these features in the data set. Figure 18.5 includes an example of an IBM SPSS software application and a file information display feature that is generated in the software. It was obtained by selecting File/Display Data File Information/Working File.

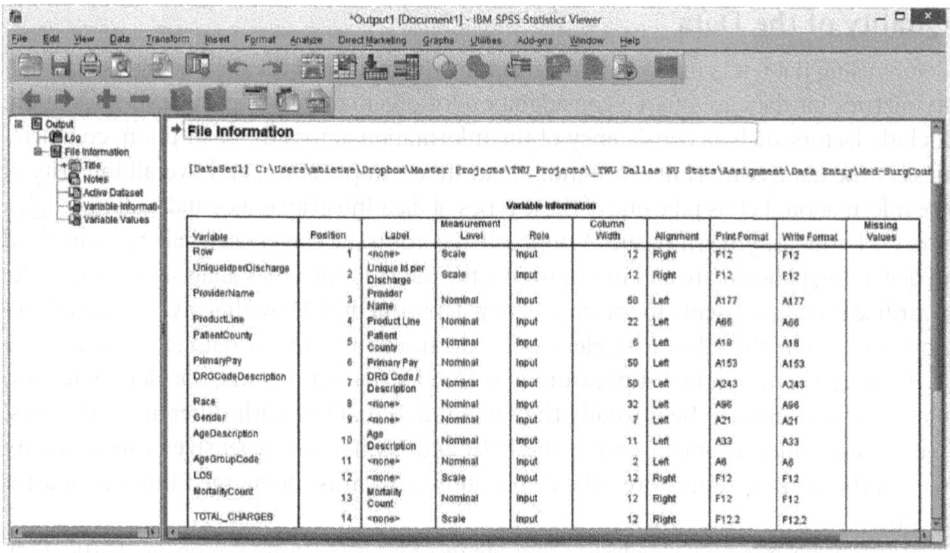

Variable	Position	Label	Measurement Level	Role	Column Width	Alignment	Print Format	Write Format	Missing Values
Row	1	<none>	Scale	Input	12	Right	F12	F12	
UniqueIdperDischarge	2	Unique Id per Discharge	Scale	Input	12	Right	F12	F12	
ProviderName	3	Provider Name	Nominal	Input	50	Left	A177	A177	
ProductLine	4	Product Line	Nominal	Input	22	Left	A66	A66	
PatientCounty	5	Patient County	Nominal	Input	6	Left	A18	A18	
PrimaryPay	6	Primary Pay	Nominal	Input	50	Left	A153	A153	
DRGCodeDescription	7	DRG Code / Description	Nominal	Input	50	Left	A243	A243	
Race	8	<none>	Nominal	Input	32	Left	A96	A96	
Gender	9	<none>	Nominal	Input	7	Left	A21	A21	
AgeDescription	10	Age Description	Nominal	Input	11	Left	A33	A33	
AgeGroupCode	11	<none>	Nominal	Input	2	Left	A6	A6	
LOS	12	<none>	Scale	Input	12	Right	F12	F12	
MortalityCount	13	Mortality Count	Nominal	Input	12	Right	F12	F12	
TOTAL_CHARGES	14	<none>	Scale	Input	12	Right	F12.2	F12.2	

FIGURE 18.5. Display file information feature in IBM SPSS.

Exploratory Data Analysis

Exploration of data can help determine whether data are accurate and complete, distributions of data, what statistical techniques might be appropriate for analyzing the data, and examining initial relationships that might exist among variables. A data exploration analysis provides a variety of visual and numerical summaries of data and can be performed by all cases, a subset of cases, or separately for groups of cases. Grouping variables are ordinal or nominal data and are often used to examine demographics of patient populations such as age distribution by groups, race, ethnicity, and gender.

To perform an exploratory data analysis, initially the analyst screens the data, examines the data file for outliers, and checks any assumptions one might have related to the data. For example, you are aware that you have a very large women's health services division with obstetrical and gynecological services outweighing all other services. Therefore, in inspecting the data, you are aware that your distribution of men to women should be an approximately 40:60 ratio. When you explore the data in a cross-tabulation (i.e., tables with rows and columns representing variables of interest) noting count and percentage of cases by age group, you determine that your assumptions appear to be accurately reflected in the data set; therefore, your data pull likely well represents the population of the facility related to gender distribution.

Graphically Examining the Data Set

You can use charts and graphs to examine data visually. Depending on the type of chart, you might add an interpolation, fit, or reference line to examine relationships in the data. An interpolation line is the fit of the line from one point to another given the distribution of the data. You can scatter plot the data to examine distribution of certain variables. Many software statistical and analytic packages have the capability of running reports on the data file. It is important that charts and graphs do not misrepresent the data and showcase what one intends the examiner to detect from the data analysis. The graphic should quickly reveal aggregate information to the reviewer in an appealing, quickly digestible manner. According to Tufte (2001), an ideal chart or graph:

- ▶ "Shows" the data
- ▶ Induces the viewer to think about the substance rather than the methodology, graphic design, the technology, or other things
- ▶ Avoids distorting what the data have to say
- ▶ Presents many numbers in a small space
- ▶ Makes large data sets coherent
- ▶ Encourages the eye to compare different pieces of data
- ▶ Reveals the data at several levels of detail
- ▶ Serves a reasonably clear purpose
- ▶ Is closely integrated with the statistical and verbal descriptions of the data set (Tufte, 2001)

Data Transformation

Data often require that we transform the data from their original source. This is typically the case in health care data analysis. When we indicate we are transforming data, we do not mean that the data take on new meaning or the original data are modified such that they no longer represent the source information. Transformation in this case is a technique used for analysis of data that requires manipulation of the original data to answer the question of interest. This could involve collapsing the data into age groups, deriving an outcome from source data, such as mapping discharge status codes to a mortality measure of "yes" or "no" or primary cesarean delivery coding data mapped to a variable noting "yes" or "no" for cesarean delivery. Table 18.1 presents an example of data transformation. This transformation involves remapping data on birth weight (scale variable) to a categorical variable with categories of "low birth weight" and "not low birth weight." Likewise, two variables are mapped into one variable with race and ethnicity (two variables) mapped into a simplified variable with White, Black, or Hispanic (three categories).

Text Data to Numeric Values

A common data transformation that is often required, particularly when analyzing data using spreadsheets or statistical packages, involves converting data from text or string data into numeric values. Often, programs have the ability to autocode data into numerics for the end user. These types of functions quickly create a numeric version of the string variable and make additional recoding of values easier. There are also recode functions in various programs that automate this process.

Data Mapping

Data mapping is an important concept and competency for an analyst to master. It is an essential element in analyzing health care data with important implications for using

TABLE 18.1 Data Transformation: Low Birth Weight × Maternal Race Cross-tabulation

			Maternal Race			Total
			White	Hispanic	African American	
Low birth weight	Not low birth weight	Count	1,229	31	149	1,409
		Percentage of total	81.9%	2.1%	9.9%	93.9%
	Low birth weight	Count	67	8	16	91
		Percentage of total	4.5%	0.5%	1.1%	6.1%
Total		Count	1,296	39	165	1,500
		Percentage of total	86.4%	2.6%	11.0%	100.0%

Note: Reflects cross-tabulation of birth weight by maternal race and ethnicity (columns) with birth weight collapsed into high and low (rows) and two variables, race and ethnicity (typically two variables), collapsed and mapped into one variable with percentages and counts reflecting corresponding statistics.

clinical data from the EHR and maximizing use of historical data as data shifts and changes with updates to code sets. "Data mapping involves 'matching' between a source and a target such as between two databases that contain the same data elements but call them by different names" (McBride, Gilder, Davis, & Fenton, 2006, p. 2). Data can map from a source A to a target B by using a translational key database to connect the two sources. These maps can be bidirectional or unidirectional. Unidirectional maps indicate a map moving one way from the source to the target and cannot be mapped back. Bidirectional maps can map both ways to and from the source. Figure 18.6 reflects types of mapping situations. An example in health care data that will require mapping is the need to map International Classification of Diseases, Ninth Revision, Clinical Modification (ICD-9-CM) to the International Classification of Diseases, 10th Revision, Clinical Modification (ICD-10-CM; Centers for Disease Control and Prevention, 2015). Our historical data for trending in many of our administrative data sets uses ICD-9-CM codes. With the shift to the ICD-10-CM on the horizon, we will need to map our historical data to the new code sets. These codes do not always have a one-to-one match. This is the case with the ICD-9-CM to ICD-10-CM maps. There are multiple ICD-10-CM codes that map from the ICD-9-CM codes (Centers for Medicare & Medicaid Services [CMS], 2014). When mapping these types of code sets with many-to-one relationships (common issue

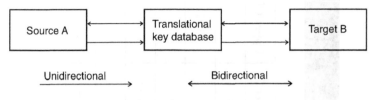

FIGURE 18.6. Data mapping.
Source: Reproduced from McBride et al. (2006).

with database analysis), challenges arise that must be addressed in the translational database. The analyst must also be very careful not to introduce errors within the analysis when using data derived from translational maps. When an analyst suspects an error has been introduced from data translations or mappings, the best way to address the issue is to track back to the original source and track forward to the data set with the suspected error.

Statistical Analysis

Inferential statistics involves deriving information from a sample data set about a given population of care and setting up a model to validly describe the population. For example, immunization rates for all children in Texas could be estimated by using observations from a sample of pediatric patients. Immunization rates for a sample of patients in a low-income clinic would not represent the immunization rate for children throughout the state of Texas, because we have introduced bias to our analysis. If we obtained the data from the state database that constituted all immunizations in the state of Texas and we were to randomly select a sample of 1,000 cases, we can reasonably consider that the sample represents the population in Texas. A random sample is a sample drawn from the population of interest where the analyst has a reasonable expectation that every member of the population has the same probability (chance) of being selected within the sample. Random samples are considered unbiased and representative of the population at large (Munro, 2005).

Parameter Estimates

Parameter estimates take on two forms, including a single number estimate or a "point estimate" and an interval estimate or range of parameters. Common point estimates are the mean, median, variance, and standard deviation. However, a common range estimate used in health care is the confidence interval (CI; Munro, 2005).

The point estimate gives us a value as an estimate of the population, whereas a confidence interval is a range of values that are likely to contain the point estimate (or parameter) within some probability. This probability is typically set at a 95% confidence interval, meaning we are 95% confident that the point estimate falls within the CI range noted. Table 18.2 provides an example of a patient safety indicator for decubitus ulcers per 1,000 inpatient admissions. The point estimate in this case is the risk-adjusted rate, and the CIs are the lower and higher bounds of the estimate. As an analyst, we would infer that the decubitus risk-adjusted rate for all of these five hospitals is somewhere between the lower and higher confidence bounds.

TABLE 18.2 Sample Data on AHRQ Indicators for Point Estimate and CI Example

AHRQ Patient Safety Indicator: Decubitus Ulcer per 1,000 Inpatient Admissions

	Numerator	Denominator	Observed Rate	Expected Rate	Rate Index	Risk-Adjusted Rate	Lower CI	Upper CI
State of Texas	15,504	557,937	27.79	27.41	1.01	23.59	23.24	23.94
Hospital A	146	5,519	26.45	28.22	0.94	21.81	18.31	25.31
Hospital B	62	4,120	15.05	25.3	0.59	13.84	9.58	18.1
Hospital C	196	8,916	21.98	25.74	0.85	19.87	16.99	22.75
Hospital D	76	3,020	25.17	22.14	1.14	26.45	21.09	31.8
Hospital E	132	3,581	36.86	27.8	1.33	30.84	26.49	35.2

AHRQ, Agency for Healthcare Research and Quality; CI, confidence interval.

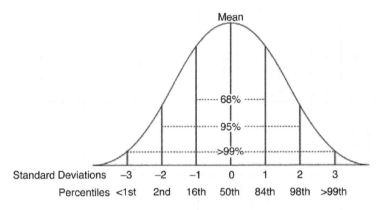

FIGURE 18.7. Normal curve.

Normal Distribution

Most distributions, although not perfectly "normal," closely approximate "normal." Figure 18.7 reflects the normal curve and parameters that the distribution reflects to constitute "a normal distribution." A normal distribution is a theoretical distribution or "bell-shaped curve" in which the mean, median, and mode converge in the center of the curve. This distribution is important for the following three reasons noted by Munro (2005): (a) Although most distributions are not perfectly normal, most variables approximate normality. (b) Many inferential statistics assume a normal distribution is present. (c) The normal curve is a probability distribution and addresses the likelihood of deriving a particular outcome when sampling from the population that is normally distributed. In many cases, health care data are not normally distributed and must be handled appropriately using nonparametric statistics or other analytic methods. We refer the reader to more advanced discussions of statistics for determining appropriate methods for analysis, but address normality as it is an important consideration for analysts to understand and consider.

Selecting the Right Statistical Test

Relationships derived from research questions to statistical tests must be understood and easily articulated by the researcher. A research question allows those interested in a given research study to have a clear understanding of the study purpose, that is, what problem the study aims to address and/or solve. However, many components of the research question, such as the independent and dependent variables, level of measure, the operational definition, the statistic, and the power analysis, are needed to correctly analyze the question. Table 18.3 illustrates the documentation of these important components. The figure reads from the left of the grid as the beginning of the process with each research question, and moves to the right with the power analysis parameters, and the targeted sample size is listed. Representing these statistical plan details ensures all team members understand steps leading to the study results.

This chapter is not intended to replace a comprehensive text on statistical methods, but instead highlights some decisions that analysts need to think through when selecting the correct statistical test. The authors also want to address differences in enumerative studies

TABLE 18.3 Statistical Analysis Plan (Template With Example)

Gray = Example

Questions/Hypotheses	Independent Variable (IV)[a]	IV Level of Data[b]	Dependent Variable (DV)[c]	DV Level of Data[d]	Covariate(s)	Operational Definitions[e]	Statistical Test	Power Analysis[f]
1. Is there a difference in patient portal use within 2 weeks of instruction based on the type of instruction provided?	Type of instruction: (a) handout with one-on-one verbal instruction (intervention group), or (b) handout alone (control group)	Nominal	Patient portal use within 2 weeks of instruction: yes or no	Nominal	Not applicable	IV: random assignment for either intervention (a) or control group (b) DV presence of a registration of the patient on the patient portal within 2 weeks of instruction	Chi square 2 × 2 analysis	88 participants in each of the two groups are needed for Power of 80%, an alpha of 0.05, and medium effect size
[Type in your actual research question 1 here]								
[Type in your actual research question 2 here]								
[Click Tab key to create more rows]								

[a]Example, intervention, and factor such as study group categories, etc.
[b]Nominal, ordinal, scale, or ratio (Pallant, 2010).
[c]Example, outcome, change over time, etc.
[d]Nominal, ordinal, scale, or ratio (Pallant, 2010).
[e]Example, score for instruments used in study, physiologic parameter such as weight in pounds, or time in minutes, etc.
[f]*Source:* G*Power software program retrieved from www.gpower.hhu.de/en.html

Source: Mari Tietze.

and analytic studies. Enumerative studies are done to develop generalizable evidence and involve hypothesis testing methods. However, analytic studies improve science and seek to improve a process. Analytic studies often predict outcomes and measure processes that impact an outcome of interest (Langley, Nolan, Nolan, Norman, & Provost, 2009). When determining which statistical test, or in the case of quality-improvement projects, which control to utilize to measure a process, the level of measurement for the independent and dependent variables is one of the first considerations. The second and equally important consideration is what one is trying to do. Are you comparing or contrasting, examining relationships or associations, or attempting to explain or predict an outcome of interest? Statistical textbooks often have visual decision trees that an analyst can use to walk through the selection process to choose the correct statistic, and we highly recommend soliciting the expertise of a biostatistician or PhD-prepared researcher to assist with these decisions. Important questions to be considered when using one of these tools or in preparation for working with a researcher and biostatistician are as follows:

▶ How many outcome variables do you have?

▶ What are the types of outcome variable(s)?

▶ How many predictor variable(s) are there?

▶ What types of predictor variable(s) are there?

▶ If a categorical predictor, how many categories are there?

▶ If a categorical predictor, are same or different participants used in each category?

▶ Do data meet assumptions for parametric tests?

It is advisable to design a tabular view of the dependent and independent variables that contains all variables and the value sets that correlate with the variables. Table 18.4 offers an example of the analytic study examining obstetrical outcomes for primary cesarean delivery, which supports the study highlighted earlier and examines the effect of inductions on primary cesarean delivery. It should be noted that the table clearly outlines the measure name, definition, including the level of measurement, the source data, and value labels (also called "value sets"). The researcher/analyst has assigned numeric values to each of the categories of data. For example, gestational age of the mother will be measured based on gestational age categories with 1 to 6 assigned to gestational weeks 37 to 42, respectively, and these data are derived from the birth certificate (BC) data files. Further, one can determine from this table that the analytic study will not include preterm or post-term deliveries. One should consider how the health outcomes model noted in Figure 18.2 helped inform the tabular view of data to fully operationalize how the researcher/analyst intends to study the outcome of primary cesarean delivery (dependent variable) while controlling for factors (independent variables) that influence the outcome (McBride, 2005).

Control Chart

Processes in health care are variable. One will always get the same result each time because of numerous contributing factors, including patients' comorbidities. There are sources of variation in all processes that can be addressed with appropriate analysis, and one

TABLE 18.4 Operational Definitions of Independent Variables Impacting Primary Cesarean Delivery-Dependent Variables

Measure Name	Definition	Source	Value Labels	Values
Nulliparity	Calculated field from the BC gravida = bclive + bcdead + 1, nulliparous is defined as gravida 1	BC data	Yes	1
			No	0
Gestational age	Calculated field from the BC estimated gestation field	BC data	37 weeks	1
			38 weeks	2
			39 weeks	3
			40 weeks	4
			41 weeks	5
			42 weeks	6
Fetal distress	Dichotomous variable	HDD	Yes	1
			No	0
Dystocia/failure to progress	Dichotomous variable	HDD	Yes	1
			No	0
Medical indication for induction	Dichotomous variable	HDD	Yes	1
			No	0
Baby's birth weight	Continuous variable	BC data		
Demographics				
Race/ethnicity	Categorical variable concatenated from HDD	HDD	White	1
			Black	2
			Hispanic	3
			Other	4

(continued)

TABLE 18.4 Operational Definitions of Independent Variables Impacting Primary Cesarean Delivery-Dependent Variables *(continued)*				
Measure Name	**Definition**	**Source**	**Value Labels**	**Values**
Payer	Field created by combining the standard and nonstandard payer codes from the HDD to represent the patient's primary payer, reduced to two categories.	HDD	Private Insurance	1
			Other	2
Maternal age	Continuous variable			11–53 years

BC, birth certificate; HDD, hospital discharge data.

Source: McBride (2005).

way of examining a process and accounting for common-cause variation involves control charts. There are two sources of variation identified in processes that are referred to as common-cause and special-cause variation. Common-cause variation is variation that is inherent in the process itself, and it is also called "noise" or random variation. Special-cause variation is variation in a process identified by one or more data points varying in an unpredictable manner from a cause that is not inherent in the process. "A signal the process has changed for better or worse" (Carey, 2003, p. 7). A process is in statistical control only if common-cause variation is present.

One way to determine whether a process in health care is in control is through use of control charts. A control chart represents a picture of a process over time. To effectively use control charts, the analyst must be able to interpret the chart. The analyst may be able to ask questions such as: What is this control chart telling me about my process? Is this picture telling me that everything is all right and there is no reason for concern or is this picture telling me that something is wrong and I should intervene? In addition, you may have changed a process over time and want to know whether the intervention had a statistical change over time. If you initiated an improvement, did you hold the gain of that improvement? Control charts help answer these important questions for health care clinicians and analysts. We refer the reader to further discussion on control charts and the selection of appropriate control charts in Chapter 21.

ANALYTICS AND BI TOOLS

There are various tools that can be applied to health care data to make sense of patterns and trends within the data set. These types of analyses are typically categorized under a BI set of applications and software products. *BI*, as defined by Adams and Garets in

Gensinger's text *Analytics in Health Care: An Introduction* is as follows: "BI refers to the processes and technologies used to obtain timely, valuable insights into business and clinical data" (Adams & Garets, 2014, p. 15). According to these two authors, BI can be broken into three categories: descriptive, predictive, and prescriptive. They base this on work originally done by the Advisory Board Company, noting these three dimensions. Within the descriptive component are reports, graphs, dashboards, drill-down reports, and alerts. Predictive analytics involves predictive models based on some outcomes such as mortality or 30-day readmissions to the hospital. Predictive analytics also includes forecasts and simulated events. However, prescriptive domains include mathematical models, linear programming, and constraint programming. Each of these domains has escalating levels of complexity and requires higher levels of competencies, with descriptive analysis noted as the most basic of analysis, but very necessary and useful; and prescriptive as some of the more advanced and more complex. Prescriptive analysis models establish possible decisions or steps in a process given a set of data or parameters presented. This area of analysis falls into the field of advanced analytics referred to as "cognitive computing," meaning the computer thinks in a way similar to how human beings process information. This area of analysis is covered more detail in Chapter 26. According to Adams and Garets, prescriptive analysis is not widely used in health care to date, but it will likely demonstrate the most impact in areas such as cognitive support for physicians and other practitioners (Adams & Garets, 2014, pp. 17–19). To accomplish generating "business intelligence," there are a number of tools and software applications within the marketplace that can be used.

Spreadsheet Applications

Common tools available to most organizations are common spreadsheet applications such as the Microsoft Excel software available on most desktop and laptop computers. Excel is an excellent tool that is used to prepare data for analysis and to explore data. It can also be used to do statistical analysis with very basic features. To perform basic statistical analysis, an add-in feature must be activated within the software. Excel can perform pivot table analyses, graphics and charts, iterative visualizations, and many other features that are useful to analysts. Graphics and charts are relatively easy to use in Excel with a point-and-click approach. Select the icon reflecting the chart desired, provide Excel with parameters you want within the chart, and the program generates graphics on an additional tab or within the working spreadsheet. To activate the Data Analysis ToolPak in Excel, the following should be performed according to instructions provided in Excel: If the Analysis Toolpak is not installed, go to the File tab and select "Options" in the left column. In the Excel Options Window, select the "Add-Ins" category on the left. Near the bottom of this window, you see Excel Add-ins already selected in a drop-down menu labeled "Manage." Click the "Go" button next to this drop-down (TechNet Magazine, 2014). A Mac version called Stats Plus is available at no cost. Figure 18.8 reflects the Excel screen image noting where these items are within the software.

Statistical Packages

Statistical packages allow extension from basic analysis to analysis, including inferential statistics. Three of the most common such software programs are IBM SPSS, SAS,

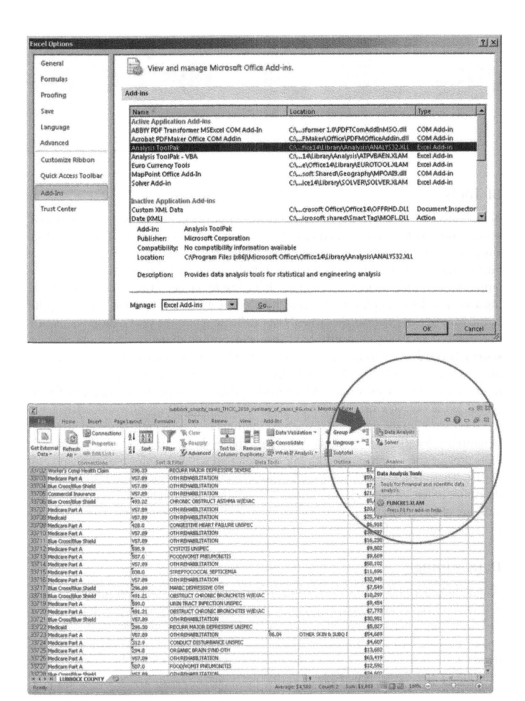

FIGURE 18.8. Add-in analysis Toolpak in Excel.

Note: Once you activate the Add-In to Excel, the data analysis package is activated.

and Stata. "R" is an open-source statistical computing program that is gaining popularity (The R Project for Statistical Computing, 2014). In addition to features that promote data cleaning, validation, and organization, these programs conduct statistical tests such as correlations, regression, *t*-test, and factor analysis, among many others.

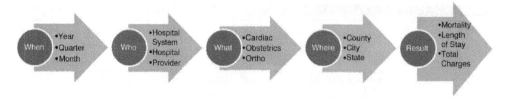

FIGURE 18.9. Setting up multidimensional analyses with BI tools.

BI Tools

BI tools are a set of software applications that typically help inform one's business as to profitability, quality, risk, and other factors that indicate how well one is doing within any given industry. Often, these tools allow multidimensional analysis that is aimed at hitting "the sweet spot" in one's data. A multidimensional business analyst thinks in terms of when, who, what, where, and result. Figure 18.9 reflects this dimensional thinking and provides examples of what might constitute a BI multidimensional strategy for health care. In this example, the "when" is an ability to report the year, quarter, or month. The "who" is an ability to stratify or filter one's report on dimensions such as hospital system, hospital, or a specific provider. The "what" would be similar functionality allowing an organization to filter or stratify using different specialty services. The "where" feature allows one to look at data and reports by patient's county, city, or state. Finally, the "what" is the outcome measures the organization seeks to determine that truly get to the "sweet spot" in the data. In this example, authors note frequently reported measures of mortality, length of stay, and total charges. The sweet spot in these types of analytic tools provide the organization with information that will help inform quality and cost of care. These types of tools are excellent for driving improvement and mining data to determine where an organization is doing well and where it might need to improve. The tools are often easy to track, trend, filter, drag, and drop by point and click of a mouse to quickly mine the data for the information needed to inform the organization.

Data Mining

Data mining is an effective way of using data to inform the business or quality strategy within an organization. There are many different tools and approaches to mining data, and the example noted earlier on multidimensional analysis is very relevant to data mining. By filtering data and examining trends, an analyst can quickly identify patterns and trends in the data that might direct the analyst to a place to look for the "sweet spot." A clinical example of that is noted next in the case study.

SUMMARY

Data analysis, an important component for understanding today's complex health care delivery system, affects provider, vendor/suppler, and payer/insurers. Given that the provider's data analysis directly affects patient care delivery, we have focused on the critical aspects for consideration. As noted in the previously described Nursing Education for Health Care Informatics (NEHI) model (McBride, Tietze, & Fenton, 2013), data management and analytics, linked with patient safety, quality, and point-of-care technology create the culminating process through which optimum health care improvement may occur. This chapter provides the specifics for supporting analytic skills development.

EXERCISES AND QUESTIONS FOR CONSIDERATION

The Excel image (Figure 18.10) comes from an existing data set of patients with type 2 diabetes who were hospitalized in 2012. The StatPak feature was used to create the associated descriptives. Using the following chart, please respond to the following questions:

1. What is the total count of case records?
2. What is the standard deviation of the total charge for hospitalization?
3. What is the median total charge?
4. What is the mode for the total charge?
5. What is the overall sum for total charges?
6. What is the maximum total charge?

Total Charges	
Mean	27,424.85594
Standard error	569.5811108
Median	19,500.92
Mode	1,531.6
Standard deviation	28,261.78593
Sample variance	798,728,544.1
Kurtosis	27.59007693
Skewness	4.193621611
Range	380,457.76
Minimum	0
Maximum	380,457.76
Sum	67,519,995.32
Count	2,462

FIGURE 18.10. Complete list of variables for total charges.
Source: Output from Microsoft Excel StatPak Add-In.

CASE STUDY

> **Activity: Describe How This Situation May or May Not Be Present in Your Organization and Why**
>
> A hospital has just been publicly reported as using its state regulatory hospital discharge data. The data have been risk adjusted to control for comordities that the patient may have entered the hospital with to effectively "level the playing field" for comparative reporting of hospitals. When your hospital's report comes, you note that you risk adjusted poorly for stroke mortality. Your hospital has just received stroke center designation and you feel confident that best practice protocols with stroke management are being followed. The analyst tracks and trends your mortality data on stroke and you note a spike in mortalities for a given quarter, which appears to be why your state public report is unsatisfactory.
>
> Drilling into the data to examine the numerators (deaths) due to stroke (denomonator and total patient population), your analyst determines that the risk of mortality has a score of 1 to 4, with 1 being a minor risk of mortality and 4 being severe. All the deaths that occurred as a result of stroke had a minor risk of mortality. Clearly, this is why the hospital did not risk adjust well, as these patients did not appear to have any risks associated with severe illness that would reasonably explain the mortalities. Next, the analyst drills further into the detailed subject-oriented data of actual patient records, followed by a full chart review to obtain the "sweet spot" that would inform improvement.
>
> Consider the following questions:
>
> 1. Would the analyst be examining aggregate, detailed data, or both in investigating this quality issue?
> 2. Would the analyst likely use a retrospective data warehouse, clinical data store, or both to investigate the mortality rate?
> 3. What type of tools or analytic approaches do you believe this analyst might use?

REFERENCES

Adams, J., & Garets, D. (2014). The healthcare analytics evolution: Moving from descriptive to predictive to prescriptive. In R. A. Gensinger (Ed.), *Analytics in healthcare: An introduction* (pp. 13–20). Chicago, IL: Health Information Management Systems Society.

Carey, R. G. (2003). *Improving healthcare with control charts: Basic and advanced SPC methods and case studies*. Milwaukee, WI: ASQ Quality Press.

Centers for Disease Control and Prevention. (2015). *International classification of diseases, tenth revision, clinical modification (ICD-10-CM)*. Retrieved from http://www.cdc.gov/nchs/icd/icd10cm.htm

Centers for Medicare & Medicaid Services. (2014). *International classification of diseases, (ICD-10-CM/PCS) transition: Frequently asked questions*. Retrieved from http://www.cdc.gov/nchs/icd/icd10cm_pcs_faq.htm

Database. (n.d.). In *Merriam-Webster's online dictionary*. Retrieved from http://www.merriam-webster.com/dictionary/database

Davenport, T. H. (2005). *Competing on analytics* (No. R0601H). Boston, MA: Harvard Business School.

Donabedian, A. (1966). Evaluating the quality of medical care. *Milbank Memorial Fund Quarterly*, 44, 166–206.

Englebardt, S. P., & Nelson, R. (2002). *Healthcare informatics: An interdisciplinary approach*. Independence, KY: Gale, Cengage Learning.

Hosmer, D., & Lemeshow, S. (2000). *Applied logistic regression* (2nd ed.). New York, NY: John Wiley & Sons.

Imhoff, C., Galemmo, N., & Geiger, J. (2003). *Mastering data warehouse design: Relational and dimensional techniques*. New York, NY: John Wiley & Sons.

Krebs, D. E. (1987). Measurement theory. *Physical Therapy*, 67(12), 1834–1839.

Langley, G. J., Nolan, K. M., Nolan, T. W., Norman, L., & Provost, L. P. (2009). *The improvement guide: A practical approach to enhancing organizational performance* (2nd ed.). San Francisco, CA: Jossey-Bass.

McBride, S. (2005). *The effect of induction of labor on the odds of cesarean delivery* (Unpublished doctoral dissertation). Texas Woman's University, Denton, TX.

McBride, S., Fenton, S., Valdes, M., & Gilder, R. (2013). *Transforming digital data into useful information. TNA-TONE Health IT Committee Educational Series*. Retrieved from http://www.texasnurses.org/?page=HITWebinars2013

McBride, S. G., Gilder, R., Davis, R., & Fenton, S. (2006). Data mapping. *Journal of the American Health Information Management Association*, 77(2), 44–48.

McBride, S. G., Tietze, M., & Fenton, M. V. (2013). Developing an applied informatics course for a doctor of nursing practice program. *Nurse Educator*, 38(1), 37–42. doi:10.1097/NNE.0b013e318276df5d

Munro, B. H. (2005). *Statistical methods for health care research* (5th ed.). Philadelphia, PA: Lippincott Williams & Wilkins.

Pallant, J. (2010). *SPSS survival manual: A step by step guide to data analysis using SPSS* (4th ed.). Maidenhead, UK: Open University Press/McGraw-Hill.

The R Project for Statistical Computing. (n.d.). *Getting started*. Retrieved from https://www.r-project.org/

Stevens, S. S. (1959). *Measurement, psychophysics and utility*. In P. Churchman & C. W. Ratoush (Eds.), *Measurement: Definitions and theories*. New York, NY: John Wiley and Sons.

TechNet Magazine. (2014). *Install the analysis toolpak for Excel 2010*. Retrieved from http://www.technet.microsoft.com/en-us/magazine/ff969363.aspx

Tufte, E. R. (2001). *The visual display of quantitative information* (2nd ed.). Chesshire, CT: Graphics Press.

Variable. (n.d.). In *Merriam-Webster's online dictionary*. Retrieved from http://www.merriam-webster.com/dictionary/variable

Waltz, C. F., Strickland, O. L., & Lenz, E. R. (2010). *Measurement in nursing and health research* (4th ed.). New York, NY: Springer Publishing Company.

CHAPTER 19

Clinical Decision Support Systems

Maxine Ketcham, Susan McBride, Mari Tietze, and Joni Padden

OBJECTIVES

1. Define clinical decision support system (CDSS) programs and discuss the importance of developing major goals and objectives to clinical decision support (CDS) programs.

2. Discuss key ingredients for successful CDSS and interventions associated with improved outcomes.

3. Describe and apply a structured methodology for using CDS interventions to improve outcomes examining the American Heart Association Million Hearts Campaign for improving cardiovascular (CV) health outcomes.

4. Describe Arden Syntax and how it is used to standardize approaches to CDS.

5. Explain common issues and barriers to appropriate use of CDS and evidence to address the barriers and common challenges.

6. Analyze CDS in light of Stages 1 and 2 of meaningful use (MU) and strategies to building CDS using patient-centered outcomes resource.

7. Discuss the importance of effective interprofessional teams and resources available to support deployment of methods described.

8. Examine case studies that provide strategies for bringing specific CDS performance improvement into organizations with a systematic and structured approach.

KEY WORDS

clinical decision support system, clinical decision support, Arden Syntax, workflow redesign, patient-centered outcomes research, Million Hearts Campaign, best practice alerts

CONTENTS

INTRODUCTION

The Office of the National Coordinator for Health Information Technology (ONC-HIT) defines *clinical decision support* (CDS) as "a process designed to aid directly in clinical decision making, in which characteristics of individual patients are used to generate patient specific interventions, assessments, recommendations, or other forms of guidance that are then presented to a decision making recipient or recipients that can include clinicians, patients, and others involved in care delivery" (HealthIT.gov, 2014, p. 1). In addition, CDS is a tool constructed within the electronic health record (EHR), triggering alerts that encourage the health care team to do the right thing at the right time with correct interventions within the clinical workflow. This simple explanation presents a challenge with CDS, because it is not always a simple thing to ensure the alerts are set up correctly in the EHR to support the clinician with an efficient process in the workflow of daily life. To do that, one must set up a process of CDS to strategically design a program using the EHR as a tool to enhance patient safety, quality, and population health. For these reasons, CDS is a key strategy within the federal Health Information Technology for Economic Clinical Health (HITECH) Act that is used for attaining meaningful use (MU) of EHRs.

CDS is one of the key strategies built into the MU guidelines and is threaded throughout the three stages of MU with escalating complexity with each stage. CDS is a tool that can be very effective at improving outcomes in many areas, including improving protocol adherence such as deep vein thrombosis (DVT) prophylaxis, cardiac mortality prevention strategies outlined in the Million Hearts Campaign, and in areas associated with the regulatory reporting requirements of quality measures. We examine some of these use cases in light of the methods described and discuss the use of CDS within the MU guidelines and the reasons for this emphasis within the federal regulations. In addition, we discuss challenges and issues that arise with inappropriate use of CDS in organizations. CDS is a powerful tool; however, without design strategies, CDS can result in misuse, creating potential patient safety and legal implications for organizations. We discuss design strategies to address these challenges through a strategic approach to CDS deployment within organizations and how to adhere to best practices to improve interventions and patient outcomes that will help mitigate these issues. Finally, we use case studies to demonstrate the use of these methods in clinical examples, which include aligning CDS with patient-centered outcomes research.

THE BASICS OF CDS

CDS tools existed prior to development of EHRs. Historical examples include practice guidelines carried in clinicians' pockets, patient cards used by providers to track a patient's treatments, and tables of important medical knowledge (Clinfowiki.org, 2015). The Oregon Health & Science University (OHSU) houses the Clinical Informatics Wiki (a.k.a. ClinfoWiki), a website devoted to topics in biomedical informatics. Many of these CDS tools continue to be relevant to the electronic age of health care, but they do so by integrating CDS within the EHRs, presenting an opportunity for the various types of decision support to be immediately available within the workflow at the time of the clinical decision-making process. CDS can be more relevant and accurate, can facilitate, and can be integrated within clinical workflow when designed well and deployed effectively. It is this innovative use of technology that increases the magnitude of CDS on patient care with respect to patient safety and quality. We examine the basics of a CDS program that helps organizations achieve success with CDS.

CDS: Definitions, Goals, and Objectives

Business decision support systems focus on financial metrics and models, whereas CDS focuses on health care outcomes and triggering clinicians to follow best practices and evidence-based guidelines. The word "support" in the term "CDS" points to the fundamental goals of CDS. CDS is an informatics term that involves technology to aid decision making, guiding the end user through complex systems to achieve a targeted outcome (Health Information and Management Systems Society [HIMSS], 2011). When used effectively, the specific build of the technology can make using a system easier and more clinically relevant for the end user. CDS is not meant to make decisions for the clinician, but rather to make clinical decisions easier or clearer by offering evidence-based choices determined by practice standards, regulatory compliance elements, current literature, and other determinants. The authors caution the end user of CDS to beware the myopic view that CDS consists of simply evidence-based order sets or hard-stop best practice alerts (BPAs). This view of CDS is short-sighted and does not allow for the full scope of what CDS can do to help clinicians and health care systems achieve higher quality standards, cost-efficient care, improved patient safety, and better compliance with regulatory reporting. CDS can help achieve these goals for an organization if the tools employed are well designed and user friendly.

The primary goal of a CDS program is to leverage data and the scientific evidence to help guide appropriate decision making. When looking at ways in which CDS tools can be leveraged in a clinical process, the CDS team needs to approach the project from a data-driven manner supported by the evidence. This requires in-depth analysis of the scientific evidence coupled with data-analysis methods to identify gaps in practice within the organization. It is equally important to identify where there are gaps in ability to report how an organization is doing with respect to patient care and whether or not recommended practice guidelines are being followed. This would constitute absence of data captured to track that information. Often, these gaps or absence of data and information tell an organization where to focus with respect to adding where a CDS tool should be. It is the role of the CDS team to identify all of the elements of a process and use data to identify areas where processes might be enhanced with the use of CDS tools to provide users with the best evidence and to support appropriate decision making and treatment decisions (HIMSS, 2014c).

For example, CDS can reinforce protocols established nationally to address patient safety, quality, and population health. Vaccination adherence is one example that is useful to consider, particularly given that vaccinations have become controversial as a public health issue, with many families electing not to vaccinate because of personal beliefs about vaccination safety (Lieu, Ray, Klein, Chung, & Kulldorff, 2015). However, there are national quality measures that health care providers and hospitals are expected to report and to perform well on with respect to adhering to vaccination protocols (National Quality Forum, 2008). In the event one's organization resides in a community with large numbers of individuals who reject vaccinations, one's institution will appear to perform poorly related to federal guidelines on vaccination unless data are captured that indicate "patient refuses vaccination." In this example, if an institution's quality goal is to achieve 100% compliance with influenza screening, vaccination, and required reporting, the CDS tools would be designed to support the entire process to reinforce quality and efficiency, not just to provide data capture for regulatory and reporting requirements. In this example, not only would the workflow of the clinicians be supported with efficiency, but also the screening tool would be designed to lead the clinician to the correct orders for the patients and to trigger the best decision on behalf of the patient given certain clinical criteria such as evidence to suggest a vaccination is necessary. The data would be captured in such a way that those patients for whom the vaccine was not indicated or who refused vaccination would also be captured so that compliance with the measure is accurate and easily reportable. In addition, when data are captured in a structured format, the reporting tools generating data from the EHR can also alert leadership when measures are not being met so that improvement strategies can be launched to address poor performance. It is not the job of the EHR or CDS to enforce compliance, but instead to make compliance with evidence-based protocols easier and more accurately reportable. Goals of a CDS program to address adherence to an influenza protocol would be to:

1. Use the relevant data and information on the patient to determine whether the patient meets the clinical requirements for vaccination

2. Note any contraindications for vaccination

3. Document reasons for not administering the vaccination for a patient meeting clinical criteria within the protocol, such as refusal of the vaccination

4. Capture the data in a structured format by the clinician to trigger the alerts based on the protocol

5. Structure data and information to document compliance with the regulatory requirements and to support quality improvement (QI)

6. Align workflow of the clinicians during assessment and treatment with efficient administration of vaccinations as necessary (Texas Health Resources, 2014)

Because the CDS tools often have unintended consequences, such as leading clinicians to think there is no alternative but what is suggested by the CDS tool, it is the responsibility of the CDS team to keep the process transparent so these kinds of pitfalls can be foreseen and avoided. If it is the intention of the tool to eliminate alternatives to a process, that too must be vetted by the clinicians during the design process. By making it easy to do the right thing at the right time, CDS tools support safe practice. However, this does not negate the need for clinicians to know what is safe or unsafe but instead helps make the safe choices clearly evident to the user within the documentation (Institute of Medicine [IOM], 2012).

STRATEGIES FOR IMPLEMENTING A SUCCESSFUL CDS PROGRAM

First and foremost, the CDS program must be strategically aligned with the mission, vision, and values of the organization (Kendall & Kendall, 2014). Successful CDS implementation requires a balance among people, process, and technology. The people aspect of this balance is not only the most important but also the most challenging. To drive the necessary changes, it is crucial to have engagement and buy-in at the top levels of the executive team and to permeate that support at all levels of the organization. Because CDS programs involve changes in process and workflow, the CDS team must involve the stakeholders who are the most impacted by the process redesign and strategically design the technology component using the EHR functionality appropriately. Key strategies for success with CDS share common themes with other success strategies and align with recommendations outlined in Chapter 8 dealing with the systems development life cycle. These strategies include the following:

1. Ensure the right stakeholders participate in the process.
2. Understand the full process before beginning to design CDS solutions and tools.
3. Recognize that documentation cannot solve problems but it can make solutions easier; conversely, it can also further exacerbate issues.
4. CDS leaders must be strong enough to do what is right instead of what is easy. Often, addressing an issue means an enormous amount of work in the background where the user only sees a slight change in the EHR.
5. Resources should be considered and justify the need for the CDS. Sometimes, it takes a complete rebuild to help address an issue.
6. Stakeholders need to be engaged throughout the process, not just at the beginning.
7. Ensure that design, vetting the build, testing, and evaluation/follow-up after installation must be done with the frontline users.
8. Ensure that leadership and the groups using the data for reporting and outcomes tracking must also be engaged in the process to verify that the strategic goals of the organization are met, as well as the needs of patients and clinicians.
9. Recognize that the CDS team needs to understand the strategic goals before designing a process with the frontline clinicians. All too often, what is done in day-to-day practice is not what is spelled out in policy or called for by regulation (Kendall & Kendall, 2014).

Characteristics and Elements of a Successful CDS Team

A successful CDS program requires builders who understand clinical relevance of the care being addressed by the CDS and relevant workflows and processes (Osheroff et al., 2012). The ideal situation is to have builders who are also clinicians and who understand the workflow. The CDS team members should mirror the roles in the organization they are designing support tools for, meaning if the team is going to support physicians, nurses, and other allied health professionals, the CDS team should have those same clinicians represented on the team. Problems quickly emerge when physicians try to design processes for nurses, or vice versa. Crucial disconnects occur when the builder and the user do not speak the same language, in this case health care-specific terminology. Even among health care providers, the terms used by a neonatal nurse may be very different from those used by a geriatric oncology nurse. Based on the authors' experience, these kinds of disconnects must be identified and eliminated.

Translation between technical information technology (IT) people and clinicians is more of an art than a science. From the experience of the authors working with interprofessional teams on CDS, a program requires leaders who have the ability to clearly translate between "IT speak" and clinical terminology. Figure 19.1 notes the importance of a team approach to the success of a program. Simple terms, such as "close," can cause huge confusion if not clearly defined in the group using the term. For example, the IT builder thinks "close" means to collapse or not see all of something. The surgeon thinks "close" means to finish the task. The nurse thinks "close" means to go to the next task. There needs to be facilitation by the CDS team to ensure every stakeholder fully understands the terms and functionality of the tools being developed and deployed. As users become more savvy with functionality and IT terminology, this process will improve

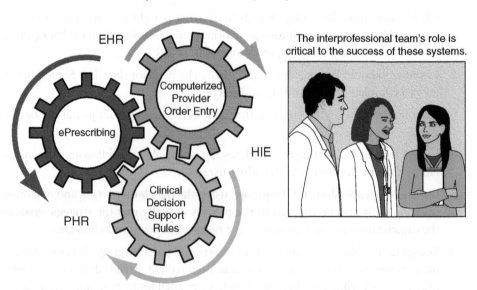

FIGURE 19.1. Interprofessional teams and CDS.

but the need to clarify so that all team members understand will always be needed. This facilitation often includes educating users as to what the systems can and cannot do. Many clinicians think the computer can do whatever they want it to do and are surprised to learn that there are limitations within any software. From the experiences of the authors, a key role of nursing informatics (NI) is to be able to clearly articulate to end users what CDS can and cannot do effectively.

For example, the group of stakeholders wants there to be a hard stop in an order. The CDS builder needs to be able to articulate that putting the hard stop in place will cause the order to function differently than an order without a hard stop. From the authors' experience, often clinicians think they want something until they learn what the downside of their request is. Once again, this is an important role that the nursing informaticist plays: Educating stakeholders on the capabilities of the system before asking them to make design decisions. Often, clinicians will ask for what is familiar to them instead of what the system is capable of doing for them. The CDS team needs to understand the goals for a project so they can recommend the best ways for the system to support the users in meeting their objectives. Mismanagement of tools, such as BPAs, will lead to fatigue and, ultimately, cause more to be missed than caught because of users ignoring alerts. The CDS team is responsible for addressing this kind of poor decision support to do a better job of making the right thing easy instead of overly relying on reminders or alerts. As sociotechnical theory would indicate, a truly successful CDS process is experienced by the end user as a seamless and unobtrusive process while still guiding the end user to the safest, best choices (IOM, 2012, p. 77).

Frameworks for Success

Bates and colleagues have outlined a framework for effective CDS that they refer to as the "10 commandments" for success. The framework is noted in Table 19.1, and it includes recommendations on timeliness, end-user needs, addressing resistance, simplicity, monitoring impact, and managing the system based on the evidence. These factors

TABLE 19.1 Success Factors for CDS

1. Speed is everything.
2. Anticipate needs and deliver in real time.
3. Fit into the user's workflow.
4. Little things can make a big difference.
5. Recognize that physicians will strongly resist stopping.
6. Changing directions is easier than stopping.
7. Simple interventions work best.
8. Ask for additional information only when you really need it.
9. Monitor impact, get feedback, and respond.
10. Manage and maintain your knowledge-based systems.

CDS, clinical decision support.

Adapted from Bates et al. (2003).

TABLE 19.2 Five-Rights Framework for Success of CDS	
Category	Definition
Right information	Evidence-based and actionable information constitute the "what" of the CDS program.
Right person	Clinicians and the patient constitute the correct individuals impacted by the CDS program, identifying the "who."
Right CDS intervention format	The tools that include documents/forms, data display, answers, order sets, algorithms, and alerts define the "how."
Right channel	The vehicle for delivering the CDS program, such as within the EHR, or supporting technology, such as smartphones or dashboards, reflect the "where."
Right point in the workflow	The process within which the clinical care is delivered that will be impacted by the CDS program comprising the workflow for redesign using CDS outlining and diagraming constitute the "when."

CDS, clinical decision support.

Source: Osheroff et al. (2012).

reinforce end-user acceptance as well as best practices for seeking best evidence to inform patient care through use of safe, efficient, and effective CDS strategies (Bates et al., 2003).

An organizing framework that includes five components has been outlined (Osheroff et al., 2012). These components involve the right information, right person, right CDS intervention format, right channel, and right timing or points in the workflow. We refer the reader to Osheroff et al.'s text as an excellent resource for designing strategic CDS programs, tools, and best practices to help an organization successfully implement a CDS program. Table 19.2 reflects these five rights and provides definitions and examples of what these rights constitute within a CDS program. These five rights address the who, what, where, when, and how of a CDS program while emphasizing the importance of clear articulation of goals and objectives that identify all five components (Osheroff et al., 2012).

TOOLS AND TYPES OF CDS

CDS encompasses a wide variety of tools, including, but not limited to, computerized alerts and reminders for providers and patients, drug–drug interaction alerts, underdose or overdose alerts based on renal or liver function or age or drug levels, actionable clinical guidelines, condition-specific order sets, focused patient data reports and summaries, documentation templates, diagnostic support, and contextually relevant reference information (HIMSS, 2014a). Table 19.3 includes a description of some of the most commonly used tools used within CDS programs.

According to Osheroff et al. (2012), another consideration for CDS is when and how the data needed to support decision making are presented. An example noted is patient-specific data of relevant labs such as the results of a patient's renal and liver function during computer provider order entry (CPOE) of medications that might be contraindicated based on certain lab results. Population-specific data are also used; for example, microbiograms, which are tables of local bacterial flora and their sensitivity and susceptibility to various antibiotics, can be used for CDS.

CDS functionalities may be deployed on a variety of platforms (e.g., mobile, cloud based, or locally installed). CDS is not intended to replace clinician or patient judgment but is deployed as a tool to assist care team members in making timely, informed, higher quality decisions. CDS is frequently not only an integrated part of the provider's EHR but may also be present in a variety of other technologies such as pharmacy systems, patients' personal health records (PHRs), or patient portals. Some providers use CDS as a "service" by securely sending patient information to a registry, implementing cloud-based CDS interventions or using forecaster programs that can provide a response back about what treatments or diagnostic testing might be appropriate for the patient (Osheroff et al., 2012).

ARDEN SYNTAX

Arden Syntax is a standardized executable format and is currently maintained by Health Level 7 (HL7). Arden Syntax has a number of advantages, including its usefulness in practical application of CDS systems, the readability of the syntax, flexibility of the standard, and its ability to be actively developed under the HL7 standards group (see Chapter 12 on standards for a discussion of this oversight function; Samwald, Fehre, de Bruin, & Adlassnig, 2012a).

Arden Syntax is considered a hybrid between classical production rules and procedural representation of clinical algorithms. Medical logic modules (MLMs) are self-contained files that organize the code into independent modules. The specific code behind the MLM can be triggered by an executable code or a time-based event (Samwald et al., 2012a). The standard was first introduced in 1989 and adopted by ASTM in 1992, followed by HL7 and ANSI (American National Standards Institute) adoption in 1999. The Arden Syntax and the MLMs make knowledge portable, whereas MLMs developed for one environment are not necessarily portable into another. Many of the EHR vendors are adopting this standard for CDS embedded into their own environments. The user of the Arden Syntax is the clinician. It provides specific links to data, trigger events, and messages that can provide time functions. This is particularly important to CDS, because so many of the triggers relate to "the time" something should or should not have happened given the parameters of the patient's condition or treatment protocols needed (Openclinical .org,[1] 2013). Figure 19.2 reflects how Arden Syntax works within a host system and

---

[1]OpenClinical is an international organization created to promote awareness and use of decision support, clinical workflow, and other advanced knowledge management technologies for patient care and clinical research.

TABLE 19.3 Types of CDS Tools With Descriptions

Types of CDS	Description
Smart documentation forms	Forms that are tailored based on patient data to emphasize data elements pertinent to the patient's conditions and health care needs
Order sets, care plans, and protocols	Structured approaches to encourage correct and efficient ordering, promote evidence-based best practices, and provide different management recommendations for different patient situations
Parameter guidance	Algorithms to promote correct entry of orders and documentation
Critiques and "immediate" warnings	Alerts that are presented just after a user has entered an order, prescription, or documentation item, to show a potential hazard, or a recommendation for further information
Relevant data summaries	A single-patient view that summarizes, organizes, and filters a patient's information to highlight important management issues
Multipatient monitors	A display of activity among all patients on a care unit, which helps providers prioritize tasks and ensures that important activities are not omitted while providers are multitasking among patients
Predictive and retrospective analytics	Analytic methods that combine multiple factors using statistical and/or artificial intelligence techniques to provide risk predictions, stratify patients, and measure progress on broad initiatives
"Info" buttons	Filtered reference information and knowledge resources within fields or "buttons" where information is provided to the end user in the context of the current data display, also referred to as metadata, or "data about data"
Expert workup and management advisors	Diagnostic and expert systems that track and advise a patient workup and management of the patient based on evidence-based protocols
Event-triggered alerts	Warnings triggered within the system based on data that alert the clinical user to a new event occurring asynchronously, such as an abnormal lab result
Reminders	Time-triggered events within the system reminding the clinical user of a task needed based on predetermined time within the system

CDS, clinical decision support.

Courtesy: HIMSS (2014a).

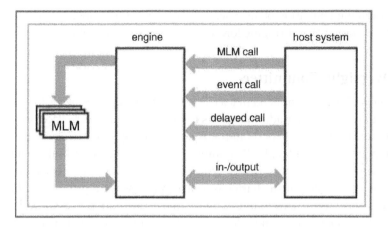

FIGURE 19.2. Arden Syntax graphical display of the structure within a host system.
Source: Samwald et al. (2012b).

the relationships among the environments. Although this syntax establishes a standard for CDS, it is very environmentally dependent, as the graphic reflects.

An example of practical and clinical application of Arden Syntax and MLM code is the calculation of body mass index (BMI) given the parameters of size, weight, and birth date. This information can further be used to trigger algorithms for clinical action and decision depending on parameters. Arden Syntax is frequently used within the certified EHR products and can be maintained by properly trained clinical informaticists to support the CDS program within institutions. This chapter does not cover in detail the application of Arden Syntax but points the reader to various resources for further understanding and application of the standard (see HL7 resources at www.hl7.org/implement/standards/).

USE OF CDSS TO ALIGN IMPROVEMENT INITIATIVES

CDS can be governed within the quality framework of the organization and used strategically to reinforce quality and patient safety initiatives within organizations. Core to a successful implementation of any quality-improvement (QI) initiative is strong leadership. This is particularly true of CDS programs, because they require commitments throughout the organization because of impacts with workflow and an ongoing investment of capital and personnel. As with any organization committed to QI, teams led by strong leaders must be brought together to develop a shared vision of quality and patient safety. This includes physician champions, the chief nursing officer, chief financial officer, chief information officer, and their staff. Accountability can then be established for the desired outcomes. Clinical champions are required to gain buy-in for the CDS effort. Champions serve as change agents, represent their groups in reviewing design and prioritizing projects, and communicate effectively to and from the clinician groups impacted by the changes (Osheroff et al., 2012). CDS programs also require stakeholders who are most impacted by the changes to clinical workflow to help in designing strategies and implementing plans. Successful CDS programs are implemented with the stakeholders, rather than bringing forced change to the stakeholders (HIMSS, 2014c).

CDS Oversight Committee

Osheroff et al. (2012) recommend that a CDS oversight committee needs to be established with the support of senior administrators to own and manage decision support workflows and functions. Members should represent a cross-pollination from the pharmacy and therapeutics committee, EHR committee, patient quality and safety, nursing unit directors, senior leadership, as well as members responsible for the CDS build. Their first actions would be to develop a charter as well as processes and procedures, hen identify committees which they need to interact with to improve care processes and workflows. For example, if the CDS program does not fall under the QI department, a key partner in the process is to engage the QI leadership and staff in the process. Conversely, if the CDS program falls under the QI department, the key to success is a strong relationship with the IT department. Another critical partner in the process is the NI content expert. It is the experience of the authors that nursing informaticists frequently lead the CDS initiative with support from physician colleagues, and the authors recommend if this is not the case, the NI content experts are important stakeholders to engage in strategizing use of CDS.

Strategy sessions should be held to determine the CDS program scope that will best support the organization's goals and programs (Osheroff et al., 2012). For example, should there just be a few tools to begin with and should one build on them as needed or start with many tools and then systematically turn off those not needed? A clear understanding of the organization's prioritized opportunities for improvement, as well as CDS functionality and review capabilities, is needed to ultimately determine which users will benefit the most from the various types of decision support tools selected for use (Osheroff et al., 2012).

Deployment of CDS Interventions

Once the executive oversight committee and the team responsible for the intervention has aligned on the CDS program strategies, the design of the intervention takes place (Osheroff et al., 2012). The design phase should be validated with all stakeholders who will be impacted by the process; the intervention should be developed followed by full testing prior to taking the intervention into the full production environment. Once the testing is complete, the intervention is ready for deployment. Evaluating and measuring impact follow the cycle of improvement.

Measuring Success of the Program

Evaluation strategies to measure impact of the CDS program are an important consideration for the team to consider. CDS program evaluation can include both quantitative and qualitative methods. It is important to strategize prior to implementation; the team will decide whether the intervention is working as expected and improving patient care (Osheroff et al., 2012).

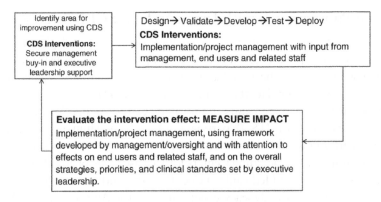

FIGURE 19.3. CDS life-cycle intervention.
Adapted from Osheroff et al. (2012, p. 45).

One qualitative evaluation strategy is to hold focus groups or survey the stake-holders most impacted by clinical workflow changes. Suggested questions to ask clinicians based on recommendations of the authors are (a) How is the process working for the nurses and physicians? (b) Does the CDS program interfere with patient care or create unintended patient safety consequences? Feedback is important to creating a continuous learning environment to inform improvement. Quantitative measures to monitor improvement are equally as important. Methods described in Chapter 22 recommend control charts and various tools for QI that should also be considered in designing quantitative evaluation strategies. Quantitative outcomes and process measures are also important to monitor for reporting to leadership on effectiveness of the program, and to share as best practices when successful programs have had a significant impact (Osheroff et al., 2012).

Another consideration for organizations that design CDS strategies is to align the program with measurement to improve pay-for-performance programs and accreditation requirements. The strategies outlined earlier follow a typical QI initiative life cycle. These strategies can be depicted in the life-cycle process reflected in Figure 19.3 (Osheroff et al., 2012).

MEANINGFUL USE AND CDS PROGRAMS

Achievement of MU-CDS is a core measure to both Stages 1 and 2 of MU. In Stage 1, providers and hospitals are required to implement one CDS rule. However, in Stage 2 of MU, there are more extensive requirements, including a connection in strategy aligned with core measures of quality within the organization. Stage 2 of MU defines CDS as an HIT functionality that builds on the foundation of an EHR to provide people involved in the care processes with general and person-specific information that is intelligently filtered and organized at appropriate times to enhance health and health care. The requirement under Stage 2 of MU is stated as follows: To meet the decision support requirements for Stage 2 of MU, there must be five CDS interventions related to four or more clinical quality measures at a relevant point in the patient care for the entire reporting period. In addition, there must be drug–drug and drug–allergy interaction tools (eHealthUniversity, 2014).

Improving Population Health Using HIT and CDS Strategies

A broader application of CDS can be seen in nationwide efforts to deploy these types of strategies to impact populations. An example of a program that constitutes a national strategy focused on improving population health outcomes that can effectively apply CDS strategies is the Million Hearts® campaign (CDC, 2011).

The Million Hearts campaign aims at improving cardiovascular health in the United States; it was launched by the U.S. Department of Health and Human Services to prevent one million heart attacks and strokes in 5 years. Partners span from across the public and private health sectors, including Centers for Disease Control and Prevention (CDC) and Centers for Medicare & Medicaid Services (CMS); health care professionals; private insurers; businesses; health advocacy groups such as the American Heart Association (AHA) and the American Stroke Association; and community organizations will support Million Hearts through a wide range of activities. The purposes are to coordinate efforts to reduce the number of people who need treatment, optimize treatment for those who need it, and realize the full value of prevention in cardiovascular health. The Million Hearts campaign is based on four tenets aligning with recommended evidence-based practice guidelines, including the following: A = aspirin use for secondary prevention (occurs in 47% of patients who could benefit), B = blood pressure (BP) control (only 46% of people with high BP have it controlled), C = cholesterol control (only 33% of people with high cholesterol have it controlled), and S = smoking cessation (only 23% of people who try to quit get help with combined nicotine replacement and behavioral therapy; CDC, 2011).

The strategies that correspond to the ABCS of the Million Hearts campaign are to prevent heart disease and stroke in participants and their families by understanding the risk and what can be done to lower or reduce them (CDC, 2011). Knowing the ABCS profile and committing to a plan that would lead to reduced risk is a key strategy for the organization. Table 19.4 provides a sample of what the overall goal and strategy for improvement might look like for a clinic that is focused on participating in a program to improve cardiovascular care using CDS (HIMSS, 2014a). A vision for the program, goals, objectives, and measurement criteria are important to establish in the planning and assessment phase of any CDS program. The stars noted in Figure 19.4 reflect compliance with indicators for meeting an MU measure. Table 19.4 outlines the measures, goals, and objectives of what a CDS program might look like related to cardiovascular care and the ABCS of the Million Hearts campaign.

CDS Intervention

Through the use of standardized clinical documentation forms and CDS alerts based on protocols, omissions in medications and better integration of multimodal approaches, such as ABCS, can be tailored to individual patient-centered needs in clinical and lifestyle change efforts to reduce CV risks. For example, if a particular patient is a smoker, the EHR would capture smoking "yes" or "no" and, subsequently, trigger the clinician to counsel the patient accordingly and provide support in smoking-cessation suggested services. When CDS tools are designed according to protocol and use certified robust EHRs, they can provide a collection of data that health care organizations can use to track and trend provider performance based on protocol adherence (HIMSS, 2014a).

TABLE 19.4 Measures of Success for a Cardiovascular CDS Improvement Program

Factor	Data Elements		
	Percentage Change	Endpoint	Metric
Aspirin prophylaxes	65% compliance or 38% improvement from current levels	Daily use of 81 mg and percentage increase among those in the cohort seen by participating clinicians	1. Population surveillance 2. ID patients failing target measure
BP*	65% compliance or a 41% improvement from current levels	Daily medication compliance and percentage increase among those in the cohort seen by participating clinicians	1. Rx refills 2. Population surveillance 3. ID patients failing measure
Cholesterol	65% compliance or a 97% improvement from current levels	Daily medication compliance and percentage increase among those in the cohort seen by participating clinicians	1. Rx refills 2. Population surveillance 3. ID patients failing measure
Smoking	17% compliance with stage of change shift or a 11% reduction in prevalence from current levels	Stage of change shift at least one level toward quitting and prevalence percentage	1. Rx nicotine replacement 2. ID patient reason for failing target
Weight control	Reduction of weight in 65% of population	1. Move 20% of obese to overweight status 2. Move 20% of overweight to normal weight 3. Sentinel changes in the program plan	1. ID patients failing target measure 2. Population surveillance 3. Self-report dashboard
Fitness	Increase in fitness in 30% of population	1. Reduce resting heart rate 2. Lower BP in 50% 3. Increase vital capacity in 50%	1. ID patients failing target measure 2. Population surveillance 3. Self-report dashboard

*MUP Configuration template/EHR Analytics.

BP, blood pressure; CDS, clinical decision support; ID, identify.

Medical Assistants

Medical assistants update patient's vital signs in structured data fields
and review or update the medical summary information

Patient Intake
- Record blood pressure
- Record height, weight, calculate BMI
- Plot and display growth chart (age appropriate)
- Record or review smoking status
- Verify, update allergy list, or **NKDA**
- Verify, update current medications, or annotate **"none"**

★ *If vital signs are not clinically relevant or appropriate*

Provider Conducts Patient Consult or Procedure

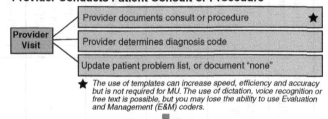

Provider Visit
- Provider documents consult or procedure ★
- Provider determines diagnosis code
- Update patient problem list, or document "none"

★ *The use of templates can increase speed, efficiency and accuracy but is not required for MU. The use of dictation, voice recognition or free text is possible, but you may lose the ability to use Evaluation and Management (E&M) coders.*

Provider Determines Patient's Care Plan

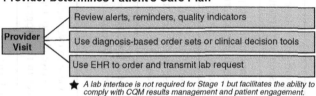

Provider Visit
- Review alerts, reminders, quality indicators
- Use diagnosis-based order sets or clinical decision tools
- Use EHR to order and transmit lab request

★ *A lab interface is not required for Stage 1 but facilitates the ability to comply with CQM results management and patient engagement.*

Provider Selects and Prescribes Medication as Needed

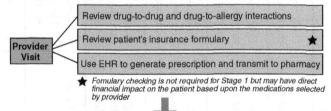

Provider Visit
- Review drug-to-drug and drug-to-allergy interactions
- Review patient's insurance formulary ★
- Use EHR to generate prescription and transmit to pharmacy

★ *Fomulary checking is not required for Stage 1 but may have direct financial impact on the patient based upon the medications selected by provider*

Patient Receives Information Before Leaving the Practice

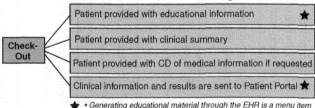

Check-Out
- Patient provided with educational information ★
- Patient provided with clinical summary
- Patient provided with CD of medical information if requested
- Clinical information and results are sent to Patient Portal ★

★ • *Generating educational material through the EHR is a menu item but makes it easier to keep up-to-date information*

• *Patient Portal is not required for Stage 1 but facilitates patient engagement and communication*

FIGURE 19.4. A workflow redesign strategy to support EHR optimization for cardiac care improvement using certified EHRs.

CQM, clinical quality measures; NKDA, no known drug allergies.

The application of CDS tied to QI also aligns with Stage 2 of MU strategies to fully enable EHRs using CDS on high-priority quality measures (HIMSS, 2014a). Certified EHRs have the ability to create clinical documentation forms to standardize the collection of important data elements in a structured data field such that CDS rules can trigger the clinician to collect the right data and intervene according to protocols outlined in Million Hearts (CDC, 2011). However, EHRs directly from the vendor do not automatically have the capacity to capture and trigger these types of adherence to evidence-based practice protocols; hence, the CDS implementation team must design and deploy the forms and CDS triggers to effectively intervene. These applications are considered more advanced implementation efforts to effectively optimize the use of these components of the EHRs and to structure the CDS and the quality reporting to work in tandem and to determine why this type of CDS application was placed in Stage 2 requirements for reaching MU. In addition to being available to trigger algorithms for the clinical alerts to providers, the structured data fields provide better ability to track and trend important data elements for quality indicators, including both process- and outcome-based indictors.

Interventions focused on integrated CDS tools can improve the appropriateness of lab and pharmaceutical intervention. EHRs, when used "meaningfully," can combine with CDS to readily present laboratory values for the clinicians to use in counseling the patient and simplify periodic monitoring of key clinical indicators that chart progress on CV risk-reduction plans. In addition, these strategies provide a powerful motivation to patients as well as trigger action in providers. Another example of how CDS tools and QI methods can support cardiovascular disease interventions is to enable EHRs to more easily collect data to evaluate the impact of QI efforts in rapid cycles of improvement. By using QI modalities combined with the EHRs, the powerful capability to impact clinical outcomes truly captures the spirit of the HITECH Act incentive program to achieve MU of technology with each patient encounter (ONC-HIT, 2013).

EHRs must be modified not only for supporting the structured data that trigger clinical alerts but also for collecting and reporting on factors that indicate the intervention has been successful for impacting the targeted population—in this case, a high-risk cardiovascular disease patient population (CDC, 2011). Providers can also incorporate clinical laboratory test results as structured data through the development of interfaces with area laboratories and hospitals that constitute an objective of Stage 1 of MU. Lab values can be used to trigger appropriate protocol, such as with high cholesterol levels triggering intervention, to further enhance cardiovascular interventions associated with the ABCS Million Hearts campaign.

Workflow Redesign

CDS protocols can effectively be "hardwired" into clinical workflows to maximize the opportunity for provider compliance with protocols driven by consistent documentation of structured data, CDS alerts for education and training, and reporting to monitor compliance. Within a CDS program focused on population health outcomes, such as cardiovascular disease adherence protocols, it is important to address current versus future state standardization of workflows. In the paper-record world, frequently, clinicians have a different workflow for the management of patients and respective patient outcomes. In the process of implementing an electronic environment to help manage patient populations, there are an equal number of options used to manage patients in the electronic environment as there are in the paper environment, but many more opportunities to standardize the delivery of care. Using best practices in clinical workflow analysis, change management, and EHR implementation to help maximize the use of EHRs and respective CDS tools, many of these barriers can be addressed. Figure 19.4 reflects the strategies of how elements essential to the Million Hearts campaign can be built into certified EHR products (Tushan, 2012). These figures reflect the work of the AHA working with the ONC to establish recommendations on how certified products can be used to reinforce clinical workflows and documentation strategies under the campaign. These workflows can be used to strategize how and when the data capture needs to occur related to the protocol, and how CDS can trigger the clinicians to adhere to documentation and workflow as outlined in Figure 19.4 (Tushan, 2012).

Education and Training to "Hardwire" Improvements

Educational intervention is also an important strategy that is used to support clinicians in maximizing the CDS and EHR functions. While training providers and clinical staff on the use of the EHR to standardize clinical documentation, CDS rule sets and custom reports are pivotal to success in a population health-based CDS program. An education campaign is recommended by the authors prior to implementation to help reinforce functionalities of the EHR system and the CDS program implemented. Standard educational campaigns have proven effective in services currently provided to the Regional Extension Centers (RECs) member providers and hospitals and similar methods will be deployed to educate providers on the utilization of clinical documentation forms, CDS, and reporting. Based on work of the authors with the RECs and preparing clinics to address the Million Hearts campaign, an educational program for a clinic might include the following elements:

▶ Review of the Million Hearts campaign and best practices related to cardiovascular disease prevention, including the ABCS protocol.

▶ Review of baseline reports on performance of ABCS measures (if available). The education program ideally should incorporate reports as to current provider adherence to the metrics in the campaign, if possible, although prior to instating the CDS and structured data often these types of reports can be collected with manual abstraction of records. Baseline measures prior to implementation and incorporation of the baselines into the education for providers help reinforce why the CDS program is needed.

▶ Train providers and clinical staff on the use of CDS and custom reports.

▶ Provide an overview of EHR functionality and opportunities to improve the quality of care and outcomes.

▶ Present a vendor-specific overview on how to maximize the use of the EHR in delivery of care. Vendor-specific education on CDS alerts may be available to utilize in combination with specific training materials that include customized forms and reports to collect structured data that are important to the cardiovascular protocol, CDS rules, and the process and outcome measures.

▶ Suggest techniques to adopt and implement new CDS rule sets clinic-wide while ensuring the highest level of compliance by all providers (CDC, 2011).

Evaluation and Monitoring for Success

Continuous surveillance of the use and nonuse of CDS and reporting of functionality is an important evaluation strategy. Utilizing specific report functionality or building reporting capability within an EHR for monitoring progress is an important development strategy (Osheroff et al., 2012). In addition, regularly recurring observational studies, focus groups with providers, and surveys can be used as qualitative methods for the CDS team to evaluate effectiveness and to improve the program in the long term. For example, if hard stops in an electronic health record of clinical decision support (EHR-CDS) strategy are enabled, they can be overridden with documentation in the record of the reason(s). These reasons can help document the compliance with the cardiovascular protocol, and if there are apparent clinical reasons for noncompliance, justification is captured in a text field for further evaluation. Along with provider debriefing, these reasons can help inform upgrades and changes in updates to the CDS tools. The CDS team brings together all stakeholders as core team participants in the organization with the primary goal of the program to fight heart disease and stroke partnered with AHA and other participating organizations across the country.

CHALLENGES AND ISSUES WITH CDS

Although the ONC endorsed certification bodies to test and certify EHRs that require CDS functionality under Stage 1 guidelines of MU (specifications), these products do not come "out of the box" ready to achieve results such as those described by the Million Hearts campaign example noted earlier. They require a significant strategy and infrastructure that is evident from the strategies described. In addition, there can be unintended consequences, including patient safety issues and legal liability concerns with CDS that are critical to consider in all organizations using CDS within EHRs (IOM, 2012).

Challenges to Implementing CDS

Implementing CDS effectively and without provider resistance presents challenges. These challenges are noted in the report by Agency for Healthcare Research and Quality (AHRQ), *Clinical Decision Support Systems: State of the Art,* to be primarily related to misalignment in the CDS intent and what the end users intended to do prior to receiving the alert, timing, and autonomy (Berner, 2009). Timing is noted as an issue in the report, indicating that providers may agree they need alerts on preventive services, but disagree on timing of when to receive the alerts within their workflow. Additional issues are speed and ease of access to alerts. The third and likely the most significant issue according to the report is the autonomy desired by clinicians related to how much control end users have over their response to the CDS. This area relates to whether the CDS alert is a "hard stop," preventing the clinicians from moving forward in the EHR until the alert is addressed, and whether it takes significant effort to override the alert (Berner, 2009, p. 8).

Features of Safe HIT to Address Challenges

The Institute of Medicine (2011) report, *Health IT and Patient Safety: Building Safer Systems for Better Care* outlines several recommendations. The report focuses on end users and recommendations as to what constitutes safety from an end-user standpoint. These recommendations are relevant to CDS programs and how the tools are deployed, which aligns with these recommendations. As noted earlier, some of the major challenges related to CDS are that the CDS does not align with end-user expectations. As a result, aligning CDS development with the IOM recommendations helps the industry design systems that are safer and more effective. The recommendations are noted as follows:

1. Retrieval simplicity that is accurate and timely with both native and imported data
2. A system that the end user desires to interact with
3. Simple and intuitive displays of data
4. Easy navigation
5. Evidence at the point of care to aid decision making
6. Enhancements to workflow with automation of mundane tasks, streamlining tasks rather than increasing physical or cognitive workload
7. Easy transfer of information to and from provider organizations
8. No unanticipated downtime (IOM, 2011)

The recommendations also indicate that the cognitive workflow and the decision-making process in health care are complex, with the need for clinicians to rapidly simulate massive amounts of data within the decision-making process in complex rapidly changing environments. The report further emphasizes the need for timely information and not a cumbersome, time-consuming, or too rigid pathway that the clinician must navigate. Further, there is an emphasis on the fact that the most vulnerable period of time for patient safety issues occurs at the initiation of new technology. This period of vulnerability further reinforces the importance of training, particularly with changes in workflow that are typical of CDS implementation. Usability guidelines are also an important consideration. To address these issues, the IOM report recommends several guidelines established by the National Institute for Standards and Technology that address design strategies in incorporating best practices in usability design, methods for evaluation and improvement, usability engineering, recommendations on organization commitments to usability, and testing guidelines related to usability and patient safety (IOM, 2011).

Legal Implications

Although there are some noted liability risks to providers who use CDSS, there could also be exposure to not acting on a CDS alert. Greenberg and Ridgely (2011) evaluated the malpractice risk associated with CDS use and concluded that the most important issue with regard to liability is whether CDS systems are well designed and well implemented. They determined that a well-designed CDS system should only provide alerts that are clinically relevant, reduce the likelihood of alert fatigue, and allow clinicians to detect adverse events. This led them to conclude that adopting a well-designed CDS system would reduce overall malpractice risk. A recent article by Kesselheim, Cresswell, Phansalkar, Bates, and Sheikh (2011) reached similar conclusions regarding the impact of reducing alert fatigue and emphasized the importance of using clinical judgment when interpreting the output of a CDS system. To further reduce liability, they also recommend stronger government regulation of CDSS and the development of international practice guidelines (Kesselheim et al., 2011).

The issue of sharing CDS content among institutions has been discussed in the context of using a Web 2.0 architecture to encourage interoperability (Wright et al., 2009). Citing other references, Wright and colleagues concluded that the patient's health care provider is responsible for making the final decision on the clinical relevance of any shared CDS content. This conclusion basically indicates that existing "hard copy" references that aid in clinical decision making are no different than electronic support documentation. However, they caution that there is little case law as precedent to address these questions (Wright et al., 2009). With this position, it could be further concluded that clinicians would be held to the same standard of care regardless of whether a CDS system is used, and as long as clinicians make the final decision the use of CDS should not increase liability risk. In other words, clinicians are held to the same level of accountability with the EHR as with the paper-based record.

Information-based liability is an important issue for all clinicians. The rapid expansion of medical information databases, EHRs, and associated medical expert systems and CDS have the potential for impacting medical malpractice (Greenberg & Ridgely, 2011). This is particularly true given that the electronic world has the ability to track actions and potentially follow the "train of thought" the clinician had given the footprint in the electronic record, which tracks clicks, routes taken through the documentation in the EHR, and whether or not the clinician responded appropriately to the protocols and CDS built into the system. Providers could potentially be held liable for failing to access a computerized medical database, failing to use available software providing decision support, or using this technology in an improper, inexpert, or inappropriate fashion with the electronic record admissible in a court of law. Likewise, nurses, hospitals, and health care systems may also be liable for staff failing to adhere to alerts. However, an area that is unclear is what actually constitutes the permanent legal record and whether or not the CDS alerts, data that trigger the alerts, the algorithms behind the alerts, and the actions that result based on the alerts are a part of that permanent record (Kesselheim et al., 2011). A well-designed CDS system should provide alerts that are clinically relevant, reduce the likelihood of alert fatigue, and allow clinicians to detect adverse events (HIMSS, 2014b).

SUMMARY

To conclude, this chapter has covered the basics of CDS definitions, types of CDS tools, and the essential elements that organizations should have in place for ensuring a successful CDS program. These elements include leadership and executive support, as well as interprofessional teams representing the stakeholders most impacted by changes to workflow. These teams are fundamental to helping design the CDS strategies. The alignment of the CDS program to fundamental strategies for QI has also been discussed along with the importance of involving departments that can help with optimizing the overall impact of the CDS intervention on patient safety and quality. The life-cycle intervention was reviewed with important steps outlined; and concerns with liability for clinicians and hospitals have been discussed. Finally, four case studies are presented.

CASE STUDY 1: OBSTETRICAL SCREENING

Problem: When a potentially laboring mother presented for an obstetric screening exam to determine whether she was truly in labor, there was no standard workflow for placement of orders necessary for the exam and no standard order set for the exam. The divergent practices in placing orders and workflows for conducting the exams caused several problems for the multiple hospital system. Problems include issues with appropriate billing and reimbursement for the exam, putting the nurse in jeopardy of practicing outside the scope of licensure, potentially missing elements of the exam needed for best patient care, and risk of violating Emergency Medical Treatment and Active Labor Act laws. To understand all of the elements needed to address the problem, the CDS team partnered with NI to learn the entire process and identify the areas in need of impact by CDS tools.

Stakeholders: The stakeholders identified for engagement in the process were the obstetrics (OB) triage nurses, the obstetricians, quality/risk department representatives, billing/finance representatives, compliance department representatives, individual member hospital nursing leadership, the CDS team, and NI. Individual and group meetings with the various stakeholder groups were conducted to get a clear understanding of all of the components needed for a successful process.

Design: CDS did an analysis of orders used for obstetrical triage across the system to find commonalities, identify differences, and see which hospitals had gaps in available orders. Comparisons were done while looking at denials for reimbursement and successful reimbursement to identify any potential missed revenue opportunities. CDS did an analysis with NI and nursing leadership to identify the appropriate scope-of-practice issues with the obstetrical triage exam screening orders and workflows. CDS and NI worked with obstetricians to ensure that appropriate care standards for the potentially laboring mother were addressed. Once the clinical workflow and necessary orders were identified, CDS and NI took the information to the other stakeholders to ensure the process met with reimbursement, quality, and legal and regulatory guidelines. A standardized system order set was built that includes all of the necessary orders for a potentially laboring mother with the verbiage necessary in the orders to qualify for maximum reimbursement. This system set replaced all of the other hospital-specific sets that had been in use. Within the approved workflow for obstetrical screening, a properly certified RN can conduct portions of the exam without contacting the physician. The order set included prechecked orders to cover these items so the nurse can easily use the order set with the fewest number of clicks and know the orders are appropriate to be placed without physician input. Depending on the results of the exam, the nurse must contact the physician to receive further orders for the laboring mother. The order set can be cleared and then reused by the nurse to place the orders being received from the physician. This prevents the nurse from having to go to multiple order sets and also allows the nurse to sign the new orders appropriately to protect

(continued)

CASE STUDY 1: OBSTETRICAL SCREENING (*continued*)

her or his licensure. The design of the order set allows for easy maintenance by the CDS team, which is very important for sustainability of use of the set, reduces the number of order sets the clinician has to search for, which is a huge satisfier for staff, and contains evidence-based orders with best practice recommendations to provide the best care for the patient.

Implementation: The implementation plan for the new obstetrical triage exam order set included training for all staff who use the set, notification of the billing and coding departments of the new orders being used, and training and support staff for the EHR. Users were very satisfied with the reduced number of clicks to get what they needed, and with the ease of use of the set. Users also indicated that "knowing they were within their scope of practice" made them more confident in using the new set. Adoption of the set was quick. Within 60 days of implementation, reimbursements increased and denials markedly decreased. Physician feedback was very positive, as the implementation led to fewer calls to the physician and the calls that were necessary were shorter and easier to manage. This allows nurses to place initial orders with reduced clicks and to be able to clear the set and use it while speaking to the physician to obtain further orders if necessary.

Outcome: Use of CDS tools to better design and build the obstetrical screening order set has resulted in increased revenue capture for all system hospitals, ease of use for all clinicians, promotion of nurses practicing within their scope of licensure, and increased satisfaction of nurses and physicians with the EHR.

CASE STUDY 2: IMMUNIZATION SCREENING

Problem: Influenza screening and vaccination are a core measure that must be reported to meet regulatory criteria and to maximize reimbursement. The criteria for influenza screening indicating the vaccine is needed change every year. If any step in the process is missed, there is a fallout that will cause the measure to not be met. During the previous year's influenza season, there had been several fallouts and missed opportunities to give the vaccine. This resulted in loss of revenue. The hospital system leadership and infection prevention department want to utilize CDS tools to help guarantee the measure will be met 100% of the time.

Stakeholders: The stakeholders identified in the process are the admission nurses, bedside nurses, quality directors, coding compliance department, individual hospital leadership, CDS team, EHR clinical documentation and orders builders, NI, the system's infection prevention director, pharmacists, physicians, and infection disease physicians. NI and the CDS team met with the various stakeholders to verify whether all of the components are necessary to meet the measures for the

(*continued*)

CASE STUDY 2: IMMUNIZATION SCREENING (*continued*)

next influenza season and reporting period. From that base of knowledge, CDS and NI developed appropriate workflows to be presented to the staff for usability testing. Once usability was vetted with the frontline staff, the entire process, including the reporting elements, were taken back to all stakeholders to verify the process will meet regulatory reporting and compliance needs.

Design: CDS and hospital leadership analyzed the missed opportunities to find commonalities and patterns. Analysis of successful vaccine workflows was done with frontline nurses and NI, highlighting what staff felt worked best and at what point in the workflow certain actions needed to occur. CDS, NI, and the system builders for clinical documentation and orders met to determine the appropriate tools to be used to help staff meet the goals set by leadership. The need to direct staff to the correct orders for vaccination if the patient screened positive for needing the vaccine was accomplished by using an actionable BPA in which the staff either had to enter the correct order or go back and correct the screening to reflect that the patient did not meet criteria for the vaccine. The choices in the screening tool were clarified to make it very easy for staff to choose the correct indications or contraindications. CDS tools based on age of the patient limited the choices available for staff to pick from based on information already entered in the system. For example, if the patient was below the age requiring screening, the screening tool would not appear for the staff to fill out. Once the order to give the vaccine was placed, other CDS tools were employed to help staff to remember to give the vaccine before the patient was dismissed home. Hard stops on printing discharge instructions were implemented to serve as a safety net for ensuring the patient was vaccinated before leaving the facility. Daily reports of compliance with the measure were made available to managers, directors, infection prevention, and hospital leadership so any fallouts could be rapidly addressed and corrected. Positive reinforcement tools were employed to let frontline staff know when they had completed a task successfully. This kind of positive reinforcement tool is highly valued by frontline staff and increases compliance as well as satisfaction. Design components included using the same language in the documentation as is used in the required reporting elements to eliminate any confusion or risk of denial. Aligning documentation choices with reporting guideline language improves reporting and shows clear compliance with measure details.

Outcome: The revised screening and ordering process increased staff satisfaction with nurses reporting increased confidence in the ability to correctly screen the patient and order the correct vaccination. The safety net of not allowing printing of discharge instructions helped reduce the number of fallouts to nearly zero. The identified fallouts were by staff who were not following the workflow and were creating intentional workarounds to the approved process. Leadership was able to rapidly identify these issues and stop them from occurring. Influenza measures for the reporting period were met at 100%.

CASE STUDY 3: NORMAL NEWBORN

Problem: Because of changes in both state law and federal regulations surrounding how physician orders must be authorized and standards related to the standing delegated order set (SDO), the leadership of the enterprise directed NI and the CDS team to look at ways to make the order sets compliant with the new regulations. The orders and process surrounding normal newborns were chosen as the test case for a new model for order sets and workflow improvement. Normal newborn orders have to include orders for the time-sensitive medications given to the infant in the first hour of life. These time-sensitive orders posed the greatest difficulty in development of an order set that would be compliant with the new regulations and that helped the nurses' practice within their scope of licensure while still being able to appropriately care for the infant. Although there are caveats in both the state and federal regulations that relate to normal newborn care, the authentication process still had to be addressed for the orders to be valid.

Stakeholders: The stakeholders in the process are the labor/delivery nurses, newborn nursery nurses, pediatricians, obstetricians, coding/compliance department, CDS, NI, hospital leadership, quality/risk department, accreditation department, and legal department.

Design: NI collaborated with CDS to develop a model for new order sets. Reasons that related to dissatisfaction with order sets were that nurses could not clearly tell what orders to place were within their scope, and the physicians disliked having to deal with purely nursing orders. Mixing nursing orders with orders that need to be initiated or signed by the physician makes most order sets too long and too cumbersome for easy utilization by users. Given both the regulatory needs and the input from users, a decision was made to break the normal newborn orders into three sets (time-sensitive set, nursing scope set, and physician set) that work together instead of one massive set. CDS did a statistical analysis of the different normal newborn sets across the system to identify commonalities, delineate differences, and determine usage of various orders. Analysis was done of established evidence and best practices related to normal newborn care to determine whether any gaps existed in the current orders that could be addressed by the new sets. Because the time-sensitive orders need to be placed and acted on potentially before a pediatrician has examined the infant, the time-sensitive set had to be designed as an SDO. State and federal rules state that SDOs must be reviewed by medical, nursing, and pharmacy leadership at least annually and be tied to a policy to be valid. The development of the time-sensitive set corresponded to creation of a system-wide policy, and NI ensured the policy and orders aligned as well as that the policy and order set were approved by all necessary committees. NI and CDS vetted the content and workflow for all three sets with the end users and system leadership, a process that took many months as each revision had to go back to all three groups for validation. The physicians were ultimately responsible for the content of the orders that required their validation and signature. The nurses and nursing

(*continued*)

CASE STUDY 3: NORMAL NEWBORN (*continued*)

leadership ensured the orders on the nursing action set were within the scope of a nurse's practice without needing authorization from a physician. The physician set contains only orders needing physician initiation or authorization that were not already ordered on the time-sensitive set. This set can be used directly by the physicians or can be done as a telephone order by the nurse with the physician if necessary. The design of the sets allowed for the correct orders to be placed at the correct time by the correct discipline. The design also supported already existing workflows surrounding the care of the normal newborn infant and is flexible enough to be used easily by both the large and small hospitals within the system. The sets utilize new functionality available for conditional orders, which allows the clinician to choose the correct order that is dependent on other assessment or history information, giving very clear direction to the staff on why the order is indicated for the patient.

Outcome: The outcome from the launch of the normal newborn order sets was overwhelmingly positive. Nurses stated that they felt much more confident that they were ordering appropriately to stay within their scope of practice. Physicians were very satisfied with the decrease in calls for orders. A minor glitch related to common practice versus recommended practice was identified surrounding orders for holding cord blood for additional testing. Many of the physicians were used to this being done automatically without orders and were unhappy when the process stopped because no order had been placed by the nurse. This concern was corrected by including an order to hold cord blood in the nurses' order set. If the physician wished to order any additional tests, the cord blood would be available.

CASE STUDY 4: EBOLA

Problem: The Ebola virus is no longer contained to the continent of Africa. Introduction of the virus to the United States called for new infection prevention measures to be developed and instituted across the nation. This new infectious disease potential in the United States necessitated the CDC and the Departments of Health in each of the states to create new screening tools and subsequent infection prevention measures. Completely new isolation and exposure precautions were mandated for any potential exposure to or risk of Ebola. All health care providers must follow the new screening guidelines to protect their patients and address the public health concerns. The new screening criteria, isolation type, and required subsequent actions need to be integrated into the EHR. Focus is on protecting the patient, the staff, and public health. Identification and containment are paramount. Hospital leadership and infection prevention staff want to leverage the EHR to help meet the new federal and state criteria related to the Ebola virus.

(*continued*)

CASE STUDY 4: EBOLA (*continued*)

Stakeholders: Stakeholders in the process are the infection prevention staff, all clinical staff in all areas (inpatient, emergency, ambulatory, outpatient clinics), CDS, EHR builders, NI, hospital and system leadership, health information management (HIM), legal, quality/risk department, and compliance department.

Design: NI leads the initiative to build and implement a new screening tool, orders, and necessary documentation for staff to safely care for the patient, themselves, and public health. NI coordinated with infection prevention and HIM to ensure the EHR builds match the paper screening tool being used for areas that do not use the EHR. The screening tool was developed to screen for Ebola and for a newly emerging disease, Middle Eastern Respiratory Syndrome Corona Virus (MERS-CoV). Development also included the ability to rapidly change the screening questions and alerts depending on what most prominent threat to public health develops. The design was intended to be broader than looking for just one disease and to be flexible in response. Because of the critical need to identify any potential exposure or risk, the screening questions were made hard stops so that the staff had to complete the entire screen. CDS tools were employed to reduce the number of questions asked that are dependent on the answers to the first three questions. If the response to any of the first three questions was positive, additional hard-stop questions would appear for the clinician to answer. CDS tools for alerts were utilized to give the clinicians reinforcement when the screen was successfully completed so they knew they were done, and to alert the staff that further actions were needed. If further actions were needed, an actionable BPA was built that would allow the clinician to do what was needed with minimal clicks and eliminated any guesswork. New orders for the new kind of isolation had to be built as did the new alerts. Links to the CDC and state websites for infection prevention are available for staff to use. For the infection prevention staff to follow and manage any potential emerging-disease patient, a new tool was built for them as well as for new reports for monitoring and compliance. Because communication among caregivers is key to safety, if the patient screened positive, alerts were fired throughout the record to ensure any clinician participating in care would be aware of the patient's infectious disease status. Great care was taken in developing tools for publicly viewable status boards so that patient privacy and confidentiality were protected. CDS safety-net features were employed to prevent any patient from being dismissed without being screened by not allowing discharge instructions to be printed. The screening tool and associated actions were tested for usability by frontline staff, both nurses and physicians. Once the workflow and documentation elements were approved by infection prevention and hospital leadership, the measures were deployed.

Outcome: Deployment of the new tool made the system compliant with the new CDC and state recommendations. Staff feedback was very positive, including comments about how easy it was to use the tool, and the staff felt confident they knew

(*continued*)

CASE STUDY 4: EBOLA (*continued*)

the steps to take if a positive screening was to occur. Because the screening was developed as more than just an Ebola screening, it was easy for staff to adopt into their workflow. Even though no Ebola patients have been identified with the new tool, several potential cases of MERS-CoV have been identified and appropriately treated. Leadership gave very positive feedback on the coordination and standardization of the tools and actions that were to span the EHR and paper workflows.

EXERCISES AND QUESTIONS FOR CONSIDERATION

Considering the four case studies presented, let us outline the life-cycle intervention for each of the programs and consider the following questions:

1. Identify the area that will be impacted by the intervention. Be specific in terms of major stakeholders involved and address management and executive leadership buy-in. Why is it important to consider executives and management for CDS interventions?

2. Examine the design, validate, develop, test, and deploy processes for each of the four case studies. How was the intervention deployed within each of the case studies? Which of the tools discussed in the chapter were used within each of the case studies?

3. In examining the four case studies, how effective were the interventions? Support your position with evaluation measures noted in each of the case studies. Are they qualitative or quantitative approaches? Could the team have improved their evaluation strategies? If so, how? If not, why not?

REFERENCES

Bates, D. W., Kuperman, G. J., Wang, S., Gandhi, T., Kittler, A., Volk, L., . . . Middleton, B. (2003). Ten commandments for effective clinical decision support: Making the practice of evidence-based medicine a reality. *Journal of the American Medical Informatics Association, 10*(6), 523–530. doi:10.1197/jamia .M1370

Berner, E. S. (2009). *Clinical decision support systems: State of the art* (No. 09-0069-EF). Rockville, MD: Agency for Healthcare Research and Quality. Retrieved from www.healthit.ahrq.gov/sites/default/ files/docs/page/09-0069-EF_1.pdf

Centers for Disease Control and Prevention. (2011). Million Hearts: Strategies to reduce the prevalence of leading cardiovascular disease risk factors. *Morbidity and Mortality Weekly Report, 60*(36), 1248–1251. Retrieved from www.cdc.gov/mmwr/preview/mmwrhtml/mm6036a4.htm

Clinfowiki.org. (2015). *Clinical decision support—History.* Retrieved from www.clinfowiki.org/wiki/ index.php/CDS#History

eHealthUniversity. (2014, September). *Clinical decision making: More than just 'alerts' tipsheet.* Retrieved from www.cms.gov/Regulations-and-Guidance/Legislation/EHRIncentivePrograms/Down loads/ClinicalDecisionSupport_Tipsheet-.pdf

Greenberg, M., & Ridgely, M. S. (2011). Clinical decision support and malpractice risk. *Journal of the American Medical Association, 306*(1), 90–91. doi:10.1001/jama.2011.929

Health Information and Management Systems Society. (2011). *So you want to do CDS: A C-level introduction to clinical decision support* (Webinar Slides No. HIMSScds2011). Chicago, IL: Author.

Health Information and Management Systems Society. (2014a). *CDS 101: Fundamental issues.* Retrieved from www.himss.org/library/clinical-decision-support/issues?navItemNumber=13240

Health Information and Management Systems Society. (2014b). *Clinical decision support: Fundamental issues.* Retrieved from www.himss.org/library/clinical-decision-support/issues?navItemNumber=13240

Health Information and Management Systems Society. (2014c). *What is clinical decision support?* Retrieved from www.himss.org/library/clinical-decision-support/what-is?navItemNumber=13238#promiseperil

HealthIT.gov. (2014). *Clinical decision support rule.* Retrieved from www.healthit.gov/providers-professionals/achieve-meaningful-use/core-measures/clinical-decision-support-rule

Institute of Medicine. (2011). *Health IT and patient safety: Building safer systems for better care* (Consensus Report). Washington, DC: Institute of Medicine of The National Academies. Retrieved from www.iom.edu/~/media/Files/Report%20Files/2011/Health-IT/HealthITandPatientSafetyreportbrief final_new.pdf

Institute of Medicine. (2012). *Health IT and patient safety building safer systems for better care.* Washington, DC: Author.

Kendall, K., & Kendall, J. (2014). *Systems analysis and design* (9th ed.). Upper Saddle River, NJ: Pearson.

Kesselheim, A. S., Cresswell, K., Phansalkar, S., Bates, D. W., & Sheikh, A. (2011). Clinical decision support systems could be modified to reduce 'alert fatigue' while still minimizing the risk of litigation. *Health Affairs, 30*(12), 2310–2317. doi:10.1377/hlthaff.2010.1111

Lieu, G., Ray, T., Klein, N., Chung, C., & Kulldorff, M. (2015). Geographic clusters in underimmunization and vaccine refusal. *Pediatrics, 135*(2), 280–289. doi:10.1542/peds.2014-2715

National Quality Forum. (2008). *National voluntary consensus standards for influenza and pneumococcal immunizations.* Retrieved from www.qualityforum.org/Publications/2008/12/National_Voluntary_Consensus_Standards_for_Influenza_and_Pneumococcal_Immunizations.aspx

Office of the National Coordinator for Health Information Technology. (2013). *HITECH programs for health information technology.* Retrieved from www.healthit.gov/policy-researchers-implementers/health-it-adoption-programs

Openclinical.org. (2013). *Arden Syntax: Methods and tools for the development of computer-interpretable guidelines.* Retrieved from www.openclinical.org/gmm_ardensyntax.html

Osheroff, J. A., Teich, J. M., Levick, D., Saldana, L., Velasco, F. T., Sittig, D. F., . . . Jenders, R. A. (2012). *Improving outcomes with CDS: An implementer's guide* (2nd ed.). Chicago, IL: Healthcare Information and Management Systems Society. Retrieved from http://www.himss.org/ResourceLibrary/ResourceDetail.aspx?ItemNumber=11590

Samwald, M., Fehre, K., de Bruin, J., & Adlassnig, K. P. (2012a). The Arden Syntax standard for clinical decision support: Experiences and directions. *Journal of Biomedical Informatics, 45*(4), 711–718. doi:10.1016/j.jbi.2012.02.001

Samwald, M., Fehre, K., de Bruin, J., & Adlassnig, K. P. (2012b). The Arden syntax standard for clinical decision support: Experiences and directions (article tools). *Journal of Biomedical Informatics, 45*(4), 711–718. doi:10.1016/j.jbi.2012.02.001

Texas Health Resources. (2014). *Vaccination protocol* (No. THRvaccine2014). Dallas, TX: Author.

Tushan, M. (2012). *Weekly webinar series for overcoming meaningful use barriers: Solutions from the field for million hearts introduction, REC experiences, and implementation into workflow* (Presentation No. ONC2012). Washington, DC: Office of the National Coordinator for Health IT.

Wright, A., Bates, D. W., Middleton, B., Hongsermeier, T., Kashyap, V., Thomas, S. M., & Sittig, D. F. (2009). Creating and sharing clinical decision support content with Web 2.0: Issues and example. *Journal of Biomedical Informatics, 42*(2), 334–346. doi:10.1016/j.jbi.2008.09.003

SECTION IV

Patient Safety, Quality,
and Population Health
(NEHI Model Component #3)

CHAPTER 20

Health Information Technology and Implications for Patient Safety

Mari Tietze and Susan McBride

OBJECTIVES

1. Discuss the implementation of the Patient Safety Act and the relationship of that Act to the national agenda to implement electronic health records (EHRs) with rapid deployment methods.

2. Discuss patient safety organizations (PSOs) and what they are designed to accomplish.

3. Describe the roles of the Agency for Healthcare Research and Quality (AHRQ) as overseer of the PSOs and the Office of the National Coordinator (ONC) to ensure safe deployment and utilization of health information technology (HIT).

4. Describe patient safety and quality issues arising from rapid deployment of EHRs.

5. Outline actions advanced practice nurses (APNs) should take when a potential or actual patient safety issue arises as a result of technology.

6. Define actions that can be taken by health care professionals to report patient safety issues appropriately.

KEY WORDS

patient safety, patient safety organizations, health information technology, errors, unintended consequences

---

CONTENTS

INTRODUCTION

Rapid deployment of electronic health records, health information exchanges, and their support technology have created fertile ground for patient safety issues to arise. This chapter discusses national issues with respect to patient safety and quality related to rapid deployment. In addition, national strategies to address patient safety under the Patient Safety and Quality Improvement Act (U.S. Congress, 2005) are reviewed, and the health care professional's role is emphasized as to when and how to act on patient safety events related to technology.

What are these unintended consequences? EHRs can offer many benefits to health care providers and their patients, including better quality of medical care, greater efficiencies, and improved patient safety. Even if these benefits are achieved, one will almost certainly face some unanticipated and undesirable consequences from implementing an EHR. These consequences are often referred to as unintended consequences (Campbell, Sittig, & Ash, 2006). They can undermine provider acceptance, increase costs, sometimes lead to failed implementation, and result in harm to patients. However, learning to anticipate and identify unintended consequences promotes effective decisions, clarifies trade-offs, and addresses problems as they arise (Campbell et al., 2006).

One example of work conducted on the topic of unintended consequences of information technology (IT) is reflected in the study by Sittig and Ash (2007). Their study collected unintended adverse consequences of EHRs from five hospitals representing 2,346 beds, having implemented an EHR system, specifically, computer provider order entry (CPOE). Practitioners provided their experiences associated with the implementation and themes emerged that helped answer the question as to what were some examples of unintended consequences (Sittig & Ash, 2007). Nine common examples follow later in this chapter.

SAFETY HISTORY RESULTING IN THE PATIENT SAFETY ACT

The safety of patients in American hospitals was called into question well over a decade ago after the release of *To Err Is Human: Building a Safer Health System*, a report by the Institute of Medicine (IOM) detailing the number of patients harmed in hospitals (Kohn, Corrigan, & Donaldson, 1999). According to the report, more people die in a given year as a result of medical errors than from motor vehicle accidents, breast cancer, or AIDS (Kohn et al., 1999). This report, among others, such as "Crossing the Quality Chasm: A New Health System for the 21st century" (Committee on Quality of Healthcare in America, 2001), created a national focus on safety in health care organizations. Advanced practice nurses are in a unique position to prevent errors by raising awareness and understanding of how and when they occur and leading teams to implement improvements to address quality concerns. According to the classic book titled *Keeping Patients Safe: Transforming the Work Environment of Nurses* (Page, 2004), nurses' close proximity to and continual observation of the patient places the profession in a position to prevent a number of errors before the patient is impacted.

A more recent IOM Report, *The Future of Nursing: Leading Change, Advancing Health,* further emphasizes the importance of nursing's role in designing safe systems that work well for patients (Cipriano, 2011). The report emphasizes nurses' close proximity to the patient, as well as the magnitude of nurses' impact as "the largest segment of the health care workforce with some of the closet, most sustained interactions with patients" (Cipriano, 2011, p. 143). A study exploring the ways that nurses in the emergency room prevent errors indicated that five themes emerged to describe methods used by nurses in identifying errors. In this emergency department setting, the themes were surveillance, anticipation, double checking, awareness of the "big picture," and experiential knowing (Henning, 2004).

Addressing the need to focus efforts on improving patient safety in the United States, Congress passed the Patient Safety Act and Quality Improvement Act 2005 (Patient Safety and Quality Improvement Act, 2005), which launched a national push for PSOs. PSOs were created in order for health care organizations to share information on patient safety events without the fear that the information might be used against them in a lawsuit. By providing confidential mechanisms in a secure environment, information on patient safety events can be collected, aggregated, and analyzed to help develop approaches to systematic errors that ail the health delivery system (AHRQ, 2014a). Given this role, PSOs are an important avenue for nurses to consider when an event occurs that either injured a patient or might have potentially injured a patient (nearmiss). Many health care organizations are associated with PSOs or work closely with a PSO to report patient safety events. Nurses should be aware of reporting mechanisms in place for their institutions, particularly as we move rapidly to deploy EHRs that impact so many critical elements of the patient care process.

PATIENT SAFETY ISSUES AND HEALTH INFORMATION TECHNOLOGY

In 2011, the IOM Committee on Patient Safety and Health Information Technology released a report titled *Health IT and Patient Safety: Building Safer Systems for Better Care* (IOM, 2011). The report outlined observations of potential HIT errors, concluding that several factors must be taken into consideration with implementation to prevent these errors from occurring. The factors included:

- ▶ Implementation strategies (fast or slow progression onto an EHR)
- ▶ The influence of the end users regarding configuration of the EHRs and training of clinicians
- ▶ Workflow using the paper record versus the new electronic system
- ▶ Availability of data for analysis of quality (IOM, 2011)

From this work, much research followed and several models for safe HIT practices have evolved.

Models of Unintended Consequences

Unintended Adverse Consequences

Much of the early research on HIT safety involved studying health care professionals, such as physicians and nurses, during and after the implementation of HIT systems in their organization. Key observations and recommendations, based on these studies, are reflected in the book titled *Clinical Information Systems: Overcoming Adverse Consequences* (Sittig & Ash, 2007). The study conducted by Campbell et al. (2006) using qualitative methods and an expert panel to gather and analyze examples of five successful CPOE sites also provided direction.

Nine unintended adverse consequences of the CPOE implementations evolved from this cumulative research. The unintended consequences apply not only to CPOE implementation but also to other HIT systems such as EHRs. The nine unintended consequences are briefly summarized here:

1. *More work for clinicians.* Example: After the introduction of an EHR, physicians often have to spend more time on documentation because they are required to (and facilitated to) provide more and more detailed information than with a paper chart. Although this information may be helpful, the process of entering the information may be time-consuming, especially at first.

2. *Unfavorable workflow changes.* Example: CPOE automates the medication and test ordering process by reducing the number of clinicians and clerical staff involved, but by doing so it also eliminates checks and counterchecks in the manual ordering process. That is, with the older system, nurses or clerks may have noticed errors, whereas now the order goes directly from the physician to the pharmacy or lab.

3. *Never-ending demands for system changes.* Example: As EHRs evolve, users rely more heavily on the software, and demand more sophisticated functionality and new features (e.g., custom order sets). The addition of new functionalities necessitates that more resources be devoted to EHR implementation and maintenance.

4. *Conflicts between electronic and paper-based systems.* Example: Physicians who prefer paper records annotate printouts and place these in patient charts as formal documentation, thus creating two distinct and sometimes conflicting medical records.

5. *Unfavorable changes in communication patterns and practices.* Example: EHRs create an "illusion of communication" (i.e., a belief that simply entering an order ensures that others will see it and act on it). For example, a physician fails to speak with a nurse about administering a medication, assuming that the nurse will see the note in the EHR and act on it.

6. *Negative user emotions.* Example: Physicians become frustrated with hard-to-use software.

7. *Generation of new kinds of errors.* Example: Busy physicians enter data in a miscellaneous section, rather than in the intended location. Improper placement can cause confusion, duplication, and even medical error.

8. *Unexpected and unintended changes in institutional power structure.* Example: IT, quality-assurance departments, and the administration gain power by requiring physicians to comply with EHR-based directives (e.g., clinical decision support alerts).

9. *Overdependence on technology.* Example: Physicians dependent on clinical decision support may have trouble remembering standard dosages, formulary recommendations, and medication contraindications during system downtimes (Campbell et al., 2006; Sittig & Ash, 2007).

Operational Model for Three Domains of Expertise

Interprofessional collaboration has been said to improve patient safety and quality outcomes and this also may be applied in the HIT environment (Interprofessional Collaborative Expert Panel, 2011). We have observed that there are three key players in the effort to manage HIT safety. They are as follows:

1. Patient safety and risk-management specialists

2. Quality-improvement specialists

3. Nursing informaticists

All three domains of expertise have made unique contributions to the end goal of improved care through EHRs and interoperability. Yet, in many organizations, these operational models work on separate departments that are not always tightly aligned.

Practical implications for department independence is an operational model that is vital to successful HIT implementations. Interdepartmental expert contributions are as follows:

▶ Quality departments maintain quality assurance and peer review protection

▶ Patient safety information has historically been maintained in risk-management departments as a result of the litigious nature of the information relating to a patient safety event resulting in injury or death

▶ HIT deployment is managed from the IT departments of most institutions

Quality departments maintain committee structure and operational procedures within health care organizations to address peer review protections with differing laws depending on the state policy. Patient safety information is particularly sensitive information to organizations and at the same time we have rapid deployment of EHRs resulting in the potential for unintended consequences. For good reason, these three departments—patient safety, quality improvement, and nursing informatics—often operate independently of one another and have different specialists with expertise in these three areas working from their particular domain of expertise.

Harrison Interactive Sociotechnical Analysis Model

Many unintended and undesired consequences of health care IT flow from interactions between the HIT and the health care organization's sociotechnical system. Factors, such as workflows, culture, social interactions, and technologies, are affected. Harrison and colleagues present a conceptual model of these processes they call *interactive sociotechnical*

analysis (ISTA). ISTA is said to capture common types of interaction with special emphasis on recursive processes, such as feedback loops, that alter the newly introduced HIT
and promote second-level changes in the social system. ISTA draws on prior studies of
unintended consequences, along with research in sociotechnical systems, ergonomics,
social informatics, technology-in-practice, and social construction of technology. The
ISTA model provides a guide for further research on emergent and recursive processes
in HIT implementation and their unintended consequences. Familiarity with the model
can also foster practitioners' awareness of unanticipated consequences that only become
evident during HIT implementation (Harrison, Koppel, & Bar-Lev, 2007). Specifically,
five interactive components of the ISTA are as follows:

1. New HIT changes the existing social system.
2. Technical and physical infrastructure mediated HIT use—interaction of new
   HIT with existing technical and physical conditions affects HIT use.
3. Social system mediates HIT use—interaction of new HIT with social system affects
   HIT use.
4. HIT use changes the social system—interaction of new HIT with social system
   affects HIT use, which then further changes the social system.
5. HIT–social system interactions engender HIT redesign—interaction of new HIT
   with the social system affects HIT use, which then leads to changes in HIT properties (Harrison et al., 2007).

As noted in Chapter 3, the arrows in the ISTA schematic show the impact of one sociotechnical subcomponent on another and correspond to the five interaction types (Harrison
et al., 2007).

Guide to Unintended Consequence Management

On the HealthIT.gov website, the Office of the National Coordinator has created a number
of resources, one of which is the *Guide to Reducing Unintended Consequences of Electronic
Health Records* (see http://healthit.gov/unintended-consequences/?q=ucguide). The guide
addresses all care settings and notes a number of common patient safety issues related
to unintended consequence of HIT. This online guide for health care providers, IT specialists, and system administrators, helps in planning and avoiding possible problems
when implementing and using an EHR. Developed to provide practical, troubleshooting
knowledge and resources for all types of health care organizations, the guide is based on
the research literature, other practice-oriented guides for EHR implementation and use,
research by its authors, and interviews with organizations that have recently implemented EHR (Jones et al., 2011).

The guide is organized into four modules:

1. Introduction to unintended consequences
2. How to avoid unintended consequences
3. Understand and identify unintended consequences
4. Remediate unintended consequences (covered later in this chapter)

Hazard Manager by Agency for Healthcare Research and Quality

The Hazard Manager is a federally funded project focused on developing and testing a software tool to capture and manage information about prospectively identified HIT hazards before they have the potential to cause harm. Rather than looking retrospectively at accidents or near misses, this tool is designed to collect structured information about potential hazards associated with specific HIT products (see Figure 20.1).

There are four main categories of hazard attributes, which include:

1. Discovery

2. Causation

3. Impact

4. Mitigation/corrective action

The beta test is being conducted under the auspices of a PSO, with three levels of security:

1. A participating health care organization can enter and see information regarding the hazard it identifies

2. Vendors will have the ability to see hazards reported by their customers

3. Health care organizations, vendors, policy makers, and researchers may request access to view aggregated, de-identified reports of hazard attributes

Stakeholders for this product include individual care delivery organizations (CDOs), organizations using the same applications (e.g., EHR user groups), HIT vendors, and policy makers.

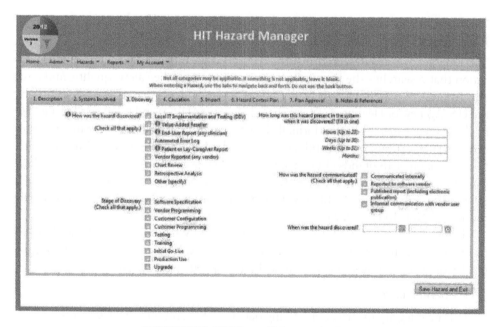

FIGURE 20.1. HIT Hazard Manager database.

HIT, health information technology.

Source: Walker, Hassol, Bradshaw, and Rezaee (2012).

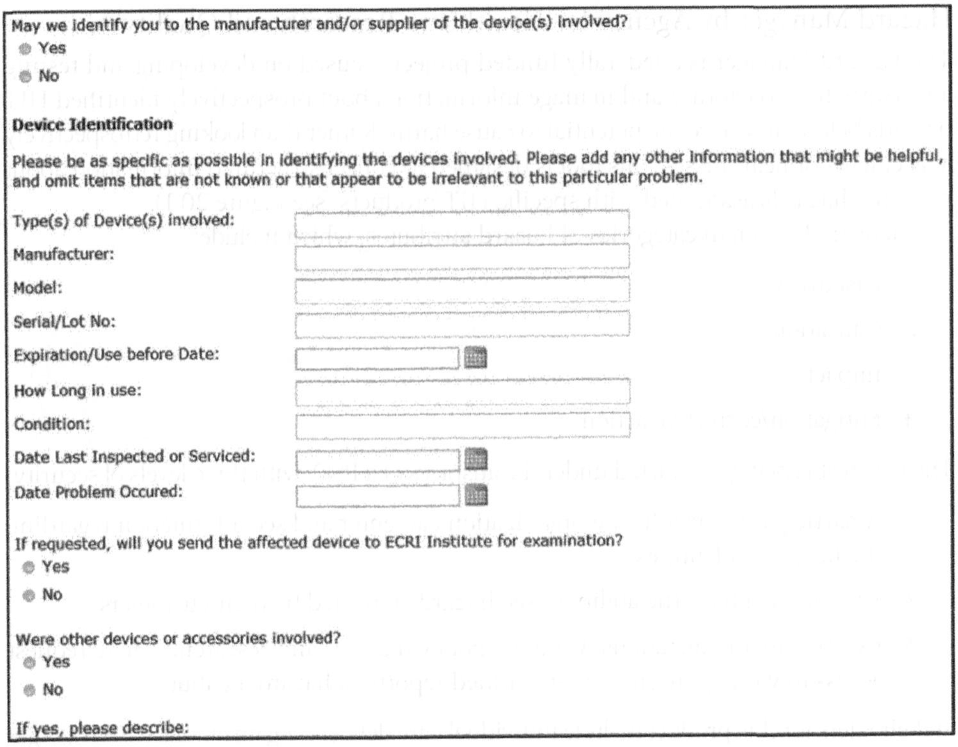

May we identify you to the manufacturer and/or supplier of the device(s) involved?
● Yes
● No

Device Identification

Please be as specific as possible in identifying the devices involved. Please add any other information that might be helpful, and omit items that are not known or that appear to be irrelevant to this particular problem.

Type(s) of Device(s) involved:

Manufacturer:

Model:

Serial/Lot No:

Expiration/Use before Date:

How Long in use:

Condition:

Date Last Inspected or Serviced:

Date Problem Occured:

If requested, will you send the affected device to ECRI Institute for examination?
● Yes
● No

Were other devices or accessories involved?
● Yes
● No

If yes, please describe:

FIGURE 20.2. Public website for error reporting; ECRI reporting page.
ECRI, Emergency Care Research Institute.
Source: ECRI Institute (2014).

Emergency Care Research Institute Annual Report of Errors

The Emergency Care Research Institute (ECRI) is an independent, nonprofit organization that researches the best approaches to improving the safety, quality, and cost-effectiveness of patient care. It is designated as an evidence-based practice center by the U.S. Agency for Healthcare Research and Quality (AHRQ) and listed as a federal PSO by the United States. In 1968 it formally began operation, focusing on research in emergency medicine, resuscitation, and related biomedical engineering studies. The Institute's first evaluation of 18 brands of manually operated resuscitators found nine to be ineffective and started ECRI as an independent evaluator and provider of medical-device-related information and guidance. ECRI provides reporting mechanisms and reports, most notably the annual "Top 10 HIT Hazards" report (Figure 20.2).

The ECRI Institute's Health Devices Group annually reviews a top-10 list of health technology hazards. In the most recent study by ECRI on patient safety and HIT, the top 10 safety hazards associated with health technology were as follows:

1. Alarm hazards

2. Data integrity incorrect of missing data in EHRs and other HIT systems

3. Mix-up of IV (intravenous) lines leading to misadministration of drugs and solutions

4. Inadequate reprocessing of endoscopes and surgical instruments

5. Ventilator disconnections not caught because of mis-set or missed alarms

6. Patient handling device use errors and device failures

7. "Dose creep": Unnoticed variations in diagnostic radiation exposures

8. Robotic surgery: Complications caused by insufficient training

9. Cybersecurity: Insufficient protection for medical devices and systems

10. Overwhelmed recall and safety alert management programs (ECRI Institute, 2014, p. 1)

Clinical Impact of HIT Error/Unintended Consequences

Data Noise and Missing the Patient Story

"The problem with EMR/EHR data is that there is so much of it." It is sometimes called "data noise" (Shaw, 2010, p. 1). Health care professionals really have to know where to look and know where to find needed information in the EMR/EHR. In health care, we have literally seconds sometimes to assess the situation and make a decision for patients (Shaw, 2010).

Thus, the notion of the number of clicks-to-information ratio has become of interest to EHR developers. Extensive click-to-information ratios can be associated with patient morbidity, poor outcomes, and even death (Minnier, 2011). There is little in the way of guidelines for appropriate click-to-information ratios. Perhaps routine information should be seven to eight clicks to information. It would seem that critical information should be two to three clicks away and/or voice activated (Minnier, 2011).

After an untoward event in which a patient's trend toward renal failure went undetected so long that it was irreversible, one hospital decided to address the problem by inventing SmartRoom technology. In retrospective review, it appeared that the patient's story and details about the patient's renal status were missed amid the noise of the EMR/EHR data. Three years later "SmartRoom as the app for the EMR" evolved as a possible solution (Shaw, 2010). The SmartRoom app:

▶ Identifies health care workers, who wear small ultrasound tags, as they walk into a patient's room; the technology displays the worker's identity and role on a wall-mounted monitor visible to patients

▶ Automatically pulls relevant, real-time patient information from the EMR and other clinical systems, including pharmacy and lab services (www.healthleadersmedia.com/content/MAG-257392/Patient-Rooms-Get-Smart)

The SmartRoom technology consists of three components:

1. A patient screen, which lets patients identify their caregivers, shows a list of the day's activities (scheduled lab tests, for instance), and can access educational materials.

2. A caregiver screen gives clinicians access to essential information, including allergies and medication regimens. This system also lets nurses and aides quickly document vital signs and complete basic tasks on a touch screen, which then updates the EMR. The system is intelligent enough to give different sets of patient data to

different categories of providers. An aide responsible for turning a patient, for instance, would be told that the patient is allergic to latex and would remind the aide to put the bed rails up. The aide would not see any details on medication dosages.

3. The SmartBoard replaces the conventional dry erase board at the nursing station. It lists patients' names and their associated caregivers, and it updates the staff on new physician orders (Cerrato, 2011).

Patient Identification Errors, Common

Wrong patient, or patient identification errors, are the most common and most worrisome of HIT errors. Recent findings by the ONC suggested that EHRs generally improve patient safety and make the process of ordering tests and medications easier, but 15% of physicians still say that an EHR led them to select the wrong medication or lab order from a list or led to a potential medication error (Bresnick, 2014). There is no industry consensus on the safest configuration of EHRs when it comes to patient identification management. For example, debate exists about how many patient records should be allowed open on the EHR at one time. A Montefiore Medical Center survey recently found that 83.5% of chief medical information officers used CPOE systems that allowed more than one patient record open at a time, but some organizations later changed the system's settings to let clinicians view only a single record (Bresnick, 2014).

A study using a "retract-and-reorder" measurement tool was used to estimate the frequency of wrong-patient electronic orders. It was then used to estimate the frequency of wrong-patient electronic orders in four hospitals in 2009. Using this tool, it was estimated that 5,246 electronic orders were placed on wrong patients. Two types of identity management tools were used to study and mitigate this situation: One was *ID-verify* and the other was *ID-reentry*. Results indicated that, compared to a control group, *ID-verify* reduced the odds of treating the wrong patient by a larger magnitude (odds ratio = 0.60, 95% confidence interval, 0.50 to 0.71; Adelman et al., 2013). These findings suggest that the challenge of patient identification exists and that studies can lead to improved outcomes (Adelman et al., 2013).

The SAFER (safety assurance factors for EHR resilience) Guide has indicated that many principles of safety must be considered for correct patient identification. The list of guidelines for the EHR included displaying the basics such as last name, first name, date of birth (with calculated age), gender, and medical record number, but having a recent photograph of the patient was also recommended (HealthIT.gov, 2014a).

Alert Fatigue

EHR systems often include decision support functionalities such as drug–drug interaction, drug–dose, drug–lab, and contraindication alerting. Several studies have identified "alert fatigue" (choosing to ignore alerts) as a common condition among clinicians using EHRs with decision support. The SAFER Guide provides a review of the relevant research literature, indicating that the majority of alerts are overridden. Multiple remediation options are available (HealthIT.gov, 2014b).

The first option would be to deactivate the alerts entirely. A more measured approach might be to convene a panel of local physicians to determine which alerts should be turned on. Perhaps the most successful approach identified in the literature is implementing tiered alerts (e.g., minor, moderate, severe). Shah and colleagues found that this kind of approach significantly increased the acceptance rate of decision support alerts (Shah et al., 2006). Lesson learned were that (a) interruptive decision support alerts can be a major source of user frustration and system inefficiency, and (b) careful consideration should be given to the type and frequency of alerts that are included in decision support systems (HealthIT.gov, 2014b).

EHR-Induced Medical Errors

EHR-induced medical errors have been studied extensively. It has been noted that they can occur for reasons such as:

1. Interfaces that do not transfer complete data from one system to another, or from medical devices to the EHR

2. Lack of coordination among different systems (e.g., emergency department systems that hold different sets of orders from the same patient)

3. Not enough data on a single screen (e.g., space for only five medications at a time when the common patient may be on 15)

4. Inconsistent nomenclature between systems (e.g., calling drugs or diagnoses by different names in different systems; Gardner, 2010)

ACTIONS FOR WHEN HIT PATIENT SAFETY ISSUES ARISE

Data Collection and Reporting

In regard to error management and prevention in health care, data collection and reporting are key components. As with any quality-improvement effort, the accuracy, consistency, and currency of the data and reporting matter greatly. Along those lines, there are levels of reporting to be considered.

Levels of Reporting

PSO reporting is the most private of all reporting for health care delivery information. The AHRQ is charged with administering the provisions of the Patient Safety Act related to PSOs. The AHRQ website has a multitude of information concerning PSOs: www.pso.ahrq.gov

▶ Important purpose of PSOs is that they protect the information reported to them in a secure environment where clinicians and health care organizations can collect, aggregate, and analyze data in order "to reduce risks and hazards of care."

▶ A complete list of AHRQ-listed PSOs is available at AHRQ's website. Congress passed the Patient Safety and Quality Improvement Act of 2005. To read the Patient Safety Act, go to www.pso.ahrq.gov/statute/pl109-41.htm.

▶ The Patient Safety Act and the Patient Safety Rule authorize the creation of PSOs to improve quality and safety through the collection and analysis of data on patient events.

▶ PSOs protect data and allow for aggregation and analysis to determine patterns and trends so that national patient safety concerns can be addressed.

▶ PSOs have standard reporting formats for several types of events, including a new reporting format for medical devices & HIT (see Figure 20.3; www.psoppc .org/web/patientsafety).

Public website blogs offer more public reporting of health care delivery information. They are available for most viewers browsing on the Internet. Information on such sites may be considered relevant but limited as a source of valid reference. An excerpt from a blog on the www.healthsystemCIO.com website is representative of public comments made about error in HIT use (see Figure 20.4). Neither the patient nor provider identifying

Event ID: _____

Initial Report Date (HERF Q1) _____

Patient Safety Event Report – Hospital:

H   **DEVICE OR MEDICAL/SURGICAL SUPPLY, INCLUDING HEALTH INFORMATION TECHNOLOGY (HIT)**

Use this form to report any patient safety event or unsafe condition involving a defect, failure, or incorrect use of a device, including an HIT device. A device includes an implant, medical equipment, or medical/surgical supply (including disposable product). An HIT device includes hardware or software that is used to electronically create, maintain, analyze, store, or receive information to aid in the diagnosis, cure, mitigation, treatment, or prevention of disease and that is not an integral part of (1) an implantable device or (2) an item of medical equipment.

For defects or events discovered prior to market approval or clinical deployment, do not use this form. If the event also involves a medication or other substance, please complete the Medication or Other Substance form in addition to this form. Narrative detail can be captured on the Healthcare Event Reporting Form (HERF). Highlighted fields are collected for local facility and Patient Safety Organization (PSO) use. This information will not be forwarded to the Network of Patient Safety Databases (NPSD).

1. **Which of the following best describes the event or unsafe condition?** CHECK ONE:

　a. ☐ Device defect or failure, including HIT
　b. ☐ Use error
　c. ☐ Combination or interaction of device defect or failure and use error
　d. ☐ Unknown

2. **What type of device was involved in the event or unsafe condition?** CHECK ONE:

　a. ☐ Implantable device (i.e., device intended to be inserted into, and remain permanently in, tissue)

　b. ☐ Medical equipment (e.g., walker, hearing aid)
　c. ☐ Medical/surgical supply, including disposable product (e.g., incontinence supply)
　d. ☐ HIT device

3. **At the time of the event, was the device placed within the patient's tissue?** CHECK ONE:

　a. ☐ Yes
　b. ☐ No
　c. ☐ Unknown

4. **Did the event result in the device being removed?** CHECK ONE:

　a. ☐ Yes
　b. ☐ No
　c. ☐ Unknown

5. **What is the name (brand or generic) of the device, product, software, or medical/surgical supply?**

_____

6. **What is the name of the manufacturer?**

_____

FIGURE 20.3. HIT reporting form and process.
Source: AHRQ (2015).

> Speaking from 13 years in the trenches of EHR-use at a variety of healthcare organizations, and applying a dash of country-boy common sense, I don't need a fancy and sophisticated, multi-year analysis to tell me that the impact is orders of magnitude higher—it's 100 times higher, at least. There are unintended consequences of EHRs upon patient safety every day in every hospital that uses an EHR.
>
> Here's a brief discussion of only four of the many patient safety events that happened under my watch, that were directly attributable to an EHR.
>
> **Missed diagnosis for soft tissue sarcoma:** In this accident, a soft tissue sarcoma went undiagnosed for at least 3 months, possibly as long as 6 months, because the radiologist's report from the Radiology Information System failed to file properly in the EHR and the referring physician *didn't know what they didn't know* and failed to follow-up on the results of the scan. The young mother of three went untreated, the cancer spread to the point that it was untreatable, and she died. The case was settled out of court for several hundred thousand dollars.

FIGURE 20.4. Blog about missed diagnosis.
Source: Sanders (2010).

information is used but one gets the sense of the magnitude of the error and the associated role of HIT.

Public websites of the *HITxChange* (www.healthitxchange.org) are also publicly available and provide HIT information that is categorized by specific user needs, such as implementation, cost management, and error reporting, to name a few. *HITxChange* is organized around implementation stages of the EHR. The website provides anonymous information about HIT errors and near errors. The information contained within the *HealthITxChange* is organized around the stages needed to plan, implement, and optimize the use of an EHR system in practice. The seven stages are preparing, business planning, selecting, contracting, implementing, assessing, and thriving (see Figure 20.5). Organizing information in this way allows implementers to access information when they need it and to plan for the upcoming stages. Within each stage, the information is further organized into four categories—people, process, technology, and other.

- ▶ *People*: This category relates to the human dimension of successful implementation, such as stakeholder buy-in.

- ▶ *Processes*: This category focuses on the activities that are necessary for development or assessment at a given stage.

- ▶ *Technology*: As its name suggests, this category focuses on aspects related to the technology (both hardware and software).

- ▶ *Other*: This category covers topics that are cross-cutting or that fall outside of the people, process, and technology categories.

The *HealthITxChange* is a nonprofit initiative that joins together health care and HIT professionals to share lessons learned and resources (referred to as pearls) for implementing EHRs in a physician office. This unique online community enables members to share and discuss HIT adoption issues with a volunteer peer network of informaticists, physicians, nurses, ancillary medical staff, administrators, vendors, and consultants. Members make

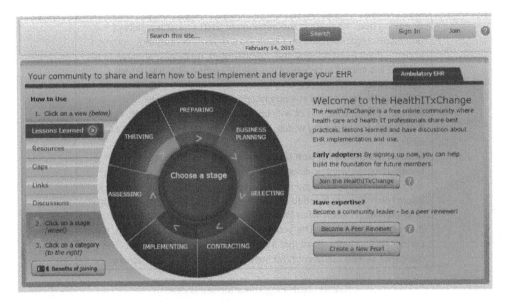

FIGURE 20.5. Home page for HealthITxChange, a public site where HIT professionals share best practices, lessons learned, and discuss EHR implementation and use.
Source: HealthITxChange.org (2014).

the community work by donating their time to share their experience and expertise through submission of pearls, participation in discussions, rating of pearls, serving as peer reviewers, and providing feedback when requested by the *HealthITxChange*.

National Trend

The national trends seem to be to align management of HIT-related errors on two fronts: risk management and patient engagement. As noted, alignment of error identification and management with the risk-management department mitigates the potential legal and regulatory components of error.

In regard to the patient engagement component of error mitigation, patient engagement has proven to be successful. For example, the Healthcare Information and Management Systems Society (HIMSS) and the National eHealth Collaborative (NeHC) have merged to form the Health Care and Promotion Fund Committee (HCPFC), which provides thought leadership on how to improve patient health through the use of IT. The HCPFC will closely align with the HIMSS-connected patient committee and connected patient community efforts.

Appendix 20.1 provides a schematic of the entire HIMSS Patient Engagement framework, which is the current platform for the previously merged NeHC University and HIMSS.

STRATEGIES TO MITIGATE HIT PATIENT SAFETY ISSUES

The ONC released a plan to address patient safety and HIT in July 2013, titled "Health Information Technology Patient Safety Action & Surveillance Plan," which outlined a number of actions that can be taken to inspire patient and provider confidence in HIT infrastructure using the best evidence available on patient safety (Office of National Coordinator for Health Information Technology, 2013). Additionally, the report discusses leveraging "existing authorities to strengthen patient safety efforts across government programs and the private sector—including patients, health care providers, technology companies, and health care safety oversight bodies" (p. 4). Specific actions by stakeholders are recommended in the report and the plan calls for coordinated effort among all government agencies, private organizations, and individuals in order to fully accomplish the plan. This report indicates there are roles and shared responsibilities for clinicians, patients and caregivers, health care delivery systems, HIT professionals/developers, federal and state agencies, and various private sector organizations. The plan is located on the HealthIT.gov website for full review. Figure 20.6 reflects all of the stakeholders, including various governmental agencies involved in promoting safety of HIT, and the relationships among organizations to fully realize the shared responsibility.

Multifaceted Options to Optimize Safety

SAFER Guide

As an action item identified in the HIT Patient Safety Action and Surveillance Plan, the ONC released a series of recommendations in the form of SAFER Guides for organizations to use in assessing their organization for optimizing the safe use of HIT in the following areas:

- ▶ High priority practices
- ▶ Organizational responsibilities
- ▶ Contingency planning
- ▶ System configuration
- ▶ System interfaces
- ▶ Patient identification
- ▶ Computer provider order entry with decision support
- ▶ Test results reporting
- ▶ Follow-up, clinician communication

Additionally, the SAFER Guides are intended to be useful to all stakeholders noted in the ONC's original plan, including EHR users, developers, PSOs, and other individuals who desire optimization and safe use of health IT (HealthIT.gov, 2014c).

Health Care Delivery Systems

A starting point for organizations to safeguard against patient safety issues arising from technology is to begin with strategic initiatives within an organization to report and address patient safety and quality issues. Using tools, such as the SAFER Guides and other assessment tools, to inform organizational strategies for improving the use of HIT is essential. For example, on release of the statistics in the IOM report related to medical errors, many organizations created plans to improve safety in U.S. hospitals through safer medication management, including technology solutions involving CPOE and barcoding medications (Kohn et al., 1999). Assessing technology along with reporting errors when they occur through appropriate channels, including the PSOs, will help to inform the

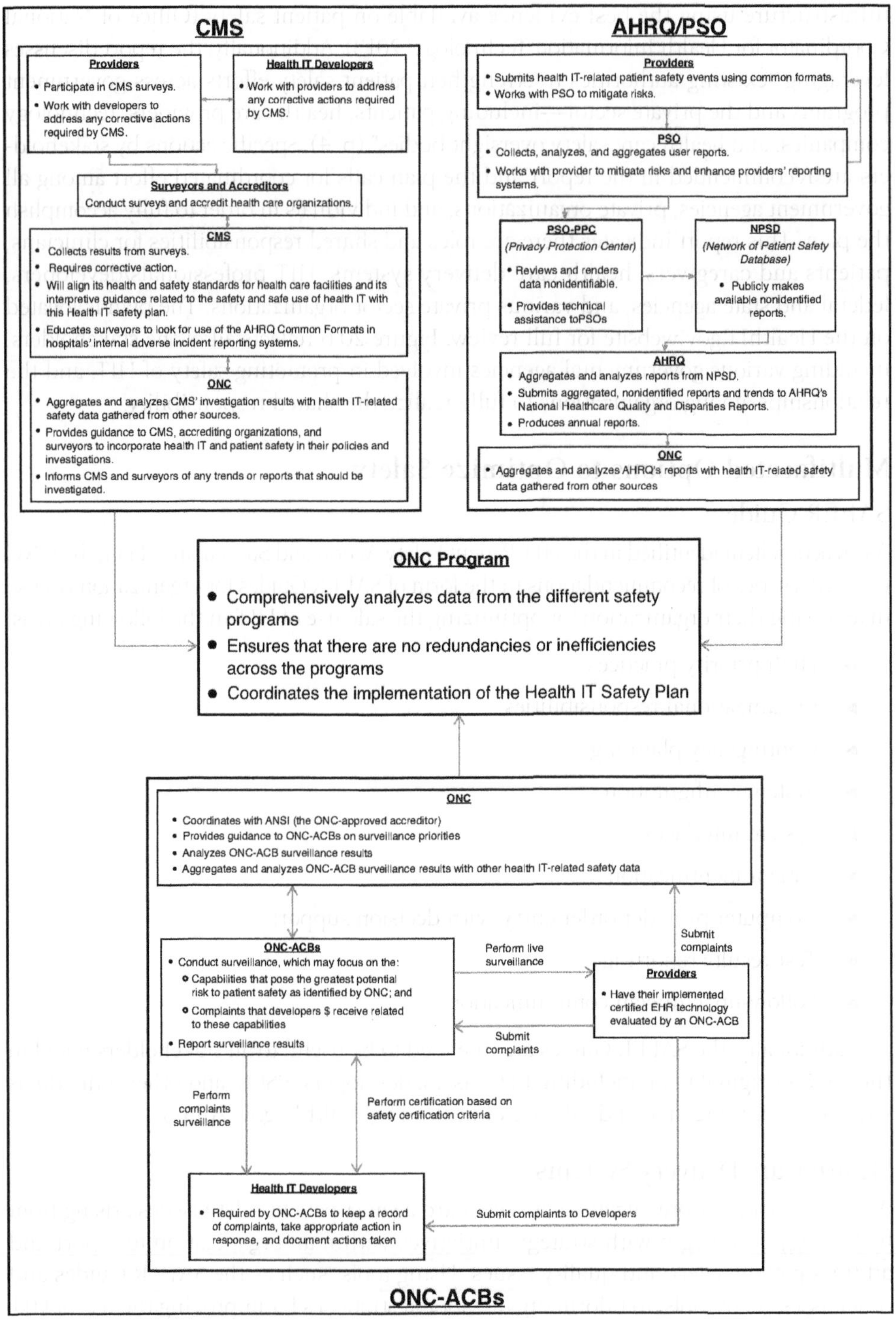

FIGURE 20.6. HIT patient safety action and surveillance plan.

ACB, authorized certification bodies; AHRQ, Agency for Healthcare Research and Quality; CMS, Centers for Medicare & Medicaid Services; ONC, Office of the National Coordinator; PPC, Privacy Protection Center; PSO, patient safety organization.
Source: Office of the National Coordinator of Health Information Technology (2013).

evidence surrounding patient safety and HIT. Many experts believe that the evidence to date on patient safety is likely "the tip of the iceberg" and that clinicians are often busy and fail to report near misses or events that related to the technology but did not create a harmful effect (HIMSS, 2011).

A critical role for health care organizations is to facilitate an environment that reinforces a "no-blame" culture, encouraging reporting of events as noted earlier, and to ensure contractual relationships with vendors foster vendor partnerships for reporting and addressing patient safety issues related to use of the EHR. Koppel and Kreda (2009) suggested that vendor contracts prohibit reporting in a commentary to the *Journal of American Medical Association*, stating:

> Healthcare information technology (HIT) vendors enjoy a contractual and legal structure that renders them virtually liability-free—"held harmless" is the term-of-art—even when their proprietary products may be implicated in adverse events involving patients. This contractual and legal device shifts liability and remedial burdens to physicians, nurses, hospitals, and clinics, even when these HIT users are strictly following vendor instructions . . . HIT vendors are not responsible for errors their systems introduce in patient treatment because physicians, nurses, pharmacists, and healthcare technicians should be able to identify—and correct—any errors generated by software faults. (Koppel & Kreda, 2009, p. 1)

TeamSTEPPS Model

The TeamSTEPPS 2.0 Core Curriculum is designed to help you develop and deploy a customized plan to train your staff in teamwork skills and lead a medical teamwork improvement initiative in your organization from initial concept development through to sustainment of positive changes. STEPPS stands for strategies and tools to enhance performance and patient safety. Comprehensive curricula and instructional guides include short case studies and videos illustrating teamwork opportunities and successes. Supporting materials include a pocket guide, CD-ROM and DVD, and evaluation tools. Instructor and Trainer workshop materials focus on change management, coaching, and implementation (AHRQ, 2014b).

TeamSTEPPS is a teamwork system designed for health care professionals that is:

► A powerful solution to improving patient safety within your organization

► An evidence-based teamwork system to improve communication and teamwork skills among health care professionals

► A source for ready-to-use materials and a training curriculum to successfully integrate teamwork principles into all areas of your health care system

► Scientifically rooted in more than 20 years of research and lessons from the application of teamwork principles

► Developed by Department of Defense's Patient Safety Program in collaboration with the AHRQ

TeamSTEPPS also provides simulation support. The purpose of this guide is to provide instruction on using simulation-based training when teaching TeamSTEPPS, as opposed to using TeamSTEPPS tools and strategies in simulation training for other purposes. The use of simulation, which has been proven to be a powerful strategy in team-based health care, affords excellent opportunities to enhance the quality of continuing education for health care professionals, as well as provide education and practice for students learning to become health care professionals. The culture of medicine has traditionally valued technical proficiency over interpersonal skills, and this may not always be the most efficacious approach to ensuring patient safety. This TeamSTEPPS simulation guide integrates critical teamwork as well as interpersonal and communication skills into simulation-based training, thereby offering strategies and tools that can improve team performance and enhance patient safety. This training course can and should be adapted to meet the needs of specific health care teams and programs. It is intended as a train-the-trainer program in which key personnel become familiar with the materials and activities so that they can offer the simulation-based TeamSTEPPS training to local health care teams. Users of this training course are encouraged to adapt and augment activities accordingly, substituting their own scenarios in the training, when applicable (American Institutes for Research, 2011).

The Leapfrog Group, an Employer-Based Safety Initiative

As a result of the 1999 report by the IOM, a group of concerned employers launched an initiative called The Leapfrog Group. This initiative led by employers was focused on market reinforcement to improve patient safety and quality through breakthrough initiatives or "Big Leaps" in hospital safety. The initial focus was on four areas: (a) CPOE, (b) evidence-based hospital referral, (c) ICU physician staffing with intensivists, and (d) NQF safety practices constituting 34 safe practices (The Leapfrog Group, 2014). Although the Leapfrog initiative has created some controversy among hospitals (Umbdenstock, 2012), the Leapfrog Group has created a CPOE evaluation tool positioned as a means for addressing the customization and monitoring of CPOE to realize the full benefit of desired safety benefits. The importance of customization is supported by the National Quality Forum and supports the requirements under meaningful use (MU; Kilbridge, Welebob, & Classen, 2006; Thompson, 2010). The latest Leapfrog tool uses simulated cases for hospitals to test the build of the EHRs for safe and efficient CPOE customizations (Leung et al., 2013). The tool can assist hospitals in prioritizing their improvement strategies and they are able to monitor progress over time by annual use of the tool to evaluate progress (L. Saldana, personal communication, February 15, 2015). The Leapfrog assessment tool and the SAFER Guides are two strategies organizations can use to facilitate safe effective use of technology to improve care.

Technology Informatics Guiding Education Reform Leadership to Transform Education

The IOM report *The Future of Nursing* is perhaps one of the best places to examine the role of clinicians with respect to improving the care we deliver. The report reinforces the importance of advanced practice graduate-prepared nurses working within interprofessional teams to transform the health care system in positive directions. The vision for the future that this report describes is one that includes promoting wellness and prevention, reliably improving health outcomes, and providing competent care across the life span, calling on patient-centric interprofessional teams as a norm for the health care industry. Further, the report examines the role of nursing in realizing this vision, and specifically notes the role of nursing in fully adopting and implementing HIT safely and effectively (IOM, 2011). Yet, explicit to technology and safety, there are no specifics about how to address the challenges we are currently seeing with HIT hazards.

A recent report by the Technology Informatics Guiding Education Reform (TIGER) Initiative Foundation titled *The Leadership Imperative: Recommendations for Integrating Technology to Transform Practice and Education* (TIGER Development Collaborative, 2014) noted key roles for clinical leaders. The report stresses the importance of clinical leaders promoting the value of HIT and emphasizes collaboration and use of evidence-based best practices, expansion of informatics competencies at all levels, promotion of shared best practices, and alignment for patient-centered outcomes. The report empha-sizes the role of stewardship within health care systems, focusing on "teamwork, col-laboration, and continuous development of and utilization of IT" to promote safety and quality of care across the United States (TIGER Development Collaborative, 2014, p. 10). This report also points to a Polarity Map model to assist in addressing patient safety challenges emphasizing the importance of balancing the positives and negatives of tech-nology. The Map recommends actions for balancing technology and practice. The exam-ple used is that if health care organizations pay too much attention to technology and not enough to impact on clinical workflow, negative outcomes occur. For further information on the TIGER team recommendations and the Polarity Map, visit the TIGER Initiative Foundation website: www.thetigerinitiative.org.

Remediating Unintended Consequences of HIT

Remediating unintended consequences is an important role of the interprofessional team and it also fully utilizes essential quality-improvement tools that are covered in subsequent chapters. These tools are noted in this section and covered more fully in the Chapter 21. The *Guide to Reducing Unintended Consequences of Electronic Health Records* is an excel-lent resource for providers and hospitals for tools and information to help understand and to use in addressing unintended consequences of HIT (Jones et al., 2011). The guide walks the end user through the process of understanding and addressing patient safety events and includes a number of useful and downloadable tools to examine the unin-tended consequences. We highlight some of the guide's recommendations.

Pinpoint the Cause

Defining the problem and gathering the evidence are critical components of remedia-tion. The root-cause analysis and the failure mode effects analysis are excellent tools for pinpointing the issues behind a patient safety and HIT event. The goal is to fully under-stand what happened and to fully document the problem with those who were immedi-ately involved in the event. Constructing a timeline that fully documents sequence of events and the timing of the occurrence helps better understand the cause. A cause-and-effect diagram presents the timeline of events that led to the problem and the indi-viduals or roles involved in the process. Figure 20.7 presents an example provided by the ONC at www.healthit.gov/unintended-consequences/content/assess-problem.html (Jones, Koppel, Wu, & Harrison, 2011a).

This process should follow with the construction of a cause-and-effect diagram, also referred to as a fishbone diagram. This cause-and-effect diagram is also a good way to

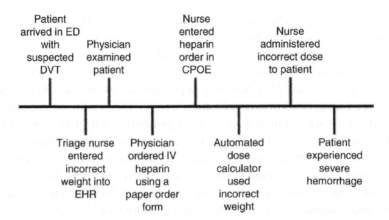

FIGURE 20.7. Timeline of events that led to the heparin overdose in the ED. www.healthit.gov/
unintended-consequences/content/assess-problem.html

CPOE, computer provider order entry; DVT, deep vein thrombosis; ED, emergency department; EHR, electronic health record.
Source: Jones et al. (2011a).

document the root cause of the problem. Within this process it is important to essentially perform an ISTA based on the ISTA framework examining all interactions of the
environment; end-user actions as to how the technology was used in workflow and the
unintended consequence; infrastructure, including the physical layout that might have
contributed to the issue; and the EHR/technology design factors that might be a contributing element to the problem. The result of this process is to develop a clearly stated
causal statement (Jones, Koppel, Wu, & Harrison, 2011b).

The National Center for Patient Safety of the U.S. Department of Veterans Affairs notes
the following in the ONC guide:

1. Clearly show the cause and effect relationship. If you eliminate the root cause or
   contributing factor you will reduce the likelihood of similar problems occurring
   in the future.

2. Use specific and accurate descriptors for what occurred, rather than negative and
   vague words. Avoid words with non-specific negative connotations or that assign
   blame (e.g., careless, poor, sloppy, etc.)

3. Identify the preceding cause(s), not the human error. Focus on systemic vulnerabilities, not human error.

4. Identify the preceding cause(s) of procedure violations. Focus on the root causes,
   not the symptoms.

5. Failure to act is only causal when there is a pre-existing duty to act. In some
   cases the absence of policies and procedures is the root cause. www.healthit.gov/
   unintended-consequences/content/assess-problem.html (Jones et al., 2011b)

Prioritize, Plan, and Execute the Remediation for a HIT
Patient Safety Issue

It is one thing to identify the cause of a patient safety event related to technology, but yet
another to actually prioritize solutions, which frequently involve establishing priorities.

The actions taken to remediate the issues should tie directly to the causal statements developed in the previous step. Using interprofessional teams to determine priority for fixes is critical to the process. The ONC website has a tool for helping teams prioritize and document the remediation plan. Noted in Table 20.1 are the elements of the tool and a brief description of what to address within that element of the remediation plan

TABLE 20.1 Remediation Plan Components for an HIT Safety Concern	
Components to Address	**Description**
Project description	Description of the problem, including why it needs remediation.
Goal statement	Identify goals and define metrics for success.
Functionality and activities requested to mediate the problem	List the key features, functions, training, or policies required to achieve the goals. If requesting modifications to an existing system, application, or database, name the system; otherwise, simply define the change needed.
Processes impacted	Note process impacted by remediation actions.
Sites and stakeholders affected	List the areas, organizations affected by the remediation.
Scope of the project	Define the scope, including date range, existing systems and/or interfaces, data specific to the remediation.
Project benefits	Describe the benefits, both financial and otherwise.
Project risks	Describe any identifiable risk associated with remediation.
Project dependencies or enablers	Describe anything that needs to occur prior to implementation to be successful.
Success factors	Describe what constitutes success.
Cost: Investment	Describe technology-related costs.
Cost: Support	Describe human being support factor costs.
Any financial benefits	List the financial benefits to the organization.

HIT, health information technology.

Adapted from the Remediation Planning tool on www.healthit.gov/unintended-consequences/content/remediate-problem.html

Source: Jones et al. (2011c).

(Jones, Koppel, Wu, & Harrison, 2011c). This remediation plan can also take the form of a project charter, which will be discussed in subsequent chapters.

The final step for remediating a patient safety concern is to actually implement the project over time and to evaluate the impact of the remediation over time. These factors should be included as measures of success in your remediation plan scope document, based on Table 20.1.

Statewide Nursing Approach for Error Mitigation

Health care professionals in all states have been affected by the rapid implementation of HIT since 2010, when EHR implementations were supported and funded through the ONC. Given that the largest population of health care professionals are nurses, the impact on nursing has been great.

In Texas, the Texas Nurses Association (TNA) and the Texas Organization of Nurse Executives (TONE) have concerns about the 300,000 practicing nurses' experience as the EHR implementations occurred. There was equal concern for the impact of patient care delivery, namely, safety and quality. As such, in 2010, the organizations partnered to create a board of directors resolution to be submitted to legislatures (Texas Nursing Association, 2010). The resolution created the statewide TNA/TONE HIT committee with the charge to study and benchmark the impact of HIT on nurses and patients. Figure 20.8 illustrates the 5-year strategic framework the committee created to address that charge.

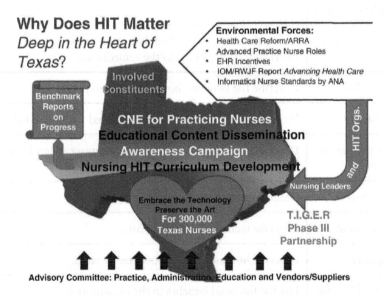

FIGURE 20.8. TNA/TONE HIT committee framework.

ANA, American Nurses Association; ARRA, American Recovery and Reinvestment Act; EHR, electronic health records; HIT, health information technology; IOM, Institute of Medicine; RWJF, Robert Wood Johnson Foundation; TIGER, Technology Informatics Guiding Education Reform; TNA, Texas Nurses Association; TONE, Texas Organization of Nurse Executives. *Source:* Mari Tietze and TNA/TONE HIT committee.

Beginning in 2011, in an effort at error mitigation, the committee delivered live and online education to nurses in Texas and around the country focused on HIT patient safety and identification of unintended consequences of the EHR. These presentations, reports, and TIGER initiative support are located at the TNA HIT special project webpage (Texas Nursing Association, 2015). Most currently, the committee is analyzing data from the statewide online survey of practicing nurses' experience using their EHRs. Preliminary results suggest that although the EHRs are proving useful, their level of maturity and potential for unintended consequences are a concern.

SUMMARY

It is evident that the introduction of HIT, such as EHRs, has benefits for patient care delivery; however, the impact of these implementations commonly introduces unintended consequences. Key components for mitigation of these have been provided, and we provide additional considerations to be used in your organization.

- ▶ Know your organization's approach to reporting and collaborate closely with the risk-management department
- ▶ Promote a "just culture" for reporting of events to increase error reporting. Know available resources to you and your organizations related to reporting patient safety issues with your EHR
- ▶ Look for the trends in your events; these types of errors are more evident by their patterns than when standing alone
- ▶ Have a link where users can report errors/issues/events/negative features easily, right there on their documentation system
- ▶ Create a culture of patient engagement/activation
- ▶ Work interprofessionally with the entire health care team

EXERCISES AND QUESTIONS FOR CONSIDERATION

Visit a clinical setting that has implemented an EHR and walk through the process of performing an ISTA based on the interactive sociotechnical framework (Figure 20.9) and tools available on the HealthIT.gov website for the *Guide to Reducing Unintended Consequences of Electronic Health Records* (Jones et al., 2011). Address the following components in your analysis:

1. Examine all interactions of the environment and end-users' actions as to how the technology is used in workflow, and document the ISTA
2. Discuss with clinicians any unintended consequences they believe might be present with the EHR
3. Note infrastructure, including the physical layout, that might contribute to inefficiency, ineffectiveness, or problems with workflow
4. Note any EHR/technology design factors within the software that might be a contributing element to the problem

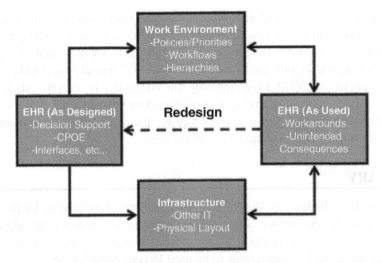

FIGURE 20.9. Sociotechnical analysis (ISTA) framework for use with EHRs. Elements of the visual flowchart of the interactive sociotechnical analysis, with four boxes linked directionally or bidirectionally; a full description of the flowchart is provided in the text.

CPOE, computer provider order entry; EHR, electronic health record; ISTA, interactive sociotechnical analysis.

Source: Jones et al. (2011b).

CASE STUDY

Consider the following case study. Your organization is a small critical access hospital (CAH) and you are the chief nursing officer (CNO) responsible for patient safety, quality, and HIT, in addition to your nursing leadership responsibilities. Your hospital is having significant financial difficulty with very tight profit margins. The EHR incentives from CMS that your organization has successfully attained have essentially kept your doors open. The implemented EHR has been considered a successful endeavor in achieving success with attaining MU Stage 1 and accessing the financial incentives associated with success. However, your organization adopted and implemented the EHR very rapidly, with what your vendor referred to as the "big bang" implementation, meaning one day your entire organization was on the paper-based record, and the following day the entire organization moved over to the EHR.

There are a number of issues with the use of the EHR, including an overdependency on old paper-based ways, maintaining a dual documentation system with some information in the electronic format and the other in the paper-based record that nurses and physicians persist in using. In your patient safety reporting, your hospital has indicated several near misses with patient safety events related to missed orders on medications and labs that you suspect is related to this dual-documentation practice. Considering lessons learned in reviewing the chapter and the tools available to you as CNO for your organization, consider the following questions:

(continued)

CASE STUDY (*continued*)

1. What is one of the first steps you will take to assess the unintended consequences of the EHR in the CAH?
2. What models are available to you to help you understand and document the problem and how will you go about using those tools?
3. What resources and tools are available to you to help you assess the issues, plan remediation, and execute a plan?

REFERENCES

Adelman, J. S., Kalkut, G. E., Schechter, C. B., Weiss, J. M., Berger, M. A., Reissman, S. H., . . . Southern, W. N. (2013). Understanding and preventing wrong-patient electronic orders: A randomized controlled trial. *Journal of the American Medical Informatics Association, 20*(2), 305–310. doi:10.1136/amia-jnl-2012-001055

Agency for Healthcare Research and Quality. (2014a). *What is a PSO?* Retrieved from http://www.pso.ahrq.gov/faq#WhatisaPSO

Agency for Healthcare Research and Quality. (2014b). *TeamSTEPPS 2.0: Core curriculum.* Retrieved from http://www.ahrq.gov/professionals/education/curriculum-tools/teamstepps/instructor/index.html

Agency for Healthcare Research and Quality. (2015). *PSO Privacy Protection Center.* Retrieved from https://www.psoppc.org/c/document_library/get_file?uuid=75912503-7bd1-4e99-a678-5dbb70008e95&groupId=10218

American Institutes for Research. (2011). *Training guide: Using simulation in TeamSTEPPS® training* (No. AHRQ 11-001 EF). Rockville, MD: Agency for Healthcare Research and Quality. Retrieved from http://www.ahrq.gov/professionals/education/curriculum-tools/teamstepps/simulation/traininggd.pdf

Bresnick, J. (2014). *AHRQ studies "wrong patient" EHR errors to improve safety.* Retrieved from https://ehrintelligence.com/2014/09/23/ahrq-studies-wrong-patient-ehr-errors-to-improve-safety

Campbell, E. M., Sittig, D. F., & Ash, J. S. (2006). Types of unintended consequences related to computerized provider order entry. *Journal of the American Medical Informatics Association, 13*(5), 547–556.

Cerrato, P. (2011). Hospital rooms get smart: IBM and University of Pittsburgh Medical Center have created smart hospital rooms that use advanced IT tools to make medical and nursing care more intelligent, faster, and safer. *InformationWeek, 2015.* Retrieved from http://www.informationweek.com/healthcare/clinical-information-systems/hospital-rooms-get-smart/d/d-id/1100822?print=yes

Cipriano, P. F. (2011). *The future of nursing: Leading change, advancing health.* (Conference Presentation No. HIMSS-2011). Chicago, IL: Healthcare Information and Management Systems Society.

Committee on Quality of Healthcare in America. (2001). *Crossing the quality chasm: A new health system for the 21st century.* Washington, DC: National Academies Press. Retrieved from http://www.nap.edu/catalog.php?record_id=10027

ECRI Institute. (2014). *Top 10 health technology hazards for 2015* (No. ECRI2015). Washington, DC: Author. Retrieved from http://www.healthleadersmedia.com/print/TEC-310879/ECRI-Institutes-Top-10-Healthcare-Tech-Hazards-for-2015

Gardner, E. (2010). Danger: EHRs can replace one set of medical errors with another. *Health Data Management, 18*(8), 30–34.

Harrison, M. I., Koppel, R., & Bar-Lev, S. (2007). Unintended consequences of information technologies in health care: An interactive sociotechnical analysis. *Journal of the American Medical Informatics Association, 14*(5), 542–549. doi:10.1197/jamia.M2384

Healthcare Information and Management Systems Society. (2011). *Investing in an EHR? How to avoid buyer's remorse, patient deaths, and physician uprisings in just 5 minutes* (No. HIMSS2011). Chicago, IL: Author. Retrieved from https://www.himss.org/files/HIMSSorg/content/files/C-SuiteIntroCSAV6.pdf

HealthIT.gov. (2014a). *SAFER guide: Patient identification, phase 1 safe HIT, #3* (No. SAFER2014). Washington, DC: Author. Retrieved from http://healthit.gov/safer/guide/sg006

HealthIT.gov. (2014b). *SAFER guide: Understanding unintended consequences, example 15: Responding to alert fatigue* (No. SAFER2014af). Washington, DC: Author. Retrieved from http://www.healthit.gov/unintended-consequences/content/example-15-responding-alert-fatigue.html

HealthIT.gov. (2014c). *Safety assurance factors for EHR resilience (SAFER)*. Retrieved from http://www.healthit.gov/safer

HealthITxChange.org. (2014). *Your community to share and learn how to best implement and leverage your EHR*. Retrieved from https://www.healthitxchange.org/Pages/landing.aspx

Henning, K. J. (2004). Overview of syndromic surveillance: What is syndromic surveillance? *Morbidity and Mortality Weekly Report, 53*(Suppl.), 5–11.

Institute of Medicine. (2011). *Health IT and patient safety: Building safer systems for better care* (Consensus Report). Washington, DC: Institute of Medicine and the National Academies Press. Retrieved from http://www.iom.edu/~/media/Files/Report%20Files/2011/Health-IT/HealthITandPatientSafetyreportbrieffinal_new.pdf

Interprofessional Collaborative Expert Panel. (2011). *Core competencies for interprofessional collaborative practice: Report of an expert panel* (No. ICEP-2011). Washington, DC: Interprofessional Education Collaborative. Retrieved from https://ipecollaborative.org/uploads/IPEC-Core-Competencies.pdf

Jones, S. S., Koppel, R., Ridgely, M. S., Palen, T. E., Wu, S., & Harrison, M. I. (2011). *Guide to reducing unintended consequences of electronic health records* (No. HHSA290200600017I). Rockville, MD: Agency for Healthcare Research and Quality. Retrieved from http://www.healthit.gov/unintended-consequences

Jones, S. S., Koppel, M. S., Wu, S., & Harrison, M. I. (2011a). *Guide to reducing unintended consequences of electronic health records, assess the problem*. Retrieved from http://www.healthit.gov/unintended-consequences/content/assess-problem.html

Jones, S. S., Koppel, M. S., Wu, S., & Harrison, M. I. (2011b). *Guide to reducing unintended consequences of electronic health records, module III understand unintended consequences*. Retrieved from http://www.healthit.gov/unintended-consequences/content/understand-unintended-consequences.html

Jones, S. S., Koppel, M. S., Wu, S., & Harrison, M. I. (2011c). *Guide to reducing unintended consequences of electronic health records, remediate the problem*. Retrieved from http://www.healthit.gov/unintended-consequences/content/remediate-problem.html

Kilbridge, P. M., Welebob, E. M., & Classen, D. C. (2006). Development of the Leapfrog methodology for evaluating hospital implemented inpatient computerized physician order entry systems. *Quality and Safety in Health Care, 15*(2), 81–84. doi:15/2/81[pii]

Kohn, L. T., Corrigan, J. M., & Donaldson, M.S. (Eds.). (1999). *To err is human: Building a safer health system*. Washington, DC: National Academies Press.

Koppel, R., & Kreda, D. (2009). Health care information technology vendors' "Hold harmless" clause implications for patients and clinicians. *Journal of the American Medical Association, 301*(12), 1276–1278.

The Leapfrog Group. (2014). *The leapfrog group fact sheet* (No. TLG2015). Washington, DC: Author. Retrieved from http://www.leapfroggroup.org/about_leapfrog/leapfrog-factsheet

Leung, A. A., Keohane, C., Lipsitz, S., Zimlichman, E., Amato, M., Simon, S. R., . . . Bates, D. W. (2013). Relationship between medication event rates and the leapfrog computerized physician order entry evaluation tool. *Journal of the American Medical Informatics Association, 20*(e1), e85–e90. doi:10.1136/amiajnl-2012-001549

Minnier, T. (2011, July). *Is there such thing as too much technology and too little patient care? Summer Institute in Nursing Informatics (SINI) presentation July 2011.* Unpublished manuscript. Retrieved from https://archive.hshsl.umaryland.edu/bitstream/10713/4001/3/Minnier,%20Tami%20SINI%20Slides.pdf

Office of the National Coordinator for Health Information Technology. (2013). *Health information technology patient safety action and surveillance plan.* (No. HHS2013). Washington, DC: U.S. Department of Health and Human Service. Retrieved from http://www.healthit.gov/sites/default/files/safety_plan_master.pdf

Page, A. (2004). *Keeping patients safe: Transforming the work environment of nurses.* Washington, DC: National Academies Press.

Patient Safety and Quality Improvement Act of 2005, Public law 109-41 (2005).

Sanders, D. (2010). *Patient safety and electronic health records.* Retrieved from http://healthsystemcio.com/2010/04/20/patient-safety-andelectronic-

Shah, N. R., Seger, A. C., Seger, D. L., Fiskio, J. M., Kuperman, G. J., Blumenfeld, B., . . . Gandhi, T. K. (2006). Improving acceptance of computerized prescribing alerts in ambulatory care. *Journal of the American Medical Informatics Association, 13*(1), 5–11. doi:M1868[pii]

Shaw, G. (2010, October). Patient rooms get smart. *Health Leaders,* p. 1-1. Retrieved from http://www.healthleadersmedia.com/print/MAG-257392/Patient-Rooms-Get-Smart

Sittig, D. F., & Ash, J. S. (2007). *Clinical information systems: Overcoming adverse consequences.* Boston, MA: Jones & Barlett.

Texas Nursing Association. (2010). Resolution on technology informatics. *Texas Nursing, 84*(2), 7–8.

Texas Nursing Association. (2015). *Texas nurses Association/Texas organization of nurse executives health IT committee web page.* Retrieved from http://www.texasnurses.org/?page=HIT

Thompson, C. A. (2010). Leapfrog group wants hospitals to monitor, not just implement, CPOE systems. *American Journal of Health-System Pharmacy, 67,* 1310–1311.

TIGER Development Collaborative. (2014). *The leadership imperative: TIGER's recommendations for integrating technology to transform practice and education* (No. TIF2014). Chicago, IL: The TIGER Initiative Foundation. Retrieved from www.thetigerinitiative.org

Umbdenstock, R. (2012). *American Hospital Association letter to the Leapfrog group.* Unpublished manuscript. Retrieved, 2015, from http://www.leapfroggroup.org/media/file/AHALettertoLeah.pdf

Walker, J. M., Hassol, A., Bradshaw, B., & Rezaee, M. E. (2012, May). *Health IT Hazard Manager beta-test: Final report* (Prepared by Abt Associates and Geisinger Health System, under Contract No. HHSA290200600011i, #14). AHRQ Publication No. 12-0058-EF. Rockville, MD: Agency for Healthcare Research and Quality.

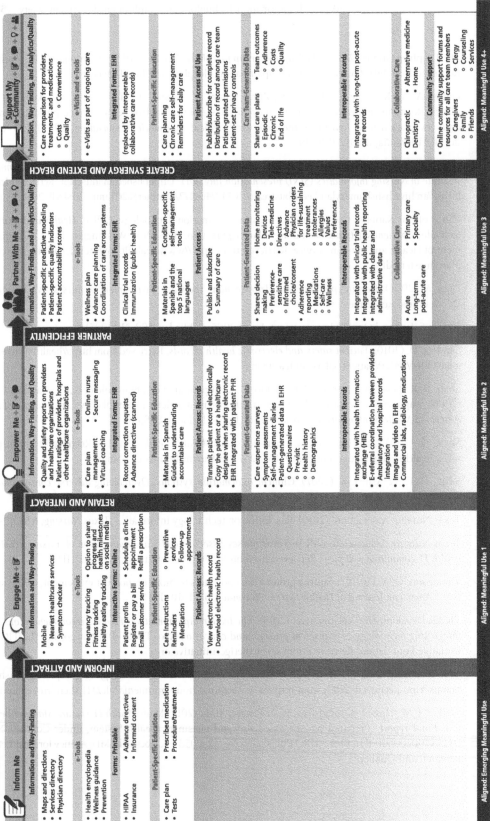

CHAPTER 21

Quality-Improvement Strategies and Essential Tools

Susan McBride, Mari Tietze, and John Terrell

OBJECTIVES

1. Discuss the fundamentals of quality improvement (QI) essential to realizing the full utilization of health information technology (HIT) beginning with strategic plans for the organization focused on quality enhancement.

2. Outline the fundamentals of fast-track process improvement and steps in the Plan-Do-Study-Act (PDSA) process.

3. Compare and contrast PDSA Cycle, Six Sigma, and Lean.

4. Describe the essential tools for QI for advanced practice nurses.

5. Define actions that can be taken by advanced practice nurses to support inter-professional teams utilizing technology and data to improve quality of the health care delivery system.

6. Examine a supply chain management and computer provider order entry (CPOE) case studies; apply methods discussed for improving efficiency, patient safety, and quality.

KEY WORDS

patient safety, quality, Plan-Do-Study-Act, control charts, run charts, Six Sigma, Lean

---

CONTENTS

INTRODUCTION

Health information technology is positioned as the panacea for the U.S. health care system that is challenged with a need to drive down costs, improve quality, and implement major change within a short period of time, with less than a decade to implement all three phases of meaningful use (MU) as originally outlined by the Office of the National Coordinator for Health Information Technology (ONC-HIT). Electronic health record (EHR) implementation and adoption comprises a core component of the national strategy to improve care and drive down costs (ONC-HIT, 2013). In addition to EHRs, we must have fundamental quality improvement strategies and tools coupled with the HIT infrastructure in order to achieve full optimization of technology for the health care industry. This chapter focuses on the fundamentals of QI and tools that all advanced practice nurses and other health professionals need in their "toolkit" to support interprofessional teams within organizations and clinical settings when utilizing technology and EHRs to improve care.

STRATEGIC PLANS FOCUSED ON QI

A starting point for organizations to safeguard against patient safety issues arising from technology and to improve quality-utilizing technology is to begin with strategic initiatives within an organization to report and address patient safety and quality. For example, upon release of the statistics in the Institute of Medicine (IOM) report related to medical errors, many organizations created plans to improve safety in U.S. hospitals through safer medication management, including technology solutions involving computer provider order entry (CPOE) and barcode electronic medication administration (Kohn, Corrigan, & Donaldson, 1999). Quality improvement initiatives related to technology are ideally aligned with overall strategic plans to improve care within the organization. These plans should align with the vision and mission of the organization, with goals and objectives to executive a plan of action. Health IT is a tool to help execute that plan. (Glaser, J. P. & Salzburg, C., 2011).

CORE CONCEPTS AND TOOLS FOR QI

There are entire textbooks that cover QI methods and the authors highly recommend supplementing this overview with other resources and textbooks on the subject. It is important that advanced practice nurses understand QI science and how to lead and implement QI projects within an interprofessional team. This section presents an overview of the fundamentals of fast track, or rapid cycle, QI methods used extensively under the Institute for Healthcare Quality Improvement (IHI) and referred to as Plan-Do-Study-Act. We also discuss Six Sigma and Lean methods and how these approaches differ from PDSA. Although these methods are not the only methods utilized to structure improvement projects, the authors selected these methods to review and discuss because we commonly see these tools utilized in the health care setting, and these methods are very relevant to our current HIT pressure to implement EHRs rapidly across the industry. Most important, these methods work very effectively when applied correctly.

The PDSA cycle, as it is often referred to, includes four phases of process. The four components collectively contribute to the successful cycle of improvement, and are a continual loop completed in short cycles to address an area of concern. The first component is planning. The planning phase is the phase of the cycle during which an issue or opportunity for improvement is identified and a plan of action needs formulating. The planning phase examines how a process might be modified in such a way as to result in improvement. The most important step in the planning process is be clear on the aim of the improvement. What is it you intend to improve? Can you measure the impact on the improvement? Do you fully understand what is occurring in the process that is creating the undesirable outcome? What data will you collect in order to measure the process you intend to improve? These are important considerations when formulating the plan for your PDSA cycle.

Workflow redesign with a current state versus future state analysis is an excellent method to use when planning an improvement surrounding implementation of technology and how that technology may be implemented to improve the process, or how the technology might be improved upon to optimize the existing technology. The planning phase includes the strategy for what will be done to improve the process and should include a thorough investigation into what the evidence suggests would be the best method to improve the area of focus. Based on that evidence, a workflow redesign strategy as discussed in Chapter 9 can be deployed. This approach involves mapping the "as is" current state, and designing a "to be" future plan to improve the overall outcome. Measures are established to gauge the effectiveness of the redesign in the planning phase and address the question of how you will know you made a difference with the redesign. Measures should be determined in the beginning of the process of planning the improvement, rather than after the improvement has been implemented. It is important to understand variation in the process related to measures prior to any improvement activity. Control charts are typically used to examine the variation in the process.

The second component is doing. The "Do" component of the PDSA cycle involves the actual implementation of the improvement. The "Do" phase is typically done on a trial or pilot basis to measure pre- and postimplementation to determine the impact on the process, and to be clear that what you thought was impacting the process is the correct assumption. You are testing your assumption in the "Do" phase.

The third component is studying. The "Study" phase of the cycle includes analyzing preliminary results. This is also referred to as the "check" phase of the improvement when the team examines and checks the results of the "Do" phase to measure the actual impact. Control charts are an excellent way in which to measure impact of the improvement on a process.

The fourth component is acting. The "Act" phase is intended to implement the improvement in the event the "Study" phase indicates a solid result, or to consider testing alternative solutions, modifying the original plan and testing again. These steps are depicted in a cycle because the team typically selects one aspect of the process to address in the short cycle; health care issues are complex, requiring multifactorial improvements that are likely to involve other aspects of the process that need improvement. Additionally, the team may elect to return to the planning phase to reconsider the alternative solutions, or select another part of the process to improve. This process results in all steps followed in a second cycle as described earlier. Figure 21.1 depicts a typical cycle for PDSA.

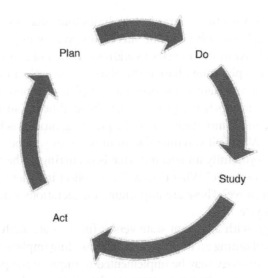

FIGURE 21.1. PDSA rapid cycle.

Basic Tools for QI

There are some fundamental tools that advanced practice nurses should consider as they construct a "toolkit" for improvement. These tools are frequently associated with measuring QI, are important to understanding the core issues relevant to the process to be improved, and are key to the proficient attainment of QI. These tools include flowcharts, check sheets, histograms, Pareto charts, cause-and-effect diagrams, scatter plots, run charts, and control charts (Table 21.1; Mears, 1995).

Flowcharts are diagrams that map workflows and processes to identify areas for improvement. Flowcharts are discussed extensively in Chapter 9 describing workflow redesign methods. Flowcharts depict steps in a process frequently referred to as workflows. Standardized symbols are used to determine the beginning and end of the process, activities and processes, direction, decisions, delays, storage, and other important aspects that you intend to depict in the process (Mears, 1995). Check sheets provide a mechanism for entering data under predetermined categories aimed at clarifying and collecting data objectively. Check sheets are often created in spreadsheets in preparation for further data analysis. Therefore, consideration should be given as to the level of measurement and how you intend to use the data you have collected. Histograms present a graphic representation of data, dividing the data in the chart in categories or groups sectioned into equal widths, with height representing the quantity (count or percentage). Histograms are used to show patterns in continuous or large discrete data sets. Pareto charts are used to identify patterns and trends, primarily looking for the most significant categories. The chart represents frequencies on the left y-axis and cumulative percentages on the right x-axis. The bars represent percentages or counts by category in descending order from left to right. Cause-and-effect diagrams visually identify the underlying cause or the potential etiology for the issue by examining relationships. The goal is to identify the root cause or primary reason for the event that occurred, and it is a common tool used to examine patient safety events. This type of tool is also referred to as a "fishbone"

TABLE 21.1 Basic Tools for QI and Common Uses	
Tool	**Common Use**
Flowcharts	To map workflows and identify areas for improvement
Check sheet	Objectively document facts and actions
Pareto diagram	Measurably identify "the problem" with data visually displayed in descending order of significance, helping to identify in an 80:20 rule in which 80% of the opportunity for improvement might be detected
Histogram	Visual depiction of continuous data, such as age, to group data into ranges of values
Fishbone diagram	Generate ideas and document a flow of events surrounding an issue
Scatter diagram	Measurably identify relationships within the events or variables
Run charts & control charts	Measure processes objectively at baseline and postimplementation of improvement

QI, quality improvement.

Source: Mears (1995).

diagram because the head of the "fish" represents the main activity or patient safety event that occurred, and the ribs are indicative of the major and minor process steps leading to the issue. Scatter plots are used to examine relationships in graphic form on *x*- and *y*-axes between variables of interest, examining the dots and the patterns that arise from the scatter of the dots. The suspected cause should be on the *x*-axis and the effect on the *y*-axis (Mears, 1995, pp. 13–17).

A run chart is a line graph often used to depict a trend or change over time. The *x*-axis reflects time and the *y*-axis examines the measurement scale, typically by count or frequency. A control chart is a line graph with separate types of charts depending on the level of measurement for continuous or discrete data. The control chart is unique from the run chart because it reflects upper and lower control limits that will help determine whether a process is in control or whether the process reflects "signal," indicating the process has changed for either better or worse. Controls charts are a very effective way to measure variance in a process (Carey, 2003). It is important to understand variation in a process prior to interrupting that process with an improvement. Control charts help to detect forms of variation that indicate the process is "in control" with common cause variation, or that the process is "out of control" with some special effect that should be understood and studied prior to modifying the process. There are various rules that the analyst applies when interpreting the control chart to detect special cause. The discussion of these rules is beyond the scope of this text, and we refer the reader to other resources and textbooks on running and interpreting control charts. Additionally, software packages that run control charts frequently have criteria built into the capability of the software that help the analyst detect a rule violation that is reflective of special cause variation.

Six Sigma

Six Sigma is a method used for measuring various processes that has an emphasis on statistical quality control, zero defects, and driving down cost. Six Sigma was originally developed by Motorola in the early 1990s (iSixSigma.com, 2014) with the primary focus of improving profitability by driving down cost through eliminating defects. The process for improvement was driven by the idea that cost reduction will result when defects are eliminated and are identified as the "cost of poor quality." Six Sigma is a program or a philosophy for QI emphasizing no tolerance for defects (Carey, 2003).

The word "sigma" refers to standard deviation that is a measure of dispersion or variance. The goal of "six sigma" is a defect-free variance (iSixSigma.com, 2014). The formula is to calculate the number of defects divided by the total number of potential defects by 1 million. This calculation reflects the total number of defects per 1 million and a conversion will convert that figure into "sigma." Six sigma is three defects per million, whereas one sigma is 691,462 defects per million. The philosophy behind the Six Sigma approach to improvement is to attain virtually no defects per million, equating to "zero defect." This is the basis for the approach of establishing a goal for safety and quality that would be aimed at achieving "six sigma," or virtually no defects or patient safety events (Carey, 2003). Six Sigma has developed a training program and certification process. The level of Six Sigma includes Greenbelts, Blackbelts, Master Blackbelts, and Champions. Many health care organizations are sending QI and HIT staff to train under the Six Sigma training program (iSixSigma.com, 2014).

Lean

Lean, of *Lean* Six Sigma, is a collection of techniques for reducing waste in a process. Waste is defined as anything that does not provide value to the customer and frequently results in decreasing the time needed to provide products or services, excess inventory, a more organized work environment, or other similar benefits. Six Sigma is a collection of techniques used to improve the quality of products and services by focusing on the reduction of variation and defects the process may produce, causing a substantial contribution to process control and increased customer satisfaction. By combining the two, Lean Six Sigma is a business management strategy that helps organizations operate more efficiently. According to many business analysts and QI experts, Lean Six Sigma is one of the most significant business performance methods developed in the history of corporate development, and it has its roots in the automobile manufacturing industry associated with the Toyota Corporation (iSixSigma.com, 2014).

Control Charts

Control charts are an important quality improvement tool to measure the process you intend to impact with the overall plan of improvement. The control chart is fundamental to the Lean Six Sigma methods, and will be reviewed in depth in this section. The type of control chart to be selected for use is determined by the level of measurement given your outcome of interest. Common indicators in health care are often dichotomous "yes" or "no" variables, and are frequently coded as 0 = "no" and 1 = "yes." This type of indicator in control-chart terminology would identify mortality or readmission as a nonconforming or defective component of the process. In this case, we measure the number of total defects over the number of total cases eligible for the outcome. Indicators, such as mortality, cesarean section, induction of labor, and readmissions within 30 days, are examples of variables in the acute care setting that fall into this level of measurement. In these types of scenarios the P-Chart is commonly used and is a fairly easy control chart to interpret. Other charts commonly used in health care include the U-Chart, C-Chart, I-Chart (also referred to as XMR), and the X-bar or S-chart. The U-Chart is a chart typically used when the nonconformity is related to a denominator that fluctuates, such as with bed days when measuring patient falls. The "U" relates to unequal area of opportunity. The C-Chart is used when there is near-equal opportunity and is very similar to the U-Chart, it is used simply to plot the count of nonconformity. An example might be total number of falls on the 7 a.m. to 3 p.m. shift on a particular hospital unit. According to Carey (2003, p. 21), the C-Chart should only be used to plot the count of events when the average does not vary by more than 20%. The I-Chart reflects actual values for a single observation with a moving range, and for that reason is also referred to as the "X-MR," meaning X has a moving range. Examples of this type of chart might be tracking profit margins or risk adjusted mortality rates. The X-Bar and S-Chart are used when each subgroup has more than one observation; X is the average tracked, whereas, S is the standard deviation. An example of the use of this type of chart in use would be to determine if the average length of stay overtime has changed for cardiac surgery patients. Figure 21.2

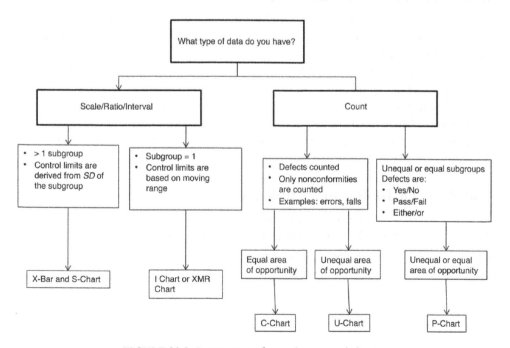

FIGURE 21.2. Decision tree for quality-control charts.
SD, standard deviation.
Source: Carey (2003).

reflects a decision tree used to determine the right control chart given the level of measurement and the outcome of interest, or variable under review. When examining mortality as a nonconformity or defect in the process, the outcome variable of interest is a count of mortalities over possible eligible cases. There is an assumed equal opportunity in the case of mortality for the patient to die (outcome = either "yes" or "no"); therefore, the decision tree noted here would indicate the P-Chart is the appropriate type of control chart to examine (Carey, 2003). Control charts using continuous data rather than attribute data are considered the more powerful in terms of ability to detect differences. Continuous data are data such as age, temperature, length of stay, and number of days until procedure, whereas attribute data are data such as "yes" and "no" outcome indicators.

Workflow Redesign: An Important Technique

Workflow redesign is an important action that can be taken and is a fundamental technique to be used by organizations to implement technology safely and effectively, as well as optimizing technologies once implemented. Workflow redesign can assist providers and hospitals in thinking through and mapping processes to target areas for improvement using technology. Workflow redesign for QI strategy was further emphasized in detail in Chapter 9. This technique, as discussed in Chapter 9, is a fundamental for addressing QI and patient safety workflow redesign within the context of a comprehensive QI strategy, and is an important tool within the "toolkit." An effective approach to QI should deploy all useful tools to be constituted as a comprehensive strategy.

Impact of QI and Workflow Redesign

The combined use of QI methodology and workflow redesign is imperative for optimum deployment of HIT for use in patient care delivery. QI consists of systematic and continuous actions that lead to measurable improvement in health care services and the health status of targeted patient groups (HRSA, 2011). As it relates to the use of HIT for patient care delivery, a solid QI program will strengthen the clinical application of the technology with techniques such as workflow redesign. Fundamental elements of quality improvement as stated by Lloyd (2004) are "listening to the voice of the customer, listening to the voice of the process, and using statistical process control methods (i.e. using data to make decisions)" (p. 13).

Use of the QI Toolkit in a Clinical Case

We now have in our QI toolkit an approach to utilize when constructing a QI project in the form of the PDSA cycle, tools to collect data, and control charts to measure impact. The following is a clinical case highlighting the use of these common process-improvement tools within an interprofessional team.

CASE STUDY 1: FOR A MATERIALS MANAGEMENT DEPARTMENT

An inpatient unit stores all of its nursing supplies in a central supply room, which is refilled daily by the Materials Management Department. A stock-out occurs when an item is needed but is unavailable in the supply room. The nurse manager has received complaints from the nursing team that stock-outs occur too frequently and in some cases led to a patient safety incident by not having the necessary supplies available in a timely manner. A Six Sigma approach is taken to focus on decreasing the frequency of theses stock-outs. The initial process flow and baseline data are provided in Figures 21.3 and 21.4.

When the flow map was brought to the team and the problem was described, several potential problems were identified:

▶ Some of the staff were not filling out the paperwork correctly because it was too time-consuming to do in real time and they often forgot what should be documented by the end of their shift.

▶ The communication between the unit and materials management took 2 days to replace used items.

▶ It was easy to write down the wrong ID code or the wrong patient chart, especially when in a hurry.

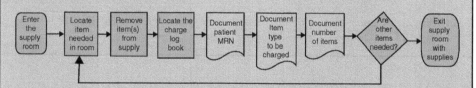

FIGURE 21.3. Initial process-flow map.

MRN, medical record number.

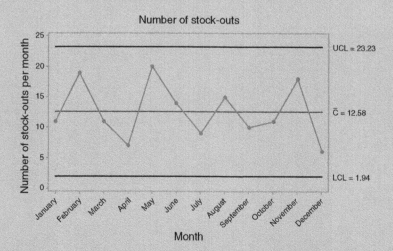

FIGURE 21.4. Control chart of number of monthly stock-outs in the supply room.

LCL, lower control limit; UCL, upper control limit.

(*continued*)

CASE STUDY 1: FOR A MATERIALS MANAGEMENT DEPARTMENT (*continued*)

After considering multiple proposed solutions with the interprofessional team, it was decided that the best solution was to use an electronic scanning system tied to the patient's electronic medical record. Figure 21.5 describes the revised process flow.

The system allowed the patients and materials to be quickly found and charged appropriately. The system also reduced stock-outs by communicating with the materials management team so they know what supplies need to be replenished at the end of the day. As a result, the nursing team spent less time retrieving supplies and was more likely to have the correct supplies, and materials used for the patients were more accurately documented in the EHR and available for future reference.

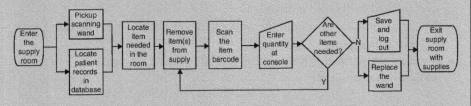

FIGURE 21.5. Future state process map once the new system connected to the EHR was installed.

CASE STUDY 2 : CPOE AND BAR CODING: TECHNOLOGY SOLUTIONS TO IMPROVE PATIENT SAFETY AND QUALITY

The workflow for ordering medications was redesigned through use of an electronic process to enter and manage the medication ordering process referred to as CPOE. *CPOE* is defined as utilization of software to support the medication ordering process of the provider. CPOE and barcoding medications have been shown to prevent medication errors in multiple studies (Agency for Healthcare Research and Quality, 2012), and, as a result, CPOE was a critical component for meaningful use Stage 1 requirements.

CPOE has helped avoid potential harm to patients through safer medication management and administration. Additionally, commentaries have called for CPOE designers to tailor alerts to maximize safety while avoiding alert fatigue. Yet, there have also been unintended consequences of CPOE systems, for example, more or new work for clinicians, unfavorable workflow issues, and/or unfavorable changes in communication patterns (Ash et al., 2007).

A typical acute care CPOE process is reflected in the workflow diagram in Figure 21.6. Hospitals and providers map processes in workflows as depicted in this figure to determine where areas of concern for patient safety might arise and to think through QI initiatives that would address the potential concerns. Workflow redesign is an important technique to adopt to address challenges with technology implementation and to optimize technology once implemented. Examine the following workflow relating to CPOE and reflect on the following questions:

1. Consider how your clinical area manages the process of medication orders. Does your organization use CPOE? Use workflow redesign methods to map your process for medication ordering and administration.
2. Compare and contrast your process to the process diagramed in Figure 21.6.
3. Consider the following questions:
   a. How does your process compare? Is it more efficient, less efficient, of better quality, or of poorer quality?
   b. Which do you believe is the better process? If one or the other is better for quality or efficiency, support your position.
   c. How will you measure the process to compare and contrast quality between your current process and the processed mapped in Figure 21.6?
   d. What control charts would you utilize to measure process over time related to CPOE quality?
   e. How would you know if the process was "in control"?

(*continued*)

CASE STUDY 2 : CPOE AND BAR CODING: TECHNOLOGY SOLUTIONS TO IMPROVE PATIENT SAFETY AND QUALITY (*continued*)

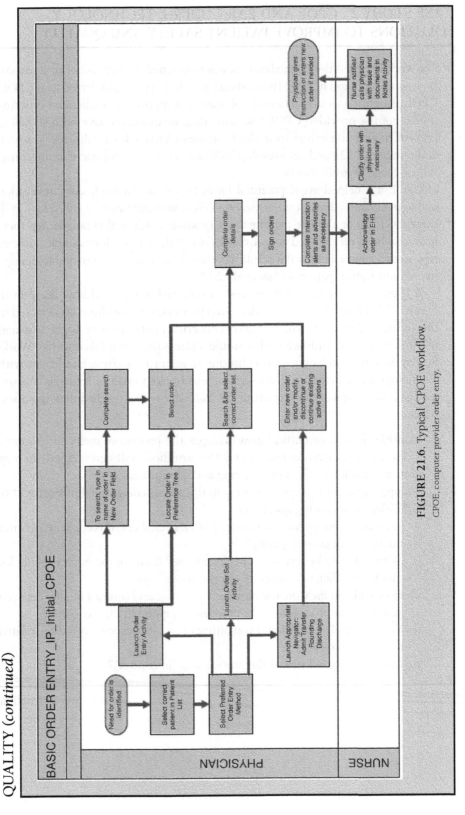

FIGURE 21.6. Typical CPOE workflow.

CPOE, computer provider order entry.

SUMMARY

To conclude, this chapter has reviewed the basic tools of QI that are well suited to use in adoption, implementation, and evaluation of HIT projects. We have described basic tools that advanced practice nurses should be proficient in using when addressing HIT in the clinical setting. A basic overview of the fundamentals of rapid-cycle QI methods, such as PDSA, have been discussed and applied to a case study on supply management. Six Sigma and Lean Six Sigma have also been described, and the importance of these methods to achieve measurable improvements in efficiency was presented. Workflow redesign and control-chart methods have been reviewed, and finally the first case study has been presented to be used by the reader to consider application of these tools to CPOE.

REFERENCES

Agency for Healthcare Research and Quality. (2012). *Computerized provider order entry.* Retrieved from June 19, 2014, http://psnet.ahrq.gov/primer.aspx?primerID=6

Ash, J. S., Sittig, D. F., Poon, E. G., Guappone, K., Campbell, E., & Dykstra, R. H. (2007). The extent and importance of unintended consequences related to computerized provider order entry. *Journal of the American Medical Informatics Association, 14*(4), 415–423.

Carey, R. G. (2003). *Improving healthcare with control-charts: Basic and advanced SPC methods and case studies.* Milwaukee, WI: ASQ Quality Press.

Glaser, J. P., & Salzburg, C. (2011). *The strategic application of information technology.* (3rd ed.). pp. 1–20. San Francisco, CA: John Wiley & Sons.

iSixSigma.com. (2014, June 20). *The history of Six Sigma.* Retrieved from http://www.isixsigma.com/new-to-six-sigma/history/history-six-sigma

Kohn, L. T., Corrigan, J. M., & Donaldson, M. S. (Eds.). (1999). *To err is human: Building a safer health system.* Washington, DC: National Academies Press.

Lloyd, R. (2004). *Quality health care: A guide to developing and using indicators.* Sudbury, MA: Jones & Bartlett.

Mears, P. (1995). *Quality improvement tools and techniques.* Spartanburg, SC: R. R. Donnelly and Sons.

Office of the National Coordinator for Health Information Technology. (2013, December 18). *How to implement EHRs.* Retrieved from http://www.healthit.gov/providers-professionals/ehr-implementation-steps

U.S. Department of Health and Human Services Health Resources and Services Adminstration. (2011). *Quality improvement.* Retrieved from http://www.hrsa.gov/quality/toolbox/methodology/quality improvement/index.html

CHAPTER 22

National Prevention Strategy, Population Health, and Health Information Technology

Andrea Lorden, Mari Tietze, and Susan McBride

OBJECTIVES

1. Describe the major drivers of quality metric development.

2. Describe differences among structure, process, and outcome metrics and how each type of metric reflects quality of health care.

3. Identify existing quality and population health metrics that are publically available and validated.

4. Describe what risk adjustment is and why it is important when reporting and interpreting quality metrics.

5. Identify public domain and other sources of data available to utilize for addressing improvement in quality and population health.

6. Use the National Prevention strategy for outlining a plan to improve population health in your organization.

KEY WORDS

population health, risk adjustment, reflection of quality care, quality metrics

---

CONTENTS

INTRODUCTION

Equipped with an understanding of meaningful use, quality of care, and basic statistical inference, we can use these together to generate metrics of health care quality. Creating and using quality metrics to inform patients, providers, and payers has challenges as unique as each of the stakeholders. It is important to achieve a level of understanding of each stakeholder's needs to develop a metric that simultaneously provides useful information to all. Further complicating the task of metric generation are the many interpretations of quality health care. In this chapter, we discuss major stakeholder needs, deconstruct quality for the purpose of measuring it, and explain relevant features of existing metrics. Finally, we discuss how existing quality metrics are applied and why risk-adjustment allows us to interpret quality metrics across providers or settings. In doing so, we meet the objectives of this chapter.

APPLICATION OF QUALITY METRICS
IN POPULATION HEALTH

With so much data available, how do we determine where to place priorities? Can we use new sources of data to improve existing metrics? And how do we disseminate the information to stakeholders? Ideally, every quality-related problem would have a metric that provided meaningful feedback. The question then becomes how specific does the measure need to be? Key stakeholders, such as patients, providers, or payers, have differing priorities that sometimes compete and sometimes complement one another. Because quality metrics are a reflection of some aspect of the provision of health care, providers on the frontline frequently identify issues, contribute to the identification of meaningful reflections of quality, and participate in the implementation process. The expertise providers bring to metric development is vital, as they ultimately are responsible for the accuracy of data collected. Additionally important to remember is that the data collected at the patient or individual level can be aggregated to reflect population health. In other words, what we do as health professionals at the individual level "adds up" and affects the health status of the community. As such, population-level health issues are important for helping us prioritize the creation of health care metrics. For the purposes of this chapter, we use the definition of "population health" offered by Kindig and Stoddart (2003). Population health is, "health outcomes of a group of individuals, including the distribution of such outcomes within the group," and "the field of population health includes health outcomes, patterns of health determinants, and policies and interventions that link these two" (Kindig & Stoddart, 2003, p. 380).

Identifying Population Health Issues

National Prevention Strategy

The Affordable Care Act's (ACA) landmark health legislation, passed in 2010, created the National Prevention Council and called for the development of the National Prevention Strategy to realize the benefits of prevention for all Americans' health. The National Prevention Strategy is critical to the prevention focus of the ACA and builds on the law's efforts to lower health care costs, improve the quality of care, and provide coverage options for the uninsured (National Prevention Council, 2014).

Although the United States provides some of the world's best health care and spent over $2.5 trillion for health in 2009, it ranks below many countries in life expectancy, infant mortality, and many other indicators of healthy living (Centers for Medicare & Medicaid Service [CMS], Office of the Actuary, National Health Statistics Group, 2011). As such, most of our nation's pressing health problems can likely be prevented.

The National Prevention Strategy aims to guide our nation in the most effective and achievable means for improving health and well-being. The strategy prioritizes prevention by integrating recommendations and actions across multiple settings to improve health and save lives. The National Prevention Strategy's vision is working together to improve the health and quality of life for individuals, families, and communities by moving the nation from a focus on sickness and disease to one based on prevention and wellness. This strategy envisions a prevention-oriented society where all sectors recognize the value of health for individuals, families, and society and work together to achieve better health for all Americans (National Prevention Council, 2014).

The National Prevention Strategy's overarching goal is to increase the number of Americans who are healthy at every stage of life. Currently, Americans can expect to live 78 years, but only 69 of these years would be spent in good health (Adams, Barnes, & Vickerie, 2008). Implementing the National Prevention Strategy can increase both the length and quality of life.

To monitor progress on this goal, the Council will track and report measures of the length and quality of life at key life stages (see Figure 22.1 for an example of baselines and targets). To realize this vision and achieve this goal, the strategy identifies four strategic directions and seven targeted priorities (see Figure 22.2). The strategic directions provide a strong foundation for all of the prevention efforts of the United States and include core recommendations necessary to build a prevention-oriented society. The strategic directions are as follows:

- ► *Healthy and safe community environments:* Create, sustain, and recognize communities that promote health and wellness through prevention.

- ► *Clinical and community preventive services:* Ensure that prevention-focused health care and community prevention efforts are available, integrated, and mutually reinforcing.

- ► *Empowered people:* Support people in making healthy choices.

- ► *Elimination of health disparities:* Eliminate disparities, improving the quality of life for all Americans (National Prevention Council, 2012, p. 7).

Every year, members of the U.S. Congress receive a summary report for the most current year comparing health status progress from previous years. The most current

Key Indicators: Goal					
Key Indicator	Aligned HP2020 Objective	Data Source	Frequency of Data Collection	Baseline (Year)	Target for 2030 (Method)
GOAL INDICATORS					
Rate of infant mortality per 1,000 live births	MICH-1.3	National Vital Statistics System, Centers for Disease Control and Prevention. National Center for Health Statistics	Annually	6.7 per 1,000 live births (2007)	4.5 per 1,000 live births (additional 15% improvement after linear extrapolation to 2030)
Proportion of Americans who live to age 25	N/A	National Vital Statistics System, Centers for Disease Control and Prevention. National Center for Health Statistics	Annually	98.3% (2007)	98.9% (additional 15% improvement after linear extrapolation to 2030)
Proportion of Americans who live to age 65	N/A	National Vital Statistics System, Centers for Disease Control and Prevention. National Center for Health Statistics	Annually	83.6% (2007)	90.6% (additional 15% improvement after linear extrapolation to 2030)
Proportion of Americans who live to age 85	N/A	National Vital Statistics System, Centers for Disease Control and Prevention. National Center for Health Statistics	Annually	38.6% (2007)	57.7% (additional 15% improvement after linear extrapolation to 2030)
Proportion of 0 to 24 year old Americans in good or better health	N/A	National Health Interview Survey. Centers for Disease Control and Prevention. National Center for Health Statistics	Annually	97.7% (2009)	97.9% (additional 15% improvement after linear extrapolation to 2030)
Proportion of 25 to 64 year old Americans in good or better health	N/A	National Health Interview Survey. Centers for Disease Control and Prevention. National Center for Health Statistics	Annually	88.6% (2009)	87.2% (additional 15% improvement after linear extrapolation to 2030)
Proportion of 65 to 84 year old Americans in good or better health	N/A	National Health Interview Survey. Centers for Disease Control and Prevention. National Center for Health Statistics	Annually	77.5% (2009)	83.3% (additional 15% improvement after linear extrapolation to 2030)
Proportion of 85+ year old Americans in good or better health	N/A	National Health Interview Survey. Centers for Disease Control and Prevention. National Center for Health Statistics	Annually	64.9% (2009)	71.7% (additional 15% improvement after linear extrapolation to 2030)

FIGURE 22.1. An example of key indicators and goals for the National Prevention Strategy.
Source: National Prevention Council (2011).

year, 2014 (National Prevention Council, 2014), indicated numerous improvements in health parameters of the nation. In the area of home, schools, community, and work environment, for example, improvements since 2012 in four impressive examples are:

- 70% increase in number of tobacco-free college campuses (774–1,343)

- 20% increase (18%–38%) in number of U.S. school districts required/recommended to test student fitness with more than 6,500 U.S. schools receiving *HealthierUS School Challenge* certification for their efforts to promote nutrition and physical activity

- 25% increase (51%–76%) in U.S. school districts offering assistance to students for mental health/social services

- 7% decrease in chronic homelessness, and an 8% decrease in homelessness among veterans, improving conditions for health and well-being (National Prevention Council, 2014, p. 5)

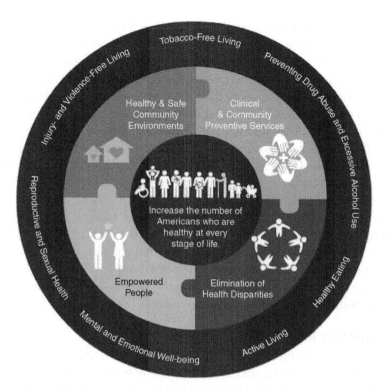

FIGURE 22.2. The National Prevention Strategy Framework.
Source: National Prevention Council (2011).

Healthy People

National priorities within the National Prevention Strategy have been largely established through the Healthy People initiative (U.S. Department of Health and Human Services, 2014c). The Healthy People initiative has its roots in the 1979 U.S. Surgeon General's report about the status of health promotion and disease prevention in the United States (U.S. Department of Health and Human Services, 2014b). Since 1979, the report has evolved into a multi year process of establishing more than 1,200 health objectives for the nation to address during each 10-year period.

Stakeholders and health experts from more than 17 federal agencies identify objectives focused on eliminating illness and premature death (U.S. Department of Health and Human Services, 2014a). Health-related data collected through a variety of health surveys and multiple agencies are used to inform and create metrics that reflect changes in the nation's health status. Examples of topics addressed by Healthy People 2020 objectives include access to health care, cancer, a variety of chronic diseases, family planning, health care-associated infection (HAI), HIV, immunization, mental health, reproduction and sexual health, substance abuse, and tobacco use, to name a few (U.S. Department of Health and Human Services, 2014c).

Community Assessment Surveys

Closer to home are community assessment programs implemented by local health departments or not-for-profit hospitals looking to fulfill their community service mission.

The local level assessment allows public health stakeholders to channel resources where the community needs are greatest. (See also Chapter 13 for more information on conducting community needs assessments.) For example, if a Middle West community's composition is very young, it is likely to benefit more from channeling its resources into an immunization program than into a global health initiative. Tools for conducting a community needs assessment can be found at the National Association of County and City Health Officials (NACCHO) website (National Association of County & City Health Officials, 2015). Additionally, population health programs, such as the Centers for Disease Control and Prevention (CDC) Healthy Communities Program, offer access to additional community assessment tools (Division of Community Health: National Center for Chronic Disease Prevention and Health Promotion, 2013).

The selection of a community assessment tool should include an examination of what each tool reflects. Although it is important to consider the needs of stakeholders during this process, the selection of an ideal assessment tool will also include considerations for underrepresented populations within the community and availability of resources to deploy the tool. By including stakeholders in the process to select an assessment tool, agencies can address concerns prior to deployment.

Payer Perspective and Accountable Care Organizations

With the passage of the Patient Protection and Affordable Care Act (PPACA) of 2010, reform of the insurance marketplace should lead to more individuals with health insurance. This translates to more individuals with insurers acting as agents in the payment for the provision of health services. Because the majority of individuals are covered by insurance, the majority of payments to providers come from insurers. Through the processing of insurance claims, payers also have access to pertinent information on services used and their associated diagnoses. Through data-mining techniques, insurers can identify the needs of their beneficiaries. For example, insurance programs, such as Medicare and Medicaid, serve specific populations; therefore, the CMS identifies the health care needs of the elderly, handicapped, poor pregnant women and their children, and other groups served by these entitlement programs.

This is important, because insurers can influence the provision of health care through payment incentives directed at benefiting the patient population served. Although more than half of insured individuals are covered by employer-based or private insurance, Medicare beneficiaries accounted for 28.4% of health insurance expenditures in 2012, and accounted for 47% of all inpatient expenditures in 2011 (CMS, 2013, 2014b; Torio & Andrews, 2013). In addition to Medicare, CMS influences payments made through the Medicaid and Children's Health Insurance Program. This places CMS in a leadership role for influencing health care through payment and nonpayment strategies. As you will see later in this chapter, CMS has used its dual role as insurer and taxpayer advocate to influence and measure the quality of health care.

Accountable care organizations (ACOs) have evolved as the most significant trend in payment structure associated with the ACA (Noble & Casalino, 2013). ACOs are said to have accountability to population health improvement and as such are critically focused on health-quality data. Some question (Figher & Shorell, 2010), however, the ability of a financial structure, such as the ACO, to be accountable for the health of the population based on financial incentives. Regardless, recent reports have suggested that ACOs have achieved cost savings while improving care for patients, with the opportunity to become even more effective (Haywood & Kosel, 2011).

ACOs, in terms of the CMS, are made up of "groups of doctors, hospitals, and other health care providers, who come together voluntarily to give coordinated high quality care to their Medicare patients" (CMS, 2014a, p. 1). More than 400 ACOs exist serving 7.3 million beneficiaries. Findings from those started in 2012 suggest that they have improved on 30 of the 33 quality measure in the last 2 years, including patients' ratings of clinicians' communication, rating of their doctor, and screening for high blood pressure. Cost savings for all of these programs have been estimated at $417 million (Cavanaugh, 2014).

Logic Model as a Framework

Before population health determination can occur, the associated data must be assessed for its ability to yield actionable results. A logic model can help with the assessment of the selected data quality-improvement plan (Watson, Broemeling, & Wong, 2009). Main components of the methodology for population health analytics entail the following:

1. Logic model to identify input, output, processes for intervention, and evaluation outcomes

2. Assessment of the targeted population health-data feeds that would support the logic model

3. Analysis of data quality status, including identification of erroneous, missing, misaligned, and immature data in regard to the logic model

4. Approach for data quality improvement aligned with logic model

5. Generation of measures based on the logic model (see Chapter 10)

An example of a primary care focused logic model that is used for the population health framework is illustrated in Chapter 10. It illustrates how the components flow to yield the desired population health outcomes (Watson et al., 2009).

Data Sources for the Future

Current trends indicate that consumer-driven health care and the engaged consumer are not only desirable but also a key strategic goal for the CDC and the Office of the National Coordinator for Health Information Technology (ONC-HIT) in efforts to adopt HIT and utilize technology to address the three-part aim. Figure 22.3 depicts several emerging areas that will provide rich new data sources to assess and intervene with populations at risk for various illness, or to target wellness-promotion campaigns.

Data Used to Identify Needs and Generate Quality Metrics

There are four basic types of data either available or soon to be available for needs assessment and quality metrics: survey data, administrative data, electronic health records (EHRs), and reporting systems.

Survey Data

Survey data, such as that used for Healthy People and community assessments, is collected through survey instruments. That is, information is collected through questionnaires

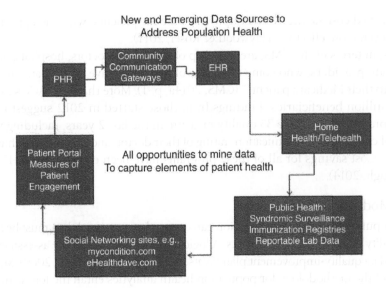

FIGURE 22.3. Potential emerging data sources for population health.
EHR, electronic health record; PHR, personal health record.

or interviews specifically designed to collect information in a statistically valid way. Survey data are not limited to individuals about themselves. They are collected from individuals about themselves, groups such as families, or organizations such as hospitals or other workplace environments. When collected through validated methods, the information is considered highly reliable. However, as most survey data are self-reported, researchers should consider the accuracy of recall by survey respondents when evaluating the data.

Numerous national surveys use complex survey design and sampling strategies to inform us about health status and health care utilization. For example, the Center for Health Statistics performs several surveys, including the National Health and Nutrition Examination Survey (NHANES), the National Health Interview Survey (NHIS), and the National Vital Statistics System (NVSS; Centers for Disease Control and Prevention and the Center for Health Statistics, 2012). Information on survey design, instruction for use of data in analysis, and data can be found at www.cdc.gov/nchs/index.htm. Other national surveys include the Behavioral Risk Factor Surveillance System (BRFSS) telephone survey by the CDC and the Medical Expenditure Panel Survey (MEPS) by the Agency for Healthcare Research and Quality (AHRQ). This is a drop in the bucket of survey data regarding health care. Chances are if the health topic is politically relevant, there is likely a survey to inform us about the topic.

Administrative Data

Another rich source of information is administrative data. Administrative data include billing information derived from insurance claims, inpatient discharges (or hospital bills), and outpatient visits (the bill for emergency room visits that do not result in being admitted to the hospital or services delivered in a hospital but not part of an overnight admission). Administrative data include documentation of clinical diagnoses and use of health services as recorded through predefined coding systems such as the International Classification of Diseases, ninth revision, Clinical Modification (ICD-9-CM;

see also Chapter 12 for more information on ICD-9-CM and ICD-10-CM), Current Procedural Terminology (CPTs), or Healthcare Common Procedure Coding System (HCPCS). The codes are assigned based on a review of the clinical record by trained coders. Diagnosis-related groups (DRGs) or major diagnostic categories (MDCs) systematically group these more specific codes into meaningful broader categories. The purpose of the DRG grouper is to facilitate payment through the prospective payment system, whereas MDCs organize diagnoses that affect similar physiological systems. Although administrative data reflect diagnoses and utilization, it is important to remember that their primary purpose is for billing. Therefore, more expensive services are likely to be identified first in the administrative record, not necessarily as events or procedures occurred chronologically or even simultaneously.

For the highly regulated hospital environment, inpatient and outpatient administrative records are required to follow state-specific formats, with nearly all states requiring some form of reporting. Although reporting requirements vary from state to state, certain elements have become standard as reflected in the Healthcare Cost and Utilization Project (HCUP) sponsored by the AHRQ. Started in 1988, hospital discharge data were collected from a sample of hospitals in eight states (HCUP, 2014). Currently, 44 states participate in the National Inpatient Sample (NIS), renamed in 2012 from the Nationwide Inpatient Sample to reflect the change from all discharges from a sample of hospitals to a sample of discharges from all participating hospitals (HCUP, 2014). The initiative to create an all-payer repository of health care costs and utilization enables the evaluation of health care by using metrics designed to reflect quality at the facility and population level.

In addition to the NIS, HCUP warehouses the State Inpatient Databases (SID), Kid's Inpatient Database (KID), Nationwide Emergency Department Sample (NEDS), State Ambulatory Surgery and Services Database (SASD), and the State Emergency Department Databases (SEDD; HCUP, 2014).

Electronic Health Records

EHRs capture detailed health information through the provider/patient interaction. This new level of detail placed into an electronic format should inform providers through timely availability of relevant patient-specific information. Specifically, matching patient diagnoses to relevant clinical best practices, EHRs support the providers through reminders for screenings or flags for out-of-range test results. Additionally, once aggregated into a longitudinal data set with other patients, researchers should be able to identify new clinical insights into disease and health care. Although not available in this aggregated form outside of provider practices, some early adaptors of the EHR are using the data they possess to identify complex patients' needs, quality problems within their practice, or track metrics identified as indicators of an effective, efficient, and even profitable practice.

Reporting Systems

Reporting systems track specific health events or predictors of health events. For example, the National Health Safety Network (NHSN) includes a national online reporting system for HAIs. In addition to collecting data from a variety of facilities, reporting systems or surveillance networks provide uniform definitions or protocols for defining cases and the population at risk. By using systems like NHSN, the data from facilities are uniform and can be used to calculate facility and area ratios that allow for appropriate comparisons between a facility and the state or national average. This type of surveillance system and data analyses allows for differentiating between quality of care issues and normal variation for outcome events.

QUALITY METRICS

Definition of Measureable Quality

Quality has been defined in numerous ways. Excellence, value, fitness, conformance, and expectation fulfillment constitute only a few of these definitions (Reeves & Bednar, 1994). Despite the inability of health care professionals to develop a consistent definition, quality continues to be a focal element when discussing, defining, and measuring successful health care. Although Donabedian's structure–process–outcome framework is only a portion of his definition of quality, it has provided health care professionals with a foundation for quality assessment. The framework provides a theoretical link to health care professionals who measure structures and processes in meaningful ways and wish to connect these to outcomes through statistical analysis. For our discussion, *quality* is defined using Donabedian's structure–process–outcome framework (Donabedian, 1980).

Structure

Structure includes the presence of facilities or materials necessary to perform health care tasks (Donabedian, 1965, 1980). Structure can include the number of operating rooms, patient beds, or appropriate stockroom storage. However, it also refers to sufficient workforce, which can be quantified in terms of number of personnel and types of training or education, including knowledge of best clinical practices.

Processes

Processes are the execution of structural knowledge, procedures, and best practices that are simultaneously accompanied by sufficient skills to perform the required tasks (Donabedian, 1965, 1980). For example, best practice congestive heart failure process measures for hospitalized patients include discharge instructions, left ventricular function assessment, smoking-cessation instruction, anticoagulant at discharge, and angiotension-converting enzyme (ACE) inhibitor or angiotension-receptor blocker (ARB) for left ventricular systolic dysfunction (CMS, 2009).

Outcomes

Outcomes are either desired or undesired results relating to improved health for the patient (Donabedian, 1965, 1980). Outcomes measures include mortality, readmission to the hospital within 30-days, nosocomial infection, or costs, to name a few. Unfortunately, outcomes are not always directly associated with the structure and process of care (Hernandez et al., 2010). That is why care must be taken when defining quality metrics and the relationships they represent.

Settings and Data Availability

Because the interaction between patient and provider occurs in a variety of settings, and the care differs significantly based on the setting, data sources frequently align with the care setting. Regardless of the type of data (survey, administrative, or EHR), the information is patient and provider specific. This translates to the need for protecting individuals' information. As such, these data sets have either restrictions to access or modifications to the data or both in order to protect individuals from being identified.

Inpatient Data

Inpatient data include information from the hospital setting for individuals who are admitted to the hospital. For quality metrics, the most common form of inpatient data is the administrative summary discharge abstract. Inpatient data can be abstracted from payer claims data as well. For most of the examples in this chapter, we use inpatient discharge summary data available from HCUP at the national level or from most state health data warehouses or health statistics departments.

Outpatient Data

Outpatient data include information regarding patients who receive care at the hospital, but are not admitted. This includes health care received in the emergency room, radiological services, and day surgeries, to name a few. Although some patients are kept overnight, if they are allocated to an observation bed, they are not considered admitted to the hospital. Therefore, the administrative billing is processed through the outpatient arm of the hospital.

Clinic or Physician Office Data

Health care provided in office or clinic settings is most frequently evaluated from payer claims data. Although there are initiatives to create local or regional all-payer claims data sets, most claims data are limited to a single payer. Limitations also exist for claims data in which beneficiaries participate in managed care (MC) programs. In fee for service (FFS) insurance programs, each time a beneficiary interacts with the health care system, a bill is submitted from the provider to the payer. This allows for tracking of diagnoses and services each time the beneficiary interacts with the health care system.

In MC programs, the payer pays a fee each month for each beneficiary in its program. In return, providers supply and direct the provision of health care to the beneficiaries. This payment structure incentivizes providers to keep beneficiaries healthy through less expensive preventive care services. However, because the billing process is no longer tied to the provision of health care, claims information for MC beneficiaries may be limited or incomplete.

Other Health Care Settings

Other health care settings include skilled nursing facilities (nursing homes), rehabilitation facilities, long-term acute care facilities, or psychiatric facilities. Although electronic health information is not readily available, these are important sources used to monitor health care delivery and associated quality outcomes.

Patient Response Data

Patient response data range from patient satisfaction surveys after discharge to the large national surveys mentioned earlier in this chapter. Patient response data are becoming increasingly important as we move toward measuring patient-centered care. This facet of quality, although not necessarily an accurate reflection of clinical quality, is important for patients to maintain dignity and encourage compliance with provider care plans.

Metric Development

Most quality metrics are reported in a form that allows comparisons across providers, facilities, or areas. Because patient populations vary among providers, facilities, and areas, most metrics are reported as rates or the number of cases per the number of patients' eligible for an outcome or per patient days of exposure. Another form of reporting is the observed outcomes to expected outcomes (O/E) ratio. A more detailed explanation of metric rates is present in the Populations Affected section, and a more detailed explanation of the O/E ratio is present in the Risk Adjustment section that follows.

To facilitate our discussion about metric development, we use an existing quality metric from AHRQ, Prevention Quality Indicator (PQI) number 9—Low Birth Weight Rate (PQI9; Health Resources and Services Administration, 2014). Although this metric uses inpatient discharge data, the principles and process can be applied to other settings and data types. The PQI and other quality indicators are described in more detail later in this chapter.

Need Identification

When a quality issue is identified through the stakeholders, a multi faceted discussion begins. For our example, barriers in access to prenatal care are considered an important population health problem (Health Resources and Services Administration, 2014). Once stakeholders agree that a quality problem exists, they must identify the populations affected, the appropriate care settings to measure, ways to minimize reporting burden while simultaneously collecting relevant data, and assuring transparency and accountability in the reporting of data.

Populations Affected

Because quality metrics are frequently expressed as rates, an important part of metric development is to identify an appropriate denominator population. Individuals with the potential of developing the outcome are selected, because in epidemiological terms they have been exposed. For our example, the "exposed" population is all babies born in hospital.

The role of the denominator population is to provide a base of comparison. For example, let us say we want to know how our state compares with other states in providing prenatal care to pregnant women. If we are from a densely populated large state, an absolute count of low-birth-weight babies may lead us to believe we are doing a poor job compared to a less populated small state likely to have fewer low-birth-weight babies simply because there are fewer babies being born there. By standardizing the way we report low-birth-weight births to a rate such as the number of low-birth-weight births per 1,000 live births, the densely populated large state may be the same or better than the less densely populated small state.

Appropriate Settings

When determining where to measure an identified need, a clear understanding of how individuals interact with the health care industry is necessary. In our example, we understand that prenatal care occurs in the office or clinic setting. However, pregnant women not receiving prenatal care will, by extension, either have limited or have no health care records prior to delivery. Therefore, as the majority of babies are born in hospitals, the best place to capture the lack of preventive prenatal care is the hospital or at the outcome level. For our example, one outcome known to be associated with lack of prenatal care is babies born with a low birth weight.

Data Availability and Reporting Burden

Once an understanding of how individuals use health care is established, we can look at the points of contact with the health care system and evaluate whether sufficient information is already collected. In our example, women presenting to deliver a baby in hospital may or may not have insurance. For women with insurance, claims data may reflect both hospitalization and prenatal care. However, this would only capture women with insurance. Additionally, obtaining claims information from multiple payers would be arduous. Because hospital discharge data is all-payer, the burden to collect information is lower. However, discharge summary data do not capture care prior to admission, and mother and baby data are not linked. Therefore, we are limited to identifying babies with low birth weight as potentially resulting from lack of prenatal care. Administrative billing data captures low birth weight through the ICD-9-CM codes used for billing purposes. Additionally, because the administrative billing would be generated regardless of outcome, administrative billing information does not produce an additional burden to providers and can be used to reflect the care provided.

Accountability and Transparency

Another advantage of using administrative data is that coding practices can be tracked to assure consistency within a provider practice area. Payers will evaluate and review bills from providers to assure they are paying for care provided. Additionally, payers have the option to deny payment for care that is unnecessary. In this way, payers influence the way care is provided and recorded.

What Should Metrics Tell Us?

Although we would like metrics to be a simple indicator of good quality care versus poor quality care, the truth is no one metric provides an absolute measure of quality care. Instead, we must look at the continuum of metrics available to identify areas of practice in which providers can improve.

About Individuals and Populations

When we evaluate a quality metric, we must always consider the underlying population. In the case of our example, PQI9, we may see an area with a higher rate of low-birth-weight babies. A couple of population considerations should include the proportion of deliveries by impoverished mothers or mothers who are in the tails of the distribution by age (extremely young or extremely old for giving birth). In combination, the information can help the community develop relevant interventions to improve access and utilization of prenatal care.

About Providers

Quality metrics can tell us several things about providers. First, a quality metric is a reflection of the population that a provider treats. Second, it is a reflection of the care provided. Providers with higher rates for adverse events who are not tied to underlying population confounders should examine their relevant structural and process of care measures to help identify areas for improvement within their practice.

Risk Adjustment

Before we can discuss adjusting for risk, we must establish a foundation that includes the key concepts of risk. Within the field of epidemiology, risk is measured a number of ways to reflect different facets of risk. For our purposes, we will generalize the epidemiological perspective to define risk as the likelihood of an individual to acquire disease. Usually expressed as a rate, we use the example of 1 in 25 hospital patients acquiring an HAI as an expression of epidemiological risk (Centers for Disease Control & Prevention, Center for Emerging and Zoonotic Infections Diseases, & Division of Healthcare Quality Promotion, 2014).

Another relevant definition of risk includes the attributes or behaviors that increase or decrease the likelihood of disease. These attributes or behaviors are thought to have a causal relationship with a given disease. For example, smoking and exposure to secondhand smoke are risk factors for lung cancer (Division of Cancer Prevention and Control & Centers for Disease Control and Prevention, 2014).

Now that we have a common understanding of risk, we can discuss attributes or behaviors that are associated with disease outcomes but are not of a causal nature. These types of variables can cause spurious statements of causality. Known in statistical terms as confounding factors, these attributes are the focus of risk adjustment.

What Is Risk Adjustment?

Risk adjustment is a statistical tool that allows us to account for confounding circumstances or factors. Using statistical methods, such as regression analyses, we can assign variation in outcomes to predictive and confounding variables. Although exact methods of risk adjustment vary based on the source of data and the specific outcome measure, the risk-adjustment process has two basic steps. First, we must identify the relevant population (see the previous section Populations Affected). The second step, typically some form of regression modeling, allows us to include relevant available predictive and confounding variables to create the most accurate picture of variation for an outcome. The process for specifying the most informative model varies according to available data and the outcome. However, age, gender, and race are the most common confounding variables, so that when available, they are included in most risk-adjustment models. Also depending on the source of data payer and facility type, they may be included in the adjustment model.

Risk adjustment also allows us to report observed over expected (O/E) ratios for comparison purposes. Once regression model coefficients are generated for the entire population (say at the state or national level), the coefficients can be applied to individual providers or geographic subpopulations to estimate the expected number of outcome events. When we report the actual number of events that are identified in the data over the number of expected events as identified through regression modeling that adjusts for confounding factors, we report the O/E ratio. This ratio, when below 1, indicates that the provider or area is performing better than the entire population. When the ratio is above 1, the provider or area is performing worse than the entire population or area, and when the ratio is near 1, the provider or area is performing similarly to the entire population.

Why Is It Important?

The purpose of risk adjustment is to account for differences in the population. By doing so, we can then observe and report differences that are attributable to provider care. With the movement toward public reporting of performance, the emphasis on risk adjustment becomes more important to providers and consumers. Risk adjustment allows us to compare outcomes among providers in like terms. More important, it helps providers identify practice areas that require change for the improved health of the patient population.

How Should Risk-Adjusted Measures Be Interpreted?

The development of most quality metrics is a rigorous peer-reviewed process. As such, considerable thought and effort have gone into creating metrics that reflect quality care and provide consumers and providers with a reasonable way to compare providers. When we look at any quality metric, we should ask ourselves three questions. First, how is the metric defined in terms of identification of cases, population examined, and confounding factors for which they have been accounted? Second, what does this metric tell us about care provided? Third, what other metrics or information should be examined to provide us with a complete picture of quality care with respect to settings and providers? Frequently, one quality metric that is out of the normal range alerts us to dig deeper as to the cause.

Major Quality Metrics

There are several sources of existing quality metrics. What follows here is a brief description of each and a link current at the time of printing. The list of metric sources is not comprehensive, but captures some of the largest metric warehouses.

National Quality Forum

www.qualityforum.org/Home.aspx
The National Quality Forum (NQF) is a nonprofit member organization whose specific purpose is to facilitate quality health care through consensus-based development and endorsement of health care quality metrics (NQF, 2014; see www.qualityforum.org/Home.aspx). As part of their services they provide a searchable quality metric database that allows filtering of results by care setting, NQF endorsement, and data source, to name a few. This is an excellent starting point if you are interested in finding existing

validated quality metrics with descriptions that include statistical details such as target population and data source.

Health and Human Services Measure Inventory

www.qualityforum.org/story/About_Us.aspx
The Health and Human Services (HHS) measure inventory is managed by AHRQ. It includes over 2,000 quality metrics sponsored or generated by eight agencies. A few of the searchable database filters include care setting, target population, and specific topics. Each metric contains a brief description of its history, data source, type of metric (structure, process, outcome), who identified the need, and the numerator and denominator definitions (see www.qualityforum.org/story/About_Us.aspx).

CMS Measures Management System

www.cms.gov/Medicare/Quality-Initiatives-Patient-Assessment-Instruments/MMS/
MeasuresManagementSystemBlueprint.html
The link given here provides an overview of the numerous CMS quality programs. Because of the numerous quality programs CMS is responsible for overseeing, accumulating all the measures in one location is difficult. However, the webpage link given at the end of this paragraph contains the link to an Excel spreadsheet that describes the 52 current quality metric databases that CMS tracks, along with relevant information on where to get more detail on the databases and the associated metrics (see www.cms .gov/Medicare/Quality-Initiatives-Patient-Assessment-Instruments/QualityMeasures/ CMS-Measures-Inventory.html).

Because of CMS's national role in health care, it is a large repository of publically available information. Although we have provided links to some basic sources of information, we recommend exploring the CMS website to better understand the role third-party payers have over the provision of health care.

National Healthcare Safety Network

www.cdc.gov/nhsn/dataStat.html
The NHSN is a voluntary national-level electronic tracking system for HAI information. Although NHSN is voluntary from a national perspective, many states require facilities to use the system to track HAIs because of the very specific definitions and uniformity achieved between facilities. Although the data are not publically available, the aggregate state and national summaries are publically available, as are the definitions employed for identification of HAIs.

Agency for Healthcare Research and Quality

http://qualityindicators.ahrq.gov/
AHRQ quality indicators are validated measures of health care quality. Derived from inpatient administrative data, the measures are delineated into four groups, Inpatient Quality (IQI), Patient Safety (PSI), Pediatric Quality (PDI), and PQI. For each metric, AHRQ provides detailed definitions along with three types of software that are free and publically available to facilitate the translation of the inpatient administrative data into

meaningful quality metrics. The software includes the WinQI software, which is Windows-compatible software, allowing the Quality Indicator rates to be calculated from data that resides on a desktop computer. The SAS® software calculates the metrics and can be used in numerous computing environments. And finally, the MONAHRQ system allows administrative data to be translated to the Quality Indicators and placed onto a website (see http://qualityindicators.ahrq.gov/).

Publicly available data for CMS and AHRQ allow providers to evaluate their patient care delivery performance as compared to their peer providers and the national benchmark. An example of the SAS code used to map variables into from a database, in this case the Texas Health Care Information Council (THCIC) database, into the AHRQ quality metrics program, is illustrated (see Appendix 22.1).

SUMMARY

In generating or interpreting quality metrics, an understanding of how health care is provided by providers, utilized by patients, and influenced by payers is necessary to correctly create or interpret any metric. Our ability to define the exposed population and adjust for the underlying population distribution enables us to compare outcomes and providers in like terms. By understanding that no single metric is an absolute measure of quality care, and that an indicator that is awry signals providers to look at their process of care, we create systematic ways for providers to improve the quality of care they provide. Improved quality of care then translates to improved population health. As part of the aforementioned NEHI (Nursing Education in Health Informatics) model (McBride, Tietze, & Fenton, 2013), population health is associated with patient safety/quality and it is therefore interlinked to point-of-care technology and data management and analytics. Together these components of care delivery, policy formation, federal regulations, and nursing informatics represent the much needed comprehensive approach to the U.S. health care system.

EXERCISES AND QUESTIONS FOR CONSIDERATION

As noted, the NQF is a nonprofit member organization whose specific purpose is to facilitate quality health care through consensus-based development and endorsement of health care quality metrics (NQF, 2014). It is considered the most comprehensive site for quality metrics (see www.qualityforum.org/Home.aspx).

On the NQF site, find three existing validated quality metrics with descriptions that would apply to your area of practice. They should include statistical details such as target population and data source. Answer the following questions/comments.

1. Can you describe each metric you selected and list the associated statistics?

2. What would be involved in having these metrics as part of the ongoing monitoring in your practice area?

3. Please comment on how you might engage your health insurance company in an ACO to be part of these metrics.

CASE STUDY

Consider the following case study.

Aims and Objectives: To evaluate the outcome of a logic model in the form of population health that addresses the complexity of community-based management of hospital readmission rates.

Background: Logic models for population health-based projects have previously been described (Chapters 10 and 13). Use the logic model provided in Chapter 10 and select a population health topic of clinical interest and design a logic model for addressing an outcome indicator or population health concern. For example, readmissions for patients with heart failure would be a suggested topic. Questions/comments to be considered are:

1. What are your data input, output, and measures of success?
2. Explain how your devised model addresses the selected population health concerns.
3. How will you assess your population or community?
4. How will you collect the data needed for your input, output, and process measures of success?

REFERENCES

Adams, P. F., Barnes, P. M., & Vickerie, J. L. (2008). Summary health statistics for the U.S. population: National Health Interview Survey, 2007. National Center for Health Statistics. *Vital Health Statistics*, *10*(238), 1–104.

Cavanaugh, S. (2014, December 22). *ACOs moving ahead [official blog for CMS]*. Retrieved from http://www.cms.gov/Medicre/Medicare-Fee-for-Service-Payment/sharedsavingsprogram/

Centers for Disease Control and Prevention and the Center for Health Statistics. (2012). *Surveys and data collection systems*. Retrieved from http://www.cdc.gov/nchs/surveys.htm

Centers for Disease Control and Prevention, Center for Emerging and Zoonotic Infections Diseases & Division of Healthcare Quality Promotion. (2014). *Data and statistics*. Retrieved from http://www.cdc .gov/HAI/surveillance/index.html

Centers for Medicare & Medicaid Services. (2009). *Roadmap for quality measurement in the traditional Medicare fee-for-service program*. Baltimore, MD: Author. Retrieved from http://www.cms.hhs .gov/QualityInitiativesGenInfo/downloads/QualityMeasurementRoadmap_OEA1-16_508.pdf

Centers for Medicare & Medicaid Services. (2013). *Medicare program—General information*. Retrieved from http://www.cms.gov/Medicare/Medicare-General-Information/MedicareGenInfo/index .html

Centers for Medicare & Medicaid Services. (2014a). *Accountable care organizations*. Retrieved from http://www.cms.gov/Medicare/Medicare-Fee-for-Service-Payment/ACO/index.html?redirect=/ACO

Centers for Medicare & Medicaid Services. (2014b). *CMS fast facts*. Retrieved from http://www.cms .gov/Research-Statistics-Data-and-Systems/Statistics-Trends-and-Reports/CMS-Fast-Facts/index.html

Centers for Medicare & Medicaid Services, Office of the Actuary, National Health Statistics Group. (2011). *National healthcare expenditures data* (No. CMSnhs2011). Washington, DC: Centers for Medicare & Medicaid Services. Retrieved from http://www.cms.gov/Research-Statistics-Data-and-Systems/Statistics-Trends-and-Reports/NationalHealthExpendData/index.html

Division of Cancer Prevention and Control, & Centers for Disease Control and Prevention. (2014). *Lung cancer.* Retrieved from http://www.cdc.gov/cancer/lung/

Division of Community Health: National Center for Chronic Disease Prevention and Health Promotion. (2013). *CDC's health communities program.* Retrieved from http://www.cdc.gov/nccdphp/dch/programs/healthycommunitiesprogram/overview/index.htm

Donabedian, A. (1965). Evaluating the quality of medical care. *Millbank Memorial Fund Quarterly, 44*(3, Part 2), 166–206.

Donabedian, A. (1980). *The definition of quality and approaches to its assessment.* Ann Arbor, MI: Health Administration Press.

Fisher, E., & Shortell, S. (2010). Accountable care organizations: Accountable to what, to whom and how. *Journal of the American Medical Association, 304*(15):1715–1716. doi:10.1001/jama.2010.1513

Haywood, T. T., & Kosel, K. C. (2011). The ACO model—a three-year financial loss? *New England Journal of Medicine, 364.* doi:10.1056/NEJMp1100950

Health Resources and Services Administration. (2014). *Prenatal—First trimester care access.* Retrieved from http://www.hrsa.gov/quality/toolbox/measures/prenatalfirsttrimester/index.html

Healthcare Cost and Utilization Project. (2014). *HCUP databases.* Rockville, MD: Agency for Healthcare Research and Quality.

Hernandez, A. F., Hammill, B. G., Peterson, E. D., Yancy, C. W., Schulman, K. A., Curtis, L. H., & Fonarow, G. C. (2010). Relationships between emerging measures of heart failure processes of care and clinical outcomes. *American Heart Journal, 159*(3), 406–413. Retrieved from http://ovidsp.ovid.com/ovidweb.cgi?T=JS&NEWS=N&PAGE=fulltext&D=medl&AN=20211302

Kindig, D., & Stoddart, G. (2003). What is population health? *American Journal of Public Health, 93*(3), 380–383. doi:10.2105/AJPH.93.3.380

McBride, S. G., Tietze, M., & Fenton, M., V. (2013). Developing an applied informatics course for a doctor of nursing practice program. *Nurse Educator, 38*(1), 37–42. doi:10.1097/NNE.0b013e318276df5d

National Association of County & City Health Officials. (2015). *Resource center for community health assessments and community health improvement plans.* Retrieved from http://www.naccho.org/topics/infrastructure/CHAIP/chachip-online-resource-center.cfm

National Prevention Council. (2011). *The National Prevention Strategy: America's plan for better health and wellness.* Retrieved from http://www.surgeongeneral.gov/priorities/prevention/strategy/index.html#The%20Priorities

National Prevention Council. (2012). *2012 annual status report* (No. NPC-2012). Washington, DC: Department of Health and Human Services, Office of the Surgeon General. Retrieved from http://www.surgeongeneral.gov/initiatives/prevention/2012-npc-status-report.pdf

National Prevention Council. (2014). *2014 annual status report* (No. NPC2014). Washington, DC: U.S. Department of Health and Human Services, Office of the Surgeon General. Retrieved from http://www.surgeongeneral.gov/initiatives/prevention/2014-npc-status-report.pdf

National Quality Forum. (2014). *About us.* Retrieved from http://www.qualityforum.org/story/About_Us.aspx

Noble, D. J., & Casalino, L. P. (2013). Can accountable care organizations improve population health?: Should they try? *Journal of the American Medical Association, 309*(11), 1119–1120. doi:10.1001/jama.2013.592

Reeves, C. A., & Bednar, D. A. (1994). Defining quality: Alternatives and implications. *Academy of Management Review, 19*(3), 419–445.

Torio, C. M., & Andrews, R. M. (2013). *National inpatient hospital costs: The most expensive conditions by payer, 2011* (HCUP Statistical Brief No. 160). Rockville, MD: Agency for Healthcare Research and Quality.

U.S. Department of Health and Human Services. (2014a). *2020 topics & objective—Objectives A–Z.* Retrieved from http://www.healthypeople.gov/2020/topicsobjectives2020/default.aspx

U.S. Department of Health and Human Services. (2014b). *History & development of health people.* Retrieved from http://www.healthypeople.gov/2020/about/history.aspx

U.S. Department of Health and Human Services. (2014c). *Objective development and selection process.* Retrieved from http://www.healthypeople.gov/2020/about/objectiveDevelopment.aspx

Watson, D. E., Broemeling, A., & Wong, S. T. (2009). A results-based logic model for primary healthcare: A conceptual foundation for population-based information systems. *Healthcare Policy, 5*(Special Issue), 33–46.

APPENDIX 22.1 VARIABLE MAPPING FOR THCIC VARIABLES INTO THE AHRQ REQUIREMENTS FOR VERSION 4.5

```
*** Record_id renamed to KEY;
format key z12.;
label key= 'KEY';
key = input(record_id,12.);

*** Assign mid-point age to in place of age category;
If pat_age = "00" then age= .038;
     else if pat_age = "01" then age = .460;
     else if pat_age = "02" then age = 2.5;
     else if pat_age = "03" then age = 7;
     else if pat_age = "04" then age = 12;
     else if pat_age = "05" then age = 16;
     else if pat_age = "06" then age = 18.5;
     else if pat_age = "07" then age = 22;
     else if pat_age = "08" then age = 27;
     else if pat_age = "09" then age = 32;
     else if pat_age = "10" then age = 37;
     else if pat_age = "11" then age = 42;
     else if pat_age = "12" then age = 47;
     else if pat_age = "13" then age = 52;
     else if pat_age = "14" then age = 57;
     else if pat_age = "15" then age = 62;
     else if pat_age = "16" then age = 67;
     else if pat_age = "17" then age = 72;
     else if pat_age = "18" then age = 77;
     else if pat_age = "19" then age = 82;
     else if pat_age = "20" then age = 87;
     else if pat_age = "21" then age = 90;
```

```
else if pat_age = "22" then age = 8.5;
else if pat_age = "23" then age = 31;
else if pat_age = "24" then age = 54.5;
else if pat_age = "25" then age = 69.5;
else if pat_age = "26" then age = 75;
```

(CONTINUED but content not displayed)

```
Array proc {25} $ princ_surg_proc_day oth_surg_proc_day_1-oth_surg_proc_day_24;
Array pr {25} prday1-prday25;

do i= 1 to 25;

    pr(i) = input(proc(i),4.);

    end;
```

RUN;

Note: This is a sample of the mapping script/code. It is not intended to be complete mapping of all THCIC data.

CHAPTER 23

Developing Competencies in Nursing for an Electronic Age of Health Care

Laura Thomas, Susan McBride, Sharon Decker, and Mari Tietze

OBJECTIVES

1. Examine the basics of competency evaluation and the current state of evaluating nursing informatics competencies.

2. Examine the relevance of simulation in nursing and clinical education and discuss the importance of fully engaging the clinician in training through simulated activity with electronic health records and other point-of-care technology.

3. Examine the HEALTH three-dimensional model developed and recommended by the International Medical Informatics Association for education in biomedical and health informatics.

4. Discuss how simulation, the HEALTH model, and quality and safety education in nursing (QSEN) competencies can combine to inform the development of strategies to prepare clinicians for the future of health care.

5. Discuss how both simulation and QSEN competencies could align to promote the goals of the Robert Wood Johnson Foundation's commitment to continuously improving health care through educational modalities.

KEY WORDS

patient safety, quality, simulation, nursing education, electronic health records, competencies

---

CONTENTS

INTRODUCTION

Competency must be defined before it can be assessed and documented (Wright, 2005). However, there is little consensus on what competency means; no agreed-on definition exists among educators, employers, and regulators (Tilley, 2008). An interprofessional definition of *competency* is "the knowledge, skills, abilities, and behaviors needed to carry out a job" (Wright, 2005, p. 7). The National Council of State Boards of Nursing (2009) defines *nursing competency* as "having the knowledge, skills and ability to practice safely and effectively" (p. 136). Defining *competency* is further complicated in the education setting with the primary focus being preparation for initial licensure, whereas in the practice setting, the focus is on developing ongoing competency (Tilley, 2008). In addition, no standards exist to identify when competency assessment should focus on general professional competency versus specialty competency. Historically, prelicensure and graduate education focused on mastering didactic information and pass–fail demonstration of skills, not competency-based evaluation (Fordham, 1987; Tilley, 2008). Recently, the focus in the literature shifted to competency-based undergraduate and graduate education in medicine and nursing (Batalden, Leach, Swing, Dreyfus, & Dreyfus, 2002; Redman, Lenburg, & Walker, 1999). Even so, implementation of competency-based education is not standard practice in the majority of educational programs (Institute of Medicine [IOM], 2003; IOM: Committee on Quality of Healthcare in America, 2001). In addition, competency-based education should include assessment of the core competencies defined by the IOM. Ongoing measurement of competency from nursing school into nursing practice is critical to professional development (Waddell, 2001). So how does one measure competency? Tracking and documenting competencies is a challenge for educators and nurse leaders. Adding the complexity of the electronic environment and the impact of the electronic health record (EHR) on clinical competency evaluation processes compounds the complexity. This chapter discusses the current state of competency evaluation for informatics and examines potential strategies for the future that can align with recommended models for developing competencies committed to defining the future role of nursing to continuously improve health care.

Evaluating Informatics Competencies

Currently, most of the evaluation methods used to examine competencies related to use of EHR in the clinical environment use levels 1 through 4 of nursing informatics competencies developed by the seminal work of Staggers, Gassert, and Curran (2002; Table 23.1). However, methods to evaluate competencies of these four levels of informatics competencies rely primarily on methods that self-report through survey instrumentation methods. Valid and reliable methods to evaluate informatics competencies measurably and objectively within simulation centers are not currently available. Basic competency recommendations for integration of informatics content into baccalaureate and graduate nursing programs have been addressed by Hunter, McGonigle, and Hebda (2013) and, more recently, by Hill, McGonigle, Hunter, Sipes, and Hebda (2014), who developed a method for self-evaluation of competencies for more advanced informatics competencies, including levels 3 and 4. Yet, methods to objectively evaluate these four levels of nursing informatics competencies in simulation centers that incorporate objective evaluation criteria are lacking.

TABLE 23.1 Four Levels of Nursing Informatics Competencies	
Level	**Description**
1	Nurses with fundamental information management and computer technology skills use existing information systems and available information to manage their practice.
2	Nurses have proficiency in their domain of interest (e.g., public health, education, administration). These nurses are highly skilled in using information management and computer technology skills to support their major area of practice. They see relationships among data elements, and make judgments based on trends and patterns within these data. Experienced nurses use current information systems but collaborate with the informatics nurse specialist to suggest system improvements.
3	Registered nurses who are prepared at least at the baccalaureate level who possess additional knowledge and skills specific to information management and computer technology. They focus on information needs for the practice of nursing, which includes education, administration, research, and clinical practice. Informatics specialists' practices are built on the integration and application of information science, computer science, and nursing science. In their practice, informatics specialists use the tools of critical thinking, process skills, data-management skills (includes identifying, acquiring, preserving, retrieving, aggregating, analyzing, and transmitting data), systems development life cycle, and computer skills.
4	Nurses are educationally prepared to conduct informatics research and to generate informatics theory. These nurses lead the advancement of informatics practice and research because they have a vision of what is possible, and a keen sense of timing to make things happen. Innovators function with an ongoing healthy skepticism of existing data-management practices and are creative in developing solutions. Innovators possess a sophisticated level of understanding and skills in information management and computer technology. They understand the interdependence of systems, disciplines, and outcomes, and can finesse situations to maximize outcomes.

Adapted from Staggers, Gassert, and Curran (2002).

SIMULATION AND EHRs

EHRs coupled with health information exchange (HIE) across care settings are poised to fundamentally transform the health care landscape. The conventional aspects of reading through a chart to obtain the full picture of a patient shift into a more complex multidimensional view of information in the electronic environment, creating a significant change in the way clinicians access, read, digest, and use the information within the health record to treat patients. The IOM and the Office of the National Coordinator for Health Information Technology (ONC-HIT) are calling on academia and industry to rethink how we train health care professionals to work in interprofessional teams to safely and effectively use EHRs.

Widespread adoption of EHRs in ambulatory and acute care settings is rapidly occurring in the United States as a result of the Medicare Incentive Program and the Health Information Technology for Economic and Clinical Health (HITECH) Act of 2009. Yet, simulation centers throughout the country are lagging behind with respect to fully implementing EHRs and employing methods for developing and evaluating competencies in critical functions such as electronic medication administration, computer provider order entry (CPOE), and the integration of the EHR within clinical workflow and decision making for clinicians. Nurses and physicians are frequently trained in computer-equipped classroom settings with as much hands-on experience as possible; however, the transferability of knowledge from this setting is ineffective when students later encounter the EHR in the practice setting.

Background

EHR use has increased dramatically over the last 10 years since President Bush's 2004 mandate to make EHRs accessible to most Americans by 2014. President Obama followed that mandate by signing the American Recovery and Reinvestment Act (ARRA) into law in 2009, which provided funding for the purchase of health information technology (HIT). As EHRs began to infiltrate the health care practice setting, it became apparent that the education of health care professionals had to change to meet the demands of a technology-rich practice environment. Recommendations stating health care professionals and graduates need to develop competencies in computer literacy and information technologies have been voiced since the 1970s (Anderson, Gremy, & Pages, 1974; Hart, Newton, & Boone, 2010; Ronald & Skiba, 1987; Staggers, Gassert, & Curran, 2001, 2002). The IOM identified the use of information technologies to improve access to clinical information and support clinical decision making as a challenge to address and resolve in an effort to improve health care delivery (Corrigan, Donaldson, & Kohn, 2001).

This ongoing integration of informatics technology has changed the provision and monitoring of health care practices. Specifically, the integration of EHRs, supported by federal infrastructure and mandates, required health care providers to develop the competencies required to appropriately use health care technologies when providing patient care. The need for students of the health sciences to develop informatics competencies to provide quality, safe care in the evolving health care environment has been identified by multiple authorities (e.g., Donahue & Thiede, 2008; Jones & Donelle, 2011; Hart, Newton, & Boone, 2010). Yet, institutions, both in academia and in practice, continue to face challenges to include funding for the initial purchase and maintenance costs of informatics technology, availability of technical support, as well as addressing limited exposure of students to EHRs, limited EHR expertise of faculty/educators, and multiple variances among EHR systems (Greenawalt, 2014; Jha et al., 2009).

Position statements and accreditation requirements related to the integration of informatics technology have been published by national agencies and workgroups. In 2003, the IOM recommended, "All health professionals should be educated to deliver patient-centered care as members of an interdisciplinary team, emphasizing evidence-based practice (EBP), quality improvement (QI) approaches, and informatics" (IOM, 2003, p. 121). In 2008, the importance of adopting EHRs in clinical practice and developing competency standards for graduating and practicing nurses was initially identified by the Technology Informatics Guiding Education Reform (TIGER) initiative. The TIGER initiative identified three components for the TIGER nursing informatics competencies model: (a) basic computer competencies, (b) information literacy, and (c) information management. Additionally, the collaborative stressed health care providers must be able to determine what information is needed, utilize the appropriate resources to find the information, use valid resources to critique the information, provide evidence-based care based on this information, and evaluate the outcomes of the process. A timeline was established that recommended all graduating nursing students and practicing nurses be able to demonstrate the established competencies by January 2013 (Gassert, 2008).

National nursing organizations also expressed the importance of preparing the current and future workforce of a technology-enhanced environment. The National League of Nursing (2008) in the position statement, *Preparing the Next Generation of Nurses to Practice in a Technology-Rich Environment: An Informatics Agenda*, stated, "It is imperative that graduates of today's nursing programs know how to interact with . . . informatics tools to ensure safe and quality care" (p. 1).

Institutions educating health care providers are challenged to explore new strategies to produce competent graduates. The American Association of Colleges of Nursing (AACN) identified use of patient care technologies for data gathering, decision support, and coordinating patient care as essential knowledge and skills for both the baccalaureate and master's education graduates. In the essentials for each level of nursing education, the AACN included competencies for the use of HIT for all nursing students (AACN, 2008, 2011a, 2011b). The QSEN competencies identified informatics as one of the five competencies for both prelicensure and graduate-level nurses. In terms of QSEN, *informatics* was defined as "use information and technology to communicate, manage knowledge, mitigate error, and support decision making" (Cronenwett et al, 2007, p. 129).

Simulation for Educating Health Care Professionals

During the past decade, multiple factors have resulted in requests from national organizations and accreditation agencies to transform the educational process for health care professionals. This demand is the result of multiple contributing factors to include changes in technology, a shortage of qualified faculty, and insufficient clinical placement opportunities for learning. National issues related to patient safety and mandates from accreditation agencies request a paradigm shift to evidence-based educational strategies, integration of competences related to health care technologies, and the integration of interprofessional teamwork skills into curricula (IOM, 2011). Simulation-based experience that combines other technologies provides a unique educational strategy to assist in the development of knowledge, skills, attitudes, and clinical judgment that are mandatory to provide safe, quality patient care (e.g. Aggarwal et al., 2010; Gaba, 2004; IOM, 2011; O'Donnell, Decker, Howard, Levett-Jones, & Miller, 2014).

Simulation-based learning requires learners to actively participate in dynamic experiences as opposed to static, traditional modes of learning. Simulation-based experiences can be conducted in various settings. These settings include a simulation center, a classroom (a case study), or in situ (the actual patient care environment). Research has demonstrated that when integrated appropriately, simulation-based education promotes (a) clinical judgment, (b) skills acquisition and retention, (c) interprofessional teamwork, and (d) has a positive impact on patient outcomes (Gaba, 2004; O'Donnell et al., 2014).

Only a few studies were identified that explored the impact of integrating EHRs into simulation-based activities to develop specific competencies. Competencies included the skills required to use electronic medical records to obtain appropriate information in a timely manner, use the information appropriately to support clinical judgments, and document care as part of the patient-care routine. For example, in one study, after nursing students participated in simulation-based virtual and high-fidelity experiences that integrated an EHR, faculty observed knowledge gained from these experiences being transferred to patient care in a subacute clinical setting (Donahoe & Thiede, 2008).

Undergraduate nursing students who participated in simulation-based experiences that integrated an EHR expressed the increased perception of self-confidence using the EHR in the acute care setting. Furthermore, these students expressed that exposure to EHRs prior to providing patient care allowed them to focus on the patient instead of the computer (Lucas, 2010). Additionally, both faculty and staff working with these students identified notable differences in the students' performance in the clinical setting. These differences included increased ease in use of the EHR system and more thorough documentation (Lucas, 2010). Friedman, Wong, and Blumenthal (2010) combined the use of classroom, online training, and simulation-based activities with standardized patients to assist health care providers to transition to the EHR without compromising patient care. Feedback from the participants indicated the experience facilitated the ability to maintain interpersonal communication with patients while using the EHR at the point of care.

Integration of EHRs in Simulation Centers

The use of simulation for the education of health care professionals has grown in recent years. Simulation centers can provide a realistic setting for learning, reducing the safety risks of testing electronic systems in the practice setting (Ammenworth et al., 2012; Brydges et al., 2015; Lamdman et al., 2014). The simulation center can accurately reflect the practice environment from the room set up to simulate patient interactions with standardized patients (Ammenworth et al., 2012). The realistic setup of the environment may provide external validity in simulation research studies (Ammenworth et al., 2012). The simulation center can also host usability testing labs, product development, human factors testing, and device development (Lamdman et al., 2014). Verification of software and system functions is essential to prevent errors in the practice setting that may harm the patient (Denham et al., 2013). Vendor software applications do not guarantee optimal use by health care providers or safe integration without using scenarios that are clinically accurate, interprofessional, and multifaceted (Denham et al., 2013). The Texas Medical Institute of Technology's EHR computer prescriber order entry (TMIT EHR-CPOE) Flight Simulator was used to detect errors after the implementation of CPOE (Denham et al., 2013). The simulator detected gaps in performance of health care providers when using CPOE. Although the flight simulator specifically addressed medication administration, it can also be used to improve the quality of CPOE data entry and prevent medication errors (Denham et al., 2013). The system software has to provide some assurance that errors will be detected, with verification through the use of simulation that can support the software's validity in practice (Denham et al., 2013).

Many schools have used academic versions of vendor software in simulation centers; however, in order to provide an accurate, realistic experience for students from multiple professions, software that replicates the complexity of the EHR in the practice setting should be utilized (Lucas, 2010). Rubbelke, Keenan, and Haycraft (2014) created a SimLab hospital and charting in Goggle Drive and found that students were able to document during nursing care within the simulated scenario; the simulation lacked barcode scanning and the time stamp feature of a complete EHR. Students found the system easy to use and similar to the EHR used in the practice setting. Faculty must be trained to use the available software and provided with teaching strategies to effectively integrate EHR use in simulation. Other studies that integrated academic software found that students felt more prepared for the clinical setting after using the EHR in simulation (Johnson & Bushy, 2011). Both studies examined the students' perceptions of their improvement in EHR competencies; however, no measurement of improvement was provided (Johnson & Bushy, 2011; Rubbelke et al., 2014). Faculty commitment to the use of the EHR is essential for successful integration (Gardner & Jones, 2012). The development of simulation scenarios, student outcomes, and learning objectives was time-consuming for faculty in both studies. The successful use of the EHR in simulation occurred when faculty champions led and supported faculty through the transition (Johnson & Bushy, 2011; Rubbelke et al., 2014). Some studies focused on the use of the EHRs for documentation (Milano et al., 2014); however, integration of decision-support modules and CPOE complicates system use (Milano et al., 2014). Nursing workflow must be considered to successfully use EHR in the simulation setting with students. Software used in academic nursing simulation may be developed specifically for that use and may not integrate all the functions of an EHR. Nurse educators in Singapore utilized a software vendor to develop an EHR that was specific to undergraduate students and focused on documentation (Kowitlawakul, Wang, & Chan, 2012). The problem with academically developed software is that it tends to be simplistic compared to the robust systems used in the health care setting (Lucas, 2010). The focus in the current studies seems to be on teaching students to document in the didactic setting rather than learning to use the software as part of the patient care workflow in simulation.

The most common method of teaching students and health care professionals to use the EHR revolves around didactic sessions in classroom-based sessions, where health care professionals sit at computer terminals and learn how to document within the software. Learning the software in the computer lab does not replicate the experience of using the EHR in a clinical setting while providing patient care. It has become apparent that technology education needs to take place within the health care professional's workflow while providing a safe environment for learning. The use of an EHR in a simulation center promotes an optimal learning environment through the use of an EHR in simulation scenarios. A survey of undergraduate nursing faculty at one university found that students were not prepared to document in the practice setting after learning paper documentation in nursing school (Lucas, 2010). Students stated they learned to document in the clinical setting rather than the simulation center. The lack of instruction in electronic documentation in simulation placed the burden on the students to learn computerized documentation while simultaneously trying to learn nursing care in the practice setting (Lucas, 2010).

Collaboration between academic and practice settings has been utilized to provide students with access and hands-on education with the type of software they will use during clinical rotations. When one practice setting is used, students may receive the learning experience they need. However, not all academic settings are affiliated with one practice setting. The use of diverse EHRs at different practice sites will not eliminate the need for student education with the EHR; however, when students learn to document in any electronic system, those skills are transferable to another electronic system. Students perceived that hands-on practice with the EHR allowed them to focus on care of the patient rather than use of the computer (Lucas, 2010).

INTERNATIONAL MEDICAL INFORMATICS ASSOCIATION ON HEALTH INFORMATICS

The International Medical Informatics Association (IMIA) updated recommendations for education in biomedical and health informatics focused on a three-dimensional model. The three dimensions are as follows: (a) professionals in health care, including physicians, nurses, and biomedical health informatics professionals (BMHI); (b) specialization in BMHI, including HIT users and specialists; and (c) stage of career progression ranging from bachelor's to doctoral degrees (Mantas et al., 2010). Learning outcomes and competencies are outlined for two foci, including IT users and the actual BMHI specialist. IMIA also recommends courses and tracks for all health care professionals to develop competencies in informatics. IMIA has developed a model based on the acronym "HEALTH." Table 23.2 outlines the key principles in the model. The model emphasizes levels of competencies needed to fully realize the benefits of HIT for improvements in health and quality of care, including an emphasis on the levels noted earlier as well as competent faculty to develop and deliver the curriculum needed.

QUALITY AND SAFETY EDUCATION IN NURSING MODEL

The Robert Wood Johnson Foundation (RWJF) funded an initiative emphasizing the importance of nursing to the future of U.S. health care underscoring the need for care to continuously improve and evolve. The QSEN initiative led by Cronenwett started with a phased approach, with phase one ending in 2007. The first phase outlined knowledge, skills, and attitudes that reinforce six quality and safety competencies: (a) QI, (b) safety, (c) teamwork and collaboration, (d) patient-centered care, (e) EBP, and (f) informatics. Table 23.3 outlines and defines the six QSEN competencies.

TABLE 23.2 IMIA HEALTH Model for Realizing the Benefits of HIT	
H	<u>Health care</u> professionals
E	Different modes of <u>education</u>
A	<u>Alternative</u> types of education in specialization of BMHI
L	<u>Levels</u> of education relating to stages of career progression
T	Qualified <u>teachers</u> to provide courses
H	Recognized qualifications for biomedical and <u>health</u> informatics positions

BMHI, biomedical health informatics professional; HIT, health information technology; IMIA, International Medical Informatics Association.

Source: Mantas et al. (2010).

TABLE 23.3 Six QSEN Competencies	
1. QI	Use data to monitor the outcomes of care processes and use improvement methods to design and test changes to continuously improve the quality and safety of health care systems.
2. Safety	Minimize risk of harm to patients and providers through both system effectiveness and individual performance.
3. Teamwork and collaboration	Function effectively within nursing and interprofessional teams, fostering open communication, mutual respect, and shared decision making to achieve quality patient care.
4. Patient-centered care	Recognize the patient or designee as the source of control and full partner in providing compassionate and coordinated care based on respect for patient's preferences, values, and needs.
5. EBP	Integrate best current evidence with clinical expertise and patient/family preferences and values for delivery of optimal health care.
6. Informatics	Use information and technology to communicate, manage knowledge, mitigate error, and support decision making.

EBP, evidence-based practice; QI, quality improvement; QSEN, quality and safety education in nursing.

Source: Smith, Cronenwett, and Sherwood (2007).

Three Levels of QSEN Competencies

The QSEN competencies approach nursing education from an integrative perspective to promote clinical reasoning in the health care setting (Benner, Sutphen, Leonard, & Day, 2010). Simulation encompasses all aspects of the three QSEN competencies: knowledge, skills, and attitudes. The use of simulation to ensure nurses are integrating the QSEN competencies into practice can be accomplished through the use of teaching and testing scenarios utilizing high- or low-fidelity manikins or standardized patients (Ironside, Jefferies, & Martin, 2009). The ability to participate in a simulated scenario whether the patient is a manikin or standardized patient (an individual trained to play the role of patient) requires application of didactic knowledge to the clinical situation. Application of evidence-based guidelines to the care provided during the scenario reinforces learning and provides a safe environment to practice clinical reasoning skills (Benner et al., 2010; Cronenwett et al., 2007; Cronenwett, Sherwood, & Gelman, 2009). Simulation centers may utilize model units to help students and nurses develop EHR skills that would be transferable to the practice setting (Sherwood & Drunkard, 2007). Scenarios can be conducted with interprofessional teams to provide opportunities for students to interact with other health care providers in patient care situations (Sherwood & Drunkard, 2007). Educators can integrate the EHR into simulated scenarios to facilitate EHR use during real-time patient care. Real-time documentation reduces errors, facilitates accurate interprofessional communication, and reduces delays in care, improving patient outcomes (Cronenwett et al., 2009; Malloch, 2007). Patient and family preferences can be incorporated through the plan of care that will be readily available to other health care professionals, improving care transitions, and promoting patient-centered care (Cronenwett et al., 2007).

When students and nurses are taught to document, it is done predominantly in a paper-based format, or alternatively as electronic documentation in a classroom setting. Many times students document after the simulated scenario to improve throughput times in the simulation lab. These methods of educating nurses in EHR documentation are ineffective in learning the real-time documentation necessary to provide patient-centered care (Cronenwett et al., 2007). Simulated scenarios that integrate documentation into the scenario teach nurses to document as part of their workflow and routine, skills that may be translated to the clinical setting. Students can receive feedback from faculty to improve the accuracy and consistency of documentation without erroneously documenting in an active patient chart. Faculty can provide structured patient care scenarios in the simulation environment to assess competencies in a predictable environment (Ironside et al., 2009). Variable types of patient scenarios can be used in conjunction with the EHR to assess students' and nurses' ability to practice safely, document appropriately, and ascertain whether the knowledge, skills, and abilities (KSAs) are met. Identification of deficiencies in KSAs can be identified and students can remediate to improve student performance (Ironside et al., 2009). Improved student and nurse performance with the EHR in simulation can improve patient outcomes and the quality of care.

Examples of Teaching Strategy Ideas by Learning Setting

As noted in Table 23.3, Cronenwett identifies six learning strategies as: (a) QI, (b) safety, (c) teamwork and collaboration, (d) patient-centered care, (e) EBP, and (f) informatics.

This section discusses the informatics example provided by Cronenwett et al. (2009) and provide teaching approaches, including classroom skills, simulation lab activities, and clinical practicum.

In terms of the informatics educational content of QSEN competencies, informatics is described as the "use of information and technology to communicate, manage knowledge, mitigate error, and support decision making" (QSEN, 2012). One way to incorporate the numerous components of QSEN strategies is to overlay the interprofessional education (IPE) collaborative competencies. The model for IPE competencies focuses on four main domains (Interprofessional Collaborative Expert Panel, 2011). As noted in previous chapters, they are: utilize informatics, provide patient-centered care, apply QI, and employ EBP.

Figure 23.1 illustrates the impact of such an approach to education, where time spent on interprofessional team activity yields faster, less costly patient care delivery solutions and EBP outcomes. Community involvement and patient engagement/activation are inherent components of the IPE collaborative effort.

One example of a teaching strategy that incorporated both informatics and IPE competencies is to use telehealth, mobile health, and/or remote patient monitoring in the teaching scenario. The various ancillary students from physical therapy (PT), occupational therapy, nutrition, nursing, behavioral/mental health, health system management, business, and so forth, after gaining an understanding of their respective roles, would then explore the informatics solutions available for the clinical case study and/or patient assignment. The PT student would contribute a PT-oriented informatics application, for example. Together the student group evaluates informatics solution options, including cost/benefits, and achieves a consensus on the optimum case study solution. In the end, this approach has proven to be a positive learning experience for students as indicated by a greater than 90% post-course satisfaction rate.

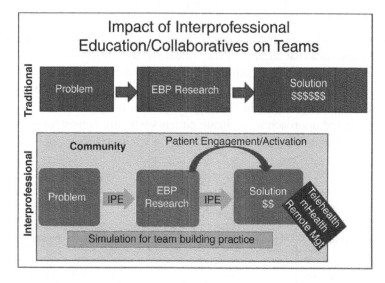

FIGURE 23.1. Comparison of traditional versus IPE approaches.

EBP, evidence-based practice.

Source: Mari Tietze.

METHODS TO FULLY IMPLEMENT EHRs INTO SIMULATION CENTERS

Fully implementing EHRs into the simulation centers across the country presents unique challenges with respect to adoption and implementation of the EHRs for use in supporting competency development for informatics. Ideally, these systems would replicate the actual clinical production environment of the EHR as the student would experience the technology within the workflow of the clinical setting. To implement an EHR within a simulation center that replicates the production environment presents unique challenges. Additionally, loading data that is representative of variability that the clinician experiences in the clinical setting presents labor-intensive requirements to load clinical scenarios within the simulation center EHR environment. If clinical production data could be de-identified and loaded in the simulation environment, the maintenance of the simulation center EHR is significantly reduced, and the data would better represent clinical conditions and the variability of complex conditions.

Fabricated clinical scenarios in the simulation lab education EHRs that are typically used today often lack clinical detail and variability. The electronic data within EHRs present unique opportunities to scramble and de-identify data within the EHR and use the data for clinical education. Yet, methods are needed to develop these types of strategies. It is conceivable that by using the detailed data within the EHR, educators would not need to go to laborious efforts to fabricate cases and manually load the data (data entry) into the EHR. This labor-intensive process is one of the major maintenance challenges preventing simulation labs across the country from fully implementing EHRs. Additionally, having faculty and staff available to support this process is difficult in current academic environments and education departments in practice settings. There are two approaches that the authors suggest could be considered in support of this process. Figure 23.2 reflects suggested strategies. In the figure, it is noted that the clinical scenarios for use in simulation need to be replicated to provide similar experiences for multiple students. For example, if you are evaluating clinical competencies on identifying and managing a potential septic patient, a query would be developed to identify cases in the production data that align with the simulated case on sepsis.

Two options to explore when loading data into a simulation environment for the EHR are considered. The goal is to create a complete simulation domain that replicates the environment clinicians experience in the clinical setting in the full production domain. Option one is the preferred approach to replicate patients who are consistent with a clinical scenario to be simulated because this option does not rely on data input in a production

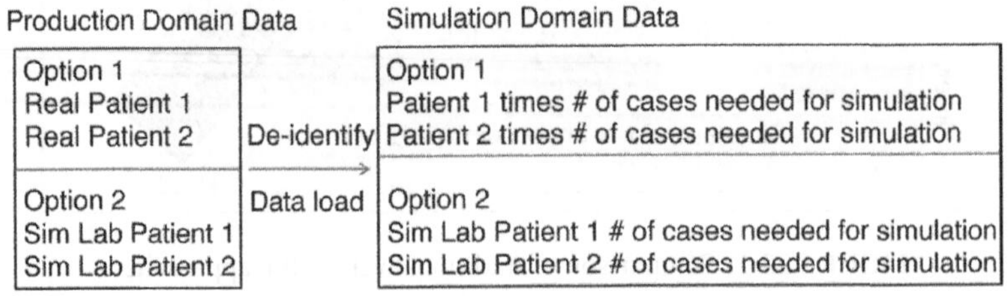

Production Domain Data		Simulation Domain Data
Option 1 Real Patient 1 Real Patient 2	De-identify	Option 1 Patient 1 times # of cases needed for simulation Patient 2 times # of cases needed for simulation
Option 2 Sim Lab Patient 1 Sim Lab Patient 2	Data load	Option 2 Sim Lab Patient 1 # of cases needed for simulation Sim Lab Patient 2 # of cases needed for simulation

FIGURE 23.2. Two methods to load clinical data in EHRs for simulation centers.

domain. For example, if the simulation experience needed is to identify and effectively react to an evolving sepsis case that resulted from a urinary tract infection (UTI), the existing clinical data could be queried to identify sepsis UTI cases. Data could be de-identified by patient, provider, and staff, and loaded within the EHR to replicate the sepsis simulation event for the number of cases needed to take the students through the simulation.

The other alternative is to set up a simulation-isolated environment in the production domain, and create the simulation cases within the production environment, replicate the number of cases needed for the number of students, and load the cases to the simulated environment. In either scenario, the data are loaded and representative of clinical cases that might be experienced. This data load could be followed by a standing order consistently delivered to the students within the EHR. The standing order could be consistently handled in the simulated EHR experience and the student would run through the series of orders, treatment, and documentation within the workflow of caring for the septic patient. Rubrics and faculty evaluation tools aligned with current methods used to assess handling of septic cases could couple with appropriate and timely use of the EHR within the scenario. In addition, the data within the simulated environment could be examined to determine whether the reporting of metrics associated with sepsis is appropriately documented for capture in the EHR. Furthermore, the evaluation of clinical reasoning skills and EHR competencies can determine whether appropriate interventions are carried out during the clinical scenario. An important consideration is the proper handling of PHI, staff, and provider data, so that no identifiable information is present in the EHR for simulation. This presents unique issues that should be addressed in accordance with methods to protect PHI through de-identification methods discussed in Chapter 14.

CASE STUDY

You are a nursing educator within a large academic medical center responsible for the annual competency evaluation of nurses within the hospital and clinics. The senior vice president for quality and safety, the chief information officer, and the chief nursing information officer requested a meeting to discuss identified issues related to the EHR documentation and patient safety issues with regard to medication orders, management of the orders within the EHR, and administration of the medications.

Events involving patient safety are increasing and the senior executives believe this is largely an issue related to competency in using the new EHR (implemented in the last 2 years). They have asked you to recommend a training and competency evaluation strategy that might affect these measures of patient safety and improve competencies related to the documentation errors they are seeing. They are taking responsibility for monitoring progress on impact, and are asking you to come back with recommendations for the education program.

After meeting with your chief nursing officer, education department staff, directors of nursing on the units, and the staff nurses, all parties agree that it would be

(continued)

CASE STUDY (*continued*)

helpful to have a training program for the EHR that simulates clinical workflow on some of the common issues concerning medication errors. You and your department are responsible for the simulation center and the following are questions for your team to consider as you design a plan for implementation of the EHR in the simulation lab:

1. What strategies will you use to fully implement the practice domain that replicates the EHR production domain with which nurses are currently working?
2. How will you identify cases related to the patient safety events that are occurring and incorporate them into the EHR to simulate what is happening and allow nurses time to practice on workflow and documentation related to these events?
3. How will you evaluate the nurses' performance and what assessment tools will you need?
4. How much time do you believe you need per nurse to run through the simulated case, and how will you manage these time constraints and the schedule in the simulation center?
5. Will you manually load data into the EHR representing the clinical data, including data that is clinically representative of the cases in which medication and documentation errors are occurring?
6. What other alternative could you consider in loading clinical data representative of the conditions related to medication and documentation errors?
7. What challenges do you identify in the data loading strategies?
8. Finally, recommend an executive summary to leadership and a project charter for the implementation of an EHR in your simulation center.

SUMMARY

This chapter has covered the challenges relating to evaluating clinical competencies with use of EHRs. We have covered the need to establish requirements involving HIT within the simulation center and discussed challenges related to adoption, implementation, and evaluation of the EHRs in the simulation centers for training health care professionals. Also covered within the chapter are the QSEN model and teaching strategies, including the emphasis on simulation as one of those teaching strategies.

As mentioned in previous chapters, the Nursing Education Health Informatics (NEHI) model allows for three related constructs to be integrated: point-of-care technology, data analytics, and patient safety/quality for population health (McBride, Tietze, & Fenton, 2013). For the QSEN competencies and in the context of informatics, the NEHI model provides the guiding framework for NEHI data analytics to be applied for EBP while NEHI point-of-care technology can be used to learn case study activities such as telehealth.

We conclude with a discussion of the current state of the science related to evaluating competencies with a case study that includes questions for consideration.

REFERENCES

Aggarwal, R., Mytton, O. T., Derbrew, M., Hananel, D., Heydenburg, M., Issenberg, B., . . . Reznick, R. (2010). Training and simulation for patient safety. *Quality and Safety in Health Care, 19*(Suppl. 2), i34–i43. doi:10.1136/qshc.2009.038562

American Association of Colleges of Nursing. (2008). *The essentials of baccalaureate education for professional nursing practice.* Retrieved from http://www.aacn.nche.edu/education/pdf/baccessentials 08.pdf

American Association of Colleges of Nursing. (2011a). *Quality and safety education for nurses (QSEN).* Retrieved from http://qsen.org/competencies/

American Association of Colleges of Nursing. (2011b). *The essentials of master's education in nursing.* Retrieved from http://www.aacn.nche.edu/education-resources/MastersEssentials11.pdf

Ammenworth, E., Hackl, W. O., Binzer, K., Christofferson, T. E. H., Jensen, S., Lawton, K., . . . Nohr, C. (2012). Simulation studies for the evaluation of health information technologies: Experience and results. *Health Information Management Journal, 41*(2), 14–21.

Anderson, J., Gremy, F., & Pages, J. (1974). *Education in informatics of health care professionals.* New York, NY: Elsevier.

Batalden, P., Leach, D., Swing, S., Dreyfus, H., & Dreyfus, S. (2002). General competencies and accreditation in graduate medical education. *Health Affairs, 21*(5), 103.

Benner, P., Sutphen, M., Leonard, V., & Day, R. (2010). *Educating nurses: A call to radical transformation.* San Francisco: Jossey-Bass.

Brydges, R., Hatala, R., Zendjas, B., Erwin, P., & Cook, D. A. (2015). Linking simulation based educational assessments and patient related outcomes: A systematic review and meta-analysis. *Academic Medicine, 9*(2), 246–256. doi:10-1097/ACM.0000000000000549

Corrigan, J. M., Donaldson, M. S., Kohn, L. T. (Eds.). (2001). *Crossing the quality chasm: A new health system for the 21st century.* Washington, DC: National Academy Press.

Cronenwett, L., Sherwood, G., Barnsteiner, J., Disch, J., Johnson, J., Mitchell, P., . . . Warren, J. (2007). Quality and safety education for nurses. *Nursing Outlook, 55,* 122–131. doi:10.1016/j.outlook.2007 .02.006

Cronenwett, L., Sherwood, G., & Gelmon, S. (2009). Improving quality and safety education: The QSEN learning collaborative. *Nursing Outlook, 57*(6), 304–312.

Denham, C. R., Classen, D. C., Swenson, S. J., Henderson, M. J., Zeltner, T., & Bates, D. W. (2013). Safe use of electronic health records and health information technology systems: Trust but verify. *Journal of Patient Safety, 9*(4), 177–189.

Donahue, B., & Thiede, K. (2008). Innovative strategies for nursing education: Enhancing curriculum with the electronic health record. *Clinical Simulation in Nursing Education, 4*(1), e29–e34. doi:10.1016/ j.ecns.2009.05.053

Fordham, A. J. (1987). Using a competency based approach in nurse education. *Nursing Standard, 19*(31), 41–48.

Friedman, C. P., Wong, A. K., & Blumenthal, D. (2010). Achieving a nationwide learning health system. *Science Translational Medicine, 2*(57), 1–3. Retrieved from http://stm.sciencemag.org/content/2/57/ 57cm29.full-text.pdf+html

Gaba, D. M. (2004). The future vision of simulation in health care [Electronic version]. *Quality and Safety in Health Care, 13*(Supp. 1), i2–i10.

Gardner, C. L., & Jones, S. J. (2012). Utilization of academic electronic health records in undergraduate nursing education. *Online Journal of Nursing Informatics, 16*(2). Retrieved from http://ojni.org/issues/?p=1702

Gassert, C. A. (2008). Technology and informatics competencies. *Nursing Clinics of North America, 43*, 507–521. doi:10.1016/j.cnur.2008.06.005

Greenawalt, J. A. (2014). Documentation in contemporary times: Challenges and successes in teaching. *Clinical Simulation in Nursing, 10*(4), e199–e204. Retrieved from http://dx.doi.org/10.1016/j.ecns.2013.11.008

Hart, J. K., Newton, B. W., & Boone, S. E. (2010). University of Arkansas for Medical Sciences electronic health record and medical informatics training for undergraduate health professionals. *Journal of the Medical Library Association, 98*(3), 212–216. doi:10.3163/1536-5050.98.3.007

Hill, T., McGonigle, D., Hunter, K., Sipes, C., & Hebda, T. (2014). An instrument for assessing advanced nursing informatics competencies. *Journal of Nursing Education and Practice, 4*(7), 104–112. doi:10.5430/jnep.v4n7p104

Hunter, K., McGonigle, D., & Hebda, T. (2013). The integration of informatics content in baccalaureate and graduate nursing education. *Nurse Educator, 38*(2), 110–113. PMID: 23608911. Retrieved from http://dx.doi.org/10.1097/NNE.0b013e31828dc292

Institute of Medicine: Committee on Quality of Healthcare in America. (2001). *Crossing the quality chasm: A new health system for the 21st century*. Washington, DC: National Academies Press.

Institute of Medicine: Committee on Quality of Healthcare in America, Board on Health Care Services. (2003). The Core competencies needed for health care professionals. In A. C. Greiner & E. Knebel (Eds.), *Health professions education: A bridge to quality* (pp. 45–67). Washington, DC: National Academies Press.

Institute of Medicine: Committee on Quality of Health Care in America, Board on Health Care Services. (2011). *Health IT and patient safety: Building safer systems for better care*. Washington, DC: National Academies Press.

Interprofessional Collaborative Expert Panel. (2011). *Core competencies for interprofessional collaborative practice: Report of an expert panel* (No. ICEP-2011). Interprofessional Education Collaborative. Retrieved from https://ipecollaborative.org/uploads/IPEC-Core-Competencies.pdf

Ironside, P., Jeffries, R., & Martin, A. (2009). Fostering patient safety competencies using multiple-patient simulation experiences. *Nursing Outlook, 57*(6), 332–337. doi:10.1016/j.outlook.2009.07.010

Jha, A. K., DesRoches, C. M., Campbell, E. G., Donelan, K., Rao, S. R., Ferris, T. G., . . . Blumenthal, D. (2009). Use of electronic health records in U.S. hospitals. *New England Journal of Medicine, 360*(16), 1628–1638.

Johnson, D. M., & Bushy, T. I. (2011). Integrating the academic electronic health record into the nursing curriculum: Preparing student nurses for practice. *Computers, Informatics, Nursing, 29*(2), 130–137. doi:10.1097/NCN.0b013e318212led8

Jones, S., & Donelle, L. (2011). Assessment of electronic health record usability with undergraduate nursing students. *International Journal of Nursing Education Scholarship, 8*(1). doi:102202/1548-923X.2123

Kowitlawakul, Y., Wang, L., & Chan, S. W. C. (2012). Development of the electronic health records for nursing education (EHRNE) software program. *Nurse Education Today, 33*, 1529–1535.

Lamdman, A. B., Redden, L., Neri, P., Poole, S., Horsky, J., Raja, A. S., . . . Poon, E. G. (2014). Using a medical simulation center as an electronic health record usability laboratory. *Journal of the American Informatics Association, 21*, 558–563. doi:10.1136/amiajnl-2013002233

Lucas, L. (2010). Partnering to enhance the nursing curriculum: Electronic medical record accessibility. *Clinical Simulation in Nursing, 6*, e97–e102. doi:10.1016/j.ecns.2009.07.006

Malloch, K. (2007). The electronic health record: An essential tool for advancing patient safety. *Nursing Outlook, 55*(3), 159–161.

Mantas, J., Ammenwerth, E., Demiris, G., Hasman, A., Haux, H., Hersh, W., . . . IMIA Recommendations on Education Task Force. (2010). Recommendations of the International Medical Informatics Association (IMIA) on education in biomedical and health informatics. *Methods of Information in Medicine, 49*, 105–120.

McBride, S. G., Tietze, M., & Fenton, M. V. (2013). Developing an applied informatics course for a doctor of nursing practice program. *Nurse Educator, 38*(1), 37–42. doi:10.1097/NNE.0b013e3182 76df5d

Milano, C. E., Hardman, J. A., Plesui, A., Rdesinski, R. E., & Biagioli, F. E. (2014). Simulated electronic health record (Sim-EHR) curriculum: Teaching EHR skills and use of the EHR for disease management and prevention. *Academic Medicine, 89*(3), 399–403. doi:10.1097/ACM.0000000000000149

National Council of State Boards of Nursing. (2009). *Report of the Continued Competence Committee.* Retrieved from https://www.ncsbn.org/section_i_2009.pdf

National League for Nursing. (2008). *Preparing the next generation of nurses to practice in a technology-rich environment: An informatics agenda.* New York, NY: Author. Retrieved from http://www.nln.org/docs/default-source/professional-development-programs/preparing-the-next-generation-of-nurses.pdf?sfvrsn=6

O'Donnell, J., Decker, S., Howard, V., Levett-Jones, T., & Miller, C. W. (2014). NLN/Jeffries simulation framework state of the science project: Simulation learning outcomes. *Clinical Simulation in Nursing, 10*(7), 373–382. Retrieved from http://dx.doi.org/10.1016/j.ecns.2014.06.004

QSEN. (2012). *Graduate-level QSEN Competencies: Knowledge, skills and attitudes.* Retrieved from http://www.aacn.nche.edu/faculty/qsen/competencies.pdf

Redman, R. W., Lenburg, C. B., & Walker, P. H. (1999). Competency assessment: Methods for development and implementation in nursing education. *Online Journal of Issues in Nursing, 4*(2), 1–7. Retrieved from http://www.nursingworld.org/MainMenuCategories/ANAMarketplace/ANAPeriodicals/OJIN/TableofContents/Volume41999/No2Sep1999/InitialandContinuingCompetenceinEducationandPracticeCompetencyAssessmentMethodsforDeve.html

Ronald, J. S., & Skiba, D. J. (1987). *Guidelines for basic computer education in nursing.* New York, NY: National League for Nursing.

Rubbelke, C. S., Keenan, S. C., & Haycraft, L. L. (2014). An interactive simulated electronic health record using Google drive. *Computers, Informatics, Nursing, 32*(1), 1–6. doi:10.1097/CIN.000000 0000000043

Sherwood, G., & Drundard, K. (2007). Quality and safety curriculum in nursing education: Matching practice realities. *Nursing Outlook, 55*, 151–155.

Smith, E., Cronenwett, L., & Sherwood, G. (2007). Current assessments of quality and safety education in nursing. *Nursing Outlook, 55*(3), 132–137.

Staggers, N., Gassert, C.A., & Curran, C. (2001). Informatics competencies for nurses at four levels of practice. *Journal of Nursing Education, 40*(7), 303–316.

Staggers, N., Gassert, C. A., & Curran, C. (2002). A Delphi study to determine informatics competencies for nurses at four levels of practice. *Nursing Research, 51*(6), 383–390.

Tilley, D. D. S. (2008). Competency in nursing: A concept analysis. *Journal of Continuing Education in Nursing, 39*(2), 58–66.

Waddell, D. L. (2001). Measurement issues in promoting continued competence. *Journal of Continuing Education in Nursing, 32*(3), 102–106.

Wright, D. (2005). *The ultimate guide to competency assessment in health care* (3rd ed.). Minneapolis, MN: Creative Health Care Management.

SECTION V

New and Emerging Technologies

CHAPTER 24

Genomics and Implications for Health Information Technology

Diane C. Seibert and Susan McBride

OBJECTIVES

1. Describe the expanding field of genomics.

2. List key elements under meaningful use (MU) and the national goals for health information technology (HIT) that may be impacted as information systems expand to include genomics.

3. Discuss implications for patient engagement, patient portals, and ethics related to HIT and genomics.

4. Review relevant national and international resources available to clinicians to support clinical decision making with respect to genetic patient information.

5. Discuss implications for current and future HIT infrastructure, including electronic health records (EHRs), health information exchanges, patient portals, and expansion of data management capacity.

KEY WORDS

genomics, genome wide association studies, HapMap Project, Genetic Information Non-discrimination Act, genomic science, epigenetics, genome, whole genome sequencing

---

CONTENTS

INTRODUCTION

The field of genomics has the potential to profoundly change the way health care is delivered and how health care systems operate. Because genomic health care is heavily dependent on data storage and interpretation, no other area of health care is better suited to electronic information management. *Genomics* is defined by the World Health Organization (WHO) as "the study of genes and their functions and related techniques" (WHO, 2014). Consumer engagement takes on new meaning when the conversation changes from discussing an individual's genome to describing how that information will be collected, stored, accessed, and used by both the engaged consumer and the clinician. We are reaching an era in health care that is often referred to as "the Era of 'Personalized Medicine'" (Masys et al., 2012, p. 419).

This chapter begins with a brief examination of important historical developments of genomic science; reviews some of the unique ethical and clinical challenges that arise when genomics is included in screening, diagnostic, and treatment plans; and introduces some of the information technology (IT) management challenges presented by the sheer size of the data sets required to accommodate genomic and family health history data. It concludes by offering a glimpse of how advanced analytics, clinical decision support (CDS), and patient portals may change clinical practice in the very near future.

BACKGROUND AND HISTORY

Technological and scientific advances in genomic science have opened up tremendous potential in personalized medicine. Consider the following: all people are 99.9% identical in genetic makeup, but differences in the remaining 0.1% hold important clues about health and disease (Centers for Disease Control and Prevention [CDC], 2014). By studying the relationship and interactions among genes, environment, and behaviors (genomic science), researchers and practitioners can learn why two people exposed to the same environmental factors don't always develop the same diseases (CDC, 2014). Personalized genomic information will help drive the shift from interventional to preventive medicine, personalizing treatments based on an individual's specific genetic makeup and his or her reactions at a microcellular level. Personalized genomic material can be used to determine an individual's disease susceptibility and expected responsiveness to medications, as well as to provide targeted interventions and preventive care (Naveed et al., 2014). Genomic advances are thought of as more of an evolution than a revolution. Offit indicates genomic medicine should not be considered a new paradigm, but instead is best viewed as incremental building on decades of scientific advances resulting in an ability to truly personalize medical practice (Offit, 2011).

History of Genetic Discovery

The basic tenets of genetic inheritance have been known since antiquity. Hippocrates and Aristotle both described the transmission of parental traits to offspring, and farmers have been selectively breeding animals for desirable traits and cross-pollinating crops for larger yields for thousands of years, so the idea that parents pass along characteristics to their children is nothing new. Unraveling the biologic mechanisms that direct genomic inheritance, however, has been painfully slow. Although DNA was first isolated in 1869 by Friedrich Miescher (Dahm, 2008), nearly a century would pass before Watson and Crick described the structure of DNA in 1953 (Pabst, Scherubel, & Minnick, 1996), and another half century would tick by before the first draft of the human genome was completed (Collins, Green, Guttmacher, & Guyer, 2003).

The Evolution of Personalized Medicine Through Genomic Advances

Over the past decade, the pace of genomic discoveries has literally exploded. Technological advances and the ability to analyze massive amounts of data on an individual's genetic makeup have driven this explosion. In 10 short years, the price of sequencing a human genome has plummeted from hundreds of millions of dollars to just a few thousand dollars; due to technological advances gene sequencing speed has doubled every 4 months, and it now takes approximately 10 days to sequence a human genome using high-capacity sequencing machines (National Human Genome Research Institute, 2013).

Scientists are now turning their attention to trying to identify what all this genomic data mean. Fifteen years before the human genome was decoded, scientists suggested that if both genomic and health data were obtained from a large number of individuals, the genetic underpinnings of complex disorders, such as hypertension or diabetes, might be unraveled (Dahm, 2008). As soon as the human genome was unveiled in 2003, an international team of geneticists began creating an international genetic map or "Haplotype Map" (HapMap), cataloguing common human genetic variants as they became known (The International HapMap Consortium, 2003, 2013).

HapMap Project

The HapMap contains a description of each gene variant, where each variant is located, and how variants are distributed across and within different populations. The data is then used to conduct genome-wide association studies (GWAS), which examine the associations between gene alterations and common diseases. From the very beginning, GWAS have had two primary goals: (a) identify gene markers that predict disease risk and (b) identify the molecular pathways responsible for the development of disease. Since the first GWAS studies were published in 2005, new molecular pathways have been described for many common diseases, including macular degeneration (a common form of blindness in older adults), type 2 diabetes, Parkinson's disease, heart disorders, obesity, Crohn's disease, and prostate cancer, and variations in antidepressant medication response.

Genomic advances proceeded at a glacial pace until the mid-1900s, gradually accelerating in the 1980s and 1990s, and then erupted onto the health care and media stage at the dawn of the 21st century. Prior to what is now called the genomic era, genomic health care was the exclusive domain of a small, committed group of genetic specialists who delivered care to an equally small community of individuals with rare single-gene disorders. Outside the confines of these genomic specialty practices, few clinicians were taught anything about genomics in their basic science or clinical specialty courses, and unless they had patients in their practice with genetic disorders (sickle cell disease, cystic fibrosis, or hemophilia), fewer still considered genetics to be relevant to their practice. Advances in genomic sequencing, the HapMap project, GWAS, pharmacogenomics (branch of pharmacology using DNA to inform drug development and testing; National Library of Medicine, 2014), and the efforts of health care organizations have all converged to make genomic information and testing more relevant and more accepted at the point of care.

CONSUMER ENGAGEMENT AND THE ERA OF PERSONALIZED MEDICINE

Tobol, in his recent text *The Patient Will See You Now*, predicts that genomics will forever reshape the practice of medicine, comparing the use of personalized genomic information to the use of Google maps for directions in the form of the geographical information system (GIS). He indicates that having your genomic information is like having multiple superimposed and integrated layers of your own GIS map, which can be used by health care providers to make decisions about your medical care. Additionally, individuals can use their personal GIS map to address risks associated with diseases for which they may be predisposed because of genetic makeup (Topol, 2015).

Genetic Testing

Genetic testing is a method for using a laboratory test to identify genetic variations associated with disease, and includes analysis for DNA, ribonucleic acid (RNA), or protein. Genetic testing can be used to confirm or rule out disease, as well as to determine the probability that an individual might develop a disease. Initial genetic tests were for screening for inherited chromosomal disorders such as cystic fibrosis. More recently, however, as genomic science has expanded, providers can identify risk for diseases such as heart disease and cancer. There are different types of testing, including diagnostic testing, predictive and presymptomatic genetic tests, carrier testing, prenatal testing, newborn screening (NBS), pharmacogenetics, and research genetic testing (National Human Genome Research Institute, 2015).

Direct-to-Consumer Testing

Once genomics became "actionable" in even small ways, consumers began pushing just as hard as researchers in an effort to learn more about their personal risks, while advancing genomic science. Within 3 years of the completion of the human genome, several direct-to-consumer (DTC) companies began marketing genetic tests directly to consumers via the Internet, television advertisements, or other marketing venues without involving health care professionals at all. Nearly simultaneously, after a 10-year effort to get the law through Congress, the Genetic Information Nondiscrimination Act (GINA) was passed and signed into law by President George W. Bush in 2008, and all aspects of the law were in effect as of November 2009. GINA was created to remove barriers to the appropriate use of genetic services by the public, while protecting individuals from misuse of genetic information in health insurance and employment (Roberts, 2010). Although there are still some significant regulatory loopholes (GINA does not cover life insurance, long-term care insurance, or disability insurance), the provision of some legal protection against genetic discrimination offered sufficient security for many people to feel comfortable enough to purchase DTC testing kits and learn more about their personal genetic code.

Important Historical Pharmaceutical Regulatory Developments

Marketing medical products (pharmaceutical agents, devices or laboratory tests) directly to consumers is an ancient practice, with door-to-door salesmen hawking medications and medical "miracle drugs" that were just as likely to cause injury as they were to cure anything. This began to change in the 19th century as advances in medical research improved knowledge of disease processes, which led to better therapies and improved outcomes. The United States Pharmacopoeia was established in 1820 to "set standards for the identity, strength, quality, and purity of medicines, food ingredients, and dietary supplements" (U.S. Pharmacopeia, 2014); and ethical drug companies only marketed and sold standardized drugs to medical professionals in keeping with the American Medical Association's (AMA) Code of Ethics, first published in 1847. Regulation of medical devices and pharmaceutical agents was initially voluntary, but in 1906 the Food and Drug Administration (FDA) was created, giving a federal agency the authority to ensure that drug labeling accurately reflected drug strength, quality, and purity. Within a decade, the passing of the Sherley Amendment and creation of the Federal Trade Commission (FTC) prohibited fraudulent therapeutic claims and restricted the marketing of therapeutic products to physicians (Greene & Herzberg, 2010). These restrictions did not completely eliminate the marketing and sale of drugs to consumers, as evidenced by the large and profitable over-the-counter (OTC) drug market. By the end of World War II, DTC advertising of OTC products was common, but still reinforced the importance of involving a physician when selecting and using a pharmaceutical agent. With the ability to create synthetic drugs, thousands of new, powerful, and effective drug products began appearing and advertisements for brand-name prescription were being marketed in consumer magazines, although always with the caveat that a physician should be involved in the decision. Over the next three decades, drug companies continued to push for permission to market directly to consumers and, in 1999, the FDA issued guidance on DTC advertising, permitting it as long as it included a discussion of the risks and benefits, and included a contact information for consumers if they wanted more information on the drug (Greene & Herzberg, 2010). All of these legislative actions and decisions led up to the current controversy over DTC genetic tests.

Since the first company began offering DTC genomic testing in April of 2008, there has been controversy over whether or not the FDA should, or can, regulate DTC genetic tests (Geels, 2007). On November 22, 2013, it became clear that the FDA does believe it can and should regulate DTC genetic tests, when it sent a letter to 23andMe, one of the biotech companies still marketing genetic testing kits to consumers, to stop marketing its "Saliva Collection Kit and Personal Genome Service" (PGS) because the spit collection tube was an unapproved medical device (Geels, 2007). In its letter, the FDA stated it was "concerned about the public health consequences of inaccurate results from the PGS device; the main purpose of compliance with FDA's regulatory requirements is to ensure that the tests work." The FDA provided examples, such as the reporting of drug metabo-lism gene variants, that could have potentially serious health implications if the test was wrong, or if patients (and providers) misinterpreted the data (U.S. Food and Drug Adminis-tration, 2013). At the time this chapter was written, 23andMe was continuing to market and sell test kits, but had stopped reporting health data to new customers, reporting only less controversial ancestry data. An excellent article by Pascal Su in the September 2013 edition of *Yale Journal of Biological Medicine* (Su, 2013) describes some of the key issues in DTC genetic testing. Consumers have become increasingly interested in DTC genetic tests because the prices have plummeted, testing is noninvasive—requiring only saliva or a cheek swab, and because results are returned via the Internet, thus increasing accessibility, convenience, and privacy. People are usually interested in DTC genetic tests for one of three reasons: (a) they are curious about their genetic makeup, (b) they are concerned about their risk for developing familial diseases (providers are often interested in this as well), or (c) because they want to learn more about their ancestry.

Risks and Benefits of DTC Genetic Testing

There are some theoretical benefits to DTC genetic testing, including empowering indi-viduals to adopt more healthy behaviors and to increase awareness of genomics among the general public. However, there are also some significant downsides to DTC genetic testing with the most obvious being increased health care costs associated with confir-matory tests, or additional screening requirements after testing. Other concerns include uncertainty regarding the clinical value of these tests when genotype-specific therapy is not yet available. Genomic testing may also aggravate health care inequity, and carries the emotional cost of confirming the presence of a deleterious mutation. Finally, genes are shared among family members, some of whom may be interested in the information, whereas other family members may not want to know (Su, 2013).

IMPLICATIONS FOR NATIONAL HEALTH CARE PLAN AND NATIONAL HEALTH INFORMATION TECHNOLOGY

Although computing power has expanded rapidly since the 1950s, doubling every 18 months or so (Guyatt & Drummond, 2002), computing power is slowly falling behind, and new IT strategies are needed. Collectively, over 2,000 DNA sequencing instruments around the globe sequence over 15 quadrillion nucleotides a year, generating *15 petabytes* of data. As the cost declines, the demand for genetic information will continue to increase, driving an increase in the number of sequencing instruments, and attendant data storage

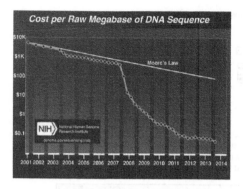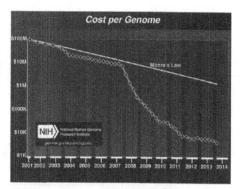

FIGURE 24.1. Declining costs of sequencing the human genome.
Source: Wetterstrand (2014).

areas needed throughout the country. Figure 24.1 reflects the diminishing cost of mapping the human genome, which is now increasing the potential for the availability of these data within the clinical practices to support diagnostic and patient care treatment decisions. Yet, electronic health records (EHRs) and regional health information exchanges (HIEs) must have the capacity to manage these data.

Data Complexity

The complexity of these data and information management will challenge the health care industry's ability to efficiently and effectively use genomic data at the point of care. Figure 24.2 depicts both the size and complexity of the data contained in one human genome. Starting at the chromosome level of microns (millionths of a meter), the authors selected Chromosome 21, showing the approximate location of the APP gene (amyloid beta precursor protein), which has been suspected of regulating the amyloid plaques that are implicated in Alzheimer's disease (DNA Learning Center, 2014). This visual provides an example of the incredible complexity and size of patient-level genomic data. In addition, science and clinical evidence in this area are evolving so rapidly and technology infrastructure must be updated with the ability to accommodate rapid updates. For example, there is evidence that over time and with age, an individual's DNA may evolve, so the technology must be capable of updating massive amounts of patient-level genomic data as well (Geigl et al., 2004).

"Certified" EHRs

As discussed in Chapters 1 and 4, MU involves three stages defined under the HITECH Act, with regulatory requirements determining what constitutes each stage of MU. In January 2013, the National Health Information Technology Policy Committee outlined priorities to be included in stage 4 MU. Tang (vice chair of the committee) stated, "It [stage 4] will involve the triad of population health, decision support, and quality measurement, including dashboards and registries." The committee outlined three priorities: (a) optimization of the current EHRs, (b) better interoperability with HIE, and (c) consumerism in health care (Sittig & Singh, 2010).

Chromosomes

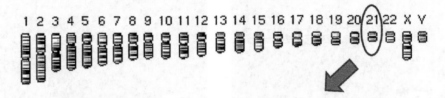

Chromosome 21 - Level of Zoom: Approximately 4 Microns (Four Millionths of a Meter)
Zoomed Out to Entire Chromosome 21, showing approximate location of the APP Gene.
(amyloid beta precursor) abnormalities associated with amyloid plaques of Alzheimer's Disease

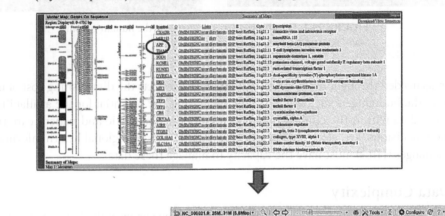

APP Gene Zoomed In to Nanometer Scale
(Billionths of a Meter).
Showing approximate 7 nanometer (seven
billionths of a meter) base pair helix range
of APP Gene on Chromosome 21.

FIGURE 24.2. National Center for Biotechnology Information depiction of Chromosome 21 with
Alzheimer's gene marker.
Source: NCBI (2014).

These three areas have tremendous implication for genomic information. To optimize
EHRs and improve health outcomes, clinicians need to have rapid, easy access to information relevant to that patient's care, including access to his or her genomic information
and family health history. Yet, current EHRs and structures established under the meaningful use requirement have a long way to go if EHR technology platforms and software
are to be capable of capturing and effectively presenting these types of data. The second
priority relating to better interoperability has implications for how much data will be
transmitted about the individual health care consumer from one clinician to another.
Patient engagement is another important consideration within the third priority.

Biorepositories

A biorepository, also called a biobank or a genebank, is a collection of biologic specimens containing genetic material gathered from living organisms (human, animal, plant, microbiological, etc.). The purpose of a biorepository is to collect, process, store, and distribute stored biologic specimens to support clinical care or scientific research. One of the earliest and perhaps the most familiar biorepository is the blood bank, but several other types of biobanks exist. Tissue banks store biologic materials, such as corneas, bone, and skin, to be used in transplant surgeries, pathologists store tissue samples removed during surgical procedures, and newborn blood specimens are stored for at least a year in all states, but may be stored indefinitely in some states. The number of biorepositories has continued to grow, as has the number of specimens contained in them. The National Institutes of Health (NIH), the Centers for Disease Control and Prevention (CDC), and the Department of Defense (DoD) all maintain large biorepositories, as do several universities and some privately held companies.

The effective use of biorepositories at the point of care is highly dependent on robust, reliable information systems. Powerful computers with large storage capacities are required to store the data, and advanced statistical and computational software is needed to classify and later rapidly retrieve appropriate information. When electronic patient records can be linked to an individual's genomic data, and genomic information becomes a routine part of health care, the promise of truly "personalized" health care will have arrived.

Genes, as well as disease risk, are shared among family members, so health records containing detailed genomic, personal, and clinical information about one family member will very likely reveal health risks for other family members. Policies need to be developed to help health care providers and systems better manage the myriad ethical, legal, and social issues that arise when genomic information is shared among related individuals. Providers will need computer-driven decision support tools to help them effectively and efficiently use this genomic information, and data must be displayed so that they can quickly be interpreted at the point of care. New electronic interfaces (a new EHR system) may be needed to effectively link genomic, clinical, and personal information in a meaningful way (Groen, Mahootian, & Goldstein, 2008).

Biorepositories also trigger decisions regarding whether or not the stored information can (or should) be used for purposes other than the original intent. For example, can residual blood spots from NBS tests be used by researchers interested in learning more about the prevalence of type 2 diabetes genes in a particular population? Biorepositories can advance genomic research in profound and powerful ways, but their use by researchers is a hotly debated topic among ethicists, clinicians, researchers, and the general public because most of the genetic "donors" have not been informed about how their biologic data are going to be used, nor have they provided informed consent for their samples to be used in research. Although EHRs hold great promise to improve health care quality, cost, and safety, the national debate is likely to be controversial, because previously de-identified genomic data can be linked to individuals and their family members.

One key advantage of associating individuals with their genetic code is the possibility of linking phenotype (e.g., the number of dental caries) with genotype (e.g., genes associated with tooth enamel), which helps advance science (and health care) for every human being. Data are continually evolving as well, so as time goes on, the genes involved in aging, for example, will become better understood, offering new therapeutic options for numerous conditions (e.g., osteoporosis, cardiovascular disease, hair loss) associated with aging. For example, data could be sorted to examine the correlation between genotype and phenotype in people with specific diseases or medication exposures. This aggregation of data can support research on a previously unimaginable scale at a very low cost because the data would all be contained within the EHR. However, many barriers to conducting this kind of research need to be addressed before this dream becomes a reality. Some of the barriers are clinical as well as technical, including the development of phenotype algorithms and data repositories capable of managing enormous volumes of data, and ability to exchange the data via HIEs. Addressing these barriers will be critical if these data are to be available and to secure critical financial, logistical, and community support (Denny, 2012). Additional barriers include appropriate storage and access to the data within the EHR.

Desired Characteristics for the Integration of Genomic Data Into the EHR

Masys et al. (2012) recommend that genomic data be integrated into the EHR and describe both the desired characteristics and current challenges posed by these recommendations given the current state of technology, workflow processes, and current resources. These recommended characteristics and implications for clinical use in EHRs include the following:

- Ability to separate clinical interpretation of primary molecular patient information
- Data compression techniques that prevent data loss
- Linkage of laboratory data to molecular information
- Response times of EHRs that are capable of displaying clinically actionable patterns or subsets of information at the point of care
- Ability to support human-viewable and machine-readable formats along with the most up-to-date genomic and epigenetic science to facilitate CDS
- Ability to store multiple genome-scale data sets over an individual's lifetime to address the changing state resulting from the normal phenomenon of aging impacting structural changes at cellular levels
- Ability to support research in genomic discovery using data within the EHR for secondary data analysis (Masys et al., 2012)

Although forward momentum is being made to incorporate genomics into EHRs, additional standards work and flexibility are required and are emphasized by Masys and colleagues, including compression and decompression requirements to maintain data integrity, and a more robust ability to update information over time.

In addition to these recommendations another consideration is the effective archive and display of family health history data within the EHR. In the family health history section of the 2014 Test Procedure for Certified EHRs, there are requirements for EHRs to include the ability to manage these types of data (Office of the National Coordinator of Health Information Technology, 2012).

EHRs operating under EHR certification standards with these requirements must have the capacity to capture the history of individual family members, but experts are still uncertain as to whether the standards are robust enough, particularly as they relate to managing the complexity of these data over time as the individual ages and science progresses (Masys et al., 2012).

Clinical Decision Support

Although clinical decision support strategies (CDSS) are ideally suited to genomics because a single genome contains hundreds of thousands of data points, interpretation requires high throughput computing power, and the most effective information emerges when individual data are compared to population data. Much more advanced data management and advanced analytics will be needed to detect patterns and trends and trigger the right rules given the sheer volume of data that needs to be analyzed. Ability to support CDS is one of the seven characteristics called for in the desiderata for genomics data in the EHR under recommendation #5, but will be challenging because of sheer data volume, and requirements to be both human- and machine-readable to present data in a way that is understandable to both (Masys et al., 2012). Despite the development challenges, genomic CDSS tools could be incredibly powerful at the point of care to prompt appropriate personalized treatment protocols based on genetic makeup of individuals. Yet, these tools are likely to appear different to the end user and operate very differently from our current CDS.

IMPLICATIONS FOR PUBLIC HEALTH: NBS

NBS programs, some of the oldest and most effective public health screening programs in the United States, have been credited with saving thousands of lives by identifying selected genetic, endocrine, and metabolic disorders that can be treated if they are identified early in life. NBS programs began in 1959 when Dr. Robert Guthrie developed a new laboratory technique, a bacterial inhibition assay (BIA), which made it possible to detect abnormally high phenylalanine levels in neonatal serum within 3 days of birth. This technological advancement was a significant improvement over the existing "wet diaper" test, which was unreliable until about 8 weeks of life, often after irreversible brain damage had already occurred (Harrison & Lyerla, 2012). The ability to identify infants with phenylketonuria (PKU) early enough to prevent brain damage generated a great deal of excitement in both the professional and lay communities. Within 2 years, every infant born in Massachusetts was being screened for PKU; by 1975, 43 states had enacted NBS laws and, by 1990, every infant born in the United States was screened for at least four disorders (PKU, congenital adrenal hyperplasia, congenital hypothyroidism, and galactosemia). The scope of NBS has steadily expanded, and most infants are now being screened for disorders that can cause disability, premature death, infectious diseases, and hearing and cardiovascular disorders. It is important to recognize that NBS is still organized and administered at the state level, and although there is much more uniformity now than there was a decade ago, each state independently determines what numbers and types of NBS tests they will offer and whether or not obtaining informed consent from parents is required. Although parental informed consent is typically required before children can be treated or included in research studies, the mandatory nature of NBS is (and always has been) controversial. The mandatory nature of NBS is based on the belief established in the 1960s that the benefits (to the child, the family, and to society) of universal early diagnosis and treatment outweighed the requirement to obtain parental informed consent.

A number of technological advances have been developed since BIA was introduced, all of which have increased the sensitivity, specificity, and scope of NBS services. The basic concept of evaluating serum analyte levels (proteins, enzymes) against predetermined cutoff values is still being used to evaluate each sample, and DNA is more and more commonly being used to evaluate abnormal NBS results ("second tier evaluation") because the genotype can confirm a suspected diagnosis, inform the prognosis, and guide treatment. Over the past decade, as gene sequencing technology has rapidly become faster, less expensive (see Figure 24.1), and more accurate, advocates have proposed that DNA-based screening replace current NBS technology because whole genome sequencing (WGS) could improve the early detection of many more disorders, helping more individuals and families. Opponents argue that WGS raises significant ethical, legal, and societal concerns that have to be addressed before moving to population screening using WGS (see case study; Knoppers, Sénécal, Borry, & Avard, 2014).

The impact of WGS on health care information systems will likely be profound. One individual's fully *sequenced* genome requires approximately 100 gigabyte of storage space, but a fully *analyzed* genome could require as much as 1 terabyte of storage space. This is emphasized in Figure 24.2, noted earlier in the chapter. Consider the visual and size of these data for one individual, multiplied by the number of individuals in a health care system. Just storing the raw data may be costprohibitive. If the information is to be useful, the data must be maintained, updated, compressed, decompressed, and presented in such a way that clinicians can rapidly access the information they need and have confidence that it is accurately presented.

BENEFITS AND CHALLENGES OF GENOMIC RESOURCES

Numerous genomic resources have been developed over the past two decades (Table 24.1), the majority of which were developed to improve access to reliable genomic information and/or improve general genomic knowledge among clinicians. In a rapidly evolving science like genomics, staying abreast of emerging information and maintaining accuracy of web-based content is a significant and ongoing challenge, and studies have shown that even well-respected, heavily used resources may contain inaccurate and/or incomplete genomic information (Levy, LoPresti, & Seibert, 2008). To compound the problem, many genomic resources are "information dense," requiring clinicians to have at least a working knowledge of genomics to fully understand the content and adequate *time* to locate, read, and absorb the information before acting (ordering a genetic or diagnostic test, selecting a particular therapy, etc.). Although most providers are now much more comfortable turning to electronic resources for information (Clarke et al., 2013), most are unwilling to

TABLE 24.1 Electronic Resources Available to Clinicians

Resource	Purpose	Weblink
Online Mendelian Inheritance in Man (OMIM)	A compendium of human genetic conditions with a searchable database.	www.ncbi.nlm.nih.gov/omim
GeneReviews	Expert-authored disease reviews, including comprehensively developed resources for medical genetics information for physicians, genetic counselors, other health care providers, and researchers.	www.genetests.org
Genetics Home Reference	A health care consumer guide to genetic information not intended for use by health care professionals other than as an educational tool for patients.	http://ghr.nlm.nih.gov
National Newborn Screening and Global Resource Center	An independent U.S. resource center for information relevant to NBS tests and genetics activities nationwide.	http://genes-r-us.uthscsa.edu/
23andMe	A health care consumer website for genetic information on ancestry.	https://www.23andme.com
The Animated Genome	What may be the largest collaboration to date between the NIH and the Smithsonian Institution, "Genome: Unlocking Life's Code" recognizes the accomplishments of the past, showcases the future, and highlights the increasing relevance of genomics in people's lives. This website offers you the opportunity to explore and learn more about the exhibit if you can't physically visit the high-tech museum exhibit in person.	http://unlockinglifescode.org/media/animations/659
The Genetic Testing Registry	The Genetic Testing Registry (GTR) provides a central location for voluntary submission of genetic test information by providers. The scope includes the test's purpose, methodology, validity, evidence of the test's usefulness, and laboratory contacts and credentials. The overarching goal of the GTR is to advance the public health and research into the genetic basis of health and disease.	www.ncbi.nlm.nih.gov/gtr

(continued)

TABLE 24.1 Electronic Resources Available to Clinicians (*continued*)

Resource	Purpose	Weblink
Why Women Are Stripey	Excellent YouTube video discussing epigenetics and X chromosome inactivation.	https://www.youtube.com/watch?v=BD6h-wDj7bw
Essential Genetic and Genomic Competencies for Nurses with Graduate Degrees	The primary purpose of this document is to identify essential genetic and genomic competencies for individuals prepared at the graduate level in nursing.	www.genome.gov/Pages/Health/HealthCareProvidersInfo/Grad_Gen_Comp.pdf
Essentials of Genetic and Genomic Nursing: Competencies, Curricula Guidelines, and Outcome Indicators, 2nd Edition	This text establishes the minimum basis for preparing the nursing workforce to deliver competent genetic and genomic-focused nursing care.	www.genome.gov/pages/careers/healthprofessionaleducation/geneticscompetency.pdf
Genetics/Genomics Competency Center	Provides high-quality educational resources for group instruction or self-directed learning in genetics/genomics by health care educators and practitioners.	www.g-2-c-2.org
Global Genetics and Genomics Community	A bilingual collection of unfolding case studies for use with students and practicing health care providers learning basic genetic/genomic concepts.	www.g-3-c.org/en
Orphanet	A reference portal for information on rare diseases and orphan drugs, intended for all audiences. Orphanet's aim is to help improve the diagnosis, care, and treatment of patients with rare diseases.	www.orpha.net/consor/cgi-bin/index.php?lng=EN

Name	Description	URL
Genetics in Primary Care Institute	Organization focused on increasing primary care provider (PCP) knowledge and skills in providing genetic-based services.	www.geneticsinprimarycare.org/Pages/default.aspx
Genetic Alliance	Brings together diverse stakeholders to create novel partnership in advocacy while integrating individual, family, and community perspectives to improve health systems. Goal is to revolutionize access to information to enable translation of research into services and individualized decision making.	https://www.youtube.com/user/geneticalliance/featured
Baby's First Test	Baby's First Test website houses the nation's newborn screening clearinghouse. The clearinghouse provides current educational and family support and services information, materials, and resources about NBS at the local, state, and national levels and serves as the clearinghouse for NBS information. This resource is dedicated to educating parents, family members, health professionals, industry representatives, and other members of the public about the NBS system. This site also provides many ways for people to connect and share their viewpoints and questions about the NBS system.	www.babysfirsttest.org
Neonatal eHandbook	The Neonatal eHandbook provides a structured approach to the clinical management of conditions regularly encountered by health professionals caring for newborns.	www.health.vic.gov.au/neonatalhandbook
Genes in Life	A site where the lay public can learn how genetics affects individuals and their families, why people should talk to health care providers about genetics, how to get involved in genetics research, and more.	www.genesinlife.org

NBS, newborn screening.

spend more than 2 to 3 minutes searching for information when they are with a patient (Drucker, 1971). If any CDSS resource is to be useful at the point of care, it must be available (preferably open access), easy to use, and return information rapidly. Genomic decision support tools are particularly challenging to develop and maintain because genetic information is emerging, and changing, constantly. The implications for clinical practice are potentially very powerful. One of the most effective ways to connect genomics to care might be to develop EHRs with capabilities to integrate family health history, personal medical and laboratory data, genomic data (if WGS has been done), and data entered at a particular visit (symptoms, physical exam findings, etc.), with the outcome of suggesting the provided, associated possible genetic risks.

ETHICAL CONSIDERATIONS

Ethical issues are perhaps as significant as the technical challenges of managing the information generated by the human genome (Badzek, Henaghan, Turner, & Monsen, 2013). The explosion of information emerging from the mapping of the human genome has presented significant challenges for law, bioethics, and biopolitical arenas, and much remains to be done in the legislative arena, particularly with respect to the bioethical promises of health care professionals to protect and balance autonomy, justice, and beneficence for patients and their families (Badzek et al., 2013).

Bridging family history information and personal genomic information among family members' EHRs raises serious legal and ethical questions about the patient–provider relationship. Consider the following: Patients have a contractual relationship with a particular provider for care (Buppert, 2012), and the patient's chart is considered a legal record of communication and activity among the provider, patient, and health care system with obligations to protect the personal health information of the patient (American Health Information Management Association [AHIMA], 2011). When EHRs are linked by genomic data, the individual's rights to privacy could potentially be nullified when a clinician with whom there is no direct relationship accesses and evaluates shared genomic information on behalf of a family member. How will patients be able to reveal their genomic information to their caregivers, and be assured there are firewalls between their information and their family members with whom the provider has no direct relationship?

Ethical considerations pose complex issues related to individual's autonomy and the capture, storage, and use of personal genomic information. The principle of autonomy supports an individual's right to choose whether or not to use DTC genomic information. Yet, in November 2013, the FDA officially denied access to the health information section on 23andMe's website to the consumer, stating they had concerns about the safety and efficacy of this genomic information. The principles of beneficence "promoting the well-being of others and non-maleficence" or "first do no harm" are relevant to the FDA's actions. Yet, 23andMe and their founders questioned the justice of the FDA's decision to suspend the health information aspect of their service to the consumer. This is only one example of some of the many ethical issues that have arisen and will continue to arise as genomics becomes fully integrated into health care systems. Many unanswered questions remain regarding genomic information. Genomic data could potentially replace all other medical and biological concepts of human identity. Many of the most challenging issues remain to be worked out, and it is unclear whether all the issues have even been identified. When and how will individuals be informed about their individual risks, based on genomic information? For example, should parents be told that their child is at slightly increased risk for an adult-onset disorder like macular degeneration at the 2-week newborn visit? Many examples of these issues exist, but for the purposes of this chapter, perhaps the most pressing concern is the safety of genomic information. Genomic information is the most detailed human "identity map in existence, its theft would constitute the most profound kind of identity theft possible" (Groen et al., 2008). So, once this genomic data is collected, stored, and linked in an EHR to an individual, are sufficient protections in place to safeguard them? Information privacy and security should be the most pressing concern for HIT professionals managing EHR systems containing genomic information on patients (Groen et al., 2008).

CASE STUDY

"Where Genomics and Clinical Care Intersect"

The case study reflects how the developments in WGS may impact the future of NBS and the potential for this expanded use of these data to inform care of the newborn. This case also amplifies many of the issues discussed in this chapter, including ethical, legal, and logistical challenges. Consider the following case study:

Sophia, a beautiful baby with bright eyes and a lusty cry, was born at 7:30 on a Thursday morning. Within a few minutes she was vigorously nursing, and by 10 a.m. was sleeping quietly in an open crib beside her mother's bed. Although Sophia appeared healthy, she had inherited a genetic disorder that might kill her in early childhood.

The Process in 2014

If Sophia was born in a state that tested for the selected genetic disorder on their NBS panel the following steps would most likely occur:

a. Just before discharge, a nurse would prick Sophia's foot with a lancet and send a small amount of her blood to the lab for testing. In almost all states this testing would be done without parental consent ("presumed consent").

b. A laboratory test (most likely tandem mass spectrometry) would be used to screen Sophia's blood for approximately 29 specific genetic disorders.

c. If one of her serum analytes was abnormal, a "2nd tier" test would be conducted to confirm the initial finding.

d. If positive, Sophia's provider and parents would be notified, educated about the condition, and a management plan would be developed to guide Sophia's treatment.

(continued)

CASE STUDY (*continued*)

If Sophia was born in a state that did not include that selected genetic disorder on their NBS panel or if she had a genetic disorder that was not one of the disorders included on any state NBS panel, Sophia's condition would remain undiagnosed until symptoms manifested.

Consider a Scenario in Which WGS Replaced the Current NBS Process

If Sophia were born in a state where WGS had replaced the technologies currently used in NBS, the following series of events might take place:

a. Just before discharge, a nurse would collect blood from Sophia's foot using a lancet, or cells from Sophia's cheek using a buccal swab, and send to the lab for testing.
b. The state NBS lab would use a WGS technology (some of the technologies currently available include nanopore, fluorophore, nanoball and pyrosequencing), to generate a complete genome sequence.
c. The laboratory could then conduct a limited analysis of Sophia's WGS data to determine whether she had acquired any disorder that needed to be identified and treated immediately (i.e., in infancy). Although WGS may not completely eliminate "2nd tier" testing, it would likely reduce it significantly.
d. Once the NBS lab had completed its analysis of a limited set of disorders, her raw data would be transferred to her health care plan. Her genomic health information would be uploaded into her EHR.

This is where many of the ethical, legal, and societal challenges with WGS really begin to emerge. Assuming Sophia's genome reveals information about health risks that manifest in adulthood, some of the key issues include:

a. Should consent be required for screening that doesn't stand to directly benefit the infant during childhood?
b. Who should be told about health care conditions that will not emerge in childhood?
c. When should information about an adult-onset health care condition be provided?
d. How much should be revealed at one time?
e. What health care professional is best positioned to discuss all the health risks that might be revealed in Sophia's genome?
f. What education will health professionals need to prepare them to handle the data and the subsequent questions?
g. What kind of education do parents need to understand genomic results?
h. Who ensures that Sophia and her family are kept informed as understanding of what genes and associated risks evolve?
i. What is the impact of "false positive" reports?

(*continued*)

CASE STUDY (*continued*)

> j. What nonhealth care risk information should be disclosed (i.e., non-paternity)?
>
> k. Should speculative (nonvalidated or poorly predictive) results be disclosed?
>
> l. Genes are shared among family members and although an infant's genomic data may help some family members (i.e., can help to inform Sophia's parent's plan for future pregnancies), it may reveal information about other family members that they may not want to know. How will this information be protected?
>
> m. What impact could WGS have on health care systems?
>
> 1. How will information systems handle the massive amount of raw data?
>
> 2. How will the information systems display genomic information to providers? What will the graphic user interface (GUI) look like?
>
> 3. Who will ensure that the interpretation (analysis) of genomic information contained in health care system databases is both accurate and continually updated?
>
> 4. How will health care systems handle the inevitable "false positive" results?
>
> 5. How long should raw data be stored? Should it be stored in the patient's file and, if so, under what conditions?
>
> 6. Should genomic information collected for health care purposes be released to legal authorities investigating criminal activity?
>
> n. Who does the data belong to: the state, the insurance company, or the individual?

SUMMARY

To conclude, we have defined and discussed genomic and epigenetic issues that present themselves to clinicians in the informatics age. We have also discussed the history of the mapping of the genome and evaluation of the science. Implications for clinicians have been highlighted in the given case study describing two separate scenarios with implications for both public health and clinical care to neonatal care. These scenarios demonstrate how genomics and personalized medicine raise significant clinical implications but also change how we manage data within the EHR, our public health system, and repositories that support both. Desirable characteristics for the EHR to shift and change to accommodate the age of genomics and epigenetics are outlined, and challenges discussed. Finally, we have highlighted the ethical issues surrounding genomics and epigenetics, demonstrating the power of the information, coupled with the responsibility for the management and use of this information.

EXERCISES AND QUESTIONS FOR CONSIDERATION

Consider content covered with respect to genomics, EHRs, the current versus future state of HIT needed, and the resultant ethical challenges and consider the following questions:

1. How do you envision that genomics and personalized medicine will change the landscape of health care? Consider the roles of the clinician, nursing informatics,

HIT professionals, and the entire interprofessional team. Outline roles and considerations for the shifts in health care delivery caused by genomics and personalized medicine.

2. Genomics and personalized medicine present numerous issues with respect to bioethical considerations. Consider the role of the FDA described in this chapter and their authority to regulate the direct sales to the consumer market, as well as the right as a consumer to have your DNA information available to you to make informed decisions about your health. Place yourself in the role of the FDA with respect to direct sales to consumer markets and consider this vantage point to protect the consumer. Now, consider you are an individual with a known familial risk for either breast cancer or colon cancer and you want to know what your personal risk is for developing the disease, yet the company you requested the information from has just been stopped from distributing that information by the FDA.

3. Consider the complexity of the technical issues related to managing and utilizing genomic data discussed in the chapter and the desirable characteristics of an EHR to fully utilize genomic information for patients (see the section "Desired Characteristics for the Integration of Genomic Data Into the EHR" in this chapter). Select one or more of the challenges and consider the aspects of the current EHR you utilize in your clinical practice setting. What would need to change in order for your EHR to meet one or more of the criteria discussed in this chapter, with respect to desirable characteristics of an EHR? Finally, how will your EHR, and how will your processing of patients, change with respect to workflow?

REFERENCES

American Health Information Management Association. (2011, February). Fundamentals of the legal health record and designated record set. *Journal of AHIMA, 82*(2). Retrieved from http://library.ahima.org/xpedio/groups/public/documents/ahima/bok1_048604.hcsp?dDocName=bok1_048604

Badzek, L., Henaghan, M., Turner, M., & Monsen, R. (2013). Ethical, legal, and social issues in the translation of genomics into health care. *Journal of Nursing Scholarship, 45*(1), 15–24. doi:10.1111/jnu.12000

Buppert, C. (2012). *Nurse practitioner's business practice and legal guide* (4th ed.). Boston, MA: Jones & Barlett Learning.

Centers for Disease Control and Prevention. (2014). *Public health genomics*. Retrieved from http://www.cdc.gov/genomics

Clarke, M. A., Belden, J. L., Koopman, R. J., Steege, L. M., Moore, J. L., Canfield, S. M., & Kim, M. S. (2013). Information needs and information-seeking behaviour analysis of primary care physicians and nurses: A literature review. *Health Information and Library Journal, 30*(3), 178–190. doi:10.1111/hir.12036

Collins, F. S., Green, E. D., Guttmacher, A. E., & Guyer, M. S. (2003). A vision for the future of genomics research. *Nature, 422*(6934), 835–847. doi:10.1038/nature01626

Dahm, R. (2008). The first discovery of DNA. *American Scientist, 96*(4), 320. doi:10.1511/2008.73.3846

Denny, J. C. (2012). Mining electronic health records in the genomics era. *PLoS Computational Biology, 8*(12), 2014-e1002823. doi:10.1371/journal.pcbi.1002823

DNA Learning Center. (2014). *Genes to cognition online*. Retrieved from http://www.dnalc.org/view/1448-APP-Gene.html

Drucker, P. F. (1971). What we can learn from Japanese management. *Harvard Business Review*, *49*(2), 110–122.

Geels, F. W. (2007). Feelings of discontent and the promise of middle range theory for STS: Examples from technology dynamics. *Science, Technology & Human Values*, *32*(6), 627–651. doi:10.1177/0162243907303597

Geigl, J. B., Langer, S., Barwisch, S., Pfleghaar, K., Lederer, G., & Speicher, M. R. (2004). Analysis of gene expression patterns and chromosomal changes associated with aging. *Cancer Research*, *64*(23), 8550–8557.

Greene, J. A., & Herzberg, D. (2010). Hidden in plain sight marketing prescription drugs to consumers in the twentieth century. *American Journal of Public Health*, *100*(5), 793–803. doi:10.2105/AJPH.2009.181255

Groen, P., Mahootian, F., & Goldstein, D. (2008). *Medical informatics: Emerging technologies, 'Open' EHR systems, and ethics in the 21st century*. Retrieved from http://www.shepherd.edu/surc/cosi/Medical%20Informatics%20and%20Ethics%20042008.doc

Guyatt, G., & Drummond, R. (2002). *Users' guides to the medical literature: A manual for evidence-based clinical practice* (1st ed.). USA: American Medical Association.

Harrison, R. L., & Lyerla, F. (2012). Using nursing clinical decision support systems to achieve meaningful use. *Computers, Informatics, Nursing*, *30*(7), 380–385. doi:10.1097/NCN.0b013e31823eb813

The International HapMap Consortium. (2003). The International HapMap project. *Nature*, *426*, 789–796.

The International HapMap Consortium. (2013). *International HapMap project*. Retrieved from http://hapmap.ncbi.nlm.nih.gov

Knoppers, B. M., Sénécal, K., Borry, P., & Avard, D. (2014). Whole-genome sequencing in newborn screening programs. *Science Translational Medicine*, *6*(229), 229. doi:10.1126/scitranslmed.3008494

Levy, H. P., LoPresti, L., & Seibert, D. C. (2008). Twenty questions in genetic medicine: An assessment of world wide web databases for genetics information at the point of care. *Genetics in Medicine*, *10*(9), 659–667. doi:10.1097GIM.0b013e318180639d

Masys, D. R., Jarvik, G. P., Abernethy, N. F., Anderson, N. R., Papanicolaou, G. J., Paltoo, D. N., . . . Levy, J. P. (2012). Technical desiderata for the integration of genomic data into electronic health records. *Journal of Biomedical Informatics*, *45*, 419–422.

National Center for Biotechnology Information (NCBI). (2014). NCBI map viewer of human genome. *Annotation release 107. Master map genes on sequence*. Retrieved from http://www.ncbi.nlm.nih.gov/projects/mapview/maps.cgi?taxid=9606&chr=21

National Human Genome Research Institute. (2013). *The 10-year anniversary of the human genome project: Commemorating and reflecting* (No. NHGRI2013). Washington, DC: Author. Retrieved from http://www.genome.gov/27555238

National Human Genome Research Institute. (2015). *Frequently asked questions about genetic testing*. Retrieved from http://www.genome.gov/pfv.cfm?pageID=19516567

National Library of Medicine. (2014). *Talking glossary of genetic terms*. Retrieved from http://ghr.nlm.nih.gov/glossary=pharmacogenomics

Naveed, M., Ayday, E., Clayton, E. W., Fellay, J., Gunter, C. A., Hubaux, J. P., . . . Wang, X. (2014). Privacy and security in the genomic era. ArXiv: 1405.1891v1. Retrieved from http:/arxiv.org/abs/1405.1891

Office of the National Coordinator for Health Information Technology. (2012). *Test procedure for §170.314.a.13 family health history*. Retrieved from http://www.healthit.gov/sites/default/files/standards-certification/2014-edition-draft-test-procedures/170-314-a-13-family-health-history-2014-test-procedures-draft-v1.0.pdf

Offit, K. (2011). Personalized medicine: New genomics, old lessons. *Human Genetics, 130*(1), 3–14. doi:10.1007/s00439-011-1028-3

Pabst, M. K., Scherubel, J. C., & Minnick, A. F. (1996). The impact of computerized documentation on nurses' use of time. *Computers in Nursing, 14*(1), 25–30. doi:PMID: 8605657

Roberts, J. L. (2010). Preempting discrimination: Lessons from the Genetic Information Nondiscrimination Act. *Vanderbilt Law Review, 63*(2), 439–439. Retrieved from http://www.vanderbiltlawreview.org/articles/2010/03/Roberts-Preempting-Discrimination-63-Vand.-L.-Rev.-439-2010.pdf

Sittig, D. F., & Singh, H. (2010). A new sociotechnical model for studying health information technology in complex adaptive healthcare systems. *Quality and Safety in Health Care, 19*(1, Suppl. 3), i68–i74. doi:10.1136/qshc.2010.042085

Su, P. (2013). Direct-to-consumer genetic testing: A comprehensive view. *Yale Journal of Biology and Medicine, 86*(3), 359–365. Retrieved from http://www.ncbi.nlm.nih.gov/pmc/articles/PMC3767220/pdf/yjbm_86_3_359.pdf

Topol, E. (2015). *The patient will see you now: The future of medicine is in your hands*. New York, NY: Basic Books.

U.S. Food and Drug Administration. (2013). *Inspections, compliance, enforcement, and criminal investigations, 23andMe, Inc. 11/22/13*. Retrieved from http://www.fda.gov/iceci/enforcementactions/warningletters/2013/ucm376296.htm

U.S. Pharmacopeia. (2014). *About USP*. Retrieved from http://www.usp.org/about-usp

Wetterstrand, K. A. (2014). *DNA sequencing costs: Data from the NHGRI Genome Sequencing Program (GSP)*. Retrieved from http://www.genome.gov/sequencingcosts

World Health Organization. (2014). *WHO definitions of genetics and genomics*. Retrieved from http://www.who.int/genomics/geneticsVSgenomics/en/

CHAPTER 25

Nanotechnology and Implications for Health Care Interprofessional Teams

Mari Tietze and Susan McBride

OBJECTIVES

1. Define *nanotechnology* and examine implications for advanced practice nurses and interprofessional teams.

2. Describe the emerging field of nanotechnology and the various applications of nanotechnology currently in use in the health care industry.

3. Discuss how nanotechnology is subject to change many aspects of how we care for patients and implications for clinical care.

4. Discuss implications for nursing informatics and technology support roles with respect to nanotechnology.

5. Examine a case study related to the use of nanotechnology in clinical care and reflect on implications for the health care industry.

KEY WORDS

nanotechnology, nanomedicine, nanomaterial, nanometer, lab on a chip, nano tattoo, nanoinformatics

CONTENTS

INTRODUCTION

Nanotechnology may change the health care industry as we know it today, particularly in terms of combining nanotechnologies with other technologies discussed throughout the text. *Nanotechnology* is defined as the research and development of materials, devices, and systems designed to function at very small micro-levels and that exhibit physical, chemical, or biological properties (California Department of Energy, 2004). The term "nano" means "very small or minute" and in terms of measurement, the nanometer (nm) is frequently designated in terms of "one billionth" or 10^{-9} (0.000000001; Dictionary.com Unabridged, 2015). At the scale size of approximately 100 nm or less, biological molecules and structures operate in living cells (National Institutes of Health [NIH], 2013). This is an important concept to grasp in terms of understanding how small nanotechnology actually is, much too small for the naked eye to see. In addition, the physiologic impact of being small enough to navigate in and out of cellular tissue allows targeted pharmaceuticals to be delivered very efficiently and effectively. This size relative to the atom is roughly 10 times the size of the atom. To provide a comparison for full comprehension, the size of DNA is 2 to 3 nm, influenza virus is 75 to 100 nm, tuberculous bacteria is 2,000 nm (2 μm), red blood cells are 7,000 to 8,000 nm (7–8 μm), and human hair is 60,000 to 120,000 nm (60–120 μm; NIH, 2014). This puts this size in perspective as to how this technology works at the micro-level to impact the human body.

It is generally known among most aspects of nanotechnology that "small size" is a common characteristic. However, some of us are knowledgeable about nanotechnology because of more practical experience. As such, a colleague recalls his first experience with a nanotechnology story as a young child; he has been fascinated with it ever since. Our colleague tells us,

> Acetylene gas, if burned in oxygen at a low enough concentration makes "carbon black" soot. That soot makes thick black spider webs that float in the air. How is that even possible for Acetylene C_2H_2 to self-assemble into long chains of carbon fibers that float around for hours, like gossamer threads and ribbons of flat black silk? I asked that question for years as a child, when I learned how to weld in my father's shop at the age of 12. I got in a lot of trouble for wasting precious acetylene by burning it at the concentration that made huge clouds of thick black soot that got all over everything. My mom was especially upset because I ended up looking like a coal miner with it all over my hair and clothes. I asked that question and no one knew the answer for sure, until Richard Smalley was able to identify Buckyball and nanotube fibers in graphite and acetylene carbon black soot, as well as diesel exhaust. (Gilder, 2015, p. 2)

Today, the health care industry is seeing nanotechnology used in a number of different ways, including advanced drug delivery systems, laboratory systems on a chip, and with other various chemicals and biodetectors (California Department of Energy, 2004). There are numerous applications of nanotechnology within the health care industry, many of which can be examined by a quick visit to www.nano.gov; new breakthroughs are occurring at a rapid pace (National Nanotechnology Coordination Office, 2015). This expansion of science through use of nanomaterials and nanotechnologies not only creates innovative solutions but also presents new challenges in terms of ethics and safety. This relatively new field dating back just 2 short decades is poised to change the way diagnostics and treatment interventions are delivered, and this has implications for the health care consumer to better manage his or her own health using new microscale devices (Staggers, McCasky, Brazelton, & Kennedy, 2008). This chapter discusses this new and emerging field of nanotechnology and profiles a few of the informatics and technology-related applications of nanotechnology in health care. In addition, implications are examined for clinicians, interprofessional teams, health care consumers, and nursing informatics (NI).

APPLICATIONS IN HEALTH CARE

Nanomedicine is defined by the NIH as "an offshoot of nanotechnology" referring to "highly specific medical intervention at the molecular scale for curing disease or repairing damaged tissues, such as bone, muscle, or nerve" (NIH, 2013, p. 1). The NIH has a program that started in 2005 that was designed specifically to address this new and emerging field of medicine. Aggressive timelines were set to address risk and benefit over a 10-year period using a unique approach to translate bench science into evidence for fairly rapid use in clinical practice. Under this program, eight nanodevelopment centers were established in the first phase of the program and four of the centers continued operation in the second half of the program. There are two major goals of the program: (a) to understand how the biological machinery inside living cells is built and operates at the nanoscale and (b) to use this information to re-engineer these structures, develop new technologies that could be applied to treating diseases, and/or leverage the new knowledge to focus work directly on translational studies to treat a disease or repair damaged tissue. Table 25.1 notes several of the NIH-funded projects under this program that are designed to translate scientific advances of nanotechnology into clinical practice (NIH, 2013).

Lab-on-a-Chip

One exciting application of nanotechnology is in the area of clinical laboratory results and reporting. Lab-on-a-chip (LOC) is a quick diagnostic laboratory test performed using nanotechnology to measure microfluidic immunoassays. The device is also referred to as an mChip or a mobile microfluidic chip ("Lab on a chip" as screening tool option, 2011). LOC tests blood for viruses, cancer, chromosomal disorders, and susceptibility to a specific disease. Figure 25.1 illustrates the small size of these chips, and Figure 25.2 illustrates the typical functional components contained with the chip (U.S. Environmental Protection Agency, 2009).

Diseases can be detected earlier with LOC than with traditional lab testing. For example, there are many types of LOC technology, with most being made of silicon, glass, and polymers that use a sample reagent liquid transport and external power sources. One example is developed by Tom Duke at the London Center for Nanotechnology that detects HIV in blood samples. This chip uses a sensor that needs only one drop of blood. Any virus particles pass between the pillars to the other end of the sensor, where they are attracted to a series of tiny cantilevers coated with antibodies. These are mini diving

TABLE 25.1 Nanotechnology NIH Projects Profiled

Use Case	Description of the Project	Application
Tunable quantum dots (QDs) for imaging cells	QDs are nanocrystals that are activated by and emit specific wavelengths of light. Drs. Andrew Smith and Shuming Nie developed a new approach to synthesize QDs that permitted unprecedented control over their preparation. The improved QDs are expected to be a highly effective tool in imaging live cells, as well as in other diagnostic applications.	Biomedical imaging and diagnostics
Light-controlled pain relief	Researchers developed a molecule that can silence pain-sensing neurons using light, opening up new avenues in pain research and the design of novel analgesics (Mourot, Tochitsky, & Kramer, 2013).	Pain relief and analgesic intervention
Nanoparticles deliver combination cargos directly to cancer targets	Investigators (Ashley et al., 2014) constructed synthetic "protocells" that were used to kill liver tumor cells without adversely affecting healthy cells. Protocells are made by enclosing highly porous silica nanoparticles to carry high concentrations and different combinations of cargo, such as drugs, small interfering RNAs, and other toxins. The cargo capacity and time course of release can be controlled by changing the pore size and chemistry of the silica core, but the protocell is designed to release the cargo only on entry into the target cell.	Targeted cancer treatment

NIH, National Institutes of Health; RNA, ribonucleic acid.

Adapted from National Institutes of Health (2015).

boards that bend when something lands on them, and deflections can be measured by bouncing a laser off them. "The more the diving boards are deflected, the more virus is present" (Jha, 2011, p. 1). This example is one of many representing the key advantages of less time, less blood, and less space needed for supplies.

Another benefit of this technology is improvement to safety. This includes the safety of the patient, health care provider, and the general public. According to an article published in *Nature Medicine*, this testing only requires microliters of blood that can be obtained from a finger stick (Chin et al., 2011). This prevents unneeded exposure to larger needles by the nurse and patient. Results are obtained within 20 minutes and require no interpretation by the tester (Chin et al., 2011). Quicker results allow for quicker treatment that can protect the public from exposure as well.

This type of laboratory chip technology also demonstrated a sensitivity of 100% and a specificity of 96%, which is as accurate as lab-based HIV testing (Chin et al., 2011). The

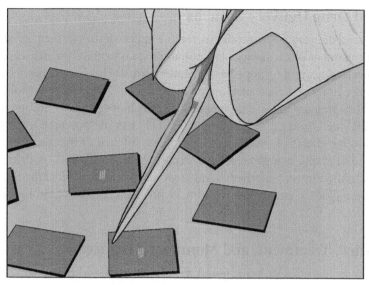

FIGURE 25.1. A comparison of the size of LOCs.

LOC, lab-on-a-chip.

Adapted from U.S. Environmental Protection Agency (2009).

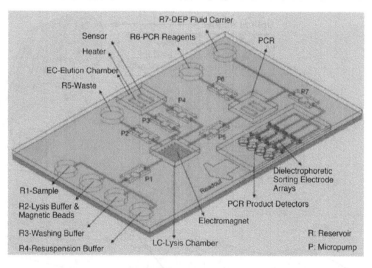

FIGURE 25.2. Detail of functional LOC components.

LOC, lab-on-a-chip.

Source: U.S. Environmental Protection Agency (2009).

portability of LOC can be useful at home. For example, one model that tests brain natriuretic peptide (BNP) levels for patients with congestive heart failure is used in rural areas and allows for patients to be more involved in their care. Testing BNP at home reduces 30-day readmissions by 25% (Komatireddy & Topol, 2012). The future advancements in lab-on-a-chip technology will always depend on two major scientific disciplines: microfluidics and molecular biology. Nanotechnology will play a key role in tying these two fields together as the technology progresses (Claussen & Medintz, 2012).

Advanced Drug Delivery Systems

Nanodrugs and delivery systems offer incredible opportunities in the prevention, diagnosis, and treatment of cardiovascular, pulmonary, and endocrine diseases as well as those of dermatology and orthopedics (O'Malley, 2010). This is possible because nanodrugs promise improved bioavailability, reduced toxicity, and enhanced solubility.

Nano-chemotherapy can be designed based on biopsy results and engineered to ignore healthy cells and target diseased cells. This has the potential to eliminate the systemic adverse effects of treatment. Nanorobots, inhaled or injected, could monitor responses to therapy, complete cellular repairs, detect disease, or deliver specific agents at specific targets. Another example would be inhaled biochips that continuously monitor glucose and release insulin in precise doses to control glucose levels (Mamo et al., 2010).

Diagnostics, Treatment, and Monitoring Devices

Nano tattoos for diabetics are being tested and evaluated in studies that will detect blood glucose levels. Figure 25.3 presents the mechanism of action for nano tattoos. The change in the glucose levels will trigger changes in coloration that can be picked up by

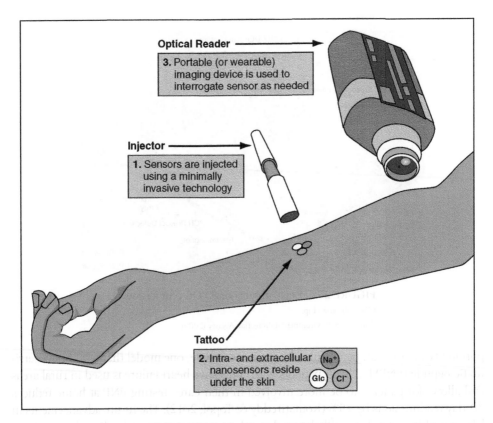

FIGURE 25.3. Nano tattoo mechanism.
Source: Saenz (2010b).

a light-monitoring device (Saenz, 2010b). In similar research in Canada, investigators are developing contact lenses for diabetics consisting of nanoparticles in a hydrogel lens that changes color depending on the glucose level in tears (Saenz, 2010a).

More recently, the concern for the safety of nano tattoos for diabetes management has been addressed (Bennett & Naranja, 2013). A checklist of bioethical and system design issues that are appropriately considered in the preclinical, precommercialization phase of nano tattoo development would benefit societal use. This can be accomplished by engaging relevant researcher, medical, patient–user and patient–advocate communities concerned with its appropriate application, as well as policy-making communities focused on effectively managing diabetes-related health care costs. The checklist of factors includes fundamental issues and is generally applicable to nanomedical inventions. The nonexclusive list of seven factors includes (a) patent scope, (b) patent thicket [cost], (c) potential patient autonomy, (d) beneficence, (e) multidimensional justice, (f) privacy, and (g) system design (Bennett & Naranja, 2013).

Regardless of the availability of nano tattoos for diabetes management, most patients with diabetes depend on handheld glucometers for monitoring glycemic level (Veiseh, Tang, Whitehead, Anderson, & Langer, 2015). These devices rely on a single sampling of blood collected through finger pricks and are typically used only a few times a day (on average four to six times a day). These patients use a wide variety of approaches to monitor their glucose levels and associated insulin delivery mechanisms. These mechanisms range from manual insulin injections to continuous glucose monitors (CGMs), all of which have their drawbacks. Given the advances in nanotechnology of the past few years, we expect nanotechnology to play an important part in improving the management of diabetes within the next decade. The emergence of Food and Drug Administration-approved nanotechnology formulations coupled with the clinical success of insulin-delivering technologies through the pulmonary route is encouraging. In our view, the greatest need and also the highest clinical potential for nanotechnology-based diabetes therapy lies in the development of robust glucose-sensitive nanoparticles and nanodevices for integration into sensors, and the development of integrated glucose-sensing and insulin-delivering nanoformulations (Veiseh et al., 2015).

Genomics and Nanotechnology Interplay

The postgenomics era has brought about new "omics" biotechnologies, such as proteomics and metabolomics, as well as their novel applications to personal genomics and the quantified self. These advances are now also catalyzing other and newer postgenomics innovations, leading to convergences between omics and nanotechnology. Nanotechnology has been utilized as a complementary component to advance proteomics through different kinds of nanotechnology applications, including nanoporous structures, functionalized nanoparticles, quantum dots, and polymeric nanostructures. As noted, these applications have led to several highly sensitive diagnostics and new methods of drug delivery and targeted therapy for clinical use (Kobeissy et al., 2014).

Some of the areas where genomics and nanotechnology have an interplay have been presented. Their applications as seen through the lens of postgenomics life sciences include (a) immunosensors for inflammatory, pathogenic, and autoimmune markers for infectious and autoimmune diseases; (b) amplified immunoassays for detection of cancer biomarkers; and (c) methods for targeted therapy and automatically adjusted drug delivery such as in experimental stroke and brain injury studies. As nanoproteomics becomes more broadly available, it is anticipated that further breakthroughs will occur in personalized and targeted medicine with the support of nanotechnology (Kobeissy et al., 2014).

IMPLICATIONS OF NANOTECHNOLOGY TO NURSING INFORMATICS AND INTERPROFESSIONAL TEAMS

Implications for Clinicians and the Health Care Consumer

One implication for clinicians is a societal fear regarding this technology as a function of the physical size of the component or material and concerns about safe use of the new products and materials involved in nanotechnology. The terms "Nanotek" and "grey goo" have been used to describe nanomaterials and have also been the subject of sci-fi movies and media concern pertaining to uncertainty about the safety of this new and emerging field of medicine for the individual patient and the environment. Nanoteck compounds are used for common sunscreens and transdermal patches as a drug delivery mechanism as with nicotine and nitroglycerin patches (Nohynek, Lademann, Ribaud, & Roberts, 2007).

Scientists are concerned that nanotechnology might follow the path that genetically engineered food has taken with consumer concerns about safety despite a large body of evidence indicating that genetically modified food is safe. In a 2003 news feature by Geoff Brumfiel in *Nature Magazine*, the following is noted: "Nanotechnology is set to be the next campaign focus for environmental groups" (Brumfiel, 2003, p. 246). The article poses the question for the reader as to whether or not scientists can mitigate concerns to secure public trust. Or will nanotechnology go the route that genetically modified foods have taken and not be trusted?

"As nursing progresses through the technological transformation, nurse leaders will be challenged to design a sustainable and humanized framework of care which continues to protect the values and brings dignity and respect for the patient" (Meetoo, 2011, p. 713). Nurses must be prepared to continue learning and adapting their practice as nanotechnology changes health care. This will include learning new ways to administer medicine and provide basic care (Delaney & Lewis, 2006). The most important thing for health care practitioners to remember is that new technology does not replace the core values that have driven nursing care since its inception.

Implications for Informatics

"Nanoinformatics" is a term used to encompass aspects of data collection, tools, and sharing, along with associated applications that are becoming a key element of nanotechnology research, nanotechnology environmental health and safety, product development, and sustainable manufacturing (Nanoinformatics Workshop 2015 Committee, 2015). Informatics is a part of nanotechnology through its computing and data-management tools (Staggers et al., 2008). Continual research on nanotechnology's impact on human health should be conducted to better address both the benefits and risks of nanotechnology.

Nanotechnology has the ability to be individualized to every person's unique health. Research is necessary to understand how nanotechnology works inside the human body as well as the potential effects it may have on the spreading of diseases and other health complications. Because nanotechnology is potentially geared toward a more customizable level of health care through nanoparticles and sensory capabilities, the standard for electronic health record (EHR) technology will need to be investigated and inevitably upgraded to incorporate advanced features. Future research of this integration must address challenges of data storage within the EHR and ways to maintain or increase privacy of patients' nanodata.

In terms of the relationship between nanotechnology and interprofessional education, practice and education core competencies in interprofessional education suggest that nanotechnology initiatives would benefit from an interprofessional education/collaborative approach (Interprofessional Collaborative Expert Panel, 2011). This is because interprofessional education competencies are geared toward optimum management of complex patient issues. One example was provided in the realm of pharmacy education where education on the biomolecular, human genome project and clinical applications of nanotechnology were integrated with the interprofessional education approach to encourage dialogue with different health professions to produce a patient-based team approach (Gong, 2013).

Safety Considerations for Nanotechnology and Nanomedicine

Safety considerations for managing the risk of nanotechnology and nanomedicine have significant implications. Nanotoxicology is a new field related to nanotechnology and nanomedicine that specifically addresses potentially toxic reactions to nanomaterials. Engineered nanomaterials (ENMs) have the potential "to cause undesirable effects, contaminate the environment and adversely affect susceptible parts of the population" (Oberdorster, 2010, p. 89). Given that the field of nanotechnology and nanomedicine is so new, little solid evidence has accumulated to determine what might constitute environmental exposure or unintentional consequences, including toxic reactions of individual patients related to dosage, dose rate, and the biokenetics of the nanomaterials.

SUMMARY

Although research is currently being conducted to understand the emerging field of nanotechnology in the health care sector, there are still areas of discussion that deserve additional research and attention. As nanotechnology is becoming an integral part of health care, both patients and practitioners are curious to better understand both the medical benefits and risks that it entails. Further critical research is needed on the impact on health and outcomes for patients and practitioners, risks involving information storage of nanodata, how to integrate nanotechnology capabilities into existing EHRs, as well as other forms of health information technology (HIT), and how to accommodate the changes in roles for patients and clinicians. Informatics related to nanomedicine, known as *nanoinformatics*, will be a key component of this needed discovery.

EXERCISES AND QUESTIONS FOR CONSIDERATION

Nanotechnology may fundamentally change the way we deliver health care by placing the patient much more in control of his or her diagnoses, treatment, and information related to his or her health and well-being. This chapter has considered several use cases reflective of these new developments with significant implications for interprofessional teams, clinical practice, consumer management of health, and roles within nursing informatics. Let us consider the content covered with respect to nanotechnology and nanomedicine and respond to the following questions:

1. Discuss implications of nanotechnology and nanomedicine in terms of changing roles for interprofessional teams. How might we begin to prepare the industry in practice and academic preparation of new health care professionals for these innovative and new technologies?

2. How will HIT and informatics roles be impacted by nanotechnology and nanomedicine?

3. Implantable devices have been the subject of sci-fi movies and fictional books; however, these new and emerging technologies are now available to us as legitimate diagnostics and treatments. How will we prepare health care consumers who have read many of these fictional stories for this new wave of technology to mitigate potential fears that these stories might have created within the health care consumer community?

4. What are some of the legitimate bioethical and safety concerns that patients and health care consumers might have and how do we address these issues within health care organizations and interprofessional teams?

5. There are many benefits to the health care consumer in terms of managing one's own health with respect to use of nanotechnologies and nanomaterials. Let us examine one or two of these benefits and compare the risks discussed in a risk–benefit analysis.

CASE STUDY

Consider the following scenario: A patient with diabetes is about to be stamped with a tattoo that will identify the patient at the molecular level; the tattoo comprises tiny particles that are configured to detect biochemical shifts in metabolism to monitor glucose levels. This is now a part of the scientific revolution related to the use of nanotechnologies and nanomaterials in the field of nanomedicine and may become a common treatment for diabetes. Tattoos used to monitor glucose levels are an example of the miniaturization of medicine. This particular patient has watched sci-fi movies, is familiar with the term "grey goo," and is fearful of the treatment approach. The physician explains to the patient that the use of the tattoo will be the best for her treatment plan. When the physician leaves the room, the

(continued)

CASE STUDY (*continued*)

patient states, "I don't know about this tattoo thing. I have never wanted a tattoo, and this sounds like some sort of sci-fi movie I watched a while back." Reflect on the following questions:

1. How would you use the bioethical checklist recommended by Bennett and Naranja to address this situation?
2. What ethical principles are at play within this scenario?
3. How might you educate the patient on what nanotechnology is and how it works to alleviate concerns?
4. What common treatments for smoking cessation and cardiac disease might you use to compare the tattoo treatment to and to explain how nanotechnology works?

REFERENCES

Ashley, J. D., Stefanick, J. F., Schroeder, V. A., Suckow, M. A., Alves, N. J., Suzuki, R., . . . Bilgicer, B. (2014). Liposomal carfilzomib nanoparticles effectively target multiple myeloma cells and demonstrate enhanced efficacy in vivo. *Journal of Controlled Release: Official Journal of the Controlled Release Society, 196,* 113–121. doi:10.1016/j.jconrel.2014.10.005

Bennett, M. G., & Naranja, R. J., Jr. (2013). Getting nano tattoos right—A checklist of legal and ethical hurdles for an emerging nanomedical technology. *Nanomedicine: Nanotechnology, Biology, and Medicine, 9*(6), 729–731. doi:10.1016/j.nano.2013.04.006

Brumfiel, G. (2003). Nanotechnology: A little knowledge. *Nature, 424*(6946), 246–248. doi:10.1038/424246a

California Department of Energy. (2004). *What is nanotechnology?* Retrieved from www.lanl.gov/mst/nano/definition.html

Chin, C. D., Laksanasopin, T., Cheung, Y. K., Steinmiller, D., Linder, V., Parsa, H., . . . Sia, S. K. (2011). Microfluidics-based diagnostics of infectious diseases in the developing world. *Nature Medicine, 17*(8), 1015–1019. doi:10.1038/nm.2408

Claussen, J. C., & Medintz, I. L. (2012). Using nanotechnology to improve lab on a chip devices. *Biochip and Tissue Chips, 2*(4), 1–1. Retrieved from http://www.omicsonline.org/using-nanotechnology-to-improve-lab-on-a-chip-devices-2153-0777-2-e117.php?aid=9488

Delaney, C. W., & Lewis, D. (2006). Nanotechnology: Is NI proactive? *Computers, Informatics, Nursing, 24*(3), 173–174. Retrieved from http://www.nursingcenter.com/lnc/journalarticle?Article_ID=644942

Dictionary.com Unabridged. (2015). *Nano.* Retrieved from http://www.dictionary.reference.com/browse/nano

Gilder, R. (2015). *Nanotechnology from a child's perspective.* Unpublished manuscript.

Gong, J. (2013). International pharmaceutical students' federation critical appraisal essay 2013: The challenge of individualized pharmaceutical care, the need for interprofessional education. *Pharmacy Education, 13,* 1–1.

Interprofessional Collaborative Expert Panel. (2011). *Core competencies for interprofessional collaborative practice: Report of an expert panel* (No. ICEP-2011). Washington, DC: Interprofessional Education Collaborative. Retrieved from http://www.ipecollaborative.org/uploads/IPEC-Core-Competencies.pdf

Jha, A. (2011). The incredible shrinking laboratory or "lab-on-a-chip." *Guardian*, *11*(28), 1–1. Retrieved from http://www.theguardian.com/science/2011/nov/28/incredible-shrinking-laboratory-lab-chip

Kobeissy, F. H., Gulbakan, B., Alawieh, A., Karam, P., Zhang, Z., Guingab-Cagmat, J. D., . . . Wang, K. (2014). Post-genomics nanotechnology is gaining momentum: Nanoproteomics and applications in life sciences. *OMICS: A Journal of Integrative Biology*, *18*(2), 111–131. doi:10.1089/omi.2013.0074

Komatireddy, R., & Topol, E. J. (2012). Medicine unplugged: The future of laboratory medicine. *Clinical Chemistry*, *58*(12), 1644–1647. doi:10.1373/clinchem.2012.194324

"Lab on a chip" as screening tool option. (2011). *AIDS Alert*, *26*(11), 128–129.

Mamo, T., Moseman, E. A., Kolishetti, N., Salvador-Morales, C., Shi, J., Kuritzkes, D. R., . . . Farokhzad, O. C. (2010). Emerging nanotechnology approaches for HIV/AIDS treatment and prevention. *Nanomedicine*, *5*(2), 269–285. doi:10.2217/nnm.10.1

Meetoo, D. (2011). Nanotechnology: Science fiction or a future reality? *British Journal of Nursing*, *20*(12), 713. doi:10.12968/bjon.2011.20.12.713

Mourot, A., Tochitsky, I., & Kramer, R. H. (2013). Light at the end of the channel: Optical manipulation of intrinsic neuronal excitability with chemical photoswitches. *Frontiers in Molecular Neuroscience*, *6*, 5. doi:10.3389/fnmol.2013.00005

Nanoinformatics Workshop 2015 Committee. (2015). *Enabling successful discovery and applications*. Retrieved from http://www.nanoinformatics.org

National Institutes of Health. (2013). *Nanomedicine overview*. Retrieved from http://www.commonfund.nih.gov/nanomedicine/overview

National Institutes of Health. (2014). *Nanotechnology safety and health program* (No. NIHnanoSaf2014). Washington, DC: U.S. Department of Health and Human Services. Retrieved from http://www.ors.od.nih.gov/sr/dohs/Documents/Nanotechnology%20Safety%20and%20Health%20Program.pdf

National Institutes of Health. (2015). *Nanomedicine*. Retrieved from https://commonfund.nih.gov/nanomedicine/index

National Nanotechnology Coordination Office. (2015). *U.S. national nanotechnology initiative*. Retrieved from http://www.nano.gov

Nohynek, G. J., Lademann, J., Ribaud, C., & Roberts, M. S. (2007). Grey goo on the skin? Nanotechnology, cosmetic and sunscreen safety. *Critical Reviews in Toxicology*, *37*(3), 251–277. doi:773426392 [pii]

Oberdorster, G. (2010). Safety assessment for nanotechnology and nanomedicine: Concepts of nanotoxicology. *Journal of Internal Medicine*, *267*(1), 89–105. doi:10.1111/j.1365-2796.2009.02187.x

O'Malley, P. (2010). Nanopharmacology: For the future-think small. *Clinical Nurse Specialist CNS*, *24*(3), 123–124. doi:10.1097/NUR.0b013e3181d828bd

Saenz, A. (2010a, January). *Nanotech contact lens monitors diabetes by changing color*. Singularity University. Retrieved from http://www.singularityhub.com/2010/01/15/nanotech-contact-lens-monitors-diabetes-by-changing-color

Saenz, A. (2010b). *Nanotechnology "tattoos" to help diabetics track glucose levels*. Singularity University. Retrieved from http://www.singularityhub.com/2010/06/10/nanotechnology-tattoos-to-help-diabetics-track-glucose-levels

Staggers, N., McCasky, T., Brazelton, N., & Kennedy, R. (2008). Nanotechnology: The coming revolution and its implications for consumers, clinicians, and informatics. *Nursing Outlook, 56*(5), 268–274. doi:10.1016/j.outlook.2008.06.004

U.S. Environmental Protection Agency. (2009). *Potential nano-enabled environmental applications for radionuclides*. Washington, DC: Author.

Veiseh, O., Tang, B. C., Whitehead, K. A., Anderson, D. G., & Langer, R. (2015). Managing diabetes with nanomedicine: Challenges and opportunities. *Nature Reviews Drug Discovery, 14*(1), 45–57. doi:10.1038/nrd4477

CHAPTER 26

"Big Data" and Advanced Analytics

Susan McBride, Cynthia Powers, Richard Gilder,
and Billy U. Philips, Jr.

1. Discuss the concept of "big data" and the impact that large volumes of data from the electronic environment and other data sources will have on the future of health care.

2. Discuss advanced techniques in data mining, "big data," and analytics implications.

3. Describe the role of the data scientist and the importance of that role to the future of health care.

4. Consider a specific use case for advanced analytics utilizing "big data" in an oncology unit examining the use of cognitive computing power through the IBM Watson project.

5. Discuss the importance of new and expanding nursing competencies and roles related to workflow redesign, advanced analytics professionals, and how advanced practices nurses are well suited for these roles.

| KEY WORDS |

big data, data mining, Watson project, data scientist, advanced analytics, unstructured data

| CONTENTS |

INTRODUCTION

The average health care worker today has more information at hand than she or he can effectively use. Electronic health records (EHRs) capture volumes of information in both structured and unstructured data fields, not just on current events and encounters but also on historical data within the record that could include years of history on any given patient and multiple encounters across care settings. Add to that images and scans, laboratory results, monitors and sensors, and the notes of all practitioners composing a comprehensive clinical picture of a person in our care and the volume of information is considerable. This trend is not just happening in health care but also in society at large. Economists predict that "big data" will be the third largest component of the U.S. gross domestic product (GDP) by 2020, accounting for a maximum of $325 billion with a long-term impact that is even greater as data become integral to every facet of wealth (Lund, Manyika, Nyquist, Mendonca, & Ramaswamy, 2013). We live in a technological and information-rich world that has just begun to affect the health care industry. "Big data" and analytics are poised to change our lives worldwide. "Big data" are defined in terms of volume, velocity, and variety, or the 3Vs (Gartner Inc., 2013). These factors result in high volumes of streaming data, which include semistructured and unstructured formats (Soares, 2015).

This chapter explores what constitutes "big data," including definitions and examples of their use in health care, and how data mining and advanced analytics techniques are currently being used in health care. It also discusses how these items will impact nursing and clinicians in the future. In addition, we explore the role of the data scientist and how new roles and competencies for health care informaticists will be paramount to future health care use of big data. Finally, we discuss the importance of how advanced practice nurses are critical to the success of operationalizing "big data" and advanced analytics in the practice setting through examination of a case study.

WHAT ARE "BIG DATA?"

There are many definitions for the term "big data," most of which relate to the size and structure of the data. Perhaps the simplest feature of "big data" is that they have outgrown conventional databases and data warehouse solutions, and they contain massive amounts of unstructured data (Sharma, 2011). These types of data are massive enough to cause problems with commodity solutions (off the shelf) for capture, storage, transfer, curation, analysis, visualization, sharing, or other operations. There are a number of different types of big data, which include indexes; images or videos; social networks, such as Twitter or Facebook; surveillance data; company records, including medical records; and data-heavy fields such as astronomy, genomics, and economics (Sharma, 2011). Another aspect of big data is the use case and whether the data are archival, transactional for mostly read-only situations, or require write operations or other manipulations. This, combined with a general explosion of the data quantity in all industries, means we need a new generation of data tools and a new nomenclature to express what is frequently referred to by the oversimplified term big data.

Depending on the resource, one can find variations in the definition of the term big data. Moore, Eyestone, and Coddington (2013) define it as "vast amounts of diverse data, both structured and unstructured, that organizations can access quickly and analyze using innovative new tools that help pinpoint opportunities to better manage and improve value" (Moore et al., 2013, p. 61). Another interesting definition for big data is "massive bodies of digital data collected from all sorts of sources that are too large, raw, or unstructured for analysis using conventional relational database techniques" (Jee & Kim, 2013, p. 79).

Although uniquely different, these definitions provide some common elements that go into describing big data. Big data occur in large quantities (volume); may present in different ways such as structured, unstructured, or transactional (variety); and are accumulated and created quickly (velocity). Although these are the basic tenets of big data as a part of its constantly changing nature, these components also present the greatest challenges to working with big data.

Big Data Are Prolific Data

Let us consider that approximately 90% of the global data that exist today have been created over the past 2 years (Jee & Kim, 2013). It is also estimated that 2.5 quintillion bytes of data are generated on a daily basis (IBM Corporate, 2011). Most individuals have no frame of reference or conceptual framework to envision how big "big" is. If one can imagine one billion DVDs stacked one on another and laid sideways from Houston, Texas, to Orlando, Florida, they would contain all the data created by humans till the year 2003. That quantified would be 5×10^{18} bytes or 5 with 18 zeros behind it! We created that amount in 2 days in 2011; by the year 2014, we created that amount in 10 minutes. These types of examples constitute massive amounts of data and information available for potential use. So, what does this explosion of "big" look like in health care? Reports say that data from the U.S. health care system alone reached 150 exabytes in 2011. At this rate of growth, big data for U.S. health care will soon reach the zettabyte (1,021 gigabytes) scale and, not long after, the yottabyte (1,024 gigabytes; Raghupathi & Raghupathi, 2014). Here is a way to comprehend this scale: 5 exabytes is the text representation of all words ever spoken by human beings; 42 zettabytes would store all human speech ever spoken if digitized as 16 kHz 16-bit audio. The yottabype is the largest unit of measurement to date in the metric system. To get some sense of how large a yottabyte of data would be, McAfee, associate director of the Center for Digital Business at the Massachusetts Institute of Technology Sloan School of Management, states: "storing a yottabyte on terabyte-size hard drives would require 1 million city-block-size data centers, as big as the states of Delaware and Rhode Island" (Scoop Staff, 2014, p. 1).

Data Storage and Processing Power

Having described the massive size of these data stores, we need to think in terms of how the industry will store and manage massive amounts of information. Today, for example, one can buy a disk drive that would store all of the world's music for about $600

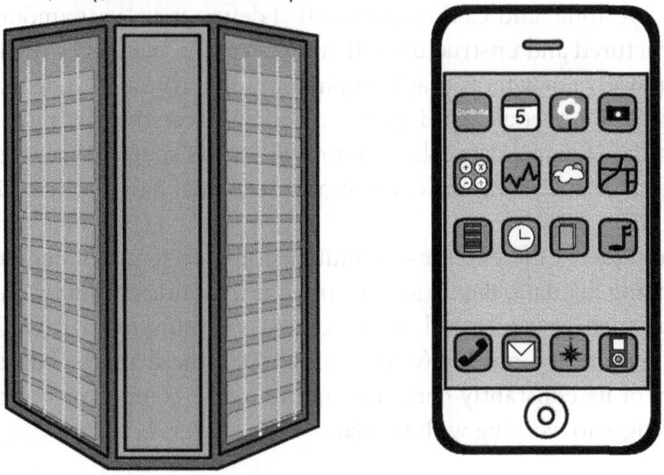

Computing is Faster and Cheaper

1975
Cray CDC-7600
Fastest Supercomputer
$5m ($32m in 2013 dollars)

2012
iPhone 4
Same speed $400

FIGURE 26.1. Cray computer compared to the speed and cost of the cell phone.

(Manyika et al., 2013). Additionally, computing has also become much faster than historical processing. For example, in 1975, the Cray CDC-7600, the world's fastest computer, was located at the University of Texas and was used by one of the authors to analyze dissertation data, cutting analytic time from 1 day to 1 second of epidemiologic analysis. Today, many of our mobile phones have processing power equal to the 1975 Cray. That Cray computer cost $5 million, which in today's dollars reflect an estimated equivalent of $32 million (Manyika et al., 2013). In contrast, a common mobile cell phone costs approximately $100 to $900 rather than millions of dollars and has computing speeds comparable to the Cray. Computing is not just faster but also much cheaper (Manyika et al., 2013). Figure 26.1 reflects the comparison of the Cray to the mobile phone. As a result of technological advances, we have storage and computing speed; it is reasonable that we can ask and answer nearly any question we might conceive at negligible costs given our advanced analytics and capability with technology. However, to do so means we must learn how to discover new knowledge by the way we ask questions. As John Naisbitt indicated in his 1982 book *Megatrends*, "We are drowning in data and starving for knowledge" (Naisbitt, 1982, p. 17). This is certainly the case in the health care industry today and is expected to get much more profound as we contemplate full use of genomic and epigenetic data.

FIVE KEY BIG DATA USE CASE CATEGORIES

There are five use cases typically seen in other industries related to the use of big data, all of which are applicable to the health care industry. These use cases include (a) data explorations and mining techniques to improve decision making; (b) extending the ability to view the health care consumer by internal and external data sources; (c) security and intelligence to lower risk, detect fraud, and monitor cybersecurity; (d) operational and clinical analysis to improve health care outcomes, quality, and cost; and (e) ability to augment data warehouse capabilities to integrate and use big data to increase efficiencies and improve outcomes. Figure 26.2 reflects the most common of the use cases for big data. Health care is one of the industries pushing the constraints of using traditional methods to manage and analyze data. The masses of unstructured textually rich data within the EHR are one of the prime examples of data that constitute big data. Mayer-Schonberger (2013) explains the phenomenon of big data as "things one can do at a large scale that cannot be done at a smaller one to extract new insights or create new forms of value" (p. 6). Examples of these new data sources considered to be big data and also creating substantial value are genomics and epigenetics.

Each one of these sources has several features that have been common techniques for decades. These include massive parallelism (common record types such as an EHR entry

The Nationwide Health Information Network

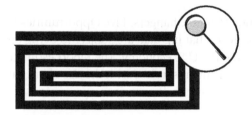

Big Data Exploration
Find, visualize, understand all big data
to improve decision making

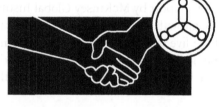

Enhanced 360° View of the Customer
Extend existing customer views
(MDM, CRM, etc) by incorporating
additional internal and external
information sources

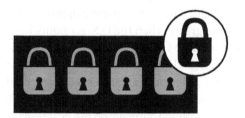

Security/Intelligence Extension
Lower risk, detect fraud and monitor
cyber security in real-time

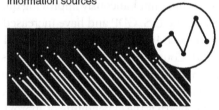

Operations Analysis
Analyze a variety of machine data for
improved business results

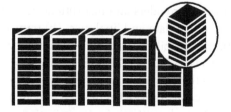

Data Warehouse Augmentation
Integrate big data and data warehouse
capabilities to increase operational efficiency

FIGURE 26.2. Use cases of big data.
CRM, customer relationship management; MDM, master data management.

for a patient) where the fields are synonymous from case to case. Each, to a greater or lesser degree, requires huge data volume storage and distribution for the purpose of manipulation through analytics or for use in high-performance computing and data mining such as pattern or thread recognition and, more recently, for machine learning algorithms. Because these use cases and these common techniques have been around, why are these use cases so prominent now and what is new about these techniques? This is a result of the fact that we are collecting and storing more data, because it has become affordable and easier to use primarily because of an increase in processing speed. In addition, unlike a decade ago, open source coding and new sources of information with widespread access to the Internet are much more common and have led to much easier, more efficient orders of magnitude and more elegant solutions in using and managing big data. Finally, commodity hardware and software have made utility-level usage available to all. We examine techniques for using big data in health care, and consider some of these use cases in large health care systems for operational and clinical analysis to improve health care outcomes using advanced analytic software in the areas of cognitive computing and data mining.

In a report by McKinsey Global Institute, "Game Changers: Five Opportunities for U.S. Growth and Renewal," the authors indicate that big data are subject to being one of the five largest opportunities for promoting the U.S. economy. The report estimates potential cost savings for health care and government services with the use of big data to be between \$135 billion and \$285 billion (Figure 26.3).

BIG DATA IN HEALTH CARE

At the forefront of health care in the United States is the unquestionable need to contain costs while simultaneously improving quality. Health care costs represent approximately 18% of the U.S. GDP and have increased at a rate greater than the U.S. economy for 31 of the past 40 years (Executive Office of the President Council of Economic Advisers, 2009). Coupled with these rising costs is the unprecedented complexity of health care information, particularly in oncology where there are significant advances being made in genomic sequencing, immunotherapy, and targeted therapies (Malin, 2013). Of significant concern is the expenditure of approximately \$95 billion annually on medical research in the United States, with only 6% of all clinical trials completed on time (American Cancer Society, 2014). In 2012, the Institute of Medicine (IOM) issued a document outlining three charges that would help address these challenges. This initiative called for the following from health care providers and institutions: (a) using tools such as computing power in the form of big data and analytics; (b) improving connectivity; and (c) improving organizational capabilities and ensuring collaboration between teams of clinicians and with patients (IOM, 2012). In essence, the IOM (2012) emphasized the need for health care systems that provided rapid, real-time data for use in routine clinical care that would lead to comparative-effectiveness research, quality improvement, safety, and the generation of new hypothesis for investigation to create learning organizations with use of data and information (IOM, 2012, pp. 55–57). These recommendations set the stage for cognitive computing power to be introduced as a potential solution. However, these systems present challenges with adoption and implementation that

Each of the Game Changers Could Substantially Raise U.S. GDP by 2020

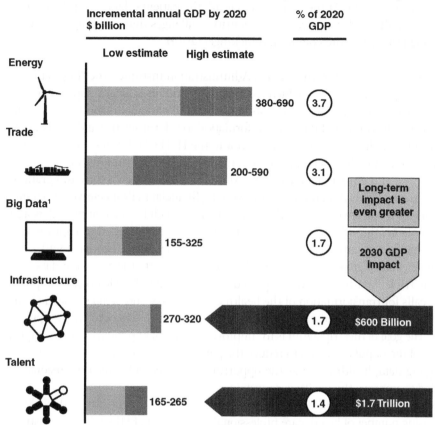

FIGURE 26.3. Big data are an economic game changer.

Note: These figures are based on a partial-equilibrium analysis that estimates only first-order effects and therefore cannot be summed to calculate the full economic impact.

[1] Figures reflect additional GDP in retail and manufacturing sectors only. Big data could also produce cost savings in government services and health care ($135 billion–$285 billion), but these do not directly translate into additional GDP.

GDP, gross domestic product.

Source: McKinsey Global Institute (2013).

require nursing expertise and leadership given the impact on clinical and operational workflows largely managed by nursing.

Improvement in health care delivery through technology has received support and reinforcement by legislation, such as the Health Information Technology for Economic and Clinical Health (HITECH) Act, passed in 2009 (HITECH Programs and Advisory Committee, 2009). In June 2014, as the HITECH Act moved into its 5th year of implementation, Dr. Karen DeSalvo, the national coordinator for health information technology (HIT) stated:

> There's great promise in what we can do with information, whether that's to improve systems around quality and safety or whether it's to advance science and/or cure and treatment for individuals with genomics at the bedside all the

way to population-level advancements. There's an array of opportunities for use of the data. At the end of the day, it's the patient's data . . . and we have to get ahead of the privacy and security challenges that are going to arise as Big Data gets more common. (Fluckinger, 2014)

Subsequently, in 2012, the Obama Administration instituted the "Big Data Research and Development Initiative," which received $200 million of federal support (Jee & Kim, 2013, p. 81). The purpose of this national initiative is to maximize the use of Big Data (massive bodies of digital data) into information to inform science and discovery in biomedical research (Jee & Kim, 2013). Prior to the HITECH Act, most of our health care data in the United States had been kept in silos within institutions, clinics, insurance companies, and government agencies. Although we continue to face integration challenges, the HITECH Act and the accompanying financial EHR Incentives Program of the Centers for Medicare & Medicaid Services (CMS), which is aimed at providers adopting and implementing EHRs, have created the infrastructure needed to capture and store electronic data at unprecedented levels of detail. This is further coupled with data from genomics and epigenetics, thus propelling health care into the era of big data.

The Triple Aim framework supported by the Institute for Healthcare Improvement (IHI) calls for transformation of the health care industry and creates a need to embrace the use of big data, analytics, and innovative tools such as cognitive computing systems. The goal of the Triple Aim is to "improve the patient experience of care, improve the health of the population, and to reduce the per capita cost of health care" (IHI, 2015). By using big data, health care has the opportunity to affect all three dimensions that are needed to improve the health care system.

With the introduction of meaningful use (MU) as outlined in the HITECH Act, an increasing number of health care professionals are utilizing EHRs to care for patients and to track patient outcomes at the point of care (HITECH Programs and Advisory Committee, 2009). There is a direct correlation between increasing EHR implementations and increased electronic data. Electronic data collected from EHRs are placed in three categories: quantitative data such as lab or pathology values (structured data), qualitative data such as text (unstructured data), and transactional data such as records of medication administration (Murdoch & Detsky, 2013). In addition to EHR data, separate databases are used in health care for research purposes, which are not necessarily integrated with the EHR. To provide a comprehensive clinical picture for patients, data from every source must be combined as health care providers use them, in real time.

With this emerging wealth of information, health care is beginning to identify how and where big data and advanced analytics can improve health care costs and help shape the reform of clinical patient care. In addition, big data analytics can serve to provide solutions in public health, such as the ability to predict future health care needs of a population or infectious disease outbreaks (Webster, 2014). Big data may also be used to improve disease detection by providing comprehensive information, trends, and comparisons that result in increased accuracy for initial diagnoses. This could result in reduced medical errors such as those resulting from misdiagnosis or omissions of care. These types of utilities for big data and advanced analytics could ultimately translate to improved patient outcomes and reduced costs. In addition, big data and cognitive computing analyses of data deliver information in "real time" to clinicians.

DATA MINING

Knowledge can be discovered by mining large data sets. In the era of gold mining there were three distinct phases of the process—prospecting for the vein, following the lode, and smelting of the ore into refined gold—so too there are three similar phases in data mining. Often, in the Gold Rush era, prospectors would find nuggets of coarse gold usually when a stream eroded a point of the vein and washed them downstream. Almost all the initial finds were by happenstance, and that is what led to major discoveries. In that era, thousands of tons of gold-containing material were leached to extract gold ore deposits that could then go to the smelter for refining and pouring into bullion bars.

In data mining, prospecting for the vein focuses on findings in the data—anomalies, correlations, patterns, or trends. Once these data nuggets are discovered, the focus is to mine the lode by determining trajectories that produce dimensionality that gives the data its characteristics features. This ultimately forms a picture of the data lode, which is a modeling function that has predictive or at least systematic valuation. Finally, the ore-rich material is smelted by removing variation and sorting causation to eliminate the noise in the data system. Here, dependencies of the data that are useful to clarifying and shaping the picture are used and graphic representations are often ways in which the data are portrayed.

Data Mining Defined

Historically, *data mining* has been defined in terms of mining data and information from large databases and is also associated with machine learning or advanced analytics techniques (Chen, Han, & Yu, 1996). *Data mining* is also defined as a method in computer science that is used to discover patterns and trends within large data sets. Data mining techniques contain many specialized classifications and subclassifications involving various methods that intersect with artificial intelligence, machine learning, statistics, and database systems (Chakrabarti et al., 2006; Clifton, 2014). In a classical work on data mining, Chen et al. (1996) classify the types of data mining in terms of the type of databases being mined, knowledge to be mined, and techniques to be utilized in mining.

Data Mining Techniques

There are a number of different techniques in data mining, which include anomaly detection, association rule learning, cluster analysis, classification, regression modeling, and summarization. All these techniques are associated with knowledge discovery within databases (Fayyad, Piatetsky-Shapiro, & Smyth, 1996). Table 26.1 reflects these techniques, definitions, and uses of these types of techniques in health care. Anomaly detection is used in public health to detect patterns and trends in disease outbreak (Wong, Moore, Cooper, & Wagner, 2002). This technique is used in some of the software used by the Centers for Disease Control and Prevention (CDC) for syndromic surveillance systems using emergency department (ED) data to detect disease outbreak from aberrations in the data (Henning, 2004). In addition, associations and relationships in health care data are often used to examine outcomes by examining relationships in variables, or they may be used in hierarchical data models. This type of data mining may also be

TABLE 26.1 Types of Data Mining Techniques		
Technique	Definition	Health Care Application
Anomaly detection	Pattern detection in identifying data errors or unusual deviation from the norm	Rule-based anomaly detection for detection of disease outbreaks
Association rule learning	Identifying association between variables	Identifies relationships in variables associated with an outcome of interest, can be preliminary work to predictive modeling
Cluster analysis	Discovering groups or structures in the data	Clusters of market segments on patient preferences by health care market
Classification	Generalizing known structure to new data or information	Classifying patient safety errors related to HIT can support taxonomy development
Regression modeling	Modeling data for prediction or explaining some phenomenon with the least amount of error as possible	Regression models are often used for predictive analytics such as predicting factors that are associated with mortality or 30-day readmissions
Summarization	Data aggregation or compacting information, including visualizations and report generation	Often used in BI tools to aggregate data in cubic views of data by category and by some outcome measure

BI, business intelligence; HIT, health information technology.

Source: Fayyad et al. (1996).

a preliminary step to building predictive models to examine variables that are predictive of some outcome of interest. The regression models fall into this type of category of data mining, but a process of association rules learning may be a first step in the process. Cluster analysis discovers groups or structures in the data, such as clusters of patients who tend to go to one hospital in a given zip code or county. Summarization is used in many of our business intelligence (BI) tools that aggregate cubic views of data or report certain outcomes. These data mining summarization tools allow an end user to drag and drop and quickly identify patterns and trends in the data based on the summarization of tables. These tools often have data visualization capability to see graphic relationships in the data as well. Figure 26.4 demonstrates this capability with the IBM Cognos BI toolset.

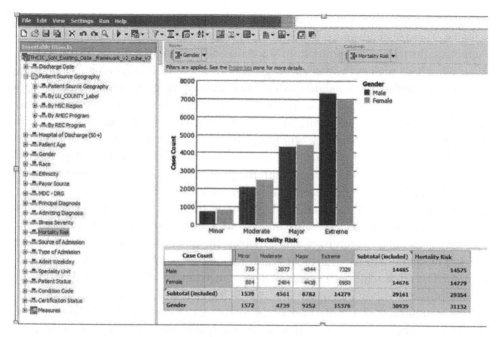

FIGURE 26.4. Data summarization BI tool.

BI, business intelligence.

Source: McBride (2012).

Advanced Data Mining Tools

There are new tools entering the market that are available in open sources that combine all these methods into one product. The IBM modeler is an example of this type of tool. According to IBM, this tool offers "an extensive predictive analytics platform that is designed to bring predictive intelligence to decisions made by individuals, groups, systems and the enterprise" (IBM, 2015). This tool combines many of the techniques noted earlier, in addition to text analyzers, data optimization tools, Bayesian and neural network compilers, chi-square automatic interaction detection (CHAID) and advanced 3D data visualization capabilities. Animation coupled with $360 \times 360 \times 360$ free rotation of visualizations greatly enhance the ability to detect subtle patterns and anomalies of interest. The IBM modeler and other similar advanced data mining tools are capable of visualizing the higher order dimensions in complex data by displaying them in the lower order dimensions of three-dimensional (3D) space. The centroids and vector sum products of n-dimensional distributions are usually invisible in terms of graphic visualization techniques that are available in common statistical suite software such as SAS, SPSS, Stata, and others. In contrast, the highly advanced graphics visualization engines of the IBM modeler and other similarly dedicated and highly specialized data mining applications not only display those hyper-dimensions as a default but also allow them to be displayed and manipulated in multiple types of graphics (3D-animated scatter plots, multidimensional Trellis arrays, multidimensional heat maps, and multidimensional probability density gradient topological maps). Visualization and manipulation of ordination in higher dimensions of data is a hallmark of data mining and a core skill of the data scientist. These über advanced exploration capabilities are what place data mining in its own class, distinct and separate from standard and archaic hypothesis testing mathematical methods such as the parametric general linear model of regression. Data mining does not ever replace the standard models, but it serves to enhance, support, and expand their application to the newly discovered phenomena that data mining techniques bring to first light. Dedicated data mining suites, such as the IBM modeler, make it possible to automate the discovery process by running the same dependent (target) variable against all available independent (predictors of the target) variables, by sample testing multiple serial predictive models of the target with the predictors, with every appropriate mathematical model available, depending on the declared level of measure (categorical, ordinal, or scale) and role (target, predictor, and both) of the entire list of variables in the data set. For a complex data set with multiple millions of rows of data observations and multiple thousands of columns of data variables, the process can take days to complete. The key resultant output of this process is a short list of the top 10 to 20 predictive modeling methods that achieved a viable model, arranged in list of best to worst in terms of scoring predictor importance, given the target being predicted, as defined when the automation is initialized. Generally, each of the top three or four models will echo the findings of each other, but each may show a completely different synoptic view of the data. The top five models may be factor analysis, cluster analysis, binary logistic regression, chi-square-automatic-interaction-detection (CHAID) analysis, and a neural network of the predicted target variable, using a similar subset of independent predictor variables. Across all five models, the list of independent variables in the models will almost always agree (with some minor variations) in terms of predictor importance. Corroboration of the same predictors across multiple different modeling methods is also a key feature that sets data mining apart from more traditional analytical approaches that focus on one method as superior to all, with subsequent rejection of any consideration of alternate methods as being applicable to development of valid and reliable predictive models that demonstrate high degrees of sensitivity, specificity, positive predictive value, and negative predictive value.

The KNIME (Konstanz Information Miner) tool is an example of an open source product that is based on the R statistical package. This analytics platform is a leading open-source platform that is downloadable from the KNIME website: www.knime.org/knime. According to the website, "KNIME, pronounced [naim], is a modern data analytics platform that allows an analyst to perform sophisticated statistics and data mining on data sets to analyze trends and predict potential results." It also has a visual workbench that combines data access, data transformation, initial investigation, powerful predictive analytics, and visualization. Figure 26.5 reflects how this workbench appears to the end user with an ability to drag and drop for managing the workflow of the data, transforming the data, and ultimately mining the data set.

SAS Enterprise Miner is yet another very sophisticated data mining tool available in the commercial market. This tool, similar to the IBM tool, has the ability to provide descriptive and predictive analytics to find patterns and trends hidden within health care data sets (SAS Institute, n.d.). All three of these tools noted earlier have the ability to manage data within workflows similar to the one noted in Figure 26.5.

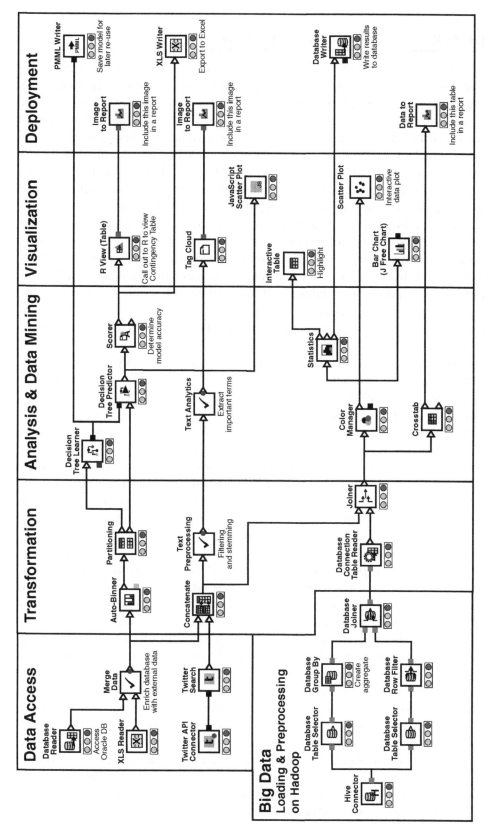

FIGURE 26.5. KNIME workbench and data workflow.

Source: www.knime.org/knime

THE ROLE OF THE DATA SCIENTIST

A new and emerging role in the health care industry is the advanced analytics profes-sional who is capable of managing and analyzing massive amounts of data and using the techniques and tools noted earlier. The average health care analyst is not capable of fully understanding and managing these types of tools and techniques without special training and a solid foundation in statistics. The *Harvard Business Review* used the term "data scientist" to describe the competencies required as "part hacker, part analyst, part communicator" (Davenport & Patil, 2012, p. 16). The job of the data scientist is focused on using analytics to solve problems, and the data scientist has the competencies to understand how to "fish out answers to important business questions from today's tsu-nami of unstructured information" (Davenport & Patil, 2012, p. 73). In this review, the case of the analysts who developed the "People You May Know" feature on Facebook is used as an example of this new skill required to support the management and analysis of big data. It is indicated that these new roles are required to exploit vast new flows of information for transforming industries (Davenport & Patil, 2012). It is further indi-cated that the rush to capitalize on these types of data is likely to face human capital constraints because of a significant lack of individuals adequately trained to work on big data and these data mining techniques and tools.

So, what does a data scientist look like and what type of work does he or she actually do? The Baylor Scott & White health care system, in their Dallas, Texas facility, has implemented a data mining lab and utilizes the IBM modeler to determine patterns and trends in the health care enterprise data. The data scientist who has oversight of this lab and helps train other analysts and researchers to utilize the tool is a master's-prepared nursing informaticist with extensive training in statistics, computer science, and biomed-ical and clinical informatics and has a solid base as a mathematician. Richard Gilder is noted in Figure 26.6 at the Baylor Scott & White health care system data mining labo-ratory. Mr. Gilder, who is a data scientist and coauthor of this chapter, is shown in front of projections of data mining graphics; he notes patterns and trends and has the ability to use data mining tools to visualize these patterns.

A typical week in the life of a data scientist is similar to driving in heavy rush-hour traffic in a major city: unpredictable. The various health care projects that the data scientist works on could be compared to traffic lanes, where many projects run simultaneously in parallel. Each project has its own lane, and each vehicle in that project convoy car-ries the next milestone in the project. It is only when the entire convoy rests safely in the parking lot after the last milestone has been passed that the objectives have been achieved or surpassed and the project is considered a success. But as we all know, every-thing can be rolling along smoothly in both directions and in all lanes on the express-way, and suddenly with no warning, a vehicle has a blowout and has to pull off to the side of the road. This event has a ripple effect on the overall traffic pattern in both directions, is disruptive, and always causes problems. In data mining, something similar happens as a direct result of the data mining process itself, and although it can be very disruptive to the normal flow of things in the health care environment where the process is occur-ring, ultimately, it is generally a very positive event with measurable outcomes such as numbers of lives saved, numbers of preventable adverse events avoided, numbers of patients returning to normal function sooner rather than later, and amounts of money

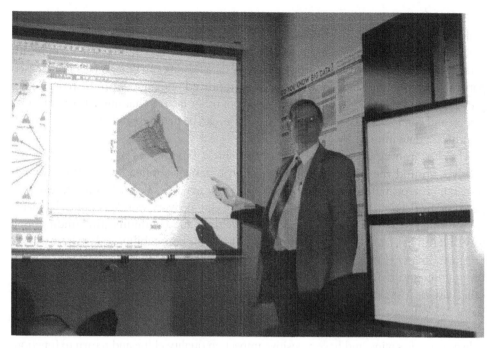

FIGURE 26.6. Baylor Scott and White data scientist and contributing author Richard Gilder in a data mining lab demonstrating some of the work done in the lab.

spent more efficiently and wisely in keeping with good stewardship, rather than inadvertently wasted through lack of timely enterprise-wide situational awareness. The chief scientific scope of work that the health care data scientist works under is known as translational research. The Baylor Scott and White Data Mining Laboratory (DML) supports the aims of translational research, supporting biomedical informatics science with state-of-the-science analytical capabilities, in an interdisciplinary collaborative environment. Translation of vast and complex data into actionable information resulting in evidence-based practices with outcomes of improved safety and quality of life is the primary mission. The DML serves as a resource to the community of health care sciences research. Translational research aspires to "re-use data" (Schaffer, 2008). Data mining requires removal of barriers around isolated data known as data silos. Data governance models within organizations can streamline and organize the removal of restrictions and barriers around data silos through hierarchical administrative oversight that trumps the subordinate individual departmental and service-line restrictions around data sources and data objects. Data mining requires data governance. Capturing and meaningfully using the data artifact stream that is constantly generated by the process of health care delivery in the environment-specific context of care is what the science of translational research aspires to do in health care data mining. The chief aim of health care data mining is identification and delivery of actionable insights to the frontline health care provider, sooner rather than later. Successful application of the data mining process to the vast, rich, complex, and chaotic streaming mixture of information-signal and artifact-noise characteristics of health care data is self-sustaining as a result of a dramatically increased demand for data mining services. Clinically significant MU of the information-signal characteristic to modulate the health care delivery process in a timely and efficient manner toward improvement, safety, and optimization for all involved, and especially the patient and the patient's family, is the heart and soul of data mining science in health care. The cost savings that result from successful data mining can be significant. Increased patient and family satisfaction resulting from improved outcomes with the reduction of preventable adverse events, and identification of other factors that impact patient satisfaction and comfort, such as environmental noise, can be detected and measured through health care data mining.

The data mining process that the data scientist experiences on an everyday basis revolves around the linchpin of MU through practical applications of translational research. The primary operational objectives of the science of translational research as practiced by data scientists in the practical health care delivery world of clinical biomedical informatics are consolidating, validating, vetting, and communicating findings in a way that can be clearly understood by those with the accountability and authority to act on them, in a safe, timely, effective, efficient, equitable, and patient-centered manner. Production and delivery of actionable insight from valuable information that would otherwise be lost as noise, confusion, and missed opportunities for improvement is the scope of work for data mining endeavors in general. In a health care data mining operation, the results of delivering actionable insight to frontline practitioners of health care delivery are life saving and have a positive impact on quality of life and return to function, which are, after all, the overarching objectives of all health care delivery.

The following illustration is provided as an example of the actual output that resulted from a typical DML project involving the public domain data provided by the CDC consisting of national birth certificate form data from more than four million birth certificate forms that were filled out in the year 2010 in the United States. The project described next requires the data scientist to perform the functions of the data mining process, and the example serves as a stepwise walk through essential cross-functional elements of the data mining process.

The problem. Every project is designed to solve a problem, and the problem for this project was that the desired analytical data set was only available for download, as an unparsed, flat text file of four million records. Let us consider that even for a modern high-end gaming machine, four million records (rows) containing 234 variables (columns) pose a severe and computationally intense challenge to even successfully open such a file in a text-editing application, such as Microsoft Word, without crashing the computer in the process. The processing time to just open and view a file such as this could take 30 to 90 minutes, and editing could take multiple hours per "find and replace" operation.

Extraction of the data from the birth certificates was the first step in the data mining process. This step was performed by the CDC. Everyone would agree that the process of filling out a birth certificate form when more than four million babies were born in the United States during 2010 was a small, but tedious part of the process of care at the point of care. The data entered into those forms, the data capture, are representative of the constant stream of data artifacts generated simply by performing the process of care. Intentionally capturing and extracting those 234 critical variables, including Apgar scores, resulted in data that could potentially be archived and made available for manipulation into normalized (observation per row and variable per column) formats for exploration and data mining far after the fact. This is also representative of the vast universe of health care data that has yet to be explored and mined for its rare and precious values. The U.S. government, through the CDC, extracted the data from each of more than four million birth certificates and aggregated the data into a single text file per birth year. Detailed instructions for the file architecture were supplied on the publicly available CDC website along with the data, and this allowed the next step in the process to be executed.

Transformation of the raw unparsed data into a normalized data set was the next step. The data set was transformed into 234 columns consisting of more than four million records, in which each row of data is equivalent to one birth certificate, and each column contains, in order, the information from each of the 234 unique fields where data were entered into the birth certificate. The data dictionary supplied field length, format, and level of measure definitions and nomenclature for each of the 234 variables.

Loading the transformed data file into a Structured Query Language (SQL) database was the next step required for further manipulation. Convenient archival storage of normalized format data renders multiple data objects of similar data formats readily available and accessible as data objects that can be included at multiple nodes in an automated stream of stored algorithms and procedures. Data mining an entire data warehouse can be performed by merging variables from multiple data objects that would otherwise never appear in the same analytical data set. Detection of subtle, yet significant patterns, anomalies, and trends through data mining algorithms is accomplished in this manner.

Exploration of the data in the IBM modeler was the next step in the data mining process when applied to the CDC birth certificate data, and the top predictive model indicated that variation in the Apgar score was a good candidate for a target variable that was being predicted and explained by several key fields in the birth certificate data. The initial CHAID (Chi-square Automatic Interaction Detector) models (Figure 26.7) indicated that an Apgar score of 7 or less was significantly higher in mothers with 36 weeks or less of gestation. A binary logistic regression (Figure 26.8) of Apgar 7 or less = 1 (yes), else = 0 (no) was manually developed based on the suggested CHAID model. The results of the trimmed model are shown next.

Conclusions and summary of the birth certificate data mining project are described next. Although the findings are not specifically actionable at a given hospital, state, or other location, some general patterns emerge for careful consideration for future research. This is also a function of the data mining process in that quite often more questions are created compared with answers delivered. The CHAID model shows the interactions among the father's age, estimated gestation, birth weight, and primary C-section delivery in terms of how they interact with each other in proportion to the target variable of Apgar 7 or less. The binary logistic regression model shows the odds ratio (the probability that Apgar is 7 or less) independently predicted by each variable in the model. According to the models, those 244,676 babies who were less than 36 weeks of gestation had 13.9% Apgar 7 or less compared with the 2,368,755 babies with more than 36 weeks of gestation who had 2.6% Apgar less than 7. This difference in Apgar 7 or less was statistically significant at $p < 0.000$, higher than 99% confidence. The odds ratio for gestation that was 36 weeks or less was 3.314, and it was also significant at better than 99% confidence. Simply stated, babies in this model with less than 36 weeks of gestation at birth were at a 313% higher risk for having a 5-minute Apgar of 7 or less. Similar statements can be made for all the variables in the model. In comparing the two models, the pattern that emerged revealed that the higher the odds ratio on the predictor variable,

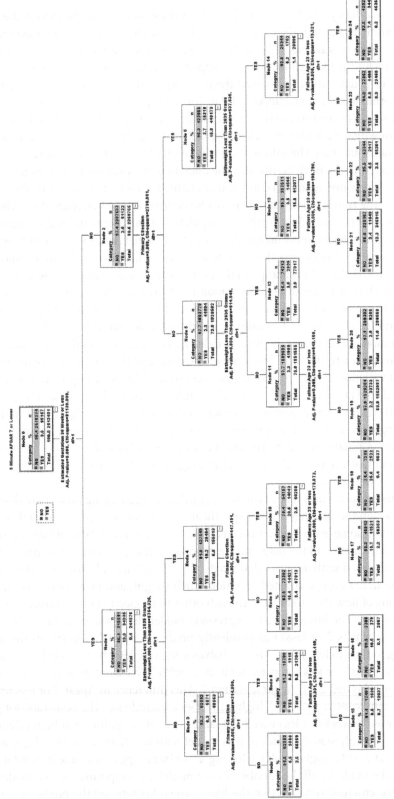

FIGURE 26.7. CHAID tree diagram.

Omnibus Tests of Model Coefficients

		Chi-square	df	Sig.
Step 1	Step	63724.554	4	.000
	Block	63724.554	4	.000
	Model	63724.554	4	.000

Model Summary

Step	-2 Log likelihood	Cox & Snell R Square	Nagelkerke R Square
1	753571.419a	.024	.090

a. Estimation terminated at iteration number 6 because parameter estimates changed by less than .001.

Classification Table a

			Predicted		
			APGAR_LTET7 5 Minute APGAR 7 or Lower		Percentage Correct
Observed			0 NO	1 YES	
Step 1	APGAR_LTET7 5 Minute	0 NO	2144733	373541	85.2
	APGAR 7 or Lower	1 YES	53648	41509	43.6
	Overall Percentage				83.7

a. The cut value is .038

Variables in the Equation

		B	S.E.	Wald	df	Sig.	Exp(B)
Step 1a	FATHERS_AGE_LTET_23	.240	.009	773.086	1	.000	1.271
	EstGestation_LTET_36	1.198	.010	14478.433	1	.000	3.314
	Birthweight_LTET2635	.823	.010	6697.506	1	.000	2.277
	PrimaryCsection	.421	.007	3229.011	1	.000	1.523
	Constant	-3.820	.005	612829.237	1	.000	.022

a. Variable(s) entered on step 1: FATHERS_AGE_LTET_23, EstGestation_LTET_36, Birthweight_LTET2635, PrimaryCsection.

FIGURE 26.8. Binary logistic regression model.

the higher it shows up in the branching of the CHAID decision tree. Father's age of 23 years or less is in the lowest of the tree branches, and it is the lowest in the odds ratio at 1.27. Babies born to fathers who are 23 years or less are at a 27% higher risk of having a 5-minute Apgar of 7 or less. These findings apply only to this data modeling exercise and could only become specifically actionable through additional analysis that would include data that are obviously missing from this data set, such as where the delivery occurred and what provider(s) were involved in management of the pregnancy. This is also an example of how data mining can inadvertently invoke controversy, and when working with data that include patient, physician, nurse, and vendor names, data mining and its findings can become extremely sensitive. A final note is that odds ratios are exponents. When all variables in the binary logistic equation are significant, they are independently predictive. Independently predictive factors can be combined, and to combine exponents, one has to multiply. Therefore, the 2,522 babies in Node 18 of the CHAID diagram who were less than 36 weeks of gestation, less than 2,635 grams of birth weight, primary C-section delivery, and born to fathers aged 23 years or less were $(3.314 \times 2.277 \times 1.523 \times 1.271)$ 14.2 times more likely to have a 5-minute Apgar of 7 or less. They were at a 1,420% higher risk of 5-minute Apgar of 7 or less. Now imagine what could happen in health care if more data mining were applied to our own regions and our own hospitals, if findings similar to these applied to patients at a higher than usual risk, and within days of appearance of a measurable risk factor that was specifically actionable? Identification of populations at risk is a best practice use case for the meaningful use of data facilitated by application of advanced data mining science to health care data. Creative and imaginative discovery of new knowledge will benefit patients and providers of care, through the science of health care data mining. This is what drives and sustains health care data mining activities and the advanced practice specialty of nursing informatics (NI).

SOFTWARE FOR ADVANCED DATA MINING ANALYTICS

There are many new advances in software for managing and analyzing big data, with unique challenges in both areas. Although this chapter does not cover a depth of products on this topic, we examine one example of a tool to depict how powerful these tools can be to the health care industry. There are a number of software packages arising in the market and in open sources to manage and analyze large volumes of data constituting big data in terms of the 3Vs, including unstructured data. One of these projects was launched by IBM in 2011. Recognizing the value as well as the challenges that big data present, IBM unveiled a cognitive computing system known as "Watson" into the world of technology. What makes Watson unique is that it is "trained to learn, based on interactions and outcomes" presented to the system (IBM Corporate, 2013a). This unique system, patterned after the human brain, has the ability not only to think but also to learn and, as such, reflects a domain of informatics referred to as "artificial intelligence." Watson uses Natural Language Processing (NLP) to process both structured and unstructured data. With this capability, cognitive computing technology can rapidly analyze large masses of data, generate insights not attainable by traditional analytics, and produce "actionable responses" based on evidence (Ventana Research, 2013). Succinctly put, cognitive systems can utilize big data to think and learn, thus processing information much faster than a human while identifying patterns, trends, and evidence-based solutions.

With approximately 80% of all health care data categorized as unstructured, this application will offer health care a tool that would assimilate valuable patient information housed in the EHR with more comprehensive analytics utilizing these additional data (Grimes, 2008). Through the power of NLP and cognitive computing, both structured and unstructured data are brought together in real time, offering clinicians trends, treatment recommendations, analysis, and quality of evidence (Malin, 2013).

WellPoint, Inc. has recently begun using IBM Watson for utilization management of evidence-based decisions by nurses to improve the quality of health care decisions (IBM Corporate, 2013b). IBM Corporate (2013a) has also been working with Memorial Sloan Kettering using IBM Watson in the field of oncology. MD Anderson Cancer Center (2013) is working with IBM to bring Watson into the clinical environment that is aimed at improving patient outcomes and advancing research discoveries. The New York Genome Center (2014) has partnered with IBM Watson in hopes of accelerating genomic medicine advances specifically for patients with glioblastoma. Because cognitive system technology is cutting edge, with its debut as recent as 2011, there is limited literature on its proven value. Health care is just beginning to identify the potential value and opportunities that cognitive computer systems technology will bring to patients, clinicians, and the bottom line.

With the increasing costs and demands in health care, the industry is in need of such tools to integrate advanced clinical decision support into tools that have the potential to aid the health care team in decision making, particularly when combined with the data from the EHR. To be effective, cognitive computing systems must first learn the information, be tested on the accuracy of what has been learned (validation), and then finally be integrated into the workflow of the health care setting. Once implemented, users begin to recognize the potential impact that these types of tools can have on quality measures and processes, such as patient wait times, treatment recommendations, preventative measures, staff efficiencies, and redesign of workflows. Using a cognitive computing system in conjunction with the EHR has the potential to improve patient care and outcomes, increase efficiency, and decrease costs. It is important to note, however, that to support big data analytics and new applications, an appropriate platform is required within the organization that provides workflow and standardized processes.

Cognitive Computing Programs for Oncology Research

With an estimated 1.7 million new cancer diagnoses in the United States in 2014 (American Cancer Society, 2014), oncology health care and research stands poised to make tremendous progress by using cognitive computing tools. Malin (2013) indicates that we are on the "cusp of transformational change" by harnessing the power of big data, advanced computer applications, and analytics. Using tools, such as the IBM Watson software, in a clinical setting will allow oncology providers the ability to review treatment options for a patient, retrieve and analyze all clinical information, view all peer-reviewed clinical articles of evidence, generate a hypothesis, and recommend weighted treatments. With this type of power and knowledge in an oncology setting, IBM Watson offers the potential to accelerate research, enhance patient care, and integrate both research and care (MD Anderson Cancer Center, 2013). Watson will assist researchers in advancing novel therapies and offering clinicians a more comprehensive view of each cancer patient.

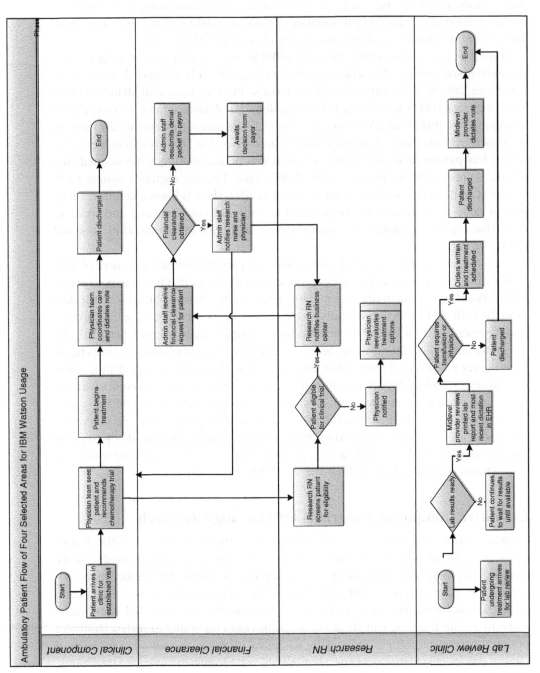

FIGURE 26.9. Basic workflow table.

Ultimately, applications, such as IBM Watson, will lead to improved patient outcomes and personalized patient care plans that are powered by big data analytics (IBM Corporate, 2013a).

A Clinical Case Utilizing IBM Watson

IBM Watson was introduced into an ambulatory oncology patient care setting to determine the effect on workflow and efficiencies. In preparation for this implementation, a project charter and a logic model were created to provide the necessary structure and direction needed for the pilot of IBM Watson, and to ensure a mechanism was in place to appropriately assess the effectiveness of this tool. A SWOT (strengths, weaknesses, opportunities, threats) analysis was completed followed by the creation of project timelines and action plans. Four areas were identified for use of IBM Watson for patient care in conjunction with the institution's EHR. Current workflows for each of the areas were captured and then validated by the institution's Office of Performance Improvement. Industrial engineers from the Office of Performance Improvement provided time measurements for each component of the workflows. This provided the baseline metrics for each of the different areas in conjunction with the current workflows. A total of 22 "touch points" on the various workflows where IBM Watson could be used were identified for the four areas prior to utilization. A total of 49 staff members and clinicians were oriented and trained on the use of IBM Watson. Approximately 30 days after implementation, the workflows and time measurements were re-examined and reviewed to identify any workflow differences and/or changes in time required to complete tasks (Figure 26.9).

This project presented a unique opportunity to utilize Lean concepts in conjunction with a project charter that focused on workflow redesign. According to Graban (2012, p. 17), "Lean is both a tool set and a management system, a method for continuous improvement and employee engagement, an approach that allows us to solve the problems that are important to us as leaders and as an organization." Baseline workflows and time metrics were initially captured in all four areas. Because Lean is also a time-based approach, any decrease in delays would be captured, resulting in improved quality and lower costs.

Ethical Considerations

As a nursing leader, reflecting on the Lean project charter for the Watson project revealed the following potential ethical considerations.

- ▶ Potential delays in patient care delivery during the implementation of the new workflow may occur.

- ▶ With new workflow that incorporates a new tool, there will be possible resistance from staff and inconsistencies of daily processes for those who do not embrace the change willingly.

- ▶ Some patient information will be housed in a "cloud." Although this is secured and has been endorsed by institutional compliance, there is the potential risk for patient medical information to be unprotected.

- ▶ Financial clearance obtained by using IBM Watson-generated evidence may not result in reimbursement.

▶ Although IBM Watson has been tested and has undergone clinical validation, there is the potential for inaccuracies caused by NLP interpretation.

▶ By using this tool, evidence-based treatment decisions will be prioritized for the health care professional to review. A potential ethical issue will be the approach that the clinician will now use. Will this replace or alter the clinician's decision?

Procedures

An education module was utilized for orientation. This module included content on IBM Watson and its potential for use, where the tool would be used and how, and the need to continue teaching the system by providing feedback. One-hour hands-on training sessions were conducted for the health care team members. A total of 49 staff members attended orientation and training. The number of individuals trained was as follows: seven physicians, eight research RNs, six fellows, 14 clinical RNs, seven MLPs (midlevel practitioners comprised of advanced practice nurses and physician assistants), and six business center staff. On completion of the training module, access was granted to the system through Google Chrome using institutionally approved security. Written instructions and tutorial videos were also made available to the staff as well as to on-site IBM staff members during week 1; three physicians who had been intimately involved in teaching and training IBM Watson volunteered to begin using the tool in clinic. This was followed by the use of the tool, respectively, by business center staff, clinical nurses, additional physicians, research nurses, MLPs, and fellows. Throughout the 30 days, two support staff members were present in the clinic to provide support and address any issues. Weekly discussions were held with the physicians, and impromptu discussions were held with the remaining clinic staff.

After approximately 30 days, the performance improvement team was scheduled to return to the clinic. Clinical staff members were informed several days prior to the team's arrival to ensure cooperation during the observation and time measurements as well as to minimize any disruptions in the clinic flow. During the preimplementation workflow, a total of eight physician clinics were observed. For the postimplementation remeasurement, only four of the original physicians observed were utilizing IBM Watson; thus, only four clinics were included in the clinical component. From the initial workflow diagrams, the performance improvement team was provided a list of touch points to re-evaluate the four areas. The number of touch points for the four areas totaled 22. For the clinical component, there were nine areas of remeasurement; for the financial clearance, there were six touch points; and for the research nurses and MLPs, there were three touch points for each component.

Workflow and Data Analysis

A postimplementation workflow evaluation with time measurements was completed by the performance improvement team after the fourth week of the IBM Watson implementation. Sufficient data were collected from the financial and clinical component from pre- and postimplementation touch points to perform an analysis. Using the midpoint salaries for this clinic's city and area, the hourly wage and hourly fringe benefits were calculated.

Initial findings demonstrated efficiencies by using IBM Watson in providing financial clearance for patients in both time and dollars. On an annual basis, approximately 725 hours of time are expected to be gained by utilizing IBM Watson in this environment. This equates to approximately $36,813 in cost savings for this one clinic. For the clinical component, approximately 253 hours of time spent by physicians and their assistants in providing patient care for oncology patients may be saved annually by using IBM Watson in this clinical setting. This equates to approximately $31,337 in annual savings based on preliminary results of this analysis. The use of IBM Watson actually added a small amount of time for the physicians and their assistants when previewing the patient, as each clinician was using both the EHR and Watson. However, a significant amount of time was saved for clinicians during the patient assessment and during treatment planning for the patient.

Nursing Resistance to New Tools

During the reevaluation, neither the research nurses nor the clinical nurses used IBM Watson while caring for patients in the clinic. Although both sets of nurses had received training that had been reinforced in the clinical setting, the nurses had chosen not to use this tool in the course of their daily routines. Feedback explanations from the clinical nurses for not utilizing IBM Watson were as follows: (a) too busy to try something different or new, (b) lack of understanding on its value, (c) no specific instructions on when to use it, and (d) it had discrepancies from information in the EHR. Although these considerations warrant further investigation, there are implications for improvement to the educational training.

The performance improvement team was unable to observe the MLPs' use of IBM Watson for either the lab review component or the research component. Both the MLPs and research nurses who were granted access were unavailable for observation and unresponsive to repeated requests to shadow them. Time constraints resulting from patient care assignments were the primary reasons given for lack of participation in the re-evaluation after implementation. Two research nurses were interviewed to obtain feedback and estimates of how IBM Watson would affect the screening of patients for clinical trial eligibility. The lack of participation by clinical and research nurses demonstrates the need for additional education and understanding for nurses on informatics, big data, and analytics. The reluctance or fear in trying new technology in clinical practice was also a factor that must be addressed and overcome. There is also a component of fear in change of role or usefulness that may have contributed to the research nurses' lack of participation in re-evaluation. Watson's potential to quickly screen a patient for clinical trial eligibility may be perceived as a career or workflow threat.

The analysis completed indicates that utilizing IBM Watson in conjunction with the EHR facilities results in increased efficiency for the clinicians and financial clearance staff through cost savings that may equate to improved patient outcomes. Clearly, workflow is affected by the use of this powerful tool; however, this is just the beginning. Although touch points were identified in each area, these are initial starting points as to how workflow can be affected. With the abilities of IBM Watson to provide treatment recommendations, patient summaries that include adverse events and predictability models, and evidence to support clinical trial recommendations, many aspects of patient care are predicted to demonstrate improved patient outcomes.

Based on the experiences of the author with this tool, components that are essential to ensuring success are as follows:

- ▶ Accurate and continuous monitoring
- ▶ Education and re-education
- ▶ Ongoing and continuous communication
- ▶ Buy-in from leadership
- ▶ Champions for every role
- ▶ Sustainability and evaluation plan

Lessons learned from this implementation were the lack of nursing and MLP champions in the clinical setting. Although clinical leadership was supportive, nurses and MLPs were both concerned about the negative impact (more time) that use of the tool would cause and confused as to how it would help them at present. Greater clarification should have occurred to explain the potential uses and purpose of IBM Watson.

Performing the postimplementation evaluation after 60 or 90 days would have most likely yielded more data and increased utilization by staff. For the financial clearance area, there were only data on five out of the six touch points; whereas for the clinical component, there were data on only four out of 10 touch points. Finally, further evaluation is needed with expanded intervals of time with implications on the importance of nursing education and buy-in. Having greater than 30 days would have allowed staff the opportunity to identify other areas for potentially using IBM Watson.

Most important, however, the use of IBM Watson in this clinical setting showed a savings of an estimated 1,895 hours annually. The dollar savings equated to these hours is estimated to be $110,453 for this one center in three areas. This supports the goals of the Triple Aim and indicates that utilization of advanced analytics, such as cognitive computing, results in efficiencies and cost savings.

IMPORTANCE OF ADVANCED PRACTICE NURSING TO OPERATIONALIZE ADVANCED ANALYTIC TOOLS

To harness the power of tools, such as IBM Watson, an appropriate platform in health care must be built. This platform must eliminate silos and provide interfaces for all databases to the big data. It must also be able to standardize and streamline processes across the health care environment to ensure continuity. For health care, this will require an enormous cultural shift and innovative approaches that include mobile access for both health care providers and patients. Re-evaluation of processes and workflows, as well as the data flow of information surrounding patient care, diagnostic, and intervention decisions, will be required to support these advances in technology and analytics.

Nursing is a primary stakeholder and a major participant within interprofessional teams for utilizing and benefiting from the use of big data, analytics, and cognitive systems such as IBM Watson. With the need to decrease costs in health care, nurses are a component of the interprofessional team needed for identifying opportunities to standardize, streamline, add value, identify inefficiencies, and improve the patient experience (IOM, 2010).

Nursing leaders are poised to lead initiatives involving big data analytic projects and adoption of implementation teams. As primary stakeholders in health care, nurses need to be at the decision-making table. Cognitive computing systems, such as IBM Watson, have the potential to transform health care with improved efficiencies and reduced costs that ultimately lead to better patient outcomes. The results from the Watson project demonstrate the feasibility and positive impact that cognitive computing tools can have on a clinical setting. The use of advanced analytics will face challenges in the health care environment with implications for nursing practice. As health care becomes more big data driven, we need to focus on overcoming the barriers that technology represents for nursing and embrace the value that it brings to caring for our patients. It is also important to note that the workflow redesign and data collection were conceived, organized, facilitated, and orchestrated by a nursing leader. This further illustrates that nursing leaders need to be both competent and confident in using and understanding advanced technology. It is vital to the advancement of the nursing profession and for improving the outcomes of our patients.

SUMMARY

We have discussed the concept of big data, defining what constitutes big data and their various uses across industries. In addition, we have discussed how big data are being used in the health care industry in innovative new ways, which include data mining techniques. These data mining techniques and tools have been reviewed in depth. To make full use of these tools, new and emerging roles will be needed, including that of the data scientist. This advanced analytic role is examined, and a "day in the life" of a data scientist is described. Finally, we have discussed a case study of the IBM Watson tool being used in a large cancer center in Texas to fully realize the transformation changes that these types of tools can provide to the nation to help realize the Triple Aim of improving care, reducing cost, and addressing population health.

EXERCISES AND QUESTIONS FOR CONSIDERATION

Let us consider the content covered with respect to the IBM Watson use case deploying cognitive computing software in an oncology unit for support of clinical and research purposes, and reflect on the following questions:

1. What are the big data under consideration in this scenario and how do you see those data being used by IBM Watson to generate value?

2. In the use case, there were resisters to change and new tools. How might the organization have mitigated that resistance?

3. What lessons can we glean from this case related to use of new and emerging technologies related to staff resistance?

4. What roles do you see the advanced practice nurse playing within the use case discussed and what implications do these roles have to the future of nursing?

REFERENCES

American Cancer Society. (2014). *Cancer facts and figures 2014*. Retrieved from http://www.cancer .org/acs/groups/content/@research/documents/webcontent/acspc-042151.pdf

Chakrabarti, S., Ester, M., Fayyad, U., Gehrke, J., Han, J., Morishita, S., . . . Wang, W. (2006). *Data mining curriculum: A proposal (version 1.0)*. Retrieved from www.kdd.org/curriculum/index.html

Chen, M., Han, J., & Yu, P. S. (1996). Data mining: An overview from a database perspective. *IEEE Transactions on Knowledge and Data Engineering*, 8(6), 866–883. doi:10.1109/69.553155

Clifton, C. (2014). *Data mining*. Retrieved from www.britannica.com/EBchecked/topic/1056150/ data-mining

Davenport, T. H., & Patil, D. J. (2012). *Data scientist: The sexiest job of the 21st century*. Retrieved from www.hbr.org/2012/10/data-scientist-the-sexiest-job-of-the-21st-century

Executive Office of the President Council of Economic Advisers. (2009). *The economic case for health care reform*. Retrieved from www.whitehouse.gov/administration/eop/cea/TheEconomicCaseforHealth CareReform

Fayyad, U., Piatetsky-Shapiro, G., & Smyth, P. (1996). From data mining to knowledge discovery in databases. *American Association for Artificial Intelligence*, 17(3), 37–54. doi:www.dx.doi.org/10.1609/ aimag.vl7i3.1230

Fluckinger, D., (2014, June). *Karen DeSalvo, M. D., discusses health data analytics, much more*. Retrieved from www.searchhealthit.techtarget.com/feature/Karen-DeSalvo-MD-discusses-health-data- analytics-much-more

Gartner Inc. (2013). *Big data*. Retrieved from www.gartner.com/it-glossary/big-data

Graban, M. (2012). *Lean hospitals: Improving quality, patient safety, and employee engagement* (2nd ed.). Boca Raton, FL: CRC Press.

Grimes, S. (2008). *Unstructured data and the 80 percent rule*. Retrieved from www.breakthrough analysis.com/2008/08/01/unstructured-data-and-the-80-percent-rule

Henning, K. J. (2004). Overview of syndromic surveillance: What is syndromic surveillance? *Morbidity and Mortality Weekly Report*, 53, 5–11.

HITECH Programs and Advisory Committee. (2009). *HITECH Act*. Retrieved from www.healthit.gov/ policy-researchers-implementers/hitech-programs-advisory-committees

IBM. (2015). *SPSS modeler*. Retrieved from www-01.ibm.com/software/analytics/spss/products/modeler

IBM Corporate. (2011). *IBM's smarter cities challenge: Syracuse*. Retrieved from http://smartercities challenge.org/city_syracuse_ny.html

IBM Corporate. (2013a). *IBM Watson: Next-generation cognitive system*. Retrieved from www.ibm.com/ innovation/us/watson

IBM Corporate. (2013b). *WellPoint, inc*. Retrieved from www.ibm.com/watson

Institute for Healthcare Improvement. (2015). *IHI triple aim initiative*. Retrieved from www.ihi.org/ Engage/Initiatives/TripleAim/Pages/default.aspx

Institute of Medicine. (2010). *The future of nursing: Leading change, advancing health*. Retrieved from http://iom.nationalacademies.org/Reports/2010/The-Future-of-Nursing-Leading-Change-Advanc- ing-Health.aspx

Institute of Medicine. (2013). *Best care at lower cost: The path to continuously learning health care in America*. Chapter 1, Introduction, and overview. Washington, DC: The National Academies Press.

Jee, K., & Kim, G. (2013). Potentiality of big data in the medical sector: Focus on how to reshape the healthcare system. *Healthcare Informatics Research, 19*(20), 79–85. doi:10.4258/hir.2013.19.2.79

Lund, S., Manyika, J., Nyquist, S., Mendonca, L., & Ramaswamy, S. (2013). *Game changers: Five opportunities for US growth and renewal*. McKinsey & Company. Retrieved from http://www.mckinsey.com/insights/americas/us_game_changers

Malin, J. (2013). Envisioning Watson as a rapid-learning system for oncology. *Journal of Oncology Practice, 9*(3), 155–157. doi:10.1200/JOP.2013.001021

Manyika, J., Chui, M., Bughin, J., Dobbs, R., Bisson, P., & Marrs, A. (2013). *Disruptive technologies: Advances that will transform life, business, and the global economy*. McKinsey Global Institute. Retrieved from http://www.mckinsey.com/search.aspx?q=Cray+computer.

Mayer-Schonberger, V., & Cukier, K. (2013). *Big data: A revolution that will transform how we live, work, and think*. New York, NY: Houghton Mifflin Harcourt.

McBride, S. (2012). *Use of state-level data by universities for improving patient safety, quality and population health*. Paper presented at the TIHCQE Conference, September 26, 2012, Lubbock, Texas.

McKinsey Global Institute. (2013). *Game changers: Five opportunities for U.S. growth and renewal*. Retrieved from http://www.mckinsey.com/insights/americas/us_game_changers

MD Anderson Cancer Center. (2013). *MD Anderson taps IBM Watson to power "moon shots."* Retrieved from http://www.mdanderson.org/newsroom/news-releases/2013/ibm-watson-to-power-moon-shots.html

Moore, K., Eyestone, K., & Coddington, D. (2013). The big deal about big data. *Healthcare Financial Management, 67*(8), 61–68. Retrieved from http://www.ncbi.nlm.nih.gov/pubmed/23957187

Murdoch, T., & Detsky, A. (2013). The inevitable application of big data to health care. *Journal of the American Medical Association, 309*(13), 1351–1352. doi:10.1001/jama.2013.393

Naisbitt, J. (1982). *Megatrends: Ten new directions transforming our lives*. New York, NY: Warner Books.

The New York Genome Center. (2014). Retrieved from http://www.nygenome.org/news/new-york-genome-center-ibm-watson-group-announce-collaboration-advance-genomic-medicine

Raghupathi, W., & Raghupathi, V. (2014). Big data analytics in healthcare: Promise and potential. *Health Information Science and Systems, 2*(3). doi:10.1186/2047-2501-2-3

SAS Institute. (n.d.). *SAS enterprise miner*. Retrieved from http://www.sas.com/en_us/software/analytics/enterprise-miner.html

Schaffer, E. (2008). *Translating translational research*. Retrieved from http://nih.gov/catalyst/2008/08.07.01/page01_translational.html

Scoop Staff. (2014). *Big data set to transform the world*. Retrieved from http://statescoop.com/big-data-set-transform-world

Sharma, A. (2011). *Big data demystified*. Retrieved from http://searchbusinessintelligence.techtarget.in/tip/Big-Data-demystified

Soares, S. (2015). *Big data integration and governance considerations for healthcare* (White Paper). Retrieved from https://tdwi.org/~/media/E0ADD3D3E5C641A78B3DAF61F984AD62.pdf

Ventana Research. (2013). *The potential of cognitive computer platforms. Sponsored by IBM* (Research Perspective). International Business Machine. Retrieved from http://www.ventanaresearch.com/research/whitePaperListing.aspx?tid=146

Webster, P. (2014). Analytics-driven health care growing in Ontario. *Canadian Medical Association Journal, 186*(2), 99. doi:10.1503/cmaj.109-4693

Wong, W., Moore, A., Cooper, G., & Wagner, M. (2002). *Rule-based anomaly pattern detection for detecting disease outbreaks.* Paper presented at the Eighteenth National Conference on Artificial Intelligence, AAAI-02. Retrieved from http://dl.acm.org/citation.cfm?id=777129

CHAPTER 27

Social Media: Ongoing Evolution in Health Care Delivery

Robert D. J. Fraser, Richard Booth,
Mari Tietze, and Susan McBride

OBJECTIVES

1. Provide explanation of the term *social media* and its relation to health and health care.

2. Outline key components and examples of social media services.

3. Discuss professional and interprofessional implications of social media.

4. Explain how practitioners can be engaged using social media.

5. Explore how social media will impact traditional informatics.

KEY WORDS

social media, network, knowledge transfer, knowledge mobilization, consumer health application

CONTENTS

INTRODUCTION

With the rise in both the power and availability of information and communication technology (ICT) over the past 2 decades, the world has witnessed revolutionary changes in how people connect, communicate, and share information. For instance, between 1997 and 2005, the percentage of Americans who reported using the Internet to search for health information rose from 41% to 80% (Rice, 2006) of the respective population. That roughly represents an increase from 46 million to 95 million people during that period (Fox, 2005). Corresponding with the increased use of the Internet for health purposes, the prevalence of broadband Internet connectivity and cellular technology also witnessed significant increases in availability and use by the U.S. population (Pew Internet & American Life Project, n.d.). These factors, combined with an emergence of new Internet technologies, afforded people the ability to dynamically interact with content and other users, fostering the rise of what is now known as Web 2.0. As Web 2.0 technologies became more standardized and embedded into all elements of the Internet after the turn of the millennium, a more meaningful neologism began to replace use of the word "Web 2.0" to describe this form of technology. The term *social media* spiked in popularity from 2009 to 2010 and has subsequently become a term used to denote not only specific Internet technology (e.g., Facebook, Twitter) but also the culture of sharing and exchange that these tools and technology afford. To date, a number of health care organizations in both the United States and abroad possess an active social media presence on the Internet. Table 27.1 outlines the total numbers of health care organizations that have a social media presence on various services, as tracked by Mayo Clinic's Center for Social Media (Mayo Clinic, 2014). Given the significant rise in popularity and use by health care organizations (and by society in general), it has become clear that social media is not a passing fad; rather, it is an ongoing and evolving evolution in communication, collaboration, and information exchange.

In its current iteration, social media tools and technology impact both individuals and organizations in various fashions. These include challenging past communication structures, clinician professionalism, and other areas where lines blur between personal and professional roles. As outlined by Swift (2013), nurses continue to hold the public's trust and play a critical role in supporting patients throughout the health care continuum by working with all age groups and populations. Given nurses' need to play an active role in health care improvement, social media tools can offer new possibilities to improve the health of individuals, quality of care delivery, and enhance disease support and monitoring outside the hospital. This chapter examines the concept of social

TABLE 27.1 Social Media Presence of Health Care Organizations Rendering Various Services							
	YouTube	Facebook	Twitter	LinkedIn	4Square	Blog	Total
Health organizations	717	1,300	1,005	653	1,084	211	6,533

media, outlines some of the common components and examples of social media, discusses the professional implications, and explains how nurses can engage meaningfully in the use of these tools.

DEFINING *SOCIAL MEDIA*

There is variation in the way in which *social media* is defined in the literature. Some authors (Kanter & Fine, 2010) take a broad approach by providing examples of services associated with the term. Others authors have left the definition broad, related to social media's core principles of connecting people and allowing content to be shared, commented on, and generated. For the purpose of this chapter, the core definition of *social media* will be the interaction among individuals during which they share, exchange, or create information and ideas across telecommunication and social networks. This simple and open definition connects social media to an evolutionary view of communication among people, which is being accelerated by the ability to generate and share information and amplified through an individual's connections and larger social network. Table 27.2 reflects the various ways in which *social media* has been defined.

ENGAGED, EMPOWERED, AND EVOLVED PATIENTS

The advancement of technology and the increased communication and sharing abilities afforded to individuals has also significantly impacted the health care sector. For instance, the term "ePatient" was likely derived from the generic term "eHealth," meaning electronic health. The term has evolved to endorse the descriptor of an engaged, empowered, and equal participant in the decision-making process of health-related matters (deBronkart, 2013). A notable ePatient, Dave deBronkart (@ePatientDave) has become a well-known advocate for patients and consumers who are actively involved and participate in their own health care. DeBronkart associates his survival of stage IV renal cancer with his active engagement in his own health care. His experience involved using social media services to connect and exchange information related to his diagnosis with experts and patients who were familiar with the specific cancer. This online presence and activity transformed his real-life health care interactions related to his checkups and knowledge of the disease, and informed his decisions about his treatment and follow-up care.

Beyond individual examples, research on the Internet that is used for health purposes has indicated that a patient's access to the Internet is changing health care information-seeking and -sharing behavior. Individuals with chronic disease are more likely to use information found through digital sources. Fox (2008) found that 75% of ePatients with chronic disease versus 55% of ePatients without chronic disease used information they found to directly affect health care decision making or behavior. Seeking information has been found to change specific behaviors of ePatients; for example, they decided to ask their physician a question or to seek a second opinion (69% of ePatients with chronic disease versus 52% without a chronic disease) and it changes the way in which patients cope with their condition or pain (57% with chronic disease versus 37% without). These trends will likely continue as a result of the growth in broadband Internet access, mobile and smartphone use, and active participation on social media services. Advanced practitioners

TABLE 27.2 Defining *Social Media*	
Reference	Definitions
Wikipedia (1,757 contributors). social media (n.d.)	"**Social media** is the social interaction among people in which they create, share or exchange information and ideas in virtual communities and networks."
Mesko (2013, p. 2)	"Internet and mobile-based digital communication: as well as the tools of the world wide web used for interactive dialogues, forming communities and supporting user-generated content. *Social media* was defined as 'a group of internet-based applications that build on the ideological and technological foundations of Web 2.0, and that allow the creation and exchange of user-generated content.'"
Nelson, Joos, and Wolf (2013, p. 10)	"Health 2.0 refers to the use of **social media**, via electronic devices, electronic health information exchange platforms, and mobile applications to promote collaboration among stakeholders and health care providers."
Kanter and Fine (2010, p. 5)	"We define **social media** as the array of digital tools such as instant messaging, text messaging, blogs, videos, and social networking sites like Facebook and MySpace that are inexpensive and easy to use. Social media enable people to create their own stories, videos and photos to manipulate them and share them widely at almost no cost."
Wilson (2014, p. 48)	"**Social media** is a collective term referring to interactions among groups of people online where information and types of media are created and shared."

must be prepared for these shifts in consumer behavior, desire for increased connectivity, and participation within their own health care. Providers and organizations who are aware of these changes are finding new ways to support their organizational goals by engaging in the use of social media.

HEALTH IMPACT OF SOCIAL MEDIA

Social media can offer advance practitioners new tools for professional development and impact. These forms of Internet technology can be used in ways that support patients and organizational outcomes, as well as in creating new opportunities for professional growth. Beyond communication and marketing strategies, the research on the impact of social media on various elements of the health care system is growing. Uses continue to expand and focus on improving health promotion, advocacy, and outcomes. For instance, social media technology is currently being used for a variety of surveillance, assessment, intervention, monitoring, and evaluation activities (Bender, Jimenez-Marroquin, & Jadad, 2011; Brownstein, Freifeld, Reis, & Mandl, 2008; Capurro et al., 2014; Heldman, Schindelar, & Iii, 2013; Innovation Cell, 2011; Neiger et al., 2012).

The use of data and information shared online has enabled health care practitioners to gain new insights into patients' health and epidemiology. For instance, the Health Department of Chicago implemented a program to search users' updates for possible cases of food poisoning and encouraged users to submit a foodborne illness form (Harris et al., 2014). This campaign solicited 193 submissions, leading to 133 restaurant inspections, 21 inspection failures, and 33 conditional passes with serious or critical issues. Another example of disease monitoring is HealthMap (http://healthmap.org/en/), a site that scrapes (automatically scans and takes information) from websites, news sources, and social networks and puts together a global perspective of infectious disease. In 2014, this website identified the spread of "mysterious hemorrhagic fever" in West Africa 9 days prior to the WHO announcing the 2014 Ebola epidemic (Zolfagharifard, 2014).

Access to Internet and adoption of smartphones has also created new opportunities for practitioners to provide specific interventions. There are growing examples of clinicians providing health care services through social media by taking advantage of mobile applications, social networking sites, and creating media for content sites (Casella, Mills, & Usher, 2014). Although far from a panacea, social media technology is currently being used in a number of nursing roles (e.g., public health; Lonergan, 2012), which has evolved traditional models of care and nurse–patient relationships.

EXAMINING KEY COMPONENTS AND FEATURES OF SOCIAL MEDIA

The broad definition of social media can be applied to a wide and growing number of platforms, services, and applications. One way to better understand similar aspects is by examining some of the key components. Understanding how these components impact users' experiences provides insights into how these may offer opportunities to health care providers.

User Profile Component

Social media platforms require users to create an account, which associates the participant with a profile. This allows the service to recognize and associate information and content with a specific individual. A profile also informs the social media platform about its users, and depending on privacy settings, information is shared with other service participants. This allows them to gather insights into the credibility, experience, and expectations of other participants. Table 27.3 reflects various services and the manner in which they handle the user profile.

Interactive Component

The interactive nature of social media reflects unique aspects of communication that have historically not been possible with more conventional modes of communication.

TABLE 27.3 User Profile Approaches by Social Media Outlets	
Social Media	**Personal Profile Approach**
Facebook	Personal profile, highlighting demographics (age, gender, etc.), preferences (music, books, etc.), relationships, and content (images, status updates, etc.)
LinkedIn	Focuses on a professional profile, similar to a résumé highlighting job experiences, skills, connections, and education
Mendeley	Allows users to share publications, professional experience, and academic areas of interest
ResearchGate	Highlights professional interests, research impact, and academic output

Commenting (i.e., leaving messages in response to others' conversations) appears to be a basic feature of most social media platforms. Although seemingly basic in nature, the ability to generate real-time comments in response to others' conversations is a paradigmatic shift afforded by social media for distributed communication. Previously, conventional media formats had to utilize postal mail, fax, or telephone to converse with an author. Comments on a news article or blog post are now common features. This allows the author to interact with the audience, as well as with others who are viewing the content, in many cases, almost in real time.

Building Connections

To facilitate building connections with other users, social media platforms provide functions that allow (and typically encourage) users to connect with others. The terminology and functionality vary across many of the platforms (e.g., "friending," "following," "linking," etc.); however, all connection building via social media platforms shares a number of similarities (e.g., enables users to follow, syndicate, or track another user's generated content). However, connecting in social media can take different forms and arrangements. Some connections create symmetrical sharing of content. For example, if user A accepts user B's request, both users share content. In other cases, it is asymmetrical, and if user C can see and receive updates and content published, user D makes that content available without user D following any content published by user C. Figure 27.1 depicts these interrelationships. Connecting with other users allows participants to determine what content they might be exposed to and extends the possible relationships that might be fostered. Table 27.4 reflects the features available with common social media platforms and how the outlet fosters building connections with other end users.

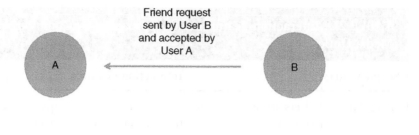

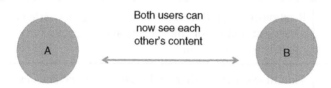

For example, Facebook friend requests operate in this type of undirected network.

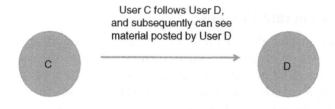

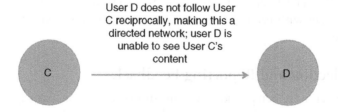

For example, Twitter can be a directed network whereby users are not required to reciprocally follow their followers.

FIGURE 27.1. Symmetrical and asymmetrical user connections.

TABLE 27.4 Interaction Features and Approaches by Common Social Media Outlets	
Social Media	**Interaction Features**
GooglePlus	Users are able to create asymmetrical relationships, following others' content. Users also selectively organize their contacts into groups, which allows them to filter how publicly content is shared (it could be shared publicly, i.e., with anyone, or selectively, i.e., shared only with family), although that does not act as a guaranteed privacy setting.
Facebook	Relationships can be symmetrical by accepting a friend request, or a user can "follow" or "like" a person or page to receive updates of publicly shared content.
Twitter	This allows users to share publications, professional experience, and academic areas of interest.

Share and Generate Content

Social media platforms also offer a variety of different mechanisms and methods to share media or to collaborate with others. Although the ability to share media among users may seem trivial in a current-day mind-set, the advent of social media technologies has significantly reduced the barrier related to costs (hosting web content) and technical skills needed to share files online. Subsequently, this has allowed users to focus on the content (e.g., health care improvement, health promotion, women's health, etc.) or medium (video, photography, text, etc.) of interest to participants, instead of the technical requirements needed to share/distribute the material mentioned earlier. Table 27.5 reflects approaches taken by social media companies to share and generate content with each of the companies competing for end users by featuring such services.

Data Collection and Reporting Feedback

Social media services often provide some measure of interaction, participation, or engagement with media content featuring the ability to track data through various reporting mechanisms. This provides feedback and insight to the user who posted something about how many visitors have seen, shared, or commented on their content, creating an incentive for that user to share it with others. It also gives the observer of the information a metric of online engagement of the media by others, conveying information about how many people have viewed or shared the content. These reporting features can be effective at better understanding the impact of the various approaches on social media. Table 27.6 reflects approaches taken toward data collection and reporting by several of the social media companies.

TABLE 27.5 Sharing Content Features by Social Media Outlets	
Social Media	**Sharing Content Features**
Flickr	Provides the ability to store and share photography. Communities are created around photography equipment being used, the subject of interest, and they provide ways to share rich content.
YouTube	Allows users to upload videos and subscribe to content channels. Users can also do basic video editing and enhancement, as well as add text captions to make content more accessible.
Google Drive	Enables users to upload and edit their own files (text documents, presentation slides, spreadsheets, etc.). It also allows select sharing and the ability to simultaneously edit individual documents.
Wikipedia	Allows registered and unregistered users to edit content, and relies heavily on volunteer efforts and contribution to a public encyclopedia. Content is now owned by a single participant and continues to evolve.
Slideshare	Focuses on sharing presentation material (slides and handouts). It allows users to share and download presentations, as well as to comment on content uploaded by others.

TABLE 27.6 Data Collection and Reporting Features of Social Media Outlets	
Social Media	**Data Collection and Reporting Features**
YouTube	Displays how many people have viewed a particular video.
Scribd	Tells users how many people have loaded (visited the URL), downloaded, or shared a document.
Google Analytics	A free tool used on many websites to track how many visitors have visited a web page, how long they have visited the page, and whether they clicked on a link or left a website.

RELATING SOCIAL MEDIA SERVICES TO HEALTH OUTCOMES

The components outlined earlier, as well as others, are combined in different ways to create unique services and platforms. Each social media platform may provide unique functionalities or access to populations of interest. Advanced health care practitioners need to examine their own objectives and consider how these services can be strategically used to support personal and/or organizational objectives.

Content Management: Wikis and Blogs in Health Care

Content management features of social media, such wikis and blogs, allow users to publish and organize information. Content is generated by a user and subsequently offered to other users who may wish to collaboratively edit or comment on published content. A blog can be used to share health care-related information and promote professional development or patient engagement. Lifeinthefastlane.com (LITFL, 2014) is an example of a blog that shares continuing-education and news related to emergency medicine, with a particular emphasis on content that is free and has open access.

Social Networks

Social networks emphasize connections and relationships of users. Social networks can focus on personal, professional, or specific interests (e.g., research, hobbies, etc.). LinkedIn is a professional network that allows users to create either an individual profile or a group. One example of this use in health care is the American Nurses Association (ANA); this group allows users to share professional information, post job opportunities, and start discussions related to nursing and health care. The ability to network with similar professionals and to connect with others for research, collaboration, or programs to improve health outcomes are ways in which LinkedIn can be used.

Bookmarking Tools

Bookmarking tools are applications available on the Internet that facilitate knowledge management of web pages by allowing users to organize and share resources with others. Diigo is a bookmarking tool that allows users to save and annotate web pages they visit (Diigo, 2014). This could be used to share educational resources and content with other health care providers as well as facilitate research and other exchange of helpful information for improving health outcomes.

Content Sharing

Content sharing allows users to upload content in various media formats. Communities can be created based on formats such as video, text, audio, and images. Additional types of specific content include education, entertainment, news, research, and health care. YouTube has been used by health care professionals to share and upload videos, with some qualified users allowed to upload videos longer than 15 minutes. The Mayo Clinic shares Medical Grand Rounds through its YouTube channel. In the Ebola public health preparedness efforts of 2014, several organizations worldwide shared content on how to effectively don and doff protective equipment. These videos were widely distributed by organizations rapidly preparing for Ebola cases as the numbers of infected individuals increased worldwide, and with cases developing within the United States.

Event Management

Event management is an approach that enables users to collaborate on event planning and organization, as well as on promotion and event ticketing. HackingHealth is an organization that organizes in-person events that gather computer programmers, clinicians, and health care administrators. Eventbrite can be used for event registration and promotion and can be used by health care organizations.

Microblogging

Microblogging is a platform for sharing short amounts of text content and weblinks. As mentioned in Table 27.1, more than 1,000 hospitals have a presence on Twitter. Twitter is an example of microblogging. Health care providers can use it to follow others in their area of practice or research, and to share ideas and resources with others. Twitter was used by the Centers for Disease Control and Prevention (CDC) to distribute information to health care professionals and the general public during the 2014 Ebola outbreak in the United States. During the crisis, Twitter users could follow the director of the CDC, Dr. Tom Frieden (@DrFriedenCDC), via Twitter, along with other CDC-operated Twitter accounts (e.g., @cdcgov, @CDCemergency).

Geolocation Services

Geolocation services focus on the location of users, enabling users to save location and associated content (comments, pictures, video) with a specific context. AEDLocator.org maps locations of automated external defibulators in the United Kingdom and Europe so as to support cardiac patients (AEDLocator, 2014).

Live Streaming

Live streaming creates a platform for broadcasting live video or audio content over the Internet. Google Hangouts can be used to stream live videos for a maximum of 10 users. This can be used to broadcast and record educational events supporting health care professionals in sharing content worldwide.

Understanding Professional Implications of Social Media to Mitigate the Risk

Professional issues are a commonly discussed risk and barrier to considering social media use by health care professionals. One possible reason is the lack of understanding of how existing rules apply to social media. Advanced health care practitioners have generally already completed their basic entry-to-practice requirements, including education related to professional issues such as legal frameworks, self-regulation, and standards of practice. The knowledge and ability to apply these requirements to their practice means they have necessary skills to consider possible ramifications of social media. As health care leaders, it is important to educate others and actively engage in creating a culture that is not only receptive toward the appropriate use of social media but also cognizant of its inherent risks. This can help prevent professional issues before they happen, which is often the cause of negative publicity for hospitals and health care professionals.

Applying Professional Filters

One way to think about social media risk is through the application of professional filters to activities and behaviors on social media. Table 27.7 outlines a hierarchy of filters that can be applied (as recommended by Fraser [2011]), such as legislative constraints, professional regulations, professional best practices, employer policies and contracts, and personal standards of professionalism. These filters can help professionals consider how they use social media. If activities or behaviors do not violate any of these filters, it may be appropriate to consider the proposed use of social media. This is where critical thinking and professional judgment are important, especially when considering and deploying social media in a clinical or professional context. If in doubt, the authors recommend being cautious with use of social media, as it can be difficult (if not impossible) to remove something from the Internet once it has been shared.

TABLE 27.7 Recommended Professional Filters to Be Applied Prior to Posting on Social Media	
Filter	**Considerations and Questions to Consider Before Posting**
Legislation	What laws apply to the situation as a result of those involved (e.g., hospital providing information, patients participating)? Privacy laws (Health Insurance Portability and Accountability Act [HIPAA] in the United States, Personal Health Information Protection Act in Ontario, Canada)
Professional regulations	What standards apply as a result of the health care providers involved? Are there nursing, medical, or other standards that need to be reviewed, such as standards for therapeutic relationships, providing medical advice, etc.?
Professional best practices	What is the ideal way to participate and positively promote your profession?
Employer policies and contracts	Does your organization have policies related to social media use? Are you allowed to access social media websites while at work, or must you declare that your views do not necessarily reflect those of your employer?
Personal standards of professionalism	What activity and content do you want to be professionally associated with?

Adapted from Fraser (2011). Used with permission

Types of Risk

Beyond the framework recommended by Fraser, it is also important for advanced health care practitioners to be aware of the subtle risks to themselves, their colleagues, or their employers. A brief overview of risks that exist when engaging in social media interactions and that should be considered prior to sharing on social media and engaging in online communication is given next.

Privacy.   In the technology era, privacy is probably one of the first things that people consider when risk is discussed. HIPAA, as discussed in Chapter 14, has 18 health identifiers that it considers personal health information (PHI). Knowledge of these 18 items is helpful in being proactive in terms of recognizing and responding to potential privacy issues related to health information. Regardless of this, social media can introduce a variety of unintended consequences related to health information breaches. For instance, given the spontaneous and networked nature of social media platforms, posting an anonymous message related to a witnessed health care situation could still inadvertently result in a breach of health information. An example of this type of risk might occur if a patient were involved in a crime that was reported in the local media. News agencies routinely scour social media platforms for insights related to current events. It is not out of the realm of possibility that the crime incident and health care interaction of the individual could be circumstantially linked together. Similarly, beyond textual information, digital photos may also be an issue for privacy violations. Posting pictures without one's consent or that have patient information (e.g., names on charts/room, patient lists on monitors) in the background are common examples of inadvertent health information breaches. With mobile devices and cell phones that are capable of spontaneous snapshots of colleagues, PHI of patients may be shared unintentionally with thousands (or millions) of people. Conscientious consideration of photos taken in the work setting and of one's coworkers needs to be thoroughly conceptualized and scrutinized prior to posting to a social media platform. These types of issues need to be openly discussed to avoid risk and to enable health care teams to fully understand the appropriate use of social media.

Copyright.   Internet access and search engines make content (e.g., text, video, pictures) easier to find and copy. This ease of accessing content does not necessarily reflect the intended copyright privileges. In the United States, the Fair Use Act and Digital Millennium Copyright Act have implications for how media is shared. Fair use may protect some uses for libraries/archives, personal use, public domain works, public interest work, and research; however, this does not necessarily mean that content can be openly shared online. Simple examples include taking copyrighted work, such as some online images, and using it in a hospital publication (e.g., patient education materials). It is important to look into what copyright license may apply, or if the owner shared it using an open standard, such as Creative Commons (http://creativecommons.org/), that clearly explains the type of rights the owner allows and expectations for use of the content. It is even possible to search for content using Creative Common's, which makes it easier to find content that can be freely used under more open copyright terms.

Exclusion and Accessibility. Even as adoption grows, there will be populations and individuals who have issues with accessing social media and related Internet technologies. It is important to balance the opportunity to reach populations that might become less accessible through traditional interactions (e.g., uninsured or undocumented individuals) and awareness of those people who will not be able to utilize social media for other reasons (e.g., language barriers, income, education). Health care providers need to consider equity and how they continue to service populations with unmet needs. Pre-implementation planning can help develop mitigation strategies such as ensuring low-literacy readability, language translation, and multiple format availability (e.g., print, DVD, posters). Both during and after project implementation, analysis of impact and participation should be completed to consider who is being reached by the project. This can allow for adjustment and development of strategies to address any of these identified issues.

Shifting Boundaries of Professional Presence and Patient Interaction

Creation of individual, professional, or organizational profiles or presence through social media changes the dynamics of individual availability and the norm related to work hours. The Internet and social media sites are available online 24 hours a day, year round. Given this level of ubiquitous presence, disclaimer information posted to a social media platform is one commonly employed method of conveying the expectations about when participants might expect a response or when new content will be published. By having disclaimer information available to users, a deeper insight and transparency into the service being offered can be conveyed. Along with official organization-sponsored social media accounts (e.g., a Facebook page operated by the CDC), individual employees may also possess personal accounts that blur the divide between their personal and professional lives. For instance, health care providers may not only post information to their personal accounts but also denote that they work for a specific health care organization. This can create concerns and reputational risk for the individual as well as for the organization (Levati, 2014) because of the ambiguity that exists as to whether the individual represents the organization in an official capacity.

Creating an Organizational Policy

Developing an organizational policy as to social media use is a proactive approach organizations (e.g., hospitals, clinics, colleges) can take to mitigate risk (Antheunis, Tates, & Nieboer, 2013). A social media toolkit from Public Health Ontario (2014) suggests that a policy should:

- ► Outline values and expectations
- ► Ensure legal and regulatory compliance
- ► Capture and support use of best practices
- ► Support consistent use, treatment, and discipline of staff
- ► Standardize decision making and reduce variation in use
- ► Protect individuals and organizations from expediency (Dhaliwal et al., 2014)

Examples of social media policies have been shared and made available through online resources such as http://socialmediagovernance.com/policies/. Development of this policy should be a process that includes various perspectives and considerations about both risks and benefits of social media to prevent an unbalanced policy. It should also be regularly revised to consider changes in internal (e.g., capacity, experiences) or external (e.g., new services, updates to regulations, case law) circumstances.

EXAMINING HOW SOCIAL MEDIA IMPACTS TRADITIONAL INFORMATICS

The rise of social media tools and technology has both changed and evolved the method of how people communicate and share information. Subsequently, virtually all areas of communication have been impacted in one way or another by social media. As outlined earlier, health care has also been significantly impacted by the presence of social media. Regardless of this, the impact of social media on the health care system (and its underpinning features) has been uniquely asymmetric to normal innovation evolution within health care. As outlined by Eysenbach (2008), patients and consumers are able to bypass or disintermediate many traditional actors and gatekeepers (e.g., nurses, physicians) within the health care system through use of network tools such as social media. Eysenbach is referring to the ability for consumers and patients to use various social media tools to connect with others to obtain information and services. Although Eysenbach qualifies that disintermediation should not be viewed in absolute terms (e.g., an individual may use both traditional and interactive mechanisms to access health information and services), social media has provided consumers with a new methodology from which to access information and services related to health.

Traditional health informatics has also been impacted by the presence of social media. Classically, health informatics tools have largely ignored or minimized the role of the patient or the consumer in their development or use. In a literature review of nursing ICT, Booth (2012) reported that focus and attention toward the consumer or patient was largely missing from the 39 studies reviewed. Advanced health care practitioners need to be aware of social media and the impact it is having on clinicians and patients. Knowledge of these concepts and possibilities can help integrate social features into traditional informatics systems implemented by health care organizations. These systems are what will shape nurses' interactions with patients, as well as with other health care professionals.

INTERPROFESSIONAL IMPLICATIONS OF SOCIAL MEDIA

The importance of interprofessional collaboration in health care delivery is evidenced by improved outcomes experienced by patients. A natural progression of this interprofessional collaboration is the application of social media. As per the definition of social media provided in this chapter, when it is applied to providers operating in an interprofessional collaborative, social media tools can allow for more rapid dissemination of complex interprofessional collaborative content (Garrett & Cutting, 2012). For example, as noted, "Interprofessional education occurs when two or more professions learn about, from and with each other to enable effective collaboration and improve health outcomes" (World Health Organization, 2010, p. 13). Given that implementation of interprofessional collaboratives has been challenging, social media has been found to facilitate the centralization of communication that is so vital to success. Blogs, Twitter, Facebook, and group discussion boards represent some of the tools used to support interprofessional collaboratives (Cain & Chretien, 2013).

SUMMARY

To conclude, this chapter has offered a review of social media and its potential to impact both health and health outcomes. Content within the chapter has included the various forms of social media outlets and companies available to health care professionals. We have also reviewed the features and content of some social media sites and have discussed approaches to be used in popular culture as well as in health care. An overview of the important filters recommended by Fraser (2011) has also been reviewed along with questions for all health care professionals to consider prior to posting to social media. We have examined the risks of posting to social media, and finally, we have also discussed implications on traditional informatics and the future of health care.

EXERCISES AND QUESTIONS FOR CONSIDERATION

When responding to the following questions, let us consider how the consumerization of technology is causing an increase in availability of information as well as in accessibility and adoption of services that have become integrated with social functions:

1. Where do individuals look for information and advice related to their health or illness? How are online services influencing this behavior?

2. Can you think of examples of when you, your family, or a friend has searched for or shared information about health experiences or goals online? If this is where consumers of health information are looking, how should health professionals engage the consumer or ensure the best information is provided?

3. The majority of health interventions and medical treatments involve risks and benefits. Discuss examples of social activities that health care providers or organizations could engage in. Then consider the potential risks that would need to be mitigated, as well as desirable outcomes.

4. Explore a health-related topic online. Try searching for a topic you are interested in (e.g., heart disease) on an Internet search engine and then search the same topic using a social media search function (e.g., http://twitter.com/search).

5. What populations of patients do you work with (e.g., diabetic, street involved, seniors) or what environment to you practice in (e.g., rural urban, primary care office, hospital)? What social networks (personal or professional) does this population use frequently?

6. How could your organization provide patient education or support through social media?

7. How could you or others in your field share your expertise and collaborate differently using social media?

REFERENCES

AEDLocator. (2014). *AEDLocator.* Retrieved from www.aedlocator.org

Antheunis, M. L., Tates, K., & Nieboer, T. E. (2013). Patients' and health professionals' use of social media in health care: Motives, barriers and expectations. *Patient Education and Counseling, 92*(3), 426–431. doi:10.1016/j.pec.2013.06.020

Bender, J. L., Jimenez-Marroquin, M. C., & Jadad, A. R. (2011). Seeking support on Facebook: A content analysis of breast cancer groups. *Journal of Medical Internet Research, 13*(1), e16. Retrieved from www.ncbi.nlm.nih.gov/pmc/articles/PMC3221337/?report=printable

Booth, R. G. (2012). Examining the functionality of the DeLone and McLean information system success model as a framework for synthesis in nursing information and communication technology research. *Computers, Informatics, Nursing, 30*(6), 330–345. doi:10.1097/NXN.0b013e31824af7f4

Brownstein, J. S., Freifeld, C. C., Reis, B. Y., & Mandl, K. D. (2008). Surveillance sans frontières: Internet-based emerging infectious disease intelligence and the HealthMap project. *PLoS Medicine, 5*(7), e151. doi:10.1371/journal.pmed.0050151

Cain, J., & Chretien, K. (2013). Exploring social media's potential in interprofessional education. *Journal of Research in Interprofessional Practice and Education, 3*(2), 1–7. Retrieved from www.jripe.org/index.php/journal/article/view/110

Capurro, D., Cole, K., Echavarría, M. I., Joe, J., Neogi, T., & Turner, A. M. (2014). The use of social networking sites for public health practice and research: A systematic review. *Journal of Medical Internet Research, 16*(3), e79. doi:10.2196/jmir.2679

Casella, E., Mills, J., & Usher, K. (2014). Social media and nursing practice: Changing the balance between the social and technical aspects of work. *Collegian Journal, 21*(2), 121–126. doi:10.1016/j.colegn.2014.03.005

deBronkart, D. (2013). How the e-patient community helped save my life: An essay by Dave deBronkart. *British Medical Journal, 1990,* 2–4. doi:10.1136/bmj.f1990

Dhaliwal, M., Davies, J., McCall, K., Brankley, L., Williams, M., & Mai, D. (2014). *Social media toolkit for Ontario public health units.* Canada, ON: Authors. Retrieved from www.wdgpublichealth.ca/sites/default/files/wdgphfiles/Social-toolkit-public-health-web-final.pdf

Diigo. (2014). *About Diigo.* Retrieved from www.diigo.com/about

Eysenbach, G. (2008). Medicine 2.0: Social networking, collaboration, participation, apomediation, and openness. *Journal of Medical Internet Research, 10*(3), e22. doi:10.2196/jmir.1030

Fox, S. (2005). *Health Information Online. PEW Interent & American Life Project.* Washington, DC. Retrieved from http://www.pewinternet.org

Fox, S. (2008). *The engaged E-patient population people turn to the Internet for health information when the stakes are high and the connection fast* (No. Pew2008). Washington, DC: Pew Research.

Fraser, R. (2011). *The nurses' social media advantage: How making connections and sharing ideas can enhance your nursing practice.* Indianapolis, IN: Sigma Theta Tau International.

Garrett, B. M., & Cutting, R. (2012). Using social media to promote international student partnerships. *Nurse Education in Practice, 12*(6), 340–345. doi:10.1016/j.nepr.2012.04.003

Harris, J. K., Mansour, R., Choucair, B., Olson, J., Nissen, C., & Bhatt, J. (2014). Health department use of social media to identify foodborne illness. *Morbidity and Mortality Weekly Report, 63*(32), 681–685. Retrieved from www.cdc.gov/mmwr/preview/mmwrhtml/mm6332a1.htm

Heldman, A. B., Schindelar, J., & Weaver, J. B. (2013). Social media engagement and public health communication: Implications for public health organizations being truly "social." *Public Health Reviews* 35(1), 1–18. Retrieved from www.publichealthreviews.eu/upload/pdf_files/13/00_Heldman.pdf

Innovation Cell. (2011). *Using social media to improve healthcare quality: Part 2.* Retrieved from www.changefoundation.ca/library/using-social-media-to-improve-healthcare-quality-part-2/

Kanter, B., & Fine, A. H. (2010). *The networked nonprofit: Connecting with social media to drive change.* San Francisco: John Wiley & Sons.

Levati, S. (2014). Professional conduct among registered nurses in the use of online social networking sites. *Journal of Advanced Nursing, 70*(10), 2284–2292. doi:10.1111/jan.12377

Life in the Fastlane. (2014). *Life in the fastlane.* Retrieved from www.lifeinthefastlane.com

Lonergan, P. (2012, May 5). Peel public health launches parenting Facebook page. *Mississauga News.* Retrieved from www.mississauga.com/news-story/3125567-peel-public-health-launches-parenting-facebook-page/

Mayo Clinic. (2014). *Social media health network: Bringing the social media revolution to health care.* Retrieved from www.network.socialmedia.mayoclinic.org/hcsml-grid/

Neiger, B. L., Thackeray, R., Van Wagenen, S. A., Hanson, C. L., West, J. H., Barnes, M. D., & Fagen, M. C. (2012). Use of social media in health promotion: Purposes, key performance indicators, and evaluation metrics. *Health Promotion Practice, 13*(2), 159–164. doi:10.1177/1524839911433467

PEW Internet & American Life Project. (n.d.). *Three technology revolutions.* Retrieved from www.pewinternet.org/three-technology-revolutions/

Public Health Ontario. (2014). *Social Media Toolkit for Ontario Public Health Units.* Toronto, Canada. Retrieved from http://www.wdgpublichealth.ca/sites/default/files/wdgphfiles/Social-toolkit-public-health-web-final.pdf

Rice, R. E. (2006). Influences, usage, and outcomes of Internet health information searching: Multivariate results from the Pew surveys. *International Journal of Medical Informatics, 75*(1), 8–28. Retrieved from http://www.sciencedirect.com/science/article/pii/S1386505605001462

Swift, A. (2013). Honesty and ethics rating of clergy slides to new low. *Gallup Politics.* Washington, DC. Retrieved from http://www.gallup.com/poll/166298/honesty-ethics-rating-clergy-slides-new-low.aspx

World Health Organization. (2010). Framework for action on interprofessional education & collaborative practice. Retrieved from http://www.who.int/hrh/resources/framework_action/en/

Zolfagharifard, E. (2014, August). Ebola was flagged by computer software HealthMap nine days before it was announced: HealthMap used social media to spot disease. *MailDaily.* Retrieved from www.dailymail.co.uk/sciencetech/article-2722164/Ebola-flagged-computer-software-nine-days-BEFORE-announced-HealthMap-used-social-media-spot-disease.html

CHAPTER 28

Electronic Clinical Quality Measures: Building an Infrastructure for Success

Susan McBride and Itara K. Barnes

OBJECTIVES

1. Define *electronic clinical quality measures* (eCQMs); discuss the importance of electronic measures to the National Quality Strategy, starting with the history of quality measures, the need to create eCQMs, and the relationship to electronic health record meaningful use (EHR-MU) requirements.

2. Describe the components of eCQMs, including foundational elements that support the delivery of the best practices of quality care by following evidence-based protocols.

3. Describe the eCQM development life cycle, including measure stewards, measure developers, and alignment of private and federal initiatives that select measures for public reporting.

4. Define and describe important building blocks for eCQMs and how they work together for implementation, including the quality data model, value sets, quality-reporting document architecture, Technical Authority for the Unified Clinical Quality Improvement Framework (Tacoma), and the health quality measures format.

5. Discuss the relationship among EHR certification, versioning of measure specifications, and the importance of vendor support with eCQM reporting.

6. Describe the importance of interprofessional teams and what characteristics align with a successful eCQM program.

KEY WORDS

electronic clinical quality measures, quality data model, value sets, quality-reporting document architecture, health quality measures format, measures application partnership, Technical Authority for the Unified Clinical Quality Improvement Framework

CONTENTS

INTRODUCTION

The success of the National Quality Strategy (NQS) hinges on the ability of providers and hospitals to successfully utilize health information technology (HIT) and data within the electronic health record to improve quality. The NQS called for under the Afford-able Care Act (ACA) focuses on promoting quality health care and improved health of patients, families, and communities. This strategy aligns with the three aims discussed in Chapters 1, 4, 19, 20, and 22, including better care, healthy communities, and lower costs. One of the primary levers that the nation is using to ensure success of this plan is to encourage the use of HIT to improve communication, transparency, and efficiency for better coordinated health and to effectively measure performance on key indicators of quality (Agency for Healthcare Research and Quality [AHRQ], 2014). Historically, hospitals and providers have been required by regulatory agencies, including the Centers for Medicare & Medicaid Services (CMS), to report measures of quality. In 2012, CMS indicated that beginning in 2014 the reporting of quality measures would shift from pro-viders and hospitals using an attestation process of reporting numerators and denomi-nators to CMS, which would require that eMeasures data be reported (CMS, 2012). Although this was the initial goal in 2012, recognizing the complexity of the process for the industry, CMS relaxed the requirements, temporarily allowing other options while the industry prepares for this reporting requirement. This process is technically intensive and has many moving parts. The purpose of this chapter is to describe the anatomy of an eMeasure; the tools and resources available to report eMeasures; review pertinent background information, including all the major stakeholders in the process; and finally, examine a case study.

UNDERSTANDING THE ANATOMY OF AN ᴇMEASURE

An eMeasure is a measurement derived from the EHR, and as such, the data within the EHR must capture and calculate the measure from a structured format. There are a num-ber of ways to classify eMeasures, including those that pertain to patients, episodes, or a proportion-based indicator. According to CMS, a *patient-based indicator* is defined as "a measure that evaluates the care of a patient and assigns the patient to a membership in one or more populations" (CMS & ONC [Office of the National Coordinator], 2014, p. 6). Episodic measures are those that evaluate the patient–provider encounter and assign the episode of care to one or more populations relevant to the encounter. Proportion-based indicators compute rates. Most of the electronic clinical quality measures for the year 2014 are proportion-based indicators and can include patient-based and episode-based indicators (CMS & ONC, 2014, p. 6). Figure 28.1 reflects an example of one of the National Quality Forum (NQF) measures for stroke with noted complexity of how an actual eMeasure is ultimately derived from the EHR data.

The capture of eMeasures does not always reflect the workflow of clinicians, and it presents challenges with reliably and validly collecting the information so that it can be extracted from the electronic environment. To analyze and report eCQMs, the electronic specifications must be developed in a manner so that the data elements, logic, and definitions for the measure are in the same format for storing and capturing the certified EHRs (Doyle, 2014). According to the NQF, a well-defined structured interoperable eMeasure will be: (a) composed of a set of common data elements aligned with the Quality Data Model (QDM); (b) encoded using a nationally recognized coding standard such as Systematized Nomenclature of Medicine (SNOMED,) ICD9/10 (International Classification of Diseases, Ninth Revision, Clinical Modification/International Classification of Diseases, Tenth Revision, Clinical Modification) codes, and RxNorm; and (c) structured logically

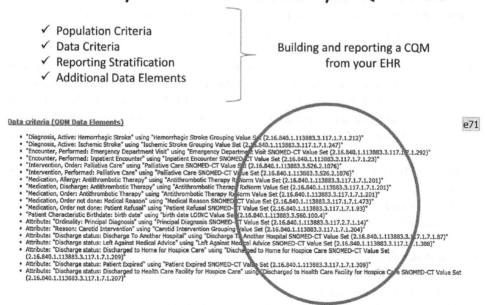

FIGURE 28.1. Stroke eMeasure example.

into a standardized expression as with the health quality measures format (HQMF) eMeasures (Eisenberg, Overage, & Johnson, 2011).

Implementing eMeasures With the Future in Mind

The focus on any implementation effort should be to capture accurate data to drive improvements and reduce costs. The goal is to avoid preventable errors and to seamlessly integrate clinical decision support (CDS) into the workflow to support clinicians in logically improving care delivery while simultaneously capturing information and data needed to ensure that quality services has been delivered. Discrete data elements are required for the capture of this information in an electronic environment. For these data to be effectively utilized for improvement, as discussed in Chapters 18 and 20, the data must be aggregated and the information should be reported using consistent measures over time to track and trend improvements. Steps recommended by Eisenberg et al. (2011) to create an eMeasure for reporting include:

1. Determining the eMeasure to be reported and the requirements for the measure
2. Identifying the content sources of the information needed to satisfy the measure
3. Considering the workflows impacted
4. Making EHR design decisions to capture the data
5. Collecting the information within a data warehouse for analysis, reporting, tracking, and trending
6. Extracting and reporting the data (Eisenberg et al., 2011)

To capture data within the EHRs, measures must be specified in terms of what and how the data are collected within the EHRs. The NQF, working through the Health Information Technology Expert Panel (HITEP), established the QDM, which is an attempt to reflect the way data are expressed in EHRs (NQF, 2012). Components of an eMeasure include the measure overview and other information about the measure that is typically located in the header of the HQMF. Population criteria are provided in enough detail within the HQMF to program the eMeasure within the EHR (CMS, 2011). The data criteria identify codes that are reflective of specific data elements needed to generate the measure. Figure 28.2 provides an example of what this looks like for a hypertension measure noting that the data steward or owner of the original measure is the American Medical Association (AMA), and the title and subsequent measure description type, and rational for the measure. There are four to five basic components of an eCQM, including (a) the initial patient population, (b) the denominator, (c) numerator, (d) exclusions, and (e) exceptions. The patient population is the specific group of patients whom the measure is intended to address. In the example noted, the population includes patients greater than or equal to 18 years of age (adults) with an active diagnosis of hypertension who have been seen for at least two or more visits by the provider. The eMeasure might be defined as follows:

Initial Patient Population =
AND: "Patient characteristic: birth date (age) > = 18 years";
AND: "Diagnosis active: hypertension";

AND: "> = 2" count(s) of:

OR: "Encounter: encounter outpatient" to determine the physician has a relationship with the patient;

OR: "Encounter: encounter nursing facility" to determine the physician has a relationship with the patient (CMS, 2013b).

The denominator is a subset of the initial patient population; in the case of the hypertension example, this would include the entire adult population by definitions noted earlier. The numerator is a subset of the denominator for whom a process or outcome of care occurs. For the hypertension indicator, the numerator is the subset of the denominator patients who had a systolic and diastolic blood pressure (BP) recorded. The eMeasure would be noted as follows:

eMeasure:

Numerator =

AND: "Physical exam finding: systolic blood pressure";

AND: "Physical exam finding: diastolic blood pressure" (CMS, 2013b).

Escalating Complexity in eCQMs From Stage 1 to Stage 2 of Meaningful Use

The quality measures under meaningful use have escalating levels of complexity while moving from Stage 1 to Stage 2 of MU. For example, the hypertension indicator noted earlier was a fairly straightforward measure indicating whether or not BP was measured for those adult patients who were hypertensive. For Stage 2 of MU, the goal is to control BP.

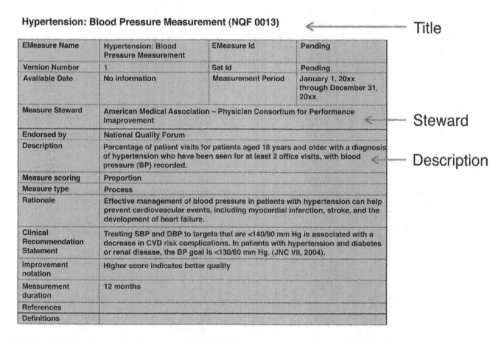

Hypertension: Blood Pressure Measurement (NQF 0013) ← Title

EMeasure Name	Hypertension: Blood Pressure Measurement	EMeasure Id	Pending
Version Number	1	Set Id	Pending
Available Date	No information	Measurement Period	January 1, 20xx through December 31, 20xx
Measure Steward	American Medical Association – Physician Consortium for Performance Imaprovement			← Steward
Endorsed by	National Quality Forum		
Description	Percentage of patient visits for patients aged 18 years and older with a diagnosis of hypertension who have been seen for at least 2 office visits, with blood pressure (BP) recorded.			← Description
Measure scoring	Proportion		
Measure type	Process		
Rationale	Effective management of blood pressure in patients with hypertension can help prevent cardiovascular events, including myocardial infarction, stroke, and the development of heart failure.		
Clinical Recommendation Statement	Treating SBP and DBP to targets that are <140/90 mm Hg is associated with a decrease in CVD risk complications. In patients with hypertension and diabetes or renal disease, the BP goal is <130/80 mm Hg. (JNC VII, 2004).		
Improvement notation	Higher score indicates better quality		
Measurement duration	12 months		
References			
Definitions			

FIGURE 28.2. Example of eMeasure in HQMF.

CVD, coronary vascular disease; DBP, diastolic blood pressure; HQMF, health quality measures format; SBP, systolic blood pressure.

Source: Centers for Medicare & Medicaid Services (2011).

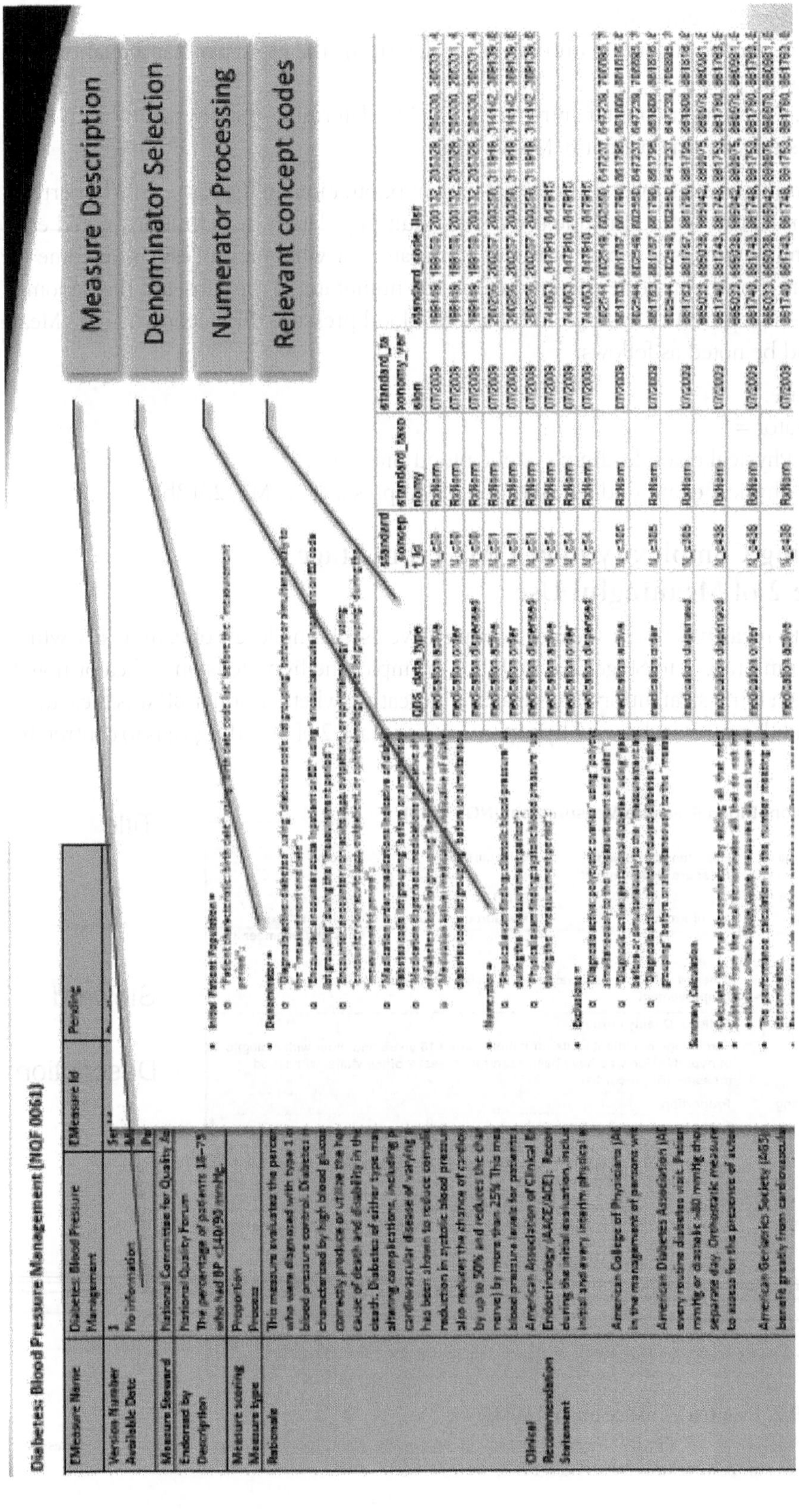

FIGURE 28.3. Hypertension measure reduced to machine-readable language.

Source: Centers for Medicare and Medicaid Services (2013a).

The complexity of the measure escalates significantly with tracking much more detailed information related to the patient with hypertension (CMS, 2013a). For example, in Figure 28.3, the NQF measure for diabetes BP management is noted in both human-readable and machine-readable language required to reduce this measure to a code that the computer would interpret. Appendix 28.1 reflects a sample of the logic map for tracking the preventive care and screening for high BP and follow-up documented with the eCQM for eligible providers as of June 2014 for the 2015 reporting year. Although on the surface tracking success with management of patients with hypertension may appear fairly simple, reducing it to machine-readable language and capturing the information within the clinical workflow is a much more complicated picture, as is evident by examining Appendix 28.1. The goal of eCQMs and efforts to improve the process is that the measure will be clear, complete, unambiguous, usable, and meaningful with data and specifications that can be consistently interpreted, implemented, and acted on by programmers and providers.

It is important to align an organization's strategies when building an eCQM program. The authors recommend creating an eCQM enterprise blueprint to outline an enterprise-wide strategy for measurement and reporting to deliver a more effective and streamlined approach for satisfying accreditation, certification, and regulatory reporting requirements. With this approach, it is important to identify all programs requiring quality measurement and reporting for the organization that may include The Joint Commission (TJC), CMS, and private payers or managed care plans. An internal inventory or list of measures that will be required for each program is the starting point. One should identify the method that will be used to report the information for each individual measure, including specifications according to versions of the actual measure, because many measures include updates and multiple versions. If there are any constraints on the measure required for submission, they too should be included in the inventory. A sample blueprint is noted in Figure 28.4; the blueprint establishes the organization's strategy for the entire process of measures required by an organization.

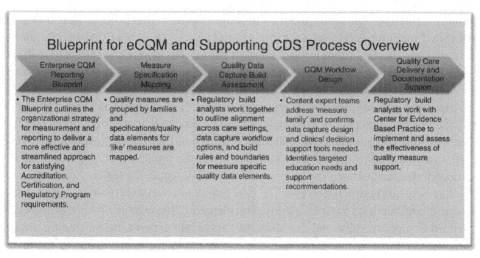

FIGURE 28.4. Blue print for eMeasures strategy.

CDS, clinical decision support; CQM, clinical quality measure; eCQM, electronic clinical quality measure.

Once complete, the full inventory should be followed by specifications mapping of the measures. This process includes mapping quality measures to grouped families of measures. For example, there may be measures relevant to specific patient populations such as the cardiovascular population. The entire clinical quality measure (CQM) inventory and grouped measures based on common focus (e.g. targeted disease state, care process, or outcome of interest) are a full reflection of the organization strategy related to quality reporting. This will be unique to the organization and should include measures from all applicable care settings. For each group, one should break the measures down to the quality data elements (including associated value sets and attributes) and then map common elements across the measures. The output is a single, comprehensive list of the elements required for the measure family. The goal of this process is to collect the data once and use the data element for many purposes to gain efficiencies across the CQM process. When commonalities are identified, the authors recommend taking the strictest of the specifications. In addition, one should attempt to include not only the electronic requirement but also any measures that may continue to rely on abstracted or state and local quality measure requirements. The goal for this mapping process is to align all measures with valid and reliable electronic specifications, thereby "eSpecifying" all measures.

Build Assessment for Capture of Quality Data

Interprofessional teams that include regulatory build analysts and clinical informaticists need to work together to outline the required alignment of measures across care settings, data capture, workflow options, EHR build rules, and boundaries for measures specific to quality data elements needed across the enterprise. It is important for the regulatory quality-reporting teams to familiarize the entire interprofessional team, including clinicians, with the foundational elements of eCQMs. It is important for the entire team to understand the required measure details so they can outline workflows needed to capture data for each required element. The team needs to both accurately and reliably capture current clinical care workflows to show where the collection of the data for eCQMs is actually occurring. Workflow and data flow are critical to this process, as is using the associated measure specifications for the foundation, including eCQM specifications, narrative specifications, and implementation guidance to define the rules and context. Once this is clearly understood and documented in workflow and data-flow diagrams, the organization can begin to confirm that the EHR and clinicians utilizing the technology are capturing data that need to be reported. EHR documentation and vendor guidance are essential components of the process and can be used to determine data-flow requirements for incorporation into the calculation engine of the specific vendor's EHR. The EHR vendor should be considered a core partner in the process of eCQM reporting. An additional documentation component is needed to link required attributes for the respective data elements within the eCQM. The final output is a comprehensive outline of workflow and build options for each quality data element. This outline of what is needed is intended to support review and discussion by the content expert teams, including clinical staff, and can be presented at the measure family level with elements linked to unique quality measures. A family of measures relates to a specific patient type (e.g., measures associated with diabetes, in which all measures related to diabetes patients can be managed and documented strategically).

Some eligible hospitals may utilize EHRs that are all inclusive, whereas others may utilize disparate EHR systems to capture some of the data points required. One example of that might be capturing hemodynamic lab data. This type of scenario may require an interface build between EHRs to obtain access to data that are necessary for CQM calculations. The following are important assessment points to be considered related to interfaced systems: Where do the data within your organization come from? What is the primary source and how does it map from one system to another when interfaces are present?

CQM Workflow and Coordinated CDS Design

Interprofessional teams, including content experts and clinical informaticists, can assist in addressing the measure family with data capture design strategies that include the use of CDS tools. It is beneficial to engage content experts to address data capture; they will consider the current workflow (as is) and document and identify modifications needed to support the quality measure in a future workflow. The interprofessional team members must have a foundational understanding of the eCQM structure and requirements, including how the quality data elements combined with the HQMF define what needs to be captured and the timing of the capture as well as how the measures should be captured. The requirement for specificity and how eCQMs differ from abstracted measures is important for the interprofessional team to discern. In addition, to help define the build and implementation strategies for the eMeasures, the interprofessional team can identify potential pain points (challenging issues to address); proactively design targeted solutions to address potential gaps; and craft initial messaging, communication, and deployment strategies for the eMeasure family. A potential pain-point might be data that are not currently or consistently captured creating challenges in data capture without resolution of the pain-point. Engaging the content expert should be done in a way that promotes improvements in the measurement process and the benefits of the transition to electronic measurement. The goal of the interprofessional team is to align standardization across the enterprise with respect to the measure definitions and data element capture to support complete, accurate, and consistent capture of quality data. The standardization process may be different by care setting or the specialty area that might support the measures. For example, tobacco assessment and cessation may be implemented in oncology clinics, family practice, and/or the acute care setting, regardless of the location where the data should be consistently captured.

CDS for eCQMs

Well-strategized and well-designed CDS can support quality improvement, and eCQMs tied to CDS are an important feature of Stage 2 of the MU strategies. CDS can be specific to the measures and directly support capture of quality data elements or guide clinicians to ensure that the measure population is appropriately identified or follow-up actions are taken as needed. Specificity is a key target, as it addresses the "who," "what," "when," "where," and "how" with as much granularity as possible (Osheroff et al., 2012). The following are important areas noted by the authors as significant CDS strategies for supporting reporting efforts of eMeasures:

▶ Order set creation can facilitate data capture

▶ Data presentation through choice lists for ordering or documentation

▶ Documentation forms and templates

▶ Reference information and guidance (general link from EHR to clinical pathway or reference clinical protocols or evidence)

▶ Reactive alerts and reminders

▶ Proactive outreach with a tie to clinical registries

The interprofessional team responsible for eCQM works cohesively with the organization's quality committee and staff responsible for oversight of CDS. As noted in Chapter 19, the CDS team often includes nursing informaticists as well as the end users. Important considerations are for this joint team effort are to establish lists and data elements to support the measure and the organization's strategy to improve care. When examining the eCQM data fields captured in the EHR, the data need to be codified appropriately for the quality data element and the associated value set, such as problem lists with active or resolved diagnoses coded in ICD-9/10 and SNOMED, or for the medication lists coded with RxNorm. Customized, locally built, and defined quality data elements may require term bindings (e.g., communication orders tagged with SNOMED codes, negations tagged with SNOMED codes). Interface for other data sources may also be required such as with interdependencies on lab or imaging results, and requirements for tagging with Logical Observation Identifiers Names and Codes (LOINC).

Validation: Quality and Accuracy of Build, Data Capture, and Measure Calculation

Validating measures for quality is an important consideration for the interprofessional teams tasked with the organization's enterprise eCQM reporting. Considerations include the validity of the build within the EHR as well as end-user data capture challenges that frequently relate to workflow. The authors recommend the following as a checklist to validate the accuracy and quality of the reporting within an organization. This is not meant to be an exclusive list to ensure quality of reporting but a starting point for an organization. Recommendations include addressing the following questions:

1. Are all term bindings in place and triggering to support quality-reporting document architecture (QRDA) files? Term binding relates to mapping data from the source system to respective value sets that at times can have multiple pathways or value sets to map.

2. Are values filing into value sets or groups to support local measure calculation?

3. Are CDS rules firing as designed to trigger the correct collection of the eMeasure?

4. Does the workflow support accurate data collection?

5. Are there data validity issues related to data capture workflow and user engagement?

To design and build codified and consistent eMeasure specifications, it is important to consider whether the value sets within and across measures align for the measures that are within the United States Health Information Knowledgebase (USHIK). The USHIK is an accessible registry and repository of health care-related metadata, specifications, and standards, and it can be accessed via the following link: https://ushik.ahrq.gov/mdr/portals (supported by AHRQ and hosted on their website). Reviewing the specifications, including the attributes at the granular level, is important for the accuracy of meeting the specifications for the eCQM—for example, determining whether quality data elements are built to support the attributes included within the quality measure, such as a measure using the presence of a laboratory order when one should be using the presence of a result for the laboratory test.

To validate eCQMs and the quality of data reported, the team typically reviews for incomplete, inaccurate, or inconsistent data that can lead to miscalculation and errors in identifying patients who are eligible for the measure. Exclusion and inclusion criteria can also be a problem with those who receive recommended care (inclusion in the measure) or those who should be considered an exception (exclusion criteria). A thorough review of the eCQM requirements against data within the EHR is necessary for assessing level of completeness, accuracy, granularity, timeliness, and currency.

The American Hospital Association (AHA) studied the impact of clinical quality indicators of MU on hospitals' reporting of eCQMs. From this study, AHA recommends using an interactive process to address challenges that an organization may encounter with the reporting of accurate eCQMs. Figure 28.5 reflects the steps that AHA noted from

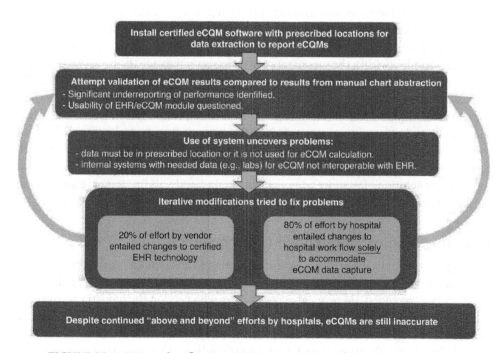

FIGURE 28.5. AHA study reflecting eCQM iterative process for hospitals.

AHA, American Heart Association; eCQM, electronic clinical quality measure; EHR, electronic health record.
Source: Eisenberg et al. (2011).

the study examining implementation of eCQMs. The figure reflects the iterative/cyclic process used to address the challenges of accurately generating the eMeasures of quality. Notable in the process is that 20% of the effort on modifications and fixes used to address accuracy challenges is completed by the vendor, whereas "80% of effort is by the hospital entailing changes to workflow solely to accommodate eCQMs" (Eisenberg et al., 2011, p. 13).

Managing for Ongoing Success

Establishing an eMeasure management approach that focuses on the full eCQM life cycle, including the build of the EHR for quality data capture, clinical workflow, CDS, performance reporting, end-user education, and annual measure updates, is important for successful enterprise eCQM strategies. The team responsible for eCQMs should expect that needs and requirements of the organization will rapidly evolve during the year. Frequent reviews of eCQM status will be required to identify issues and manage change, including version updates, correcting errors, and supporting end users in capturing accurate and valid data. This should be supported by a team that can react quickly to prioritize needs, model solutions, deploy plans, and define measures of success.

Responsibilities of a High-Functioning eCQM Team

The eCQM team should include clinicians, regulatory content experts with technical expertise, as well as end users, who are the ones most affected by the process. Regulatory content experts with technical expertise would be staff who fully understand the meaningful use requirements as well as other quality reporting regulatory requirements. In addition, these staff need to fully grasp the quality data reporting technical architecture and specifications required. The team should be established and have executive support and high visibility within the organization to effectively manage the measure packages with approaches that are customized to suit continually evolving measure demands. The team should also include representation from each group that touches the measure from initial build, implementation, and data capture through the reporting and validation stage. Responsibilities of the interprofessional team to maintain quality and validity of the eCQMs include reviewing the EHR build to capture data; creating performance reports on the measures; supporting CDS to assess effectiveness; identifying gaps; designing targeted solutions for addressing gaps or quality and validity issues; and crafting messaging, communication, education, and deployment strategies to address issues.

Guarding Against Unintended Consequences

Although studies indicate quality-measures reporting that is publically available to health care consumers fosters transparency and consumer choice and can improve the quality of services provided, there are also researchers who caution the industry to consider the unintended consequences of public reporting of quality indicators (Berwick, James, & Coye, 2003; Fung, Lim, Mattke, Damberg, & Shekelle, 2008; Marshall, Shekelle, Leatherman, & Brook, 2000). Werner and Asch (2005) indicate that reporting and monitoring quality based on "target" rates for health care interventions may discount patient preferences and clinical judgment. Further, in a study assessing attitudes of hospitals toward public reporting, Lindenauer et al. (2014) report that the study findings reveal that hospital leaders indicated that measures reported on the Hospital Compare website strongly influenced local planning and improvement efforts. These researchers also report that leaders expressed concern about adequacy of risk adjustment and unintended consequences of public reporting, including neglect of other clinical important areas. In addition, these leaders believed that these indicators were not fully reflective of quality (Lindenauer et al., 2014). These findings could be viewed as problematic from the standpoint of focusing all of the attention on quality and improvement solely on requirements, particularly in light of the challenges of elevating the eCMQs across the nation. The likelihood that these measures will drive improvements that are focused solely on priority areas within the national strategy's aims may or may not be a good fit for all areas of the United States. However, the concern about adequate risk adjustment might be better addressed with better clinical data coming from the EHRs. This will depend on the quality and validity of the data and will require that organizations follow strategies such as those discussed within the chapter. It will also require the commitment of organizations to strategize quality and improvement priorities based on what is needed, both locally and within their organizations, and not only on federal quality-reporting requirements.

QUALITY-REPORTING INITIATIVES

To fully understand the eMeasures landscape, it is important to revisit a bit of history related to the evolution of quality reporting. In 1986, TJC started the process of defining national quality measures with the testing and evaluation of six measures for hospital performance included in the Indicator Measurement System. This initiative was the foundation for the ORYX® initiative established in 1998, requiring performance reporting from hospitals (TJC, 2012). In addition, in 1989, the National Committee for Quality Assurance (NCQA) working with health maintenance organizations (HMOs) established the HMO Employer Data and Information Data Set. This initiative was expanded in 2007 under the Healthcare Effectiveness Data and Information Set (HEDIS). HEDIS included physicians and physician groups (NCQA, n.d.). CMS officially began its quality measures of reporting in 1997 with data collection on the first set of standardized measures reflecting the managed care plans of NCQA's HEDIS measure set. Subsequently, CMS expanded on that effort with incrementally more complex and comprehensive quality-reporting initiatives. Currently, CMS has measure sets that reflect the performance of hospitals, nursing homes, home health agencies, dialysis facilities, prescription drug plans (through Medicare Advantage), and, more recently, physician reporting through the Physician Quality Reporting System (PQRS; Goodrich, Garcia, & Conway, 2012). Most of these efforts were based on manually abstracted information that was very labor intensive or from claims data that lack depth of clinical information. With the expansion of EHRs, the industry has an unprecedented volume of granular data on patient care processes and outcomes that can generate eMeasures. However, this transition to eMeasures is technically challenging and requires the coordination of many organizations to harmonize measure sets that consistently and validly report on quality, efficiency, and population health. The remainder of this chapter reviews this transition and discusses how organizations can prepare to report eMeasures to CMS through certified electronic health record technology (CEHRT) starting in 2014 with Stage 2 of MU. As a component of federal certification requirements, the CEHRT must be able to calculate and report on specific measures based on specifications outlined within the certification rule-making process (Office of the National Coordinator for Health IT, 2015).

Alignment of Measures

One of the challenges the industry faces is alignment of measures across measures, particularly with the value sets that are detailed beneath the measure itself. A value set is the detailed vocabulary underneath the measure that comprises the details of how to define the measure (e.g., SNOMED-CT codes[1]). In 2001, CMS along with TJC started this process of aligning measure sets under the 7th Scope of Work (CMS, 2014c[2]). In 2003, after this initial alignment work, CMS and TJC pressed to align all hospital measures under the National Hospital Inpatient Quality Measures (NHIQM) initiative (TJC, 2015). This initiative was followed by the NQF and contracted by the Department of Health and Human Services (HHS) to provide consensus-based measures with the role of recommending prioritization, endorsement services, and maintenance of valid and reliable quality measures. CMS has various statutory requirements under many programs and environments authorizing the collection of performance measures dating back more than 15 years. To explain eMeasures, ONC has created a glossary of terms that can be found on the HealthIT.gov website (HealthIT.gov, 2015). This will be a helpful document to refer to as one begins to grasp the complexity of the eMeasures reporting mechanism that is under development within the United States.

The ACA specifically calls for the alignment of quality measures with MU, particularly with the PQRS measures for eligible providers under the Centers for Medicare & Medicaid Services Electronic Health Record (CMS-EHR) Incentive Program (The Patient Protection and Affordable Care Act, 2010). The goal was to align endorsement with development of national quality measures that were consistent with the NQS. Figure 28.6 reflects the three aims as well as the six priorities for the NQS. In 2011, the NQF played a significant role under the Health Information Technology for Economic and Clinical Health Act to "retool" 113 PQRS measures for eligible providers from paper-based abstracted measures to eMeasures (Doyle, 2014). Of these 113 measures, 44 were selected and confirmed in the final rules of the EHR-MU Incentive Program (CMS, 2013b).

Value-Based Purchasing

The ACA is an attempt to realign the payment structure to incentivize improvements in quality while simultaneously driving down costs. To realign the payment model,

---

[1]SNOMED-CT is a comprehensive clinical terminology. See www.nlm.nih.gov/research/umls/Snomed/snomed_main.html

[2]CMS Scope of Work is a contractual arrangement with quality improvement organizations (QIOs) to address the charge for health care quality improvement. See www.cms.gov/Medicare/Quality-Initiatives-Patient-Assessment-Instruments/QualityImprovementOrgs/index.html?redirect=/qualityimprovementorgs

1. **BETTER CARE:** Improve the overall quality of care, by making health care more patient-centered, reliable, accessible, and safe.

2. **HEALTHY PEOPLE/HEALTHY COMMUNITIES:** Improve the health of the U.S. population by supporting proven interventions to address behavioral, social, and environmental deteminants of health in addition to delivering higher-quality care.

3. **AFFORDABLE CARE:** Reduce the cost of quality health care for individuals, families, employers, and goverments.

NATIONAL QUALITY STRATEGY'S SIX PRIORITIES:

1. Making care safer by reducing harm caused in the delivery of care.
2. Ensuring that each person and family are engaged as partners in their care.
3. Promoting effective communication and coordination of care.
4. Promoting the most effective prevention and treatment practices for the leading cardiovascular disease.
5. Working with communities to promote wide use of best practices to enable healthy living.
6. Making quality care more affordable for individuals, families, employers, and governments by developing and spreading new health care delivery models.

FIGURE 28.6. National Quality Strategy—triple aim and six priorities.
Source: DHHS (2013).

the industry is required to shift from the traditional fee-for-service payment model for U.S. health care to a value-based purchasing model. Within the value-based purchasing models, measures of quality are required to substantiate payments based on quality. This shift to a value-based purchasing model started with hospitals, because hospitals constitute the largest proportion of health care expenses in the United States. Payment reform under a value-based purchasing model creates financial incentives based on the quality of services provided on a subset of measures that are expected to constitute "value" (CMS, 2014b). Table 28.1 reflects additional important events, programmatic infrastructure, and the associated timeline of these programs that were important events for the transition to eMeasures. These were essentially stepping stones to establish an infrastructure within state and federal initiatives to support this movement to eMeasures, which was designed to capture the triple aims and six priorities of the NQS.

TABLE 28.1 Important Building Blocks for Transition to eMeasures	
Timeline	Important Initiative
2003	Medicare Modernization Act expanded coverage for seniors to include prescription drug coverage and other expansions
2004	ONC was established
2005	Deficit Reduction Act allowed states to pursue innovative ideas
2003–current	NQF initiatives retooling paper measures to eMeasures
2010, July	44 of 113 measures published in the CMS-EHR Incentive Program Final Rule
2010	ACA

ACA, Affordable Care Act; CMS-EHR, Centers for Medicare & Medicaid Services electronic health record; eMeasures, electronic measures; NQF, National Quality Forum; ONC, Office of the National Coordinator.

Source: Doyle (2014).

MAJOR STAKEHOLDERS IN THE ᴇMEASURE DEVELOPMENT PROCESS

There are a number of stakeholders involved in setting the industry standards for eMeasures, and this helps in fully comprehending the complexity of the development process by outlining the roles of each of these stakeholders. Table 28.2 reflects the major stakeholders in this process. Developing and fully capitalizing on eMeasures requires many stakeholders, including providers, federal agencies, measures developers, and standards organizations; all of these components also include partnerships between private and public entities. In addition, the health care consumer or patient plays an important role as the ultimate stakeholder and recipient of the end product and goal of better care, better health, and reduced cost. CMS sets the agenda and manages the process for the eCQMs; however, CMS depends on other organizations to enable this process to work smoothly. For example, the ONC publishes all EHR standards and certification criteria that play a major role in coordinating standards that are built into the certification of EHRs. To be certified, the EHRs must develop the roadmap, requiring that the vendors play a key role in understanding and testing eMeasures with feedback to both CMS and ONC. Health Level Seven International (HL7), discussed in Chapter 12, establishes important building blocks for the eMeasures, including the QRDA and the HQMF. This is essentially the framework within which the measures reside within the EHR. Measures application partnership (MAP) is a public–private partnership convened by the NQF to provide recommendations to the HHS on the selection of performance

TABLE 28.2 Major Stakeholders for eMeasures	
Stakeholder	**Role in the eCQM Development Process**
CMS	CMS manages the MU programs, including managing eCQM selection and development.
CMS measures management contractor	Contractor provides technical support to measure developers in understanding the CMS-MMS blueprint processes, identifying measures for harmonization purposes, and interpreting NQF processes as they relate to measure development, endorsement, and maintenance.
eMIG	eMIG works to develop standards that measure developers use in creating new quality measures and retooling current paper-based CQMs.
Federal regulators	Several federal offices support CMS in posting the measure for public comment and confirming the final version published in the *Federal Register.*
Health caregivers	These are providers of health care, including doctors, nurses, and other medical professionals.
HL7	HL7 is a standards development organization dedicated to providing a comprehensive framework and standards for the exchange, integration, sharing, and retrieval of electronic health information. Both the QRDA and the HQMF are published by HL7.
MAP	MAP is a public–private partnership that reviews performance measures for potential use in federal public reporting and performance-based payment programs while working to align measures being used in public- and private-sector programs.
NLM	NLM manages the VSAC, which publishes value sets for use in the eMeasure development process.
NQF	The NQF is a nonprofit organization that reviews, endorses, and recommends health care quality measures. It convenes the MAP, a public–private partnership that reviews measures for potential use in public reporting and performance-based programs while also working to align measures being used in public- and private-sector programs.
ONC-HIT	ONC publishes regulations on EHR standards and certification criteria.

(continued)

TABLE 28.2 Major Stakeholders for eMeasures *(continued)*	
Stakeholder	**Role in the eCQM Development Process**
Patients and the general public	Recipients of health care and those who are a part of the health care system
TEP	A group of experts (typically clinicians, statisticians, quality improvement methodologists, or pertinent measure developers) who provide technical input to the measure contractor on the development, selection, and maintenance of measures for which CMS contractors are responsible

CMS, Centers for Medicare & Medicaid Services; CMS-MMS, Centers for Medicare & Medicaid Services Measures Management System; CQM, clinical quality measure; eCQM, electronic clinical quality measure; EHR, electronic health record; eMeasure, electronic measure; eMIG, eMeasures Issue Group; HL7, Health Level Seven International; HQMF, health quality measures format; MAP, Measure Applications Partnership; MMS, Measures Management System; NLM, National Library of Medicine; NQF, National Quality Forum; ONC, Office of the National Coordinator; ONC-HIT, Office of the National Coordinator for Health Information Technology; QRDA, quality reporting data architecture; TEP, technical expert panel; VSAC, Value Set Authority Center.

Adapted from Javellana (2014).

measures for public reporting and performance-based payment programs. During the previous year, the MAP addressed 199 unique measures for use in more than 20 federal health programs (NQF, 2014). The MAP has also developed a framework that "promotes system alignment of performance measures" and "families of measures that cut across multiple layers of the healthcare system" (Goodrich et al., 2012, p. 468).

An additionally important organization is the National Library of Medicine (NLM), which plays a significant role in data standards, including establishing the value sets within the measures, such as the SNOMED-CT codes (U.S. National Library of Medicine, 2014). The NQF is a private-sector organization and, as noted earlier, it is an organization contracted to HHS that plays the role of reviewing, endorsing, and recommending health care quality measures to support the NQS. The NQF is also the convener for the MAP and plays a significant role in working to align measures being used in both public- and private-sector programs. In addition to organizations and structures noted, a number of technical expert panels (TEPs) were also convened to help address challenges within the process (Javellana, 2014).

TOOLS AND RESOURCES IN THE ᴇMEASURE DEVELOPMENT LIFE CYCLE

The development for eCQMs for use in CMS programs follows a life cycle development process reflected in Figure 28.7. This process begins with the selection of a measure and the conceptualized indicator of quality. This concept analysis is followed by a specification for the measure that operationalizes how the measure will actually be derived

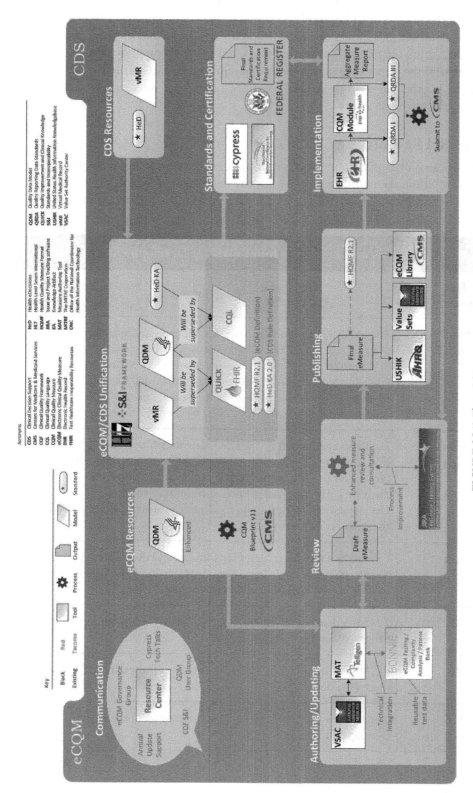

FIGURE 28.7. The eCQI ecosystem.
Source: The Mitre Corporation (2014).

from the electronic environment. Once specifications are distributed, the measure is tested in the field prior to full implementation to attempt to eliminate any issues with specifications and interpretation of those specifications by vendors programming the measures within the EHRs. This implementation phase is followed by measure use and evaluation of those measures to determine the ultimate impact of the measure on the industry. In other words, did the measure make a difference with respect to the target population (Javellana, 2014)?

Tools and Resources

There are a number of notable tools and resources that constitute some of the "moving parts" in the reporting process within the development life cycle process. Table 28.3 reflects these tools, and a few of these components are described in terms of the

TABLE 28.3 Tools and Resources for eCQMs for Development and Testing	
Tools and Resources	**Description**
CMS-MMS and blueprint	A standardized approach to the development and maintenance of the quality measures used in CMS quality initiatives and programs, the MMS provides a set of business processes and decision criteria that CMS-funded measure developers (or contractors) follow to develop, implement, and maintain quality measures. The blueprint requirements align with those cited by the NQF for endorsement.
CMS measures inventory	Database maintained by the CMS Measures Management contractor that contains details on the measures and measure concepts created for use in CMS programs along with status of the measures (e.g., archived, future, current, implemented). Developers can request input to identify measures and concepts that may require harmonization.
Cypress	Cypress is a tool for testing EHRs-MU and EHR modules. It is open source, freely available for use or adoption, and is the official testing tool for the 2014 EHR Certification program.
eCQM library	CMS maintains a list of eCQMs in use with CMS programs on its program website.
HQMF	HQMF is the industry (HL7) standard for representing a CQM as an electronic document.
MAT	The MAT is a publicly available, web-based tool for measure developers to create e-Measures.

(continued)

TABLE 28.3 Tools and Resources for eCQMs for Development and Testing *(continued)*	
Tools and Resources	**Description**
NQF-QPS	This is an online tool that allows users to search for NQF-endorsed measures.
QDM	The QDM is an information model that clearly defines concepts used in quality measures and clinical care and is intended to enable automation of EHR use. It provides a way to describe clinical concepts in a standardized format so that individuals (i.e., providers, researchers, measure developers) monitoring clinical performance and outcomes can clearly and concisely communicate necessary information.
QRDA	QRDA is the standard for transmitting/reporting health care quality measurement information. QRDA Category I reports individual patient-level data, whereas QRDA Category III reports aggregate data from multiple patients. QRDA reports are then able to be transmitted from certified vendor systems to CMS and other quality organizations.
VSAC	The VSAC currently serves as the central repository for the official versions of value sets that support MU 2014 CQMs. The VSAC provides search, retrieval, and download capabilities through a web interface and APIs.

APIs, application program interfaces; CMS, Centers for Medicare & Medicaid Services; CMS-MMS, Centers for Medicare & Medicaid Services Measures Management System; CQMs, clinical quality measures; eCQMs, electronic clinical quality measures; EHR, electronic health record; EHRs-MU, electronic health records meaningful use; HL7, Health Level Seven International; HQMF, health quality measures format; MAT, measure authoring tool; NQF-QPS, National Quality Forum Quality Positioning System; QDM, quality data model; QRDA, quality reporting document architecture; VSAC, Value Set Authority Center.

Adapted from Javellana (2014).

relationship within the development cycle. The Centers for Medicare & Medicaid Services Measures Management System is essentially the blueprint for CMS with respect to the development and maintenance of the measures for CMS and its quality initiatives and programs. The blueprint is divided into sections, including measurement development concepts; measure life cycle; eMeasure life cycle; and the tools, appendices, and forms for use by the various contracting organizations under CMS that comprise the measure developers (CMS, 2014a). The inventory is a database that contains all of the details related to the measures, including current as well as historical measures. Cypress is the testing tool for measures that includes not only the eCQMs but also all MU measures.

The eCQM library is a website that maintains a list of the eCQMs for providers and hospitals, including the current and prior measures (see www.cms.gov/Regulations-and-Guidance/Legislation/EHRIncentivePrograms/eCQM_Library.html). The Measure Authoring Tool (MAT) is used by all measure developers for eMeasures. The QDM, as stated earlier, is essentially the model that defines concepts used in the measures and captures the spirit of the measure in a standardized approach. However, the QRDA is the technical standard for transmission and includes detail-level (QRDA Category I) and aggregate data (QRDA Category III). The primary purpose of QRDA is the standardization and full support of interoperability between vendors and the CMS submission process. The Value Set Authority Center (VSAC) is the repository for the value sets for the various measures, and it supports developers and users with search, retrieval, and download capabilities. In addition, on its website in support of eCQMs, the ONC has a number of helpful materials that provide resources and educational materials on each of these components (Javellana, 2014).

To fully grasp how these organizations, tools, and resources fit together, the Mitre Corporation is the host of Technical Authority for the United Clinical Quality Improvement Framework (Tacoma). As such, it has created a visual depiction of the eMeasures development cycle and all of the various components in that process. Figure 28.7 reflects the electronic clinical quality improvement (eCQI) ecosystem that walks the reader through the eCQM life cycle from authoring of the measure all the way to implementation. Many of the tools, resources, and stakeholders involved in the process have been discussed. This visual gives the reader an overview of the complexity of the process for moving an eMeasure from concept to full implementation. A high-level overview of the developmental life cycle is also noted in Figure 28.8.

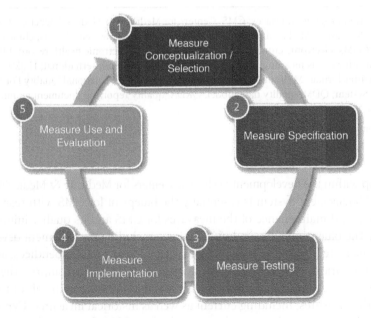

FIGURE 28.8. eCQM development life cycle.

Source: Javellana (2014).

CASE STUDY

You are the chief nursing quality officer for a large integrated delivery system and have been designated as the lead executive in charge of all regulatory reporting for quality measures, which also include the meaningful use of electronic clinical quality measures (MU-eCQMs). Your organization has successfully attested to the quality metrics under the MU process and you must now prepare your organization for eCQM reporting. Your organization is resource constrained and frequently prioritizes efforts based on federal and regulatory requirements rather than based on its needs. In fact, you are aware that you have significant quality and safety concerns that fall outside of the current set of quality indicators that your current EHR vendor has certified to report in the eCQMs to meet the MU requirements. Considering the information presented in the chapter, design your strategy for preparing your organization for eCQMs and reflect on the following questions:

1. What type of team will you put together to oversee the development and deployment of the eCQM reporting?
2. How will you ensure that the information reported is accurately reported on behalf of the organization?
3. What resources are available to you to better understand the process for eCQM development and deployment?
4. How will your organization utilize CDS to reinforce and align electronic quality improvement methods and measurement?
5. How will you balance the needs of the organization with eCQM reporting of federal reporting requirements and the local needs of your organization with respect to your quality concerns?

SUMMARY

To conclude, this chapter has covered the transformation underway regarding measurement and monitoring of the NQS using quality measures derived from EHRs. Quality measures are moving from an abstract-based and claims-encounter process to a much more complex electronic reporting mechanism. The transition of the industry from a manual process of data collection to a more advanced eMeasures mechanism for reporting and monitoring of quality using data from certified EHRs presents many challenges.

This chapter has discussed the stakeholders involved in the process and many tools and resources that constitute the "moving parts" of eMeasures development. The electronic quality improvement ecosystem is discussed and reflected visually for the reader to grasp the magnitude of the development underway to fully capitalize on eCQMs. The chapter also has presented recommendations based on the authors' experiences in the field with techniques used to develop and deploy an interprofessional team across an enterprise to ensure a successful eCQM development and reporting strategy. Finally, a case study has been presented related to challenges with eCQMs to help the reader consider strategies to validate and address quality concerns when eCQMs do not seem to be accurately reflective of practice within the organization.

REFERENCES

Agency for Healthcare Research and Quality. (2014). *National quality strategy stakeholder tool kit.* Retrieved from www.ahrq.gov/workingforquality/nqs/nqstoolkit.htm#priorities

Agency for Healthcare Research and Quality. (2015). *USHIK: United States health information knowledgebase.* Retrieved from https://ushik.ahrq.gov/mdr/portals

Berwick, D. M., James, B., & Coye, M. J. (2003). Connections between quality measurement and improvement. *Medical Care, 41*(1), 30–38. Retrieved from www.intermountainhealthcare.org/qualityandresearch/institute/Documents/articles_connections.pdf

Centers for Medicare & Medicaid Services. (2011). *The CMS EHR incentive programs: What you need to know about the clinical quality measures.* Retrieved from www.cms.gov/Regulations-and-Guidance/Legislation/EHRIncentivePrograms/downloads/CQM_Webinar_Slides.pdf

Centers for Medicare & Medicaid Services. (2012). *2014 Clinical quality measures tipsheet: Criteria for reporting clinical quality measures.* Retrieved from www.cms.gov/Regulations-and-Guidance/Legislation/EHRIncentivePrograms/Downloads/ClinicalQualityMeasuresTipsheet.pdf

Centers for Medicare & Medicaid Services. (2013a). *Additional information regarding EP clinical quality measures for 2014 EHR incentive programs.* Retrieved from www.cms.gov/Regulations-and-Guidance/Legislation/EHRIncentivePrograms/Downloads/EP_MeasuresTable_Posting_CQMs.pdf

Centers for Medicare & Medicaid Services. (2013b). *EHR incentive programs: The official website for the Medicare and Medicaid electronic health records (EHR) incentive programs.* Retrieved from www.cms.gov/Regulations-and-Guidance/Legislation/EHRIncentivePrograms/index.html

Centers for Medicare & Medicaid Services. (2014a). *CMS measures management system.* Retrieved from www.cms.gov/Medicare/Quality-Initiatives-Patient-Assessment-Instruments/MMS/MeasuresManagementSystemBlueprint.html

Centers for Medicare & Medicaid Services. (2014b). *Hospital value-based purchasing.* Retrieved from www.cms.gov/Medicare/Quality-Initiatives-Patient-Assessment-Instruments/hospital-value-based-purchasing/index.html

Centers for Medicare & Medicaid Services. (2014c). *Quality improvement organizations.* Retrieved from www.cms.gov/Medicare/Quality-Initiatives-Patient-Assessment-Instruments/QualityImprovementOrgs/index.html?redirect=/qualityimprovementorgs

Centers for Medicare & Medicaid Services. (2015). *eCQM library.* Retrieved from www.cms.gov/Regulations-and-Guidance/Legislation/EHRIncentivePrograms/eCQM_Library.html

Centers for Medicare & Medicaid Services and Office of the National Coordinator. (2014). *Electronic clinical quality measure logic and implementation guidance and technical release notes* (Release Notes No. Version 1.9). Centers for Medicare & Medicaid Services. Retrieved from www.cms.gov/Regulations-and-Guidance/Legislation/EHRIncentivePrograms/Downloads/eCQM_LogicGuidance_v19_July2014.pdf

Doyle, B. (2014). *eMeasures transition* (White Paper). Encore Health Resources. Retrieved from www.encorehealthresources.com/wp-content/uploads/2014/02/eMeasures-Transitions-Feb2014_Q.pdf

Eisenberg, F., Lasome, C., Advani, A., Martins, R., Craig, P. A., & Sprenger, S. (2011). *A study of the impact of meaningful use clinical quality measures* (Study Report). American Hospital Association. Retrieved from www.aha.org/content/13/13ehrchallenges-report.pdf

Eisenberg, F., Overage, M., & Johnson, l. (2011). *Implementing electronic measures (eMeasures) in hospitals* (Presentation). Washington, DC: National Quality Forum.

Fung, C. H., Lim, Y. W., Mattke, S., Damberg, C., & Shekelle, P. G. (2008). Systematic review: The evidence that publishing patient care performance data improves quality of care. *Annals of Internal Medicine, 148*(2), 111–123. doi:10.7326/0003-4819-148-2-200801150-00006

Goodrich, K., Garcia, E., & Conway, P. (2012). A history of and a vision of CMS quality measurement programs. *Joint Commission Journal on Quality and Patient Safety, 38*(10), 465–470. Retrieved from www.ncbi.nlm.nih.gov/pubmed/23130393

HealthIT.gov, ECQI Resource Center. (2015). *Glossary of eCQI Terms.* Retrieved from https://ecqi .healthit.gov/content/glossary-ecqi-terms

Javellana, M. (2014, December). *Developing electronic clinical quality measures (eCQMs) for use in CMS programs.* Paper presented at the Centers for Medicare & Medicaid Services Presentation on MAP-eCQM.

The Joint Commission. (2012). *Key historical milestones.* Retrieved from www.jointcommission.org/ assets/1/18/sigw_Vision_paper_web_version.pdf

The Joint Commission. (2015). *Core measure sets.* Retrieved from www.jointcommission.org/core_ measure_sets.aspx

Lindenauer, P. K., Lagu, T., Ross, J. S. Pekow, P. S., Shatz, A., Hannon, N., . . . Benjamin, E. M. (2014). Attitudes of hospital leaders toward publicly reported measures of health care quality. *Journal of the American Medical Association Internal Medicine, 174*(12), 1904–1911. doi:10.1001/jamainternmed .2014.5161

Marshall, M. N., Shekelle, P. G., Leatherman, S., & Brook, R. H. (2000). The public release of performance data: What do we expect to gain? A review of the evidence. *Journal of the American Medical Association, 283*(14), 1866–1874. doi:10.1001/jama.283.14.1866

The Mitre Corporation. (2014). Technical Authority for the Unified Clinical Quality Improvement Framework (Tacoma) Overview HL7 Meeting Presentation January 20–24, 2014. Retrieved from https:// www.hl7.org/documentcenter/public_temp_A6E10ED2-1C23-BA17-0C83431EC72201AF/wg/cqi/ HL7_Tacoma-Jan_2014_WGM.pdf

National Committee for Quality Assurance. (n.d.). *HEDIS & performance measurement.* Retrieved from www.ncqa.org/HEDISQualityMeasurement.aspx

National Quality Forum. (2012). *Guide for reading eligible provider and hospital eMeasures.* Retrieved from www.qualityforum.org/Projects/e-g/eMeasures/Guide_for_Reading_EP_and_Hospital_Measures .aspx

National Quality Forum. (2014). *MAP 2015 considerations for implementing measures in federal programs* (Technical Report-Draft for MAP Clinician Workgroup Review). Retrieved from http://public .qualityforum.org/MAP/MAP%20Clinician%20Workgroup/MAP%20Clinician%20Programmatic% 20Deliverable%20DRAFT%2012%205%202014.pdf

Office of the National Coordinator for Health IT. (2015). Comprehensive list of certified health information technology. Retrieved http://oncchpl.force.com/ehrcert

Osheroff, J. A., Teich, J. M., Levick, D., Saldana, L., Velasco, F. T., Sittig, D. F., . . . Jenders, R. A. (2012). *Improving outcomes with CDS: An implementer's guide* (2nd ed.). Chicago, IL: HIMSS.

The Patient Protection and Affordable Care Act, Pub. L. No. 118–148. (2010). Retrieved from www.gpo.gov/fdsys/pkg/PLAW-111publ148/pdf/PLAW-111publ148.pdf

U.S. Department of Health and Human Services. (2013). *2013 Annual progress report to Congress: National strategy for quality improvement in health care.* Retrieved from www.ahrq.gov/workingfor quality/nqs/nqs2013annlrpt.htm

U.S. National Library of Medicine. (2014). *SNOMED clinical terms.* Retrieved from www.nlm.nih.gov/research/umls/Snomed/snomed_main.html

Werner, R. M., & Asch, D. A. (2005). The unintended consequences of publicly reporting quality information. *Journal of the American Medical Association, 293*(10), 1239–1244. doi:10.1001/jama.293.10.1239

APPENDIX 28.1 HYPERTENSION ᴇCQM: JUNE 2014 UPDATE FOR ᴇREPORTING FOR THE 2015 REPORTING YEAR

2014 eCQM Flow
Measure Identifier: CMS22v3
Preventive Care and Screening: Screening for High Blood Pressure and Follow-Up Documented

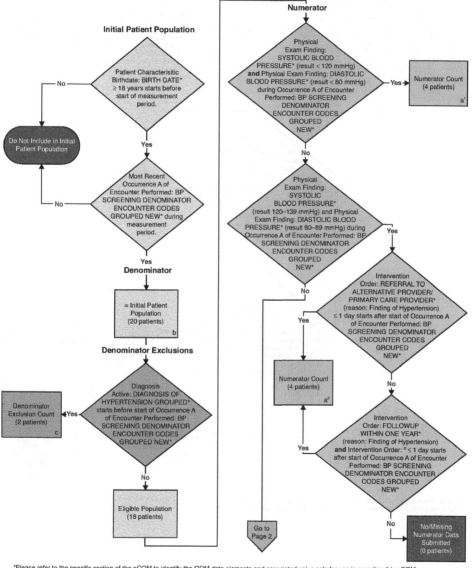

*Please refer to the specific section of the eCQM to identify the QDM data elements and associated value sets for use in reporting this eCQM.
ᵠFor a listing of appropriate interventions, please refer to the QDM data elements and associated value sets as specific data elements have not been listed.

2014 eCQM Flow
Measure Identifier: CMS22v3
Preventive Care and Screening: Screening for High Blood Pressure and Follow-Up Documented

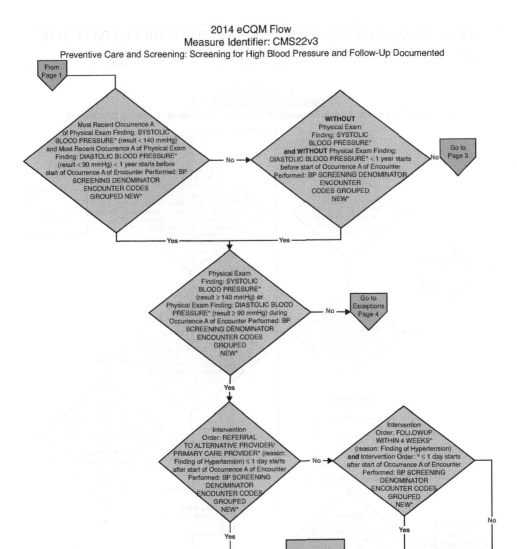

*Please refer to the specific section of the eCQM to identify the QDM data elements and associated value sets for use in reporting this eCQM.
¥For a listing of appropriate interventions, please refer to the QDM data elements and associated value sets as specific data elements have not been listed.

2014 eCQM Flow
Measure Identifier: CMS22v3
Preventive Care and Screening: Screening for High Blood Pressure and Follow-Up Documented

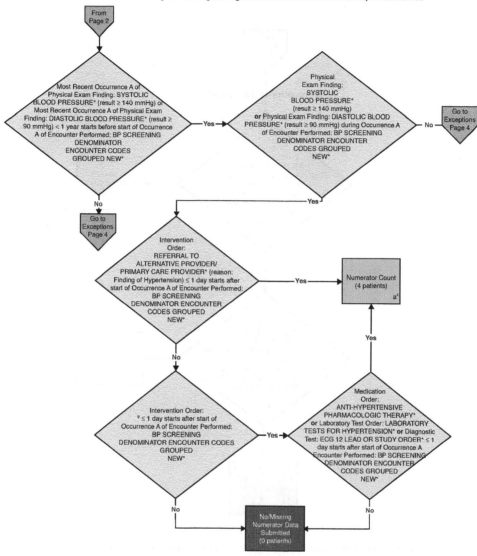

*Please refer to the specific section of the eCQM to identify the QDM data elements and associated value sets for use in reporting this eCQM.
ᵠFor a listing of appropriate interventions, please refer to the QDM data elements and associated value sets as specific data elements have not been listed.

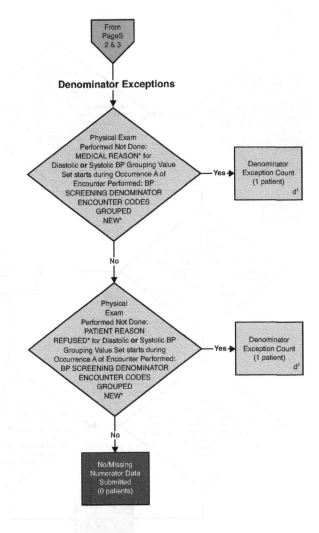

2014 eCQM Flow
Measure Identifier: CMS22v3
Preventive Care and Screening: Screening for High Blood Pressure and Follow-Up Documented

*Please refer to the specific section of the eCQM to identify the QDM data elements and associated value sets for use in reporting this eCQM.

SAMPLE CALCULATION:

Performance Rate =

$$\frac{\text{Numerator } (a^1 + a^2 + a^3 + a^4 = 16 \text{ patients})}{\text{Denominator } (b = 20 \text{ patients}) - \text{Denominator Exclusions } (c = 2 \text{ patients}) - \text{Denominator Exceptions } (d^1 + d^2 = 2 \text{ patients})} = 100.00\%$$

Source: CMS (2015).

CHAPTER 29

Interprofessional Application of Health Information Technology in Education

Mari Tietze, Cindy Acton, and Stacey Brown

OBJECTIVES

1. Describe exemplars in which interprofessional education/collaboration (IPE/C) are used to delivery health care services.

2. Explore how the role of health information technology (HIT) will support the future application of IPE/C education and delivery of health care services.

3. Discuss the relationship between IPE/C and HIT for delivery of health care services.

4. Describe the processes needed for teaching the delivery of IPE/C-based health care services in the future.

5. Utilize a toolkit to define steps in implementing an IPE/C program.

KEY WORDS

interprofessional education, interprofessional practice

CONTENTS

INTRODUCTION

The purpose of this chapter is to discuss exemplars of health care delivery in an inter-professional education/collaboration context. It also explores what is on the horizon for IPE/C. The chapter is presented in the context of health information technology as it relates to IPE/C.

A century after Flexner, Goldmark, and Welsh-Rose revolutionized postsecondary education for health professionals, two significant reports from the *Lancet* and the Institute of Medicine (IOM) sought to similarly redesign the education of health professionals for the 21st century. The independent Lancet Commission led by Julio Frenk and Lincoln Chen released *Health Professionals for a New Century: Transforming Education to Strengthen Health Systems in an Interdependent World*. The IOM produced *The Future of Nursing: Leading Change, Advancing Health* (IOM, 2010). Both these reports provide high-level visions for the health professions, but rely on educators to identify the best relevant practices and mechanisms for expanding proven, improved approaches to integrated health professional education. Considering the importance of interprofessional education (IPE) to the safe and effective delivery of health care, the IOM created an ongoing, evidence-based forum for multidisciplinary exchange on innovative health professional education initiatives. Known as the Global Forum on Innovation in Health Professional Education (National Academy of Sciences, 2015), this forum not only convenes stakeholders to highlight contemporary issues in health professional education but also supports an ongoing, innovative mechanism to grow and evaluate new ideas—a mechanism that is multifocal, multidisciplinary, and global (Cuff, 2013).

The work of the Global Forum has been reflected throughout the previous chapters in this book. For example, discussion about roles in Chapter 2 included content about the expert panel on IPE and related the use of information technology (IT) in those roles. Similarly, discussion about patient safety and quality in Chapter 20 included content about how the integration of IPE-skilled health professional teams tends to yield greater efficiency and more positive outcomes than those who are not IPE skilled. The association of IPE to consumer/patient engagement and activation is such that IPE-skilled health professionals are additive to the engagement/activation model in that these professionals can enhance patient engagement/activation efforts compared with the traditional involvement of health professionals. Finally, data analytics and clinical decision support systems (CDSS) are strengthened when IPE-skilled team members are doing the work to build and use these tools. These component relationships along with the Nursing Education Health Informatics (NEHI) model (McBride, Tietze, & Fenton, 2013) provide the context for managing the IT of the future.

History of IPE

The IPE movement became active in the mid-1990s. Many of the pioneers were foundations, such as the John A. Hartford Foundation, Robert Wood Johnson Foundation (RWJF), and Josiah Macy, Jr. Foundation. Each foundation identified the need for professional collaboration. In addition, the IOM presented alarming rates of multiple problems facing the nation related to quality care. The IOM laid out visions of how systems must change in practice, *To Err Is Human: Building a Safer Heath System* (IOM, 2000), *Crossing the Quality Chasm: A New Health System for the 21st Century* (Committee on

Quality of Healthcare in America, 2001), and in education, *Health Professions Education: A Bridge to Quality* (IOM, 2003).

By 2005, professional organizations solidified the IOM vision of focusing on interprofessional collaborative practice as the primary means to address international quality problems. Significant among the practices were the Canadian Interprofessional Health Collaborative (CIHC) and the American Interprofessional Health Collaborative (AIHC). Both organizations teamed together to form the Collaborating Across Boarders (CAB) initiative to accelerate the already rising IPE movement.

Between 2005 and 2012, accrediting agencies and professional organizations redefined competencies of individual health care professional education curricula. Professional organizations, in particular the World Health Organization and IPE/C, created sentinel reports defining IPE and identifying core competencies for interprofessional collaborative practice. Today, the reports serve as foundational documents for all health professions chartering a course of IPE.

The United States has begun building resources to support IPE. In 2012, the Health Resources and Services Administration (HRSA) of the U.S. Department of Health and Human Services awarded the University of Minnesota $4 million over 5 years to establish a national coordinating center for IPE and collaborative practice, the National Center for Interprofessional Practice and Education. In addition, the Josiah Macy, Jr. Foundation, RWJF, Gordon and Betty Moore Foundation, and John A. Hartford Foundation have collectively committed a maximum of $8.6 million in grants over 5 years to support and guide the National Center for Interprofessional Practice and Education.

Defining IPE and the Significant Role of Ethics

"IPE occurs when students from two or more professions learn about, from and with each other to enable effective collaboration and improve health outcomes" (World Health Organization, 2010, p. 7). The other report that supports IPE effort is that of the expert panel (Interprofessional Collaborative Expert Panel [ICEP], 2011). The report, for example, illustrated that a community- and population-oriented approach is central to the IPE model (see Figure 29.1). The report emphasizes that teamwork, communication value/ethics, and roles are the actions of the IPE-skilled health professionals from the trajectory of prelicensure through practice.

It has been suggested that the challenges of health systems are fundamentally ethical. These ethical principles consider health and health care a right. These principles support balance in the distribution of resources for health to both individuals and populations. Thus, cooperation is seen as the central tenet in achieving this principle (ICEP, 2011). Figure 29.2 illustrates the four competency domains of IPE; Competency Domain 1: Values/ethics for interprofessional practice clearly addresses this issue. The background and rationale of related ethics are an important, new part of crafting a professional identity, one that is both professional and interprofessional in nature. As noted, these values and ethics are patient centered with a community/population orientation, grounded in a sense of shared purpose to support the common good in health care, and reflect a shared commitment to creating safer, more efficient, and more effective systems of care.

The relationship between the four main competencies of the IPE model and the work of the IPE team is illustrated in Figure 29.3. Providing patient-centered care is core of the

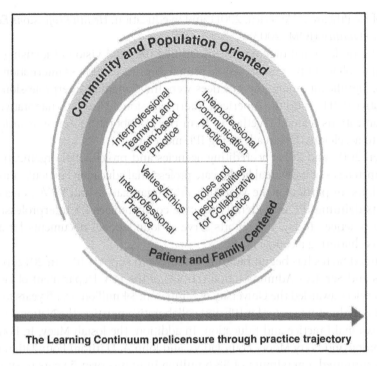

FIGURE 29.1. Interprofessional collaborative practice domains.
Source: ICEP (2011).

Competency Domain 1:	Values/Ethics for Interprofessional Practice
Competency Domain 2:	Roles/Responsibilities
Competency Domain 3:	Interprofessional Communication
Competency Domain 4:	Teams and Teamwork

FIGURE 29.2. Interprofessional collaborative practice competency domains.
Source: ICEP (2011).

competencies supported by the other three competencies: utilize informatics, employ evidence-based practice, and apply quality improvement.

RELATIONSHIP BETWEEN IPE AND HIT

As noted, *informatics* is one of the concepts of the interprofessional model suggested by the expert panel (ICEP, 2011). In addition, ubiquitous in today's health care delivery environment, informatics is a key facilitator, for example, in support of both communication

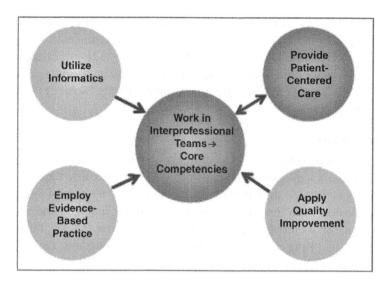

FIGURE 29.3. Interprofessional teamwork and IOM core competencies.
Source: ICEP (2011).

and simulation. Apart from the faculty and students, patients and their families benefit from interprofessional IT.

Stakeholders

Patients/Families

Engaging patients and families in quality-improvement efforts is becoming more commonplace as studies indicate that engaged patients/families yield better outcomes more efficiently and at less cost (Hibbard & Greene, 2013). Technology can facilitate this process, especially when used in an interprofessional team. This multifaceted approach to using the technology among IPE professionals as well as with patients in support of their medical management is ideal. One example of such a program is the Partnership for Patients program created by the Centers for Medicare & Medicaid Services (CMS; CMS, 2014) where providers partner with patients in shared decision-making models supported by technologies.

Providers

Providers such as nurses, physicians, and health care organizations can also benefit from interprofessional collaborative practice supported by technology. Some providers use the interprofessional approach of psychiatric care delivery long with IT (Akroyd, Jordan, & Rowlands, 2014). Others have similarly experienced such success through rapid response teams in the emergency department (ED; Allen, Jackson, & Elliott, 2015). In other situations, faculty have benefited from use of technology in interprofessional teaching (King et al., 2012; Paquette-Warren et al., 2014; Pfaff, Baxter, Jack, & Ploeg, 2014; Pulman, Scammell, & Martin, 2009).

Another such example is seen in postacute care services such as home health and remote patient monitoring for patients in their homes. CareCycle Solutions provides case managers from nursing, physical therapy, and respiratory therapy backgrounds who work together collaboratively in a virtual environment supported by a data warehouse and a decision support system. From day 1, the training of these professionals is interprofessional and involves technology. In addition, CareCycle Solutions utilizes information from their data warehouse to support business decisions involving accountable care organizations (ACOs) and other health care insurance entities (Noble & Casalino, 2013; Torres & Loehrer, 2014).

Suppliers/Vendors

The role of technology vendors in IPE/C is to understand the needs of these initiatives. An example of technology applied to interprofessional practice is to have an application available locally to provide the interprofessional information needed (Youm & Wiechmann, 2015). Vendors can support communication efforts among providers engaged in interprofessional collaborative practice by using a smartphone (Djukic, Fulmer, Adams, Lee, & Triola, 2012; King et al., 2014; Peluchette, Karl, Coustasse, & Emmett, 2012; Smith, 2014; Youm & Wiechmann, 2015).

Team Practice/Simulation

Progress in stabilization and accessibility of information and communication technology have allowed for more widespread use by the organizations, as well as by the general public. One of those advancements has been in the area of simulation methodologies in education. Sometimes called e-learning technologies, they can prove beneficial to both faculty and students (Carbonaro et al., 2008; King et al., 2012). In these scenarios, interprofessional team process skills development, pedagogical integrity, as well as instructor/faculty balance between face-to-face and online interaction and student perspectives can be assessed.

Usability testing of IT is another aspect of simulation that supports interprofessional practice. One example is the medical simulation center for an electronic health record (EHR) laboratory (Landman et al., 2014). This approach is becoming an important component of safety testing of IT; however, it is also a viable approach used to engage multiple disciplines and department staff in testing. Once such a laboratory is set up, it can be used by all stakeholders, thereby favorably addressing issues such as return on investment (ROI), cost, and benefits.

CONSIDERATIONS FOR THE FUTURE

As discussed, many organizations exist with the focus of advancing IPE/Cs, and those should continue to be followed as sources to advance IPE initiatives. In addition, at least three organizations represent efforts to infuse IT into interprofessional-based education.

Organizations to Support the Process

The Technology Informatics Guiding Education Reform Initiative

Technology Informatics Guiding Education Reform (TIGER) is an interprofessional organization that is focused on providing educational support for the advancement of

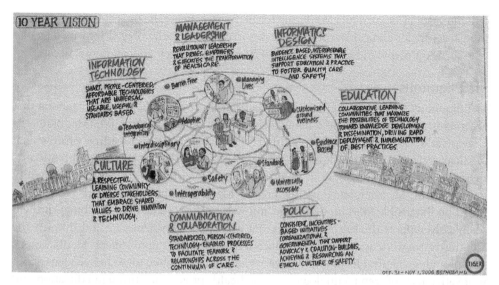

FIGURE 29.4. Ten-year vision of the TIGER initiative includes interdisciplinary education.
Source: Tiger Development Collaborative (2015a).

technology used for optimal health care delivery (TIGER Development Collaborative, 2015a). As noted in the "core" section of the 10-year vision (Figure 29.4), TIGER is interdisciplinary.

TIGER also provides the Virtual Learning Environment (VLE) website (TIGER Development Collaborative, 2015b). The TIGER VLE, powered by the Healthcare Information and Management Systems Society, is a dynamic and unique one-stop portal for academic professionals, students, adult learners, and clinical educators. The VLE contains vetted resources that are reflective of core international competencies to take one from A to Z in HIT. This personalized learning experience is designed to expand skillsets in a self-paced format. On the VLE Home page, one may integrate readily available HIT modules and resources into the current curriculum.

Health Informatics Technology Scholars

The Health Informatics Technology Scholars (HITS) program at the University of Kansas involves the School of Nursing and collaborates with the schools of nursing at the University of Colorado Denver, Johns Hopkins University, and Indiana University, in partnership with the National League for Nursing (NLN; University of Kansas Medical Center, 2013). Collectively, they present the HITS Program, which is supported by a 5-year, $1.5 million HRSA grant in partnership with the Office of Health Information Technology (OHIT). The purpose of the HITS project is to develop, implement, disseminate, and sustain a faculty development collaborative (FDC) initiative to integrate information technologies in the nursing curriculum and to expand the capacity of collegiate schools of nursing to educate students for the 21st century.

Project goals are to transform teaching and learning in the 21st century to merge informatics, telehealth, simulation, and e-learning to create powerful learning environments. Another goal is to improve nursing education and practice by developing a faculty that will integrate IT in curricula to educate future practitioners. The project will also expand infrastructure for clinical learning processes to educate a cadre of well-informed faculty who focus on real-world applications of technologies in their education practices.

MedBiquitous

MedBiquitous represents a group of educator and private industry organizations that are interested in developing and using technical standards to deliver IPE (MedBiquitous Consortium, 2015). Founded by Johns Hopkins Medicine and leading professional medical societies, the MedBiquitous Consortium is the American National Standards Institute-accredited developer of IT standards for health care education and quality improvement. Members are creating a technology blueprint for the health professions. Based on Extensible Markup Language and web services standards, this blueprint will seamlessly support the learner in ways that will improve patient care and simplify the administrative work associated with education and quality improvement. MedBiquitous also provides a neutral forum for educators and industry alike to exchange ideas about innovative uses of web technologies for the health professions through education and quality improvement.

Accreditation of Interprofessional Health Education

Accreditation of IPE is commonly discussed among advocates. The suggestions ranged from acknowledgment that a lack of consistent standards exists (Zorek & Raehl, 2013) to acknowledgment that separate academic organizations include interprofessional, inter-disciplinary, and/or team work standards as a part of their overall standards (Miller, 2014) to acknowledgement of prescribed standard guidelines with associated metrics (Accreditation of Interprofessional Health Education, 2014). Regardless of the source, given the evolving nature of the national and international IPE initiatives, it is important to be connected with these organizations and to actively share practices.

"Education to Practice" Toolkit

The Michigan-based "Education2Practice" website, supported by the statewide Michigan Health Council, is representative of open-access sharing for the advancement of IPE initiatives (Michigan Health Council, 2014). Among the website pages organized in the framework of "Learn, Do, Share," one can find a toolkit used to support implementation of IPE initiatives. Figure 29.5 illustrates the toolkit categories. Once selected, the category displays documents and other sources of information. For example, in the "Interprofessional Clinical Record" toolkit category, one can find a document for team members that tracks all the patient treatment plans in one location rather than in disparate medical records locations.

Interprofessional Informatics Program Efforts

Health Resources and Services Administration

The Health Resources and Services Administration (HRSA) division of the U.S. Department of Health and Human Services (HHS) has provided a report to guide the IPE activities of the nation. In the report, all four recommendations are directed toward linkages among the IPE educators, practitioners, policy makers, and the community (HRSA,

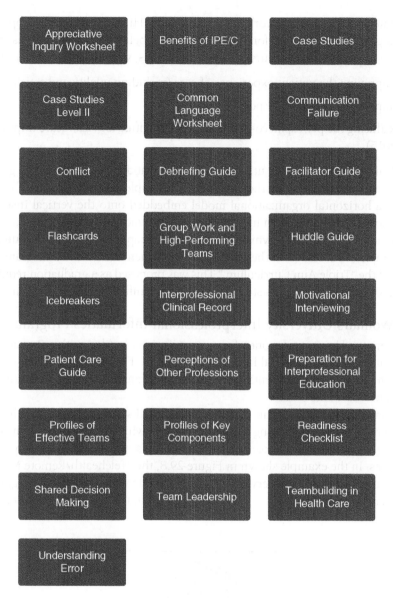

FIGURE 29.5. Education-to-practice toolkit provided by the Michigan Health Council.

IPE/C, interprofessional education/collaboration.

Source: Michigan Health Council (2014).

2014). In support of this effort, the HRSA has awarded millions of dollars to support advancement of IPE collaborative initiatives; however, in review of the challenges of the grant recipients, the greatest challenge is consistently that of engaging the other departments and/or disciplines. This observation is documented in several reports on the topic (Hall & Zierler, 2015; Paquette-Warren et al., 2014; Pfaff et al., 2014).

At least one organization has succeeded in accomplishing such implementations by integrating the IPE activities with the organization's existing Triple Aim initiative (Brandt, Lutfiyya, King, & Chioreso, 2014). The Triple Aim of the Institute for Healthcare

Improvement (IHI) is a framework developed by the IHI that describes an approach for optimizing health system performance. It is IHI's belief that new designs must be developed to simultaneously pursue three dimensions, which we call the "Triple Aim:"

- ► Improving the patient experience of care (including quality and satisfaction)
- ► Improving the health of populations
- ► Reducing the per capita cost of health care (Institute for Healthcare Improvement, 2015)

The University of Arkansas utilized a five-pillar model (see Figure 29.6) guided by the office of IPE to incorporate the university's IHI Triple Aim initiative (Wilbur, 2014). This was a horizontal organizational model embedded onto the vertical institutional organizational chart. Each team includes individuals who have an institutional perspective, objective, and influence, which allows them to map initiatives and resources. One early example of success from the curriculum implementation/evaluation team was the creation of the "Triple Aim Curriculum." This was proposed as a graduation requirement for all 2,800 health professions students as all were unified by the Triple Aim.

Texas Woman's University Interprofessional Informatics Program

Texas Woman's University is one of the organizations funded with a 3-year grant to implement an interprofessional informatics program. Figure 29.7 illustrates how students from numerous departments and/or disciplines can unite and work together before graduation.

They have an online program that uses Blackboard software to work with students from other departments, creating a "bridge" through which students can come together in an integrated part of Blackboard to work on group assignments, group papers, or on case studies. In the example shown in Figure 29.8, the "Telehealth/Remote Monitoring in Post-acute Delivery of Care Services" IPE course is offered through the College of Nursing. Students from physical therapy (PT), occupational therapy (OT), nutrition, and so

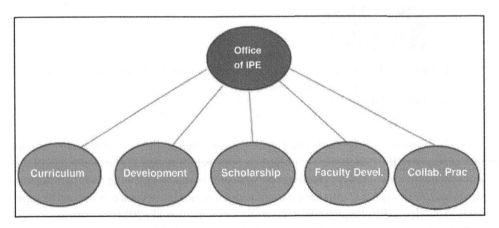

FIGURE 29.6. University of Arkansas five-pillar IPE model.

IPE, interprofessional education.

Source: Wilbur (2014).

Learning Together
So They Can Work Together

Nursing
Physical Therapy
Occupational Therapy
Nutrition/Food Science
Health Systems Management/Finance
Medicine
Dentistry
Other

Interprofessional
Students, Faculty,
and Staff

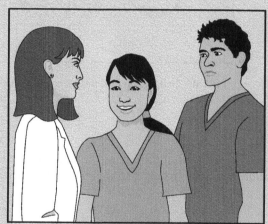

Support

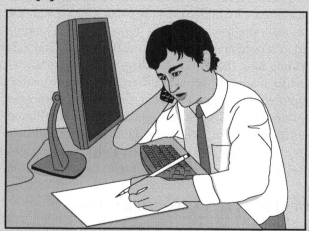

Office of
Technology

Working Together

FIGURE 29.7. Texas Woman's University Interprofessional Informatics program.

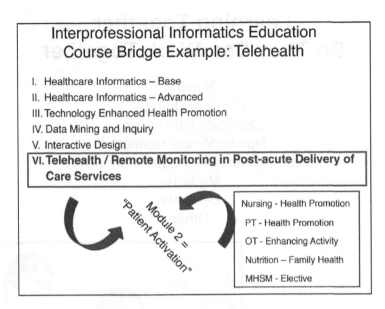

FIGURE 29.8. Example of the telehealth bridge course (curved arrows).
Source: Mari Tietze.

forth may also enroll in the course through their own departments and join the rest of the students via the "bridged Module 2 Patient Activation," which is the integrated section of Blackboard.

SUMMARY

Most experts, including the conference sponsors and the IPE/C panel, believe that to deliver high-quality, safe, and efficient care, and to meet the public's increasingly complex health care needs, the educational experience must shift from one in which health profession students are educated in silos to one that fosters collaboration, communication, and a team approach to providing care. The goal of this chapter is to energize readers to pave the way for a future in which interprofessional health teams provide care that leads to better health outcomes, improved patient experiences of care, improved efficiency, and increased job satisfaction for health professionals. Aligned with the NEHI model, as depicted in previous chapters (McBride et al., 2013), the IPE/C initiative supports optimum point-of-care technology, data analysis, and patient safety and quality for population. This alignment then facilitates the overall process and increases favorable outcomes.

EXERCISES AND QUESTIONS FOR CONSIDERATION

Define a few of the beginning steps needed to implement an IPE/C for a postacute care, remote-patient-monitoring setting. Health care professionals have a background in PT, OT, nursing, and finance. One toolkit that is readily available is that provided by the Michigan Health Council (see Figure 29.5). Utilize that toolkit located at the link http://education2practice.org/view-toolkit to define your steps:

1. How would you review the benefits of IPE/C with the team?

2. How would you use a "Huddle Guide" to support communication among the team?

3. Motivational interviewing is a common technique for engaging patients appropriately in their care process. Use the appropriate toolkit item to get the IPE team organized to consistently initiate this type of interviewing with patients.

4. What would be an appropriate clinical records document to be used by all team members?

5. Select one more toolkit item to successfully engage the IPE team in a given care delivery scenario.

CASE STUDY

The University of Washington is developing exportable educational programs to help students learn effective interprofessional communication. One focus of that training is interprofessional error disclosure. The training employs a combination of didactic presentations, role modeling demonstration of a clinical scenario using a standardized patient by an interprofessional group of faculty, and practice learning using simulation methods. Students from medicine, nursing, pharmacy, and dentistry are exposed to evidence-based information regarding the value of openness and honesty with patients and families when an error resulting in harm has occurred in their care, and they are instructed in the types of communication that patients expect to receive, including apologies. Students reflect on the scenario, including attending to the feelings associated with this difficult conversation.

Next, interprofessional groups of students can practice conducting an error disclosure in a simulation case scenario to immerse themselves in practical learning. During that scenario, they may identify how their professions may be involved in creating safer environments to avoid such a hypothetical error in the future.

This example included many opportunities for evaluating specific behavioral learning objectives/competencies, especially around interprofessional values/ethics and communication. Competency development in the domain of values/ethics stresses placing patients or communities at the center of care; building a trusting relationship with patients, families, and other team members; acting with honesty and integrity; managing ethical conflicts that are specific to interprofessional caregiving; and respecting the diversity of individual and cultural differences among patients, families, and team members. Competency development in the domain of interprofessional communication emphasizes using respectful language; organizing and communicating information with patients, families, and health team members in an understandable form; choosing effective communication tools and techniques; and communicating effectively in difficult situations (ICEP, 2011, p. 29).

REFERENCES

Accreditation of Interprofessional Health Education. (2014). *AIPHE interprofessional health education accreditation standards guide, phase 2*. Retrieved from www.caot.ca/pdfs/PIF/AIPHE%20Interprofes sional%20Health%20Education%20Accreditation%20Standards%20Guide_EN.pdf

Akroyd, M., Jordan, G., & Rowlands, P. (2014). Interprofessional, simulation-based technology-enhanced learning to improve physical healthcare in psychiatry: The RAMPPS course. *Health Informatics Journal.* doi:1460458214562287 [pii]

Allen, E., Jackson, D., & Elliott, D. (2015). Exploring interprofessional practices in rapid response systems: A case study protocol. *Nurse Researcher, 22*(3), 20–27. doi:10.7748/nr.22.3.20.e1305

Brandt, B., Lutfiyya, M. N., King, J. A., & Chioreso, C. (2014). A scoping review of interprofessional collaborative practice and education using the lens of the triple aim. *Journal of Interprofessional Care, 28*(5), 393–399. doi:10.3109/13561820.2014.906391

Carbonaro, M., King, S., Taylor, E., Satzinger, F., Snart, F., & Drummond, J. (2008). Integration of e-learning technologies in an interprofessional health science course. *Medical Teacher, 30*(1), 25–33. doi:10.1080/01421590701753450

Centers for Medicare & Medicaid Services. (2014). *Partnership for patients.* Retrieved from www .partnershipforpatients.cms.gov/

Committee on Quality of Healthcare in America. (2001). *Crossing the quality chasm: A new health system for the 21st century.* Washington, DC: National Academies Press. Retrieved from www.nap .edu/catalog.php?record_id=10027

Cuff, P. A. (2013). *Interprofessional education for collaboration: Learning how to improve health from interprofessional models across the continuum of education to practice: Workshop summary* (No. 13486). Washington, DC: The National Academies Press.

Djukic, M., Fulmer, T., Adams, J. G., Lee, S., & Triola, M. M. (2012). NYU3T: Teaching, technology, teamwork: A model for interprofessional education scalability and sustainability. *Nursing Clinics of North America, 47*(3), 333–346. doi:10.1016/j.cnur.2012.05.003

Hall, L. W., & Zierler, B. K. (2015). Interprofessional education and practice guide no. 1: Developing faculty to effectively facilitate interprofessional education. *Journal of Interprofessional Care, 29*(1), 3–7. doi:10.3109/13561820.2014.937483

Health Resources and Services Administration. (2014). *Transforming interprofessional health education and practice: Moving learners from the campus to the community to enhance population health* (No. HRSAipe2014). Washington, DC: U.S. Department of Health and Human Services. Retrieved from www.hrsa.gov/advisorycommittees/bhpradvisory/acicbl/reports/thirteenthreport.pdf

Hibbard, J. H., & Greene, J. (2013). What the evidence shows about patient activation: Better health outcomes and care experiences; fewer data on costs. *Health Affairs (Project Hope), 32*(2), 207–214. doi:10.1377/hlthaff.2012.1061

Institute for Healthcare Improvement. (2015). *IHI triple aim initiative: Better care for individuals, better health for populations, and lower per capital costs.* Retrieved from http://www.ihi.org/engage/initiatives/ tripleaim/Pages/default.aspx

Institute of Medicine. (2000). *To err is human: Building a safer health system* (No. ERR-1999). Washington, DC: Author. Retrieved from www.iom.edu/~/media/Files/Report%20Files/1999/To-Err-is-Human/To%20Err%20is%20Human%201999%20%20report%20brief.pdf

Institute of Medicine. (2003). Current educational activities in the core competencies. In A. C. Greiner & E. Knebel (Eds.), *Health professions education: A bridge to quality* (pp. 75–91). Washington, DC: National

Academies Press. Retrieved from www.nap.edu/catalog/10681/health-professions-education-a-bridge-to-quality

Institute of Medicine. (2010). *The future of nursing: Leading change, advancing health* (No. FoN2011). Washington, DC: IOM/Robert Wood Johnson Foundation. Retrieved from www.iom.edu/Reports/2010/The-Future-of-Nursing-Leading-Change-Advancing-Health.aspx

Interprofessional Collaborative Expert Panel. (2011). *Core competencies for interprofessional collaborative practice: Report of an expert panel* (No. ICEP-2011). Interprofessional Education Collaborative. Retrieved from www.ipecollaborative.org/uploads/IPEC-Core-Competencies.pdf

King, S., Carbonaro, M., Greidanus, E., Ansell, D., Foisy-Doll, C., & Magus, S. (2014). Dynamic and routine interprofessional simulations: Expanding the use of simulation to enhance interprofessional competencies. *Journal of Allied Health, 43*(3), 169–175.

King, S., Chodos, D., Stroulia, E., Carbonaro, M., MacKenzie, M., Reid, A., . . . Greidanus, E. (2012). Developing interprofessional health competencies in a virtual world. *Medical Education Online, 17,* 1–11. doi:10.3402/meo.v17i0.11213

Landman, A. B., Redden, L., Neri, P., Poole, S., Horsky, J., Raja, A. S., . . . Poon, E. G. (2014). Using a medical simulation center as an electronic health record usability laboratory. *Journal of the American Medical Informatics Association, 21*(3), 558–563. doi:10.1136/amiajnl-2013-002233

McBride, S. G., Tietze, M., & Fenton, M., V. (2013). Developing an applied informatics course for a doctor of nursing practice program. *Nurse Educator, 38*(1), 37–42. doi:10.1097/NNE.0b013e318276df5d

MedBiquitous Consortium (2015). *MedBiquitous standards make it easier to track professional achievements, access learning and measure improvements.* Retrieved from www.medbiq.org/

Michigan Health Council. (2014). *Michigan's hub for interprofessional education and collaborative care: E2P toolkit.* Retrieved from www.education2practice.org/view-toolkit

Miller, D. (2014). *Integrating interprofessional education in higher education through accreditation standards* (No. IPE2014). Okemos, MI: Michigan Health Council. Retrieved from www.education2practice.org/reports/integrating-interprofessional-education-higher-education-through-accreditation-standards

National Academy of Sciences. (2015). *Global forum on innovation in health professional education.* Retrieved from www.iom.edu/Activities/Global/InnovationHealthProfEducation.aspx

Noble, D. J., & Casalino, L. P. (2013). Can accountable care organizations improve population health?: Should they try? *Journal of the American Medical Association, 309*(11), 1119–1120. doi:10.1001/jama.2013.592

Paquette-Warren, J., Roberts, S. E., Fournie, M., Tyler, M., Brown, J., & Harris, S. (2014). Improving chronic care through continuing education of interprofessional primary healthcare teams: A process evaluation. *Journal of Interprofessional Care, 28*(3), 232–238. doi:10.3109/13561820.2013.874981

Peluchette, J., Karl, K., Coustasse, A., & Emmett, D. (2012). Professionalism and social networking: Can patients, physicians, nurses, and supervisors all be "friends?" *Health Care Manager, 31*(4), 285–294. doi:10.1097/HCM.0b013e31826fe252

Pfaff, K., Baxter, P., Jack, S., & Ploeg, J. (2014). An integrative review of the factors influencing new graduate nurse engagement in interprofessional collaboration. *Journal of Advanced Nursing, 70*(1), 4–20. doi:10.1111/jan.12195

Pulman, A., Scammell, J., & Martin, M. (2009). Enabling interprofessional education: The role of technology to enhance learning. *Nurse Education Today, 29*(2), 232–239. doi:http://dx.doi.org/10.1016/j.nedt.2008.08.012

Smith, K. A. (2014). Healthcare interprofessional education: Encouraging technology, teamwork, and team performance. *Journal of Continuing Education in Nursing, 45*(4), 181–187.

TIGER Development Collaborative. (2015a). *TIGER initiative; about.* Retrieved from www.thetiger initiative.org/

TIGER Development Collaborative. (2015b). *TIGER virtual learning environment (VLE) powered by HIMSS.* Retrieved from www.thetigerinitiative.org/virtuallearning.aspx

Torres, T., & Loehrer, S. (2014). ACOs: A step in the right direction. Accountable care may achieve better care at lower cost. *Institute of Healthcare Improvement 29*(4), 62–65.

University of Kansas Medical Center. (2013). *HITS: Health Information Technology Scholars program advancing health information technologies through faculty empowerment.* Retrieved from www.hits-colab.org/

Wilbur, L. (2014). *The University of Arkansas' five-pillar plan for an institutional triple aim culture.* Retrieved from www.nexusipe.org/news/university-arkansas%E2%80%99-five-pillar-plan-institutional-triple-aim-culture

World Health Organization. (2010). *Framework for action on interprofessional education & collaborative practice.* (No. WHO/HRH/HPN/10.3). Geneva, Switzerland: Author.

Youm, J., & Wiechmann, W. (2015). The med AppJam: A model for an interprofessional student-centered mHealth app competition. *Journal of Medical Systems, 39*(3), 34. Epub 2015 Feb 15. doi:10.1007/s10916-015-0216-4

Zorek, J., & Raehl, C. (2013). Interprofessional education accreditation standards in the USA: A comparative analysis. *Journal of Interprofessional Care, 27*(2), 123–130. doi:10.3109/13561820.2012.718295

INDEX